T4-BBV-821

The Future of Bioethics

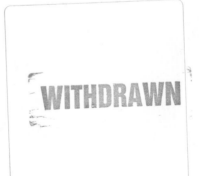
WITHDRAWN

The Future of Bioethics

International Dialogues

EDITED BY

Akira Akabayashi

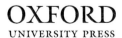

OXFORD

UNIVERSITY PRESS

OXFORD
UNIVERSITY PRESS

Great Clarendon Street, Oxford, OX2 6DP,
United Kingdom

Oxford University Press is a department of the University of Oxford.
It furthers the University's objective of excellence in research, scholarship,
and education by publishing worldwide. Oxford is a registered trade mark of
Oxford University Press in the UK and in certain other countries

© The several contributors 2014

The moral rights of the author have been asserted

First Edition published in 2014

Impression: 2

All rights reserved. No part of this publication may be reproduced, stored in
a retrieval system, or transmitted, in any form or by any means, without the
prior permission in writing of Oxford University Press, or as expressly permitted
by law, by licence, or under terms agreed with the appropriate reprographics
rights organization. Enquiries concerning reproduction outside the scope of the
above should be sent to the Rights Department, Oxford University Press, at the
address above

You must not circulate this work in any other form
and you must impose this same condition on any acquirer

Published in the United States of America by Oxford University Press
198 Madison Avenue, New York, NY 10016, United States of America

British Library Cataloguing in Publication Data
Data available

Library of Congress Control Number: 2013943974

ISBN 978–0–19–968267–6

Printed and bound in Great Britain by
CPI Group (UK) Ltd, Croydon, CRO 4YY

Links to third party websites are provided by Oxford in good faith and
for information only. Oxford disclaims any responsibility for the materials
contained in any third party website referenced in this work.

Preface

Evolving and cutting-edge medical technologies, such as developments in neuroscience and regenerative medicine, show exceptional promise in improving human health. However, they also engender unprecedented ethical, legal, and social problems that require both global and local responses.

Issues related to new technologies are further confounded by the effect of globalization on social change, made possible by astounding developments in information technology and transportation. These changes affect bioethics in two ways. They lead to issues around the movement of people and populations, in particular the migration of patients and care workers across continents, and those caused by enormous international medical research studies involving participants from many countries and cultures. Second, global issues call for global efforts and global solutions. Mobilization of humankind's ethical wisdom is required to address these in a manner that transcends cultural and national differences. Establishing culturally and ethically informed dialogue is the critical first step toward resolving these diverse problems.

This is the first book on bioethics that presents a genuine engagement between scholars and practitioners from East and West: the first book in the discipline of bioethics for the globalized world of the future. We address the emerging issues in bioethics. We aim to set the agenda for the future, focusing on new developments and their potential for change.

Most studies in bioethics advocating East–West dialogue have either attempted cross-cultural comparison or proposed Eastern philosophical paradigms as a counter to Western ideas. The tacit premise of previous writing on East–West dialogue is therefore a strain of relativism. From the Eastern perspective, Western views are treated as a cultural construct that should be referenced as models, but are not appropriate to be utilized in their existing form. To Westerners, Eastern interpretation represents ways of thinking that should be recognized but can never truly be understood in their complexity within Western cultures. For this reason, Asians place Western conceptions of bioethics on the critical chopping block, and approach them as something to be overcome. In contrast, although Westerners occasionally comment on current conditions in Asian countries, they rarely fully engage with bioethical discussions led by Asian researchers, and neither express agreement nor fully critique such views. In a globalized world, simply maintaining a respectful distance from other cultures is no longer sufficient.

The time has come for us to engage actively with different cultural perspectives, rather than hearing them and rather than listening attentively to them. The most prominent characteristic of this collection's development derives from the way in which the book has been developed. First, the contributors met to discuss and identify the issues at the cutting edge of bioethics. Then the leading researchers offered primary topic articles (PTAs). Next, researchers from various countries wrote commentaries to which the PTA authors replied. At each stage, the contributors communicated with each other to ensure genuine engagement while revising their contributions in light of ongoing dialogue. The commentary authors included leading researchers as well as promising, relatively young researchers. Thus, the book aims not only at a cross-cultural dialogue, but a dialogue between researchers of different generations.

The book comprises two parts. Part I looks at bioethical issues that arise from new medical technologies such as regenerative medicine, enhancement, research ethics, and synthetic biology. Part II addresses challenging dilemmas that result from the globalization of social change, such as transplantation tourism, public health ethics, care in the aging society, and professionalism.

One can imagine, from a glance at the table of contents and contributing authors, what an important contribution this collection will be. Therefore a lengthy preface is unnecessary. I hope that the readers will enjoy this honest dialogue between researchers from both the East and West.

While these 21 chapters do not cover all topics that are likely to arise over the course of this century, they cover particularly challenging issues faced by current researchers. Dialogue must span both local and global levels. This, to me, is "the future of bioethics."

July 2013
Akira Akabayashi

University of Tokyo

Acknowledgements

I would first like to express my appreciation to the editorial advisory board members, Drs. Arthur Caplan, Alastair Campbell, Tony Hope, Tom Murray, and Julian Savulescu. Especially, this book could not have been published without the help of Tony and Julian, who provided valuable editing assistance and advice.

I would also like to thank Drs. Keiichiro Yamamoto, Hitoshi Arima, Satoshi Kodama, and Deborah Zion for their comments and insightful suggestions.

This book was supported in part by grants from the University of Tokyo Global Center of Excellence (GCOE) Program funded by the Japanese Ministry of Education, Culture, Sports, Science and Technology, and the Uehiro Foundation on Ethics and Education.

Contents

WITHDRAWN

Section C: Emerging Problems in Research Ethics

Section D: Synthetic Biology and Chimera

Part II. Globalization and Bioethics

Section A: Organ Transplant

Section B: Public Health Ethics

Section C: Care in the Aging Society

Section D: Rethinking Medical Professionalism

List of Abbreviations

AAHRPP	Association for the Accreditation of Human Research Participants Program
ADR	Alternative Dispute Resolution
AFM	French Muscular Dystrophy Association
AJOB	American Journal of Bioethics
AMA	Australian Medical Association
AMANET	African Malaria Network Trust
ARV	antiretroviral treatment
ASBH	American Society of Bioethics and Humanities
ASC	somatic or 'adult' stem cell
ASPD	antisocial personality disorder
BAC	Bioethics Advisory Committee (of the Singapore government)
CCTP	Conditional Cash Transfer Program
CEA	cost-effectiveness analysis
CER	comparative effectiveness research
CF	cystic fibrosis
CHRB	Convention on Human Rights and Biomedicine
CML	chronic myelogenous leukemia
CMS	Centers for Medicare and Medicaid Services
CNS	central nervous system
COI	conflict of interest
COPD	chronic obstructive pulmonary disease
CPMC	Coriell Personalized Medicine Collaborative
DALY	disability-adjusted life year
DBS	deep brain stimulation
DOI	Declaration of Istanbul
DTC	direct to consumer
ELSI	ethical, legal, and social issues
EOPJ	equal opportunity-based principle of justice
EPO	erythropoietin
ES	embryonic stem

ESC	embryonic stem cell
ESRD	end-stage renal disease
EU	European Union
FDA	Food and Drug Administration
FERCAP	Forum for Ethical Review Committees in the Asian Western Pacific Region
fMRI	functional magnetic resonance imaging
GATS	Global Agreement on Trade in Services
GRID	gay-related immunodeficiency disease
HCT/Ps	human cells, tissues, and cellular and tissue-based products
hES	human embryonic stem
HMO	Health Maintenance Organization
HOTA	Human Organ Transplant Act 1987 (Singapore)
HSC	hematopoietic stem cell
ICER	incremental cost-effectiveness ratio
ICMS	International Cellular Medicine Society
ICOB	Informed Cohort Oversight Board
ICU	intensive care unit
IP	intellectual property
iPS	induced pluripotent stem
IRB	institutional review board
IRENSA	International Research Ethics Network for Southern Africa
JCAHO	Joint Commission on Accreditation of Healthcare Organizations
JCI	Joint Commission International
JMA	Japan Medical Association
JME	Journal of Medical Ethics
JPMA	Japan Pharmaceutical Manufacturers Association
JSIM	Japanese Society of Internal Medicine
JST	Japan Society for Transplantation
LTC	long-term care
MHLW	Ministry of Health, Labor, and Welfare (Japan)
MOH	Ministry of Health (China)
MSC	mesenchymal stem cell
MT	moral technology
MTERA	Medical (Therapy, Research and Education) Act 1972 (Singapore)
NCB	Nuffield Council on Bioethics
NCC	Japanese National Cancer Center

NECTAR	Network of European CNS Transplantation and Restoration
NHI	national health insurance
NHS	National Health Service
NICE	National Institute for Health and Clinical Excellence
NOTA	National Organ Transplant Act 1984
NOTU	National Organ Transplant Unit
NSFC	National Natural Science Foundation of China
OHRP	Office for Human Research Protections
ONT	Spanish National Transplant Organization
OPO	Organ Procurement Organization
OPTN	Organ Procurement and Transplantation Network
PB	procreative beneficence
PD	Parkinson's disease
PGD	preimplantation genetic diagnosis
PhRMA	Pharmaceutical Manufacturer Association
pmp	per million population
QALY	quality-adjusted life year
RCT	randomized controlled trial
SARETI	South African Research Ethics Initiative
SCNT	somatic cell nuclear transfer
SCNT	somatic cell nuclear transfer
SDM	substitute decision maker
SIDCER	Strategic Initiative for Developing Capacity in Ethical Review
SSRI	selective serotonin reuptake inhibitor
STS	science, technology, and society study
TB	tuberculosis
TEC	Transplant Ethics Committee
TRREE	Training and Resources in Research Ethics Evaluation
TTS	The Transplantation Society
UK	United Kingdom
UNESCO	United Nations Educational, Scientific and Cultural Organization
UNOS	United Network for Organ Sharing
US	United States
USADA	US Anti-Doping Agency
USPHT	United States Public Health Task Force
VE	virtue ethics

WADA   World Anti-Doping Agency
WHO   World Health Organization
WMA   World Medical Association

List of Contributors

AKIRA AKABAYASHI University of Tokyo, Japan

YOHEI AKAIDA University of Tokyo, Japan

HITOSHI ARIMA Yokohama City University, Japan

ATSUSHI ASAI Kumamoto University, Japan

MARK P. AULISIO Case Western Reserve University, USA

JING BAI National Center for Women and Children's Health, China CDC, China

TOM L. BEAUCHAMP Georgetown University, USA

CARL BECKER Kyoto University, Japan

ARIC BENDORF Centre for Values, Ethics and the Law in Medicine, Australia

EDWARD J. BERGMAN University of Pennsylvania, USA

NANCY BERLINGER Hastings Center, USA

MICHAEL C. BRANNIGAN College of Saint Rose, USA

DANIEL CALLAHAN Hastings Center, USA

ALASTAIR V. CAMPBELL National University of Singapore, Singapore

ARTHUR L. CAPLAN New York University, USA

BENJAMIN CAPPS National University of Singapore, Singapore

LEONARDO D. DE CASTRO National University of Singapore, Singapore

JACQUELINE J. L. CHIN National Singapore University, Singapore

NORMAN DANIELS Harvard University, USA

ANGUS DAWSON University of Birmingham, UK

NICOLE M. DEMING Case Western Reserve University, USA

THOMAS DOUGLAS University of Oxford, UK

MICHAEL DUNN University of Oxford, UK

H. TRISTRAM ENGELHARDT Jr., Rice University, USA

RUIPING FAN City University of Hong Kong, China

AUTUMN FIESTER University of Pennsylvania, USA

MICHAEL K. GUSMANO Hastings Center, USA

YOSHINORI HAYASHI Ritsumeikan University, Japan

ANITA HO University of British Columbia, Canada

SORAJ HONGLADAROM Chulalongkorn University, Thailand

TONY HOPE University of Oxford, UK

TOMOHIDE IBUKI National Center of Neurology and Psychiatry, Japan

YASUTAKA ICHINOKAWA University of Tokyo, Japan

TAKASHI IKEDA Meiji University, Japan

AKIRA INOUE Ritsumeikan University, Japan

KOHJI ISHIHARA University of Tokyo, Japan

TAICHI ISOBE University of Tokyo, Japan

BRUCE JENNINGS Center for Humans and Nature, USA

AMAR JESANI Centre for Studies in Ethics and Rights, Mumbai, India

D. GARETH JONES University of Otago, New Zealand

YASUHIRO KADOOKA Kumamoto University, Japan

GREGORY KAEBNICK Hastings Center, USA

KATSUNORI KAI Waseda University, Japan

OSAMU KANAMORI University of Tokyo, Japan

IAN KERRIDGE The Centre for Values, Ethics and the Law in Medicine, Australia

TAKANOBU KINJO University of the Ryukyus, Japan

SATOSHI KODAMA Kyoto University, Japan

ILHAK LEE Yonsei University, Korea

DONNA L. LUEBKE MetroHealth System, USA

TAMRA LYSAGHT National University of Singapore, Singapore

SHUNZO MAJIMA Hokkaido University, Japan

KAREN J. MASCHKE Hastings Center, USA

MICHELLE L. MCGOWAN Case Western Reserve University, USA

CATHERINE MILLS University of Sydney, Australia

NOZOMI MIZUSHIMA University of Tokyo, Japan

FARHAT MOAZAM Center of Biomedical Ethics and Culture, SIUT, Pakistan

JONATHAN D. MORENO University of Pennsylvania, USA

MASAHIRO MORIOKA Osaka Prefecture University, Japan

THOMAS MURRAY Hastings Center, USA

TAKAHIRO NAKAJIMA University of Tokyo, Japan

EISUKE NAKAZAWA University of Tokyo, Japan

MASATOSHI NARA Keio University, Japan

YUKIHIRO NOBUHARA The University of Tokyo, Japan

JUSTIN OAKLEY Monash University, Australia

KANTARO OHASHI Kobe College, Japan

TAKETOSHI OKITA Osaka University, Japan

TARO OKUDA Nanzan University, Japan

KOJI OTA University of Tokyo, Japan

JI-YONG PARK Yonsei University, Korea

MICHAEL PARKER University of Oxford, UK

INGMAR PERSSON University of Gothenburg, Sweden and University of Oxford, UK

RACHEL PHETTEPLACE Case Western Reserve University, USA

RENZONG QIU Chinese Academy of Social Sciences & Peking Union Medical College, China

MALA RAMANATHAN Sree Chitra Tirunal Institute for Medical Sciences and Technology, India

JAMES SABIN Harvard University, USA

OSAMU SAKURA The University of Tokyo, Japan

RYOJI SATO Monash University, Australia, Japan

TOMOKO SATO University of Tokyo, Japan

JULIAN SAVULESCU University of Oxford, UK

SUSUMU SHIMAZONO Sophia University, Japan

YOSUKE SHIMAZONO Osaka University, Japan

DOUGLAS SIPP RIKEN Center for Developmental Biology, Japan

ROBERT SPARROW Monash University, Australia

PETER A. SY University of the Philippines, Philippines

KYOKO TAKASHIMA University of Tokyo, Japan

DANIEL FU-CHANG TSAI National Taiwan University, Taiwan

WILHELM VOSSENKUHL Ludwig Maximilians-University, Germany

CAMERON R. WALDMAN Hastings Center, USA

ZHAOCHEN WANG Peking Union Medical College, China

MIRIAM WEISS Case Western Reserve University, USA

KEIICHIRO YAMAMOTO University of Tokyo, Japan

STUART J. YOUNGNER Case Western Reserve University, USA

XIAOMEI ZHAI Chinese Academy of Medical Sciences / Peking Union Medical College, China

PART I

Progress of Biomedical Technologies and Ethics

SECTION A

Regenerative Medicine

1.1

Primary Topic Article
The Ethics of Regenerative Medicine: Broadening the Scope beyond the Moral Status of Embryos

Tamra Lysaght and Alastair V. Campbell

Introduction

Regenerative medicine is a broad field of research and clinical application that encompasses a wide range of medical biotechnologies and practices, including cell-based therapies, stem cell research, gene technology, and tissue engineering (Greenwood et al. 2006). However, the field has mainly come to the attention of bioethicists through the prominence of stem cell research and related technologies, such as somatic cell nuclear transfer (SCNT) or research cloning. Unfortunately, much of the bioethical discussion has tended to focus narrowly around issues concerning embryonic stem cell research and, in particular, the moral status of human embryos. While we do not claim that questions over the moral status of embryos are unimportant issues for bioethicists, we do suggest that a fixation on them alone has come at the cost of many other important issues being overlooked or, at the very least, under-examined.

Even within stem cell research itself, many questions have arisen that remain largely unexamined. These include: the exploitation of women (Dodds 2004; Waldby 2008); the commodification of human tissues (Dickenson 2002; Waldby and Mitchell 2006); the accessibility of stem cell banks (Bok, Schill, and Faden 2004); the efficacy of informed consent processes (Parry 2006; Caulfield, Ogbogu, and Isasi 2007; Haimes and Taylor 2009; Provoost et al. 2010); the presentation of science (Holm 2002; Hauskeller 2005b; Lysaght and Kerridge 2010) and constructions of trust in public discourse (Jones and Salter 2003); the ownership of immortal cell lines (Glasner 2005; Mackenney and Capps 2010); and the construction of disability and illness (Goggin and Newell 2004; Tate and Pledger 2007). Although these issues have all been raised in relation to stem cell research, none has received robust attention from bioethicists. This disparity is exacerbated when stem cell research is viewed from within the broader context of regenerative medicine.

Part of the problem may lie in how the ethics of regenerative medicine is framed. For instance, the introduction of a recent volume entitled *The Bioethics of Regenerative Medicine* claimed that:

Regenerative medicine goes to the very core of the moral and metaphysical understandings that ask what it is to be human. If one is to remake what it is to be human, one should know what goals are appropriate and what constraints should apply. (King-Tak 2009: 3)

Here the issues are framed as being fundamentally moral and metaphysical. It is also assumed that the goal of regenerative medicine is indeed "to remake what it is to be human." Six of the eleven papers in this book address issues pertaining to the moral status of human embryos, with the remainder examining aspects of life extension or enhancement through the lens of various posthumanist/humanist perspectives. While some of the authors make important contributions to the metaphysical debates around embryonic stem cell research and genetic engineering, we find the presentation of the ethical issues very limiting. Furthermore, many of the contributions are located within and dichotomized by the debate around theological and secular traditions in bioethics (e.g. Engelhardt 2009; Lo 2009). We find this to be a very narrow way to approach a field that is likely to have far more practical repercussions than the analysis suggests. We also suggest that the analysis not only offers little in terms of policy and practice, but indeed, contributes to a polarization of the debates in public discourse.

As an alternative, we concur with King, Coughlin, and Furth's (2009) conclusion that long-standing fundamental issues lie at the heart of regenerative medicine relating to the nature of medical research, the relationship between research and practice, and the protection of human research subjects. They suggest that the ethical issues raised by regenerative medicine are the same as those brought up in other first-in-human studies and by clinical trials enrolling patients as research subjects. Such issues will include, but are in no way limited to, the rights and welfare of patients, financial and nonfinancial conflicts of interest, costs of and equitable access to medical technologies, distributive justice, and the role of public–private partnerships in biomedical research. These are issues in which bioethicists from across a range of disciplines are likely to find common ground and to move beyond what is arguably the incommensurability of the debates around embryonic research. Therefore, it is within this framing that we approach the ethics of regenerative medicine and argue that it should take priority in bioethical discussions around this emergent field of biomedical research and practice.

Regenerative medicine: research and practice

Before we examine some of the ethical issues, it is important first to present a definition of, and to clarify the current state of the art in, regenerative medicine.[1] According to Greenwood et al. (2006: 63), regenerative medicine is defined as:

An emerging interdisciplinary field of research and clinical applications focused on the repair, replacement, or regeneration of cells, tissues, or organs to restore impaired function resulting from any cause, including congenital defects, disease, and trauma. It uses a combination of several

---

[1] The following reflects the state of the art at the time this paper was written in 2010. While some technical statements may now be obsolete, they do not alter the central argument of the paper.

technological approaches that moves it beyond traditional transplantation and replacement therapies. These approaches may include, but are not limited to, the use of stem cells, soluble molecules, genetic engineering, tissue engineering, and advanced cell therapy.

Put more simply, regenerative medicine replaces or regenerates human cells, tissue, or organs, with the purpose of restoring or establishing normal function (Mason and Dunnill 2008). While emerging from conventional practices of surgical implantation, organ transplantation and tissue replacement, the field is distinguished from these traditional approaches in that "its goal is not just to replace what is malfunctioning, but to provide the elements required for *in vivo* repair, to devise replacements that seamlessly interact with the living body, and to stimulate the body's intrinsic capacities to regenerate" (Greenwood et al. 2006: 62–3). The boundaries that distinguish regenerative medicine from its preceding practices are not sharply defined. However, for the purposes of our analysis, we will observe these distinctions with an understanding that some overlap may exist, particularly around the various stem cell- and cellular-based approaches.

As an emerging area of medicine, many of its applications are still in the research and development phase, although some cell-based products have successfully made it into the clinic. Two skin substitute products have been approved in the US by the Food and Drug Administration (FDA): Dermagraph® for the treatment of diabetic foot ulcers (Shire Regenerative Medicine 2012) and Apligraf® for both diabetic foot ulcers and venous leg ulcers (Organogenesis 2008). Both products combined have been used to treat in excess of 300,000 patients (Mason and Manzotti 2010). Another skin product called ReCell® is a point-of-care autologous cell harvesting, processing, and delivery technology that has regulatory approvals in Europe, China, and Australia and is currently undergoing FDA clinical trials in the US (Dolphin 2009). Far from "remaking what it is to be human," these applications offer patients relatively simple and effective treatments for a variety of wounds.

Another application that has been put into clinical practice is bone marrow cell transplant. Hematopoietic stem cell (HSC) transplantation has been in clinical use experimentally for over 50 years and, for the last two decades, has been used routinely in the treatment of certain types of malignant and nonmalignant disorders of the blood and immune systems (Storb 2003). It is a procedure in which progenitor cells are administered to a patient to reconstitute normal bone marrow function (Powell, Hingorani, and Kolb 2009). HSCs are somatic cells that may be sourced either from the patient in autologous stem cell transplants or from a donor in allogeneic stem cell transplants. The cells are typically harvested from the bone marrow, although umbilical cord blood has proven to be a rich alternative source of HSCs (Gluckman 2000).

Besides HSCs, somatic or "adult" stem cells (ASCs) have also been isolated from many other mature tissues including the lungs (Engelhardt et al. 1995), skin (Watts, Lo Celso, and Silva-Vargas 2006), liver (Brill, Zvibel, and Reid 1999), brain and central nervous system (Stemplea and Anderson 1992; McKay 1997; Gage 2002), pancreas (Jones and Sarvetnick 1997), adipose tissue (Zuk et al. 2002), and the heart (Beltrami et al. 2003). ASCs are multipotent in that they have the capacity to develop into multiple tissues within a single cell lineage (Verfaillie, Pera, and Lansdorp 2002). Gaining access to these tissues to isolate the cells and grow them in clinically useful numbers has, however, been a major hurdle for the clinical application of many ASCs (Schwartz and Bryant

2008: 50). Hence, blood- and bone marrow-derived cells remain the most common source of stem cell-based therapies.

A few ASC-derived products have, nonetheless, made it to the clinic. For example, there is Osteocel® Plus, which is an allogeneic bone matrix containing viable mesenchymal stem cells approved for homologous use in musculoskeletal defects; and autologous limbal stem cell therapies are currently undergoing development for corneal burns (Mason and Manzotti 2010). One recent success story involved the autologous transplant of a trachea engineered from mesenchymal stem cell-derived chondrocytes into a patient with end-stage bronchomalacia (Macchiarini et al. 2008). Other proposed approaches have included the use of bone marrow-derived cells in treating patients with myocardial infarcts (Bartunek et al. 2010), spinal cord injury (Rossi and Keirstead 2009), multiple sclerosis (Pasquini et al. 2010), and Parkinson's disease (Wijeyekoon and Barker 2009). While some promising pre-clinical and Phase I/II results have been reported, these approaches have yet to be rigorously tested in large-scale double-blind randomized clinical trials. Thus, the clinical role for ASCs beyond their current uses in the reconstitution of bone marrow function remains uncertain.

Stem cells from embryonic sources are considered to have enormous potential in regenerative medicine. Human embryonic stem cells (ESCs), which are derived from the inner cell mass of human blastocysts, are valued as a highly efficient source of pluripotent stem cells; meaning that they have an ability for unlimited self-renewal and may be differentiated into almost any tissue type (Conley et al. 2004). The pluripotency of these cells is demonstrated by teratoma formation following injection into immunodeficient mice. However, they have yet to be tested in human studies.

In the US, Geron recently commenced Phase I safety studies of human ESC-derived oligodendrocyte progenitor cells in patients with complete thoracic spinal cord injury (Geron 2010), and another company has received FDA permission to begin Phase I/II trials with ESC-derived retinal pigment epithelial cells to treat dry age-related macular degeneration (Advanced Cell Technology 2011). However, concrete results from these trials are likely to take some time and may not be readily applicable to other applications. Thus, while ESCs have potential applications in pharmacological studies and drug discovery, and are likely to have significant impacts on the understanding of biology and disease morphology, many technical and scientific obstacles remain before more widespread clinical application of ESCs becomes feasible (Singec et al. 2007; Addis, Bulte, and Gearhart 2008; Rossi, Jamieson, and Weissman 2008). An attractive option, therefore, has been to seek out alternative sources of pluripotent stem cells.

One alternative means of deriving pluripotent stem cells is through the reprogramming of somatic cells back to an undifferentiated state. At present, reprogramming can be achieved using one of four methods, although only two are considered to have possible clinical applications (Yin et al. 2009). SCNT creates blastocysts that are clones of the original cell from which ESC lines can be derived. The feasibility of this procedure as an alternative source of pluripotent cells, however, remains in question because, subsequent to the false claims of Woo Suk Hwang (Normile, Vogel, and Couzin 2006), no one has successfully produced a human ESC line from SCNT yet. Legal and regulatory difficulties in accessing the human oocytes needed for the procedure have also limited the viability of this path in reproductive medicine.

The other method is to introduce genetic materials that induce cells into a pluripotent-like state. While these induced pluripotent stem (iPS) cells hold great clinical promise, ongoing safety concerns, such as tumorigenicity and retroviral gene removal, will need to be addressed before they can be tested in human studies (Ehnert et al. 2009; Hanna, Saha, and Jaenisch 2010). More recently, studies have suggested that cells may be induced to trans-differentiate from one germ layer into another, thereby circumventing the need for the stem cell intermediary (Vierbuchen et al. 2010). However, although promising, the current state of the art suggests that many technical issues remain unresolved (Hanna, Saha, and Jaenisch 2010). Therefore, use of these sources of stem cells is likely to be confined to the laboratory for some time to come.

As this overview suggests, regenerative medicine is a field that includes, but is much broader than, stem cell research. Even as an area within the field, stem cell science is far more complex than the bioethical debates around embryonic research would seem to otherwise indicate. With some aspects moving away from basic research and into translational clinical research, there is a need for bioethicists to shift their attention from the debate about sources to how regenerative medicine is being put into practice. In particular, there is a strong imperative to examine the interface between research and practice. While we do not claim to produce an exhaustive list of issues, the following section provides an overview of what should be considered within the ethical domain of regenerative medicine. We will then focus on one particular issue that has emerged with the use of autologous stem cells outside the context of clinical trials.

The ethics of regenerative medicine: a brief overview

While it is debatable whether the goals of regenerative medicine have much to do with "remaking humankind," it is reasonable to view the field in terms of its potential to extend human life by repairing, replacing, or regenerating damaged cells and organs. As such, issues around life extension will likely be relevant matter for debate in regenerative medicine. Likewise, where boundaries around what is considered as "treatment" are blurred, the debates around human enhancement could have relevance to the ethics of regenerative medicine (King, Coughlin, and Furth 2009). We suggest, however, that the greater part of the ethical discourse should focus on how this field translates from research to practice.

As the central focus of regenerative medicine is on the use of human cells (Mason and Dunnill 2008), it is reasonable to assume that the ethical debates will focus on issues pertaining to stem cell- and cell-based therapies. While new strategies of deriving pluripotent cell lines are emerging, they are unlikely to remove completely the need for embryonic stem cell lines (Hyun et al. 2007), at least in the short to medium term (Sipp 2009). It is thus also reasonable to assume that moral questions pertaining to the creation and destruction of human embryos and fetuses in research will continue to feature in ethical discussions around regenerative medicine. Specifically, questions over the moral status of human embryos, and whether it is sufficient to protect them from use in research (Strong 1997; Holm 2005), are likely to remain on the agenda for some time.

Similarly, SCNT is also likely to remain a topic of interest to bioethicists. Setting aside questions of moral status, this technology continues to raise concerns over the acquisition of, and trade in, human oocytes (Waldby 2008). Strategies to circumvent shortages in human oocytes have been put forward, such as using animal eggs to create human admixed embryos. However, this strategy undoubtedly will raise health and safety concerns, if and when products generated from these entities are to be used in humans (Haddow et al. 2010). Furthermore, this approach is unlikely to avoid questions around moral status (Streiffer 2005). Thus, neither strategy is likely to resolve the ethical debates around this research.

The latest development that purportedly addresses these issues is induced pluripotency. iPS cells are often cited as the scientific solution to the "ethical dilemmas" that plague human ESC and SNCT research (Rao and Condic 2008). However, while iPS research may reduce the need for destructive embryo research and the need for a supply of human oocytes, it might not resolve concerns surrounding the *creation* of human life, and may indeed create new problems as use of the technology becomes more widespread (Lysaght and Kerridge 2010). Besides the safety concerns surrounding retroviral gene transfer, complex issues pertaining to ownership and informed consent emerge from the fact that pluripotent cell lines can be propagated indefinitely (Mackenney and Capps 2010) and may also be differentiated into gametes that could be used to create human embryos, both for research and for reproduction (Aalto-Setälä, Conklin, and Lo 2009). Questions around the interests that tissue providers ought to retain in these cells are in need of further inquiry.

Related issues arise in the context of human tissue banking. Cell-based regenerative medicines are likely to rely heavily on samples that are collected and stored in tissue repositories such as umbilical cord blood banks, stem cell banks, biobanks, and on-site hospital facilities. Issues that have been raised in relation to these facilities relate to questions of ownership, the provision of informed consent and withdrawal options, the privacy of donors, maintenance of confidentiality, the fair and equitable access of recipients to stored tissues, and the marketing practices of private operators (Sugarman, Reisner, and Kurtzberg 1995; Sugarman et al. 1997; Elger et al. 2008). The interests of tissue providers must be considered since collection can be invasive and painful, depending on the tissue type and quantity being obtained, and consideration of the health impacts and risks of side effects on recipients should be paramount (Giacomini, Baylis, and Robert 2007). Thus, as reliance on these facilities increases, so too will the need to address their impacts, both on tissue providers and on recipients.

Informed consent is a familiar issue that is relevant to most, if not all, aspects of regenerative medicine. Obtaining informed consent to collect and store samples is significantly complicated by the prospects of using stored tissues to generate disease-specific cell lines and pluripotent stem cell-derived gametes (Hyun 2008). Even cellular-based therapies that do not involve stem cells may present problems in obtaining informed consent. For example, the cells used in skin substitute products, such as Apligraf®, are derived from neonatal foreskins (Wilkins et al. 1994). While these cells apparently were obtained for commercial use under informed consent, others have argued that taking foreskins from living donors for commercial application should be prohibited because it contravenes the American Medical Association's guidelines on "The Use of Minors as Organ and Tissue Donors" as well as international laws pursuant to the "European Convention on Human Rights and Biomedicine" (Svoboda, Van Howe, and Dwyer 2000: 125–6). While we have no comment on the legality of this particular practice, suffice it to say that bioethical debate around gaining informed consent from tissues sources for cellular-based therapies is warranted, particularly when biological resources are sourced from minors.

As the basic research in regenerative medicine begins to develop into clinical trials, there will be a need to focus greater attention on the design and implementation of experimental studies. While relevant to all clinical research, we believe this is the area that has received the least amount of attention when it comes to ethical discussions around regenerative medicine, and undeservedly so. King, Coughlin, and Furth (2009) provide an excellent overview of some of the issues pertaining to research design and implementation that are due particular attention when conducting clinical studies in regenerative medicine. These matters include the distinctive reverse trajectory of regenerative medicines that emphasize standardization and large-scale production from the outset rather than during the later phases of clinical trials, which is how traditional drug development typically progresses. While the costs of treatment may potentially be reduced, and more patients may be provided with greater access to the technology, King, Coughlin, and Furth (2009) suggest that this trajectory may also expose individual participants to greater risks and decreased efficacy, as the trials progress.

King, Coughlin, and Furth (2009: 14) also raise the under-addressed questions relating to first-in-human trials with subjects drawn from patients with limited treatment options. As demonstrated by Geron's Phase I safety study with human ESC-derived oligodendrocyte, it often will be necessary that first-in-human trials are conducted with patient populations. These populations have particular vulnerabilities as the patient-subjects may be terminally ill, moderately to severely impaired or seriously injured, and will be presented with options where great uncertainty surrounds the risks of harm and potential efficacy of the treatment, which may also be irreversible. There are risks that promising research may be moved into human studies too quickly and that participants and researchers alike may be more susceptible to the "therapeutic misconception." The provision of adequate information about the inherent uncertainties of early-phase studies, alternative options, and the potential irrevocability of certain choices will thus be critical in mitigating the potential harms.

We can examine some of these challenges in the design and implementation of early-phase human studies by analyzing the paradigms being employed by clinics that offer interventions with autologous adult stem cells outside the context of clinical trials. Such treatments typically involve, or are claimed to involve, the isolation of bone marrow or adipose-derived stem cells that are then injected into another part of the patient's body for indications that lack clear scientific or clinical validation. While the effectiveness of these treatments is questionable, they nonetheless fall within the domain of regenerative medicine because the procedures are aimed at using human cells to repair and restore function of impaired organs. As these procedures have not yet been demonstrated as effective in clinical trials, we argue that acceptable norms of clinical research ought to apply in their design and implementation, and that bioethicists, regulators, and policymakers should be concerned with the ethical issues that have not yet been fully addressed.

Unproven stem cell-based interventions under-addressed ethics

In recent years, there has been an explosion of clinics offering unproven stem cell-based interventions. These interventions are generally offered by privately owned clinics and marketed directly to the consumer via the Internet (Kiatpongsan and Sipp 2009). They are typically targeted at an improbable range of indications that may include, but are not limited to, Alzheimer's disease, autism, cardiovascular diseases, cerebral palsy, Down syndrome, critical limb ischemia, diabetes (types 1 and 2), HIV/AIDS, erectile dysfunction, infertility, epilepsy, liver disease, macular degeneration, multiple sclerosis, arthritis, Parkinson's disease, spinal cord injuries, and stroke (Regenberg et al. 2009). While stem cells may one day be useful in the treatment of some of these conditions, such as multiple sclerosis, spinal cord injury, and acute myocardial infarcts, many others lack clear scientific rationale, and none of them has been demonstrated to be safe or effective in formal clinical trials (Lau et al. 2008). The current lack of evidence to support the efficacy and safety of these treatments, therefore, suggests that they are experimental in nature.

Despite the experimental status of these interventions, they are generally offered at hefty fees, and without demonstrated safety and efficacy. Moreover, they are not covered by public medical benefits schemes or private health insurers to offset the high costs. Treatments can cost in excess of US $20,000 and fees do not include travel expenses, which can be significant where clinics are located overseas (Lau et al. 2008; Regenberg et al. 2009). Many operate in countries, such as the Bahamas, China, Ukraine, and Mexico, which have weak regulatory infrastructures to monitor the claims that are made by these clinics (Kiatpongsan and Sipp 2009). Thus, the term "stem cell tourism" is often used to refer to the movement of patients seeking out these treatments across international borders.

Much of the existing literature found on these stem cell clinics focuses on this dimension of tourism. Numerous commentaries have been published in the policy forums of scientific journals raising alarms over the increasing number of offshore clinics offering unproven stem cell treatments (e.g. Braude, Minger, and Warwick 2005; Nelson 2008; Eliza 2009; Kiatpongsan and Sipp 2009). The *American Journal of Bioethics* (AJOB) recently published open peer commentaries on two articles targeted at stem cell tourism. In one article, Zarzeczny and Caulfield (2010) point to the ethical and legal obligations that physicians may have toward their underage patients where their parents intend to taken them abroad for unproven stem cell treatments. In another, Murdoch and Scott (2010) warn against being paternalistic toward patients travelling to access treatments that may, if nothing else, provide them with hope.

Amongst the commentaries on these articles, there was general agreement with the authors that appropriate regulation is needed (Dolan 2010; McMahon and Thorsteinsdóttir 2010; Sipp 2010a), although the difficulties in implementing effective trans-national regulatory mechanisms were also noted (Shalev 2010). Some commentators argued that professional societies and organizations have a greater role to play in monitoring and enforcement (Caplan and Levine 2010; Crozier and Thomsen 2010; Devereaux and Loring 2010) and that clinicians, scientists, and health professionals needed to engage more directly in open dialogue with patients about the uses and limits of stem cells (Levine 2010; Regenberg 2010; Reimer, Borgelt, and Illes 2010). Others offered comments on hope and the need for more empirical research into the role it plays driving the stem cell tourism industry (Feudtner 2010; Guest and Anderson 2010). Another commentator suggested that the legal obligations owed by physicians to their minor patients might also extend to their incompetent adult patients (Chandler 2010).

Another of the commentaries, however, took a critical view of what they suggested was "stem cell exceptionalism" (Hauskeller and Wilson-Kovacs 2010). They argued that justifications are needed if standardized norms of evidence-based medical research are to apply to stem cell tourism and not to other largely unregulated, high-risk activities that involve trans-national travel, such as cosmetic surgery and gambling. This argument is based on both the practical realities of implementing regulation into legislative instruments across different localities (Wilson-Kovacs, Weber, and Hauskeller 2009) and on Murdoch and Scott's (2010: 18) point that some of these clinics may operate in countries that lack the appropriate economic, scientific, and logistical infrastructure to support standardized clinical trials. Some of these clinics also may be more focused on pursuing medical innovation to treat patients than conducting clinical research. Thus, both groups of authors caution against being overzealous in attempts to regulate offshore stem cell clinics.

Another important reason against implementing indiscriminate legislation against the fraudulence and charlatanry of some stem cell clinics is that it could stifle legitimate medical research and innovation (Lindvall and Hyun 2009). While effective measures are in place in many countries through advertising legislation to prevent false and fraudulent claims within national borders, they do not prevent, and may even encourage, travel to offshore clinics in less regulated markets (Kiatpongsan and Sipp 2009). Although these are important issues, we will not concern ourselves further with the movement of patients to offshore destinations for unproven stem cell treatments. Rather, we focus on the claim that stem cell treatments should be viewed as innovative medical procedures and so not as experimental research. This is the position of the International Cellular Medicine Society (ICMS), which is a professional organization in the United States that aims to advance "adult cell-based medical therapies" (http://www.cellmedicinesociety. org/). The implication of this claim is that the use of adult stem cells for non-validated indications would not need to be conducted under standardized norms of clinical research nor approved by the relevant national regulatory authorities.

The regulatory context of autologous stem cells

To unpack this claim, it is helpful to first assess whether the use of autologous stem cells is a medical procedure or something else. Centralised authorities, such as the Food & Drug Adminstration (FDA) in the United States, generally regulate the marketing of medicinal drugs, devices, and biologics, but not medical procedures. For example, surgical techniques and organ transplants are not regulated by the FDA, and physicians can prescribe drugs for "off label" use without formal approval (Deyo 2004). Thus, doctors can innovate in these areas without the need to undergo formal clinical trials, although they may be overseen by an institutional review board (IRB) and, over time, may publish results in peer-review journals which may (or may not) lead to formal clinical studies before becoming accepted by the profession as the standard of care. However, whether the use of autologous stem cells would fall into this category remains unclear.

Under the FDA's regulation of human cells, tissues, and cellular and tissue-based products (HCT/Ps), the uses of peripheral or umbilical cord blood stem cells for autologous use or in a first- or second-degree blood relative are exempted from premarket approval as a 361 product (FDA 2007b). For HCT/Ps to be exempt from premarket approval, they must meet all of the conditions stated in Section 1271.10 of the Food and Drugs code (FDA 2007a): These rules state that HCT/Ps must be:

1) Minimally manipulated, and
2) Intended only for homologous use, and
3) Not combined with another article (except for water, sterilizing, preservation or storage agents), and
4) Either:
   a. Have no systemic or metabolic effect, or
   b. Be for autologous use, allogeneic use in first–second-degree blood relative or reproductive use.

Under these criteria, the use of autologous stem cells for the treatment of blood malignancies is exempt from FDA approval. In this procedure, cells from the peripheral blood or bone marrow are removed from the patient prior to administering lethal doses of chemotherapy. Hematopoietic stem cells are purified and stored until they are returned to the patient to replenish and restore bone marrow function. The cells are not combined with anything other than the sterilizing and storage agents; they are minimally manipulated; and their use is homologous (i.e. taking bone marrow/blood cells out to replace bone marrow/blood cells). Hence, clinics undertaking this procedure for these purposes in the United States only need medical licenses.

HCT/Ps that do not meet these criteria are classified as biologics and are regulated under section 351 of the code (FDA 2007a). Products that the FDA has already determined to be biologics include allogeneic placental-derived cells for use in bone defects because it is non-homologous use, in combination with another article, and has a systemic effect (FDA 2010). Another is umbilical cord stem cells treated with enzyme to increase engraftment because the processing constitutes more than minimal manipulation. The position of ICMS is that the autologous use of stem cells from bone marrow for any indication should be exempt from these regulations because of the minimal manipulation that is involved in their isolation, storage, and so on (ICMS 2009). Hence, they have adopted a model developed by the assisted reproductive industry in the US, which is not regulated at the federal level and has its own accreditation criteria.

However, it is doubtful whether using autologous bone marrow or peripheral stem cells to treat conditions such as SCI or myocardial infarcts could be considered as "homologous use." In 2010, the FDA sought an injunction against a company in the US, whose medical director is founder of the ICMS, that claimed to use autologous bone marrow-derived mesenchymal stem cells to treat bone fractures, torn tendons, and other ailments (Cyranoski 2010). The FDA's position was that the cells are an adulterated drug product because they are more than minimally manipulated and intended for non-homologous use (FDA 2008).

Should the FDA be successful, stem cell clinics in the US will have to apply for a biologics license before marketing unapproved treatments, which are issued only after safety and efficacy of the product's intended use can be demonstrated. If the injunction is not granted, then this will potentially enable clinics to market autologous stem cell transplants for *any* purpose without regulatory oversight, both in the US and abroad.[2]

Given the regulatory context, it is difficult to see how an argument which calls for proper regulatory and peer oversight of novel stem cell treatments could be viewed as "exceptionalism." Indeed, it would appear that strong justifications would be needed if one were to argue that the norms of clinical research should apply to other approaches in regenerative medicine but not to adult stem cells. The "specialness" of adult cells is presumed to lie in the fact that they are from "adult" tissues and not embryos, which have tumorigenic properties. Their autologous use is also presumed to carry fewer risks than those associated with the immunogenic properties of allografts. However, recent reports of deaths occurring after transplant of fetal neural stem cells (Amariglio et al. 2009) and in autologous bone marrow cells for non-homologous uses (Kim 2010; Mendick and Palmer 2010) undermine these assumptions. Therefore, exempting clinics that offer stem cell treatments from the rigors of scientifically driven clinical research is unjustified, and this is so, even if these norms are more reflective of an ideal than an actual practice (cf. Hauskeller and Wilson-Kovacs 2010).

Moreover, regulation of autologous stem cells need not necessarily hamper innovative research. In 2008, a trachea engineered from autologous mesenchymal stem cell-derived chondrocytes was transplanted into a woman with end-stage bronchomalacia (Macchiarini et al. 2008). According to one of the collaborators, this procedure was planned and executed within a very short amount of time and with no grant application, pre-clinical testing, or regulatory validation (Hollander 2010). Instead, they proceeded with special permission from the relevant regulatory bodies of the two countries involved on the basis that their time frame would not allow them to obtain the necessary approvals and that the procedure might significantly improve the patient's quality of life. Thus, provided there is adequate flexibility and training within the regulatory authorities (Capps and Campbell 2010), there is scope for expediency in human experimentation with stem cells.

Paying for science

Another qualifying feature that distinguishes this trachea case from other unproven stem cell-based interventions is that the patient bore no special costs for the procedure. The costs of a chartered airplane to fly the trachea and surgeons to the patient were met by the University of Bristol (Hollander 2010). This raises questions about the view that it is acceptable to charge patients to participate in what are, essentially, unsupervised and unstructured human experiments. The clinical guidelines of the ICMS explicitly endorse the use of "pay-for-trial" research (ICMS 2009: 22), as well as not criticizing clinics that charge patients exorbitant fees. Such an endorsement of putting all the costs onto the patient, whether in treatment or in clinical trials, if it begins to spread, would signal a paradigm shift in how research is done and wholly alter the relationship between researchers and their research subjects.

---

[2] In 2012, the US District Court of Columbia found in favour of the FDA. Although as of 2013, this decision remained under appeal.

There is a conundrum here: if a treatment is unproven, then it must be experimental; but if subjects are paying to participate in an experimental study, can it really be called research? The payment suggests that it is treatment! However we resolve this conundrum, it is clear that there is an unfair asymmetry in the share of risks and benefits between researchers and participants when the patient-subject bears the costs of conducting the research. If clinical studies are successful, then both the participants and medical researchers potentially benefit: the researcher gets to publish positive results while making some money, and although the patient has had to pay for her participation, she potentially gets the therapeutic benefits. However, if the treatment is unsuccessful, then the patient is not only out of pocket but is potentially harmed by the treatment regimen while the researcher profits. Either way, the patient-subject bears the bulk of the risks and costs while the researcher assumes none.

It is unlikely that many clinical researchers would entertain the notion of charging patients to participate in their research, since this could make the relationship highly exploitative. The FDA does allow for payment by patients for experimental technologies in some instances. For example, although pharmaceutical companies generally pay for the cost of the trials needed to gain FDA approval for investigational drugs, they are permitted to charge patients for these drugs if used in treatment but *not* at a profit (Steinberg, Tunis, and Shapiro 1995). It is unclear how these rules would apply to autologous stem cells that are classified as biologics. In any case, it is reasonable to question the implications of charging patients to be research subjects, not just for regenerative medicine, but for research more generally.

Some may argue that charging patients to participate in medical experiments is the only way research will progress fast enough to help the many sick and dying patients who are in immediate need of treatments, particularly in countries that lack the scientific, economic, and logistical resources needed to conduct clinical trials (Murdoch and Scott 2010). However, such a rationale implies that the research is always therapeutic. While the moral justification for biomedical science may be to (eventually) generate therapeutic benefits, the main purpose of scientific research is to produce generalizable knowledge (Belmont Report 1979).

Charging patients to take part in research under the pretense that they are being treated not only conflates the duties of the physicians with those of researchers: it is also likely to exacerbate drastically the therapeutic misconception amongst patients. This misconception occurs when research subjects fail to appreciate the distinction between the imperatives of clinical research and treatment, and thereby incorrectly attribute therapeutic intention to research (Lidz and Appelbaum 2002). A patient who pays considerable fees for a treatment should rightly expect that the primary intention of clinicians is to provide a therapeutic service. However, the therapeutic intent that the act of payment implies undoubtedly overshadows the experimental orientation of the unproven stem cell treatments. Thus, it is just as misleading to call these pay-for-trial types of services "research" as "therapies."

Another problem that may exacerbate the therapeutic misconception is the language that is employed to describe these so-called stem cell treatments, not just by the clinics marketing them, but also by those studying and commentating on the phenomena. Terms such as "stem cell treatment," "stem cell therapy," "stem cell transplant," or "stem cell clinic" may imply that the intervention has some sort of therapeutic benefit when efficacy has yet to be demonstrated. Even using the term "stem cell" can be presumptive as the heterogeneity of cell populations makes it difficult to ascertain precisely what is being used in these purported treatments (Lau et al. 2008). Even the terms 'treatment' and 'therapy' can be misleading. However, pinning down appropriate nomenclature is challenging. The more precisely the nature of specific procedures is described, the less recognizable it becomes to a lay audience.[3] We don't offer any solutions to this problem, but recognize it as an issue that requires more discussion.

Another term we find problematic is "stem cell tourism." This term is misleading and somewhat limiting given the fact that many of these clinics also operate in the highly regulated markets of the United States and the European Union (Regenberg et al. 2009), where a large part of their customer base reside.[4] It is arguable that the term also puts the blame on the tourist (or patient) rather than the clinics and physicians who provide the services. When conventional medicine reaches its outer limits, patients have ethical motivations for pursuing treatments elsewhere (Murdoch and Scott 2010) and so they should not be the focus of critical inquiry. Physicians, clinical scientists, and other health-care providers are invested with an enormous amount of trust and authority, and so it is not only entirely justifiable, but an imperative, that their activities are held to the highest ethical standards, regardless of where they are located.

Bioethical and policy implications

As we look ahead to the developments in medicine over the coming decades, there is no doubt that regenerative medicine will gain more and more prominence. It is a pity, then, that the bioethics literature is so sparse up to this point, and, especially, that the polarized debate on embryonic stem cells has masked a whole set of other ethical concerns, summarized in the previous sections. Moreover, the lack of bioethical discussion is matched by a failure of governments and regulatory agencies to perceive and meet the challenges presented by these rapidly emerging developments.

Given the expansion of stem cell research over the last decade or more, it is surprising that most major jurisdictions, though tightening up some controls on experimental medicine, have not matched this with proper ethical monitoring of clinical applications and of the unclear boundary between the two. "Translational Clinical Research" is beyond doubt one of the policy buzzwords of our era, with its accompanying slogan "from bench to bedside" drawing massive public and private investment into areas such as regenerative medicine. But the ethical risks in these developments are either not properly anticipated, or are deliberately ignored, in the interests of national commercial success (the Hwang case is the paradigmatic example of this). True, some national regulatory agencies have begun to take action against clinics for making false or misleading claims (Kiatpongsan and Sipp 2009) and are more consistently utilizing the existing legal frameworks that regulate medical and biological technologies (Cyranoski 2010). However, it seems that serious debate is still needed about how to implement

---

[3] We owe this point to Douglas Sipp (personal communication).
[4] We owe this point to Douglas Sipp (personal communication).

appropriate regulation to protect research subjects and patients from undue harm and exploitation without impeding scientific progress to the bedside. For its part, we find that bioethics has, on the whole, failed to provide much in terms of moral guidance on the issues. How has this happened?

As we have already noted, attention to date around stem cell research has largely focused on the moral issues raised by the creation and destruction of human embryos. While these issues are not unique to stem cell research—they had previously received considerable attention in relation to the use of human embryos in research around assisted reproductive technologies—they were thrust (back) into the limelight following the cloning of Dolly the sheep (Wilmut et al. 1997) and isolation of the first ESC line from human blastocysts (Thomson et al. 1998). Focus on these issues reflected national and international regulatory disputes over the permissibility of this research and (specifically in the United States) whether such research ought to be classed as ineligible for federal funding.

As many regulators around the world have settled on policies that attempt to balance the need to protect nascent human life against the duty to promote beneficial medical outcomes (Hauskeller 2005a), the ESC debates appear to have subsided somewhat. However, given the fervour with which they were pursued in the first decade of this century, it is tempting to speculate on the implications that they may have had for the proliferation of unproven stem cell-based interventions. We would explain this as follows. In response to fiercely held opposition to ESC research, many advocates promoted the potential medical and therapeutic utility of this research. Claims that ESCs could be used for a range of currently untreatable illnesses and conditions were often made with great enthusiasm, such that proponents were sometimes criticized for "hyping" or overselling the research. These were followed by the counterclaims of opponents making equally hyperbolic assertions about the actual and potential utility of ASCs. Thus, both *advocates* and *opponents* of ESC research may have unwittingly encouraged understandings in the public discourse that "stem cells" not only hold great promise but that the miracle cures they might produce are just around the corner.

While it is likely that other narratives and social conditions are playing important roles in driving patients toward the dubious promises of stem cell treatments (Dolan 2010), it is instructive to reflect on how the bioethical debates may have contributed to the current context. The high profile and credibility of some of the scientific, political, medical, and bioethical actors both supporting and opposing ESC research have undoubtedly made it easier for unscrupulous operators to market unproven treatments in the ethical vacuum created. In particular, this bioethical focus on the moral status of embryos may have distracted attention away from other equally, if not more, important issues and so may have led to a hiatus in proper scrutiny and regulation of the regenerative medicine industry as a whole.

Unfortunately, then, the philosophical depth of many of the discussions of this new feature of medical research and practice has been depressingly shallow. Libertarians and consequentialists have lined up on one side and their opponents have been caricatured as unthinking dogmatists, driven by partisan, often religious, concerns. When this happens, the participants in the debate talk past each other and policymakers have nowhere to turn for guidance, as they seek to update laws and regulations. Yet there could have been common ground, if the proponents on both sides had seen their common concern for the effective defense of the vulnerable and for the promotion of social justice in health care. We have tried to identify this common ground in the detailed specification of the ethical issues that emerge if we get out of the "heat" of the debate about the status of human embryos. In this cooler atmosphere, we would argue, a reflective and critical bioethical analysis could have clear political relevance.

While it is perhaps not immediately apparent that the role of bioethics should be a political one, in actuality it is difficult to argue that it is not. In many jurisdictions, bioethics has been installed into the political system with an array of national bioethical advisory committees providing high levels of government with normative advice on policy development (Salter and Salter 2007). Whether this advice translates into morally sound policy or merely acts as a means of legitimating existing policy preferences is highly debatable (Jasanoff 2005; Campbell 2008). Bioethical advice that comes in the form of contestable philosophical argument is the most problematic. This contestability was demonstrated by the now defunct President's Bioethics Council set up by President Bush on clearly ideological lines (Charo 2007). This body was recently replaced by President Obama with a commission that "offers practical policy options" and is aimed at consensus building (Wade 2009). We do not suggest that, within the discipline, metaphysical debate should not continue to play an important role in shaping our understandings of fundamental principles and concepts. However, in order to stay relevant in changing political climates, bioethicists would do well to follow the President's lead and look for ways to forge agreements and make more meaningful contributions to the public good.

Conclusion

This chapter was not intended to provide an exhaustive analysis of the bioethical issues raised by the use of unproven stem cell treatments. Rather, we wanted to place these activities within the broader field of regenerative medicine and provide an overview of the ethical and regulatory issues that are presented by them. In the spirit of this volume, we hope that bioethicists of the future will focus greater attention on these and other issues that are likely to emerge as the translational science of regenerative medicine enters clinical practice. For if it is not the place of bioethicists to grapple with these issues and make practical contributions that generate the best ethical outcomes, then it is not clear whose role it would be. This commitment will involve moving beyond the contested philosophical issues surrounding human embryos and the meaning of life, and toward the more practical issues that arise in the translational sciences. We are not saying that bioethics should be *merely* pragmatic: theoretical and normative discussion will always be required. However, we need to be sure that our critical analysis both starts and ends in the whole range of dilemmas that medicine engenders and that it tries to foresee the new challenges that will emerge from scientific advance.

References

Aalto-Setälä, K., Conklin, B. R., and Lo, B. (2009). "Obtaining Consent for Future Research with Induced Pluripotent Cells: Opportunities and Challenges," *PLoS Biology*, 7(2): e42.

Addis, R. C., Bulte, J. W. M., and Gearhart, J. D. (2008). "Special Cells, Special Considerations: The Challenges of Bringing Embryonic Stem Sells from the Laboratory to the Clinic," *Clinical Pharmacology and Therapeutics*, 83(3): 386–9.

Advanced Cell Technology. (2011). "Advanced Cell Technology Receives FDA Clearance for Clinical Trials Using Embryonic Stem Cells to Treat Age-Related Macular Degeneration," January 3, http://www.advancedcell.com/news-and-media/press-releases/advanced-c ell-technology-receives-fda-clearance-for-clinical-trials-using-embryonic-stem-cells-to-tre/ (accessed January 7, 2011).

Amariglio, N., et al. (2009). "Donor-Derived Brain Tumor Following Neural Stem Cell Transplantation in an Ataxia Telangiectasia Patient," *PLoS Med*, 6(2): e1000029.

Bartunek, J. et al. (2010). "Cells as Biologics for Cardiac Repair in Ischaemic Heart Failure," *Heart*, 96(10): 792–800.

Belmont Report. (1979). "Ethical Principles and Guidelines for the Protection of Human Subjects of Research," *The National Commission for the Protection of Human Subjects of Biomedical and Behavioral Research*, April 18, http://www.hhs.gov/ohrp/humansubjects/guidance/belmont. html (accessed November 19, 2010).

Beltrami, A. P. et al. (2003). "Adult Cardiac Stem Cells are Multipotent and Support Myocardial Regeneration," *Cell*, 114(6): 763–76.

Bok, H., Schill, K. E., and Faden, R. R. (2004). "Justice, Ethnicity, and Stem-Cell Banks," *The Lancet*, 364(9429): 118–21.

Braude, P., Minger, S. L., and Warwick, R. M. (2005). "Stem Cell Therapy: Hope or Hype?" *BMJ*, 330(7501): 1159–60.

Brill, S., Zvibel, I., and Reid, L. M. (1999). "Expansion Conditions for Early Hepatic Progenitor Cells from Embryonal and Neonatal Rat Livers," *Digestive Diseases and Sciences*, 44(2): 364–71.

Campbell, A. V. (2008). "Public Policy and the Future of Bioethics in Asia," *Asian Bioethics Review*, Inaugural Edition (December): 24–30.

Caplan, A., and Levine, B. (2010). "Hope, Hype and Help: Ethically Assessing the Growing Market in Stem Cell Therapies," *The American Journal of Bioethics*, 10(5): 24–5.

Capps, B., and Campbell, A. V. (2010). "Contested Cells: An Introduction," in B. Capps and A. Campbell (eds), *Contested Cells: Global Perspectives on the Stem Cell Debate*. London: Imperial College Press, 1–54.

Caulfield, T., Ogbogu, U., and Isasi, R. M. (2007). "Informed Consent in Embryonic Stem Cell Research: Are We Following Basic Principles?" *Canadian Medical Association Journal*, 176(12): 1722–5.

Chandler, J. (2010). "Stem Cell Tourism: Doctors' Duties to Minors and Other Incompetent Patients," *The American Journal of Bioethics*, 10(5): 27–8.

Charo, A. (2007). "The Endarkenment," in L. A. Eckenweiler and F. G. Cohn (eds), *The Ethics of Bioethics*. Baltimore: Johns Hopkins University Press, 95–107.

Conley, B. J. et al. (2004). "Derivation, Propagation and Differentiation of Human Embryonic Stem Cells," *The International Journal of Biochemistry and Cell Biology*, 36(4): 555–67.

Crozier, G. K. D., and Thomsen, K. (2010). "Stem Cell Tourism and the Role of Health Professional Organizations," *The American Journal of Bioethics*, 10(5): 36–8.

Cyranoski, D. (2010). "FDA Challenges Stem-Cell Clinic," *Nature*, 466: 909.

Devereaux, M., and Loring, J. F. (2010). "Growth of an Industry: How U.S. Scientists and Clinicians Have Enabled Stem Cell Tourism," *The American Journal of Bioethics*, 10(5): 45–6.

Deyo, R. A. (2004). "Gaps, Tensions, and Conflicts in the FDA Approval Process: Implications for Clinical Practice," *Journal of the American Board of Family Medicine*, 17(2): 142–9.

Dickenson, D. (2002). "Commodification of Human tissue: Implications for Feminist and Development Ethics," *Developing World Bioethics*, 2(1): 55–63.

Dodds, S. (2004). "Women, Commodification, and Embryonic Stem Cell Research," in J. M. Humber and R. F. Almeder (eds), *Biomedical Ethics Reviews: Stem Cell Research*. Totowa: Humana Press, 151–74.

Dolan, T. (2010). "A Three-Pronged Management Strategy to Stem Cell Tourism," *The American Journal of Bioethics*, 10(5): 43–5.

Dolphin, W. (2009). "Avita Develops a Growth Culture," *PcW BioForum*, July–September, www.avitamedical.com/?ob=3&id=217 (accessed October 27, 2010).

Ehnert, S. et al. (2009). "The Possible Use of Stem Cells in Regenerative Medicine: Dream or Reality?" *Langenbeck's Archives of Surgery*, 394(6): 985–97.

Elger, B. et al. (eds). (2008). *Ethical Issues in Governing Biobanks: Global Perspectives*. Hampshire: Ashgate.

Eliza, B. (2009). "Stem-Cell Experts Raise Concerns about Medical Tourism," *The Lancet*, 373(9667): 883–4.

Engelhardt, H. T. (2009). "Regenerative Medicine after Humanism: Puzzles Regarding the Use of Embryonic Stem Cells, Germs-Line Genetic Engineering and the Immanent Pursuit of Human Flourishing," in I. King-Tak (ed.), *The Bioethics of Renegerative Medicine*. Dordrecht: Springer, 13–46.

Engelhardt, J. F. et al. (1995). "Progenitor Cells of the Adult Human Airway Involved in Submucosal Gland Development," *Development*, 121(7): 2031–46.

FDA. (2007a). "Code of Federal Regulations: Food and Drugs," Title 21, Volume 8, August, http://www.fda.gov/BiologicsBloodVaccines/GuidanceComplianceRegulatoryInformation/Guidances/Tissue/ucm073366.htm (accessed November 20, 2010).

FDA. (2007b). "Regulation of Human Cells, Tissues, and Cellular and Tissue-Based Products (HCT/Ps): Small Entity Compliance Guide," August, http://www.fda.gov/BiologicsBloodVaccines/GuidanceComplianceRegulatoryInformation/Guidances/Tissue/ucm073366.htm (accessed November 20, 2010).

FDA. (2008). "Regenerative Sciences, Inc.," July 25, http://www.fda.gov/BiologicsBloodVaccines/GuidanceComplianceRegulatoryInformation/ComplianceActivities/Enforcement/UntitledLetters/ucm091991.htm (accessed November 18, 2010).

FDA. (2010). "Tissue Reference Group Annual Reports," http://www.fda.gov/BiologicsBloodVaccines/TissueTissueProducts/RegulationofTissues/ucm152857.htm (accessed November 18, 2010).

Feudtner, C. (2010). "Taking Care of Hope," *The American Journal of Bioethics*, 10(5): 26–7.

Gage, F. (2002). "Discussion Point Stem Cells of the Central Nervous System," *Current Opinion in Neurobiology*, 8(5): 671–6.

Geron. (2010). "Geron Initiates Clinical Trial of Human Embryonic Stem Cell-Based Therapy," October 11, http://ir.geron.com/phoenix.zhtml?c=67323&p=irol-newsArticle&ID=1636150&highlight= (accessed December 7, 2012).

Giacomini, M., Baylis, F., and Robert, J. (2007). "Banking on It: Public Policy and the Ethics of Stem Cell Research and Development," *Social Science and Medicine*, 65(7): 1490–500.

Glasner, P. (2005). "Banking on Immortality? Exploring the Stem Cell Supply Chain from Embryo to Therapeutic Application," *Current Sociology*, 53(2): 355–66.

Gluckman, E. (2000). "Current Status of Umbilical Cord Blood Hematopoietic Stem Cell Transplantation," *Experimental Hematology*, 28(11): 1197–205.

Goggin, G., and Newell, C. (2004). "Uniting the Nation? Disability, Stem Cells, and the Australian Media," *Disability and Society*, 19(1): 47–60.

Greenwood, H. et al. (2006). "Regenerative Medicine: New Opportunities for Developing Countries," *International Journal of Biotechnology*, 8(1–2): 60–77.

Guest, J., and Anderson, K. (2010). "Hopes and Illusions," *The American Journal of Bioethics*, 10(5): 47–8.

Haddow, G. et al. (2010). "Not 'Human' Enough to Be Human but Not 'Animal' Enough to Be Animal: The Case of the HFEA, Cybrids, and Xenotransplantation in the UK," *New Genetics and Society*, 29(1): 3–17.

Haimes, E., and Taylor, K. (2009). "Fresh Embryo Donation for Human Embryonic Stem Cell (hESC) Research: The Experiences and Values of IVF Couples Asked to Be Embryo Donors," *Human Reproduction*, 24(9): 2142–50.

Hanna, J., Saha, K., and Jaenisch, R. (2010). "Pluripotency and Cellular Reprogramming: Facts, Hypotheses, Unresolved Issues," *Cell*, 143(4): 508–25.

Hauskeller, C. (2005a). "Introduction," in W. Bender, C. Hauskeller, and A. Manzei (eds), *Crossing Borders: Cultural, Religious, and Political Differences Concerning Stem Cell Research*. Munster: Agenda Verlag, 9–24.

Hauskeller, C. (2005b). "The Language of Stem Cell Science," in W. Bender, C. Hauskeller, and A. Manzei (eds), *Crossing Borders: Cultural, Religious, and Political Differences Concerning Stem Cell Research*. Munster: Agenda Verlag, 39–60.

Hauskeller, C., and Wilson-Kovacs, D. (2010). "Traveling across Borders: The Pitfalls of Clinical Trial Regulation and Stem Cell Exceptionalism," *The American Journal of Bioethics*, 10(5): 38–40.

Hollander, A. P. (2010). "A Case Study of Experimental Stem Cell Therapy and the Risks of Over-Regulation," in B. Capps, and A. Campbell (eds), *Contested Cells: Global Perspectives on the Stem Cell Debate*. London: Imperial College Press, 57–62.

Holm, S. (2002). "Going to the Roots of the Stem Cell Controversy," *Bioethics*, 16(6): 493–507.

Holm, S. (2005). "Embryonic Stem Cell Research and the Moral Status of Human Embryos," *Reproductive BioMedicine Online*, 10(Supplement 1): 63–7.

Hyun, I. (2008). "Stem Cells from Skin Cells: The Ethical Questions," *Hastings Center Report*, 38(1): 20–2.

Hyun, I. et al. (2007). "New Advances in iPS Cell Research Do Not Obviate the Need for Human Embryonic Stem Cells," *Cell Stem Cell*, 1(4): 367–8.

ICMS. (2009). "ICMS Clinical Guidelines," April, http://cellmedicinesociety.org/component/content/category/44?layout=blog (accessed December 7, 2012).

Jasanoff, S. (2005). *Designs on Nature: Science and Democracy in Europe and the United States*. Princeton, NJ: Princeton University Press.

Jones, E. M., and Sarvetnick, N. (1997). "Islet Regeneration in IFNgamma Transgenic Mice," *Hormone and Metabolic Research*, 29(6): 308–10.

Jones, M., and Salter, B. (2003). "The Governance of Human Genetics: Policy Discourse and Constructions of Public Trust," *New Genetics and Society*, 22(1): 21–41.

Kiatpongsan, S., and Sipp, D. (2009). "Monitoring and Regulating Offshore Stem Cell Clinics," *Science*, 323(5921): 1564–5.

Kim, T.-H. (2010). "Concerns Grow over Stem Cell Therapies," *The Korea Times*, October 16, http://www.koreatimes.co.kr/www/news/tech/2010/10/129_75215.html (accessed November 19, 2010).

King, N. M. P., Coughlin, C. N., and Furth, M. (2009). "Ethical Issues in Regenerative Medicine," *Wake Forest Intellectual Property Law Journal*, 9(3): 215–38.

King-Tak, I. (ed.). (2009). *The Bioethics of Regenerative Medicine*. Dordrecht: Springer.

Lau, D. et al. (2008). "Stem Cell Clinics Online: The Direct-to-Consumer Portrayal of Stem Cell Medicine," *Cell Stem Cell*, 3(6): 591–4.

Levine, A. D. (2010). "Insights from Patients' Blogs and the Need for Systematic Data on Stem Cell Tourism," *The American Journal of Bioethics*, 10(5): 28–9.

Lidz, C. W., and Appelbaum, P. S. (2002). "The Therapeutic Misconception: Problems and Solutions," *Medical Care*, 40(Supp 9): V55–63.

Lindvall, O., and Hyun, I. (2009). "Medical Innovation Versus Stem Cell Tourism," *Science*, 324(5935): 1664–5.

Lo, P.-C. (2009). "Secular Humanist Bioethics and Regenerative Medicine," in I. King-Tak (ed.), *The Bioethics of Renegerative Medicine*. Dordrecht: Springer, 47–62.

Lysaght, T., and Kerridge, I. H. (2010). "Rhetoric, Power and Legitimacy in Public Discourse: A Critical Analysis of the Public Discourse Surrounding the Review of Embryo Research and Cloning Legislation in Australia in 2005–6," in B. J. Capps, and A. Campbell (eds), *Contested Cells: Global Perspectives on the Stem Cell Debate*. Lodnon: Imperial College Press, 189–206.

Macchiarini, P. et al. (2008). "Clinical Transplantation of a Tissue-Engineered Airway," *Lancet*, 372(9655): 2023–30.

Mackenney, J., and Capps, B. (2010). "New Developments in Stem Cell Science: iPS Cells and the Challenge to Consent," in B. Capps, and A. Campbell (eds), *Contested Cells: Global Perspectives on the Stem Cell Debate*. London: Imperial College Press, 207–40.

Mason, C., and Dunnill, P. (2008). "A Brief Definition of Regenerative Medicine," *Regenerative Medicine*, 3(1): 1–5.

Mason, C., and Manzotti, E. (2010). "Regenerative Medicine Cell Therapies: Numbers of Units Manufactured and Patients Treated between 1988 and 2010," *Regenerative Medicine*, 5(3): 307–13.

McKay, R. (1997). "Stem Cells in the Central Nervous System," *Science*, 276(5309): 66–71.

McMahon, D., and Thorsteinsdóttir, H. (2010). "Regulations *Are* Needed for Stem Cell Tourism: Insights From China," *The American Journal of Bioethics*, 10(5): 34–6.

Mendick, R., and Palmer, A. (2010). "Baby Death Scandal at Stem Cell Clinic Which Treats Hundreds of British Patients a Year," *The Telegraph*, October 23, http://www.telegraph.co.uk/news/worldnews/europe/germany/8082935/Baby-death-scandal-at-stem-cell-clinic-which-treats-hundreds-of-British-patients-a-year.html (accessed November 18, 2010).

Murdoch, C. E., and Scott, C. T. (2010). "Stem Cell Tourism and the Power of Hope," *The American Journal of Bioethics*, 10(5): 16–23.

Nelson, B. (June 2008). "Stem Cell Researchers Face Down Stem Cell Tourism," *Nature Reports Stem Cells*, DOI:10.1038/stemcells.2008.89, http://www.nature.com/stem-cells/2008/0806/080605/full/stemcells.2008.89.html.

Normile, D., Vogel, G., and Couzin, J. (2006). "South Korean Team's Remaining Human Stem Cell Claim Demolished," *Science*, 311(5758): 156–7.

Organogenesis. (2008). "Organogenesis, Inc. Announces Apligraf® Cell Therapy Reimbursed in Switzerland," http://www.organogenesis.com/products/bioactive_woundhealing/apligraf.html (accessed October 20, 2010).

Parry, S. (2006). "(Re)Constructing Embryos in Stem Cell Research: Exploring the Meaning of Embryos for People Involved in Fertility Treatments," *Social Science and Medicine*, 62(10): 2349–59.

Pasquini, M. C. et al. (2010). "Hematopoietic Stem Cell Transplantation for Multiple Sclerosis: Collaboration of the CIBMTR and EBMT to Facilitate International Clinical Studies," *Biology of Blood and Marrow Transplantation*, 16(8): 1076–83.

Powell, J. L., Hingorani, P., and Kolb, E. A. (2009). "Hematopoietic Stem Cell Transplantation," *eMedicine*, http://emedicine.medscape.com/article/991032-overview (accessed October 26, 2010).

Provoost, V. et al. (2010). "Patients' Conceptualization of Cryopreserved Embryos Used in Their Fertility Treatment," *Human Reproduction*, 25(3): 705–13.

Rao, M., and Condic, M. L. (2008). "Alternative Sources of Pluripotent Stem Cells: Scientific Solutions to an Ethical Dilemma," *Stem Cells Dev*, 17(1): 1–10.

Regenberg, A. C. (2010). "Tweeting Science and Ethics: Social Media as a Tool for Constructive Public Engagement," *The American Journal of Bioethics*, 10(5): 30–1.

Regenberg, A. C. et al. (2009). "Medicine on the Fringe: Stem Cell-Based Interventions in Advance of Evidence," *Stem Cells*, 27(9): 2312–19.

Reimer, J., Borgelt, E., and Illes, J. (2010). "In Pursuit of 'Informed Hope' in the Stem Cell Discourse," *The American Journal of Bioethics*, 10(5): 31–2.

Rossi, D. J., Jamieson, C. H. M., and Weissman, I. L. (2008). "Stems Cells and the Pathways to Aging and Cancer," *Cell*, 132(4): 681–96.

Rossi, S. L., and Keirstead, H. S. (2009). "Stem Cells and Spinal Cord Regeneration," *Current Opinion in Biotechnology*, 20(5): 552–62.

Salter, B., and Salter, C. (2007). "Bioethics and the Global Moral Economy," *Science, Technology, and Human Values*, 32(5): 554–81.

Schwartz, P. H., and Bryant, P. J. (2008). "Therapeutic Uses of Stem Cells," in K. R. Monroe, R. B. Miller, and J. S. Tobis (eds), *Fundamentals of the Stem Cell Debate: The Scientific, Religious, Ethical and Political Issues*. Berkeley, CA: University of California, 37–62.

Shalev, C. (2010). "Stem Cell Tourism: A Challenge for Trans-National Governance," *The American Journal of Bioethics*, 10(5): 40–2.

Shire Regenerative Medicine (2012). "Dermagraft® Product Fact Sheet," http://www2.dermagraft.com/wp-content/uploads/2012/11/DG-1007-010-DG_Fact_Sheet.pdf (accessed January 2, 2013).

Singec, I. et al. (2007). "The Leading Edge of Stem Cell Therapeutics," *Annual Review of Medicine*, 58: 313–28.

Sipp, D. (2009). "Gold Standards in the Diamond Age: The Commodification of Pluripotency," *Cell Stem Cell*, 5(4): 360–3.

Sipp, D. (2010a). "Hope Alone Is Not an Outcome: Why Regulations Makes Sense for the Global Stem Cell Industry," *The American Journal of Bioethics*, 10(5): 33–4.

Steinberg, E. P., Tunis, S., and Shapiro, D. (1995). "Insurance Coverage for Experimental Technologies," *Health Affairs*, 144: 143–58.

Stemplea, D. L., and Anderson, D. J. (1992). "Isolation of a Stem Cell for Neurons and Glia from the Mammalian Neural Crest," *Cell*, 71(6): 973–85.

Storb, R. (2003). "Allogeneic Hematopoietic Stem Cell Transplantation: Yesterday, Today, and Tomorrow," *Experimental Hematology*, 31(1): 1–10.

Streiffer, R. (2005). "At the Edge of Humanity: Human Stem Cells, Chimeras, and Moral Status," *Kennedy Institute of Ethics Journal*, 15(4): 347–70.

Strong, C. (1997). "The Moral Status of Preembryos, Embryos, Fetuses, and Infants," *Journal of Medicine and Philosophy*, 22(5): 457–78.

Sugarman, J. et al. (1997). "Ethical Issues in Umbilical Cord Blood Banking," *JAMA*, 278(11): 938–43.

Sugarman, J., Reisner, E. G., and Kurtzberg, J. (1995). "Ethical Aspects of Banking Placental Blood for Transplantation," *JAMA*, 274(22): 1783–5.

Svoboda, J. S., Van Howe, R. S., and Dwyer, J. G. (2000). "Informed Consent for Neonatal Circumcision: An Ethical and Legal Conundrum," *Journal of Contemporary Health Law and Policy*, 17: 61–134.

Tate, D. G., and Pledger, C. (2007). "An Integrative Conceptual Framework of Disability: New Directions for Research," in A. E. Dell Orto and P. W. Power (eds), *The Psychological and Social Impact of Illness and Disability*. New York: Springer, 22–36.

Thomson, J. A. et al. (1998). "Embryonic Stem Cell Lines Derived from Human Blastocysts," *Science*, 282(5391): 1145–7.

Verfaillie, C. M., Pera, M. F., and Lansdorp, P. M. (2002). "Stem Cells: Hype and Reality," *American Society of Hematology Education Program Book*, Issue 1: 369–91.

Vierbuchen, T. et al. (2010). "Direct Conversion of Fibroblasts to Functional Neurons by Defined Factors," *Nature*, 463(7284): 1035–41.

Wade, N. (2009). "Obama Plans to Replace Bush's Bioethics Panel," *New York Times*, June 17, http://www.nytimes.com/2009/06/18/us/politics/18ethics.html?_r=1&scp=1&sq=President%27s%20Council%20on%20Bioethics&st=cse (accessed November 19, 2010).

Waldby, C. (2008). "Oocyte Markets: Women's Reproductive Labour in Embryonic Stem Cell Research," *New Genetics and Society*, 27(1): 19–31.

Waldby, C., and Mitchell, R. (2006). *Tissue Economies: Blood, Organs and Cell Lines in Late Capitalism* Durham, NC: Duke University Press.

Watts, F. M., Lo Celso, C., and Silva-Vargas, V. (2006). "Epidermal Stem Cells: An Update," *Current Opinion in Genetics and Development*, 16(5): 518–24.

Wijeyekoon, R., and Barker, R. A. (2009). "Cell Replacement Therapy for Parkinson's Disease," *Biochimica et Biophysica Acta (BBA): Molecular Basis of Disease*, 1792(7): 688–702.

Wilkins, L. M. et al. (1994). "Development of a Bilayered Living Skin Construct for Clinical Applications," *Biotechnology and Bioengeering*, 43(8): 747–56.

Wilmut, I. et al. (1997). "Viable Offspring Derived from Fetal and Adult Mammalian Cells," *Nature*, 385(6619): 810–13.

Wilson-Kovacs, D. M., Weber, S., and Hauskeller, C. (2009). "Stem Cells Clinical Trials for Cardiac Repair: Regulation as Practical Accomplishment," *Sociology of Health and Illness*, 32(1): 89–105.

Yin, H. et al. (2009). "Cell Reprogramming for the Creation of Patient-Specific Pluripotent Stem Cells by Defined Factors," *Frontiers of Agriculture in China*, 3(2): 199–208.

Zarzeczny, A., and Caulfield, T. (2010). "Stem Cell Tourism and Doctors' Duties to Minors: A View From Canada," *The American Journal of Bioethics*, 10(5): 3–15.

Zuk, P. A. et al. (2002). "Human Adipose Tissue Is a Source of Multipotent Stem Cells," *Molecular Biology of the Cell*, 13(12): 4279–95.

1.2

Commentary
Stem Cell Clinical Research: The Biology Determines the Ethics

Douglas Sipp

In their study of ethical tensions in the development and implementation of the emerging field of regenerative medicine, Lysaght and Campbell argue persuasively that it is time for the discussion of ethical, legal, and social issues (ELSI) surrounding stem cell research to expand beyond the now-familiar territory of the moral status of human blastocysts, cloning, species-crossing embryo constructs, and monochrome contrasts of dignity and utility. They introduce and examine a new set of issues that will inevitably need to be more fully addressed in order for regenerative clinical applications to be developed in a responsible, ethical, and scientifically responsible manner. These include questions of informed consent, both on the part of tissue donors and patient-subjects; risk–benefit balance assessment in "no-option" patients; and the controversial practice of commercialization of un- and under-regulated stem cell treatments.

I applaud their pioneering spirit in moving beyond the recent history of stem cell ethics to address issues of more practical concern that have already begin to emerge on the horizons. At the same time, I would hope to see them deepen their analysis in light of the rapid advances in recent years in the translation of stem cell research to clinical applications, both licit and illicit.

One area in which more in-depth work needs to be done is how the nature of cell-based treatments, in which thousands to billions of cells are transplanted or reimplanted into a patient with the expectation that they will either functionally integrate into and repair the patient's tissue over long periods, or affect modulatory responses through the secretion of molecular factors, such as cytokines, over shorter periods, distinguishes such approaches from other established clinical practices, such as surgical operations, small-molecule pharmaceutical compounds, medical devices, vaccines, and monoclonal antibodies and other biomolecular approaches. Such differences may be of great importance not only in the design of clinical research trials, but in the calculation of risk–benefit balances and the provision of informational resources used in obtaining informed consent.

Living cells are distinct from all of the above therapeutic modalities for a number of reasons. The expectation in many proposed clinical applications is that cells will functionally integrate and survive, possibly for the lifetime of the patient, which is fundamentally different from expectations for molecular compounds. Surgical procedures and medical devices also produce lifelong effects, but do not show the dynamism, heterogeneity, and stochastic behavior that populations of living cells do. Vaccines are perhaps more similar, in that they result in permanent or long-lasting effects on the patient's immune system, which is comprised of living cells and tissues, but the administration of a vaccine antigen still does not involve the introduction of quantities of cells, and indeed is expected to be cleared from the body within days by the triggered immune response.

Clearly, the transplantation of cells intended to remain biologically active for decades is a profoundly different paradigm from the administration of a drug compound that will be metabolized and eliminated over the course of hours or days, or the implantation of a medical device designed to be biologically inert. This has profound implications for the design of clinical trials, for example, in that patient-subjects may be unable to withdraw easily once they have received a transplant, which is a fundamental privilege enjoyed by human research subjects in drug trials. Along similar lines, given the potential survival of transplanted cells over the life of the recipient, and the current uncertainty over the long-term stability and toxicity of cellular grafts, trials and subsequently therapies will need to be engineered with an inbuilt "exit strategy," such as an inducible suicide gene, or be subject to years, perhaps decades, of follow-up to exclude late-onset adverse effects.

The potential longevity of cellular transplants is not the only distinguishing characteristic of cell-based treatment modalities. Stem cells in particular are known to behave in ways that simultaneously make them both attractive and risky candidates for therapeutic use. Stem cells are operationally defined by two hallmark characteristics: self-renewal and differentiation. They also have the capacity to proliferate or to generate highly proliferative progeny, and in some cases to migrate to sites of injury or tumors, and to promote angiogenesis. Differentiation, proliferation, migration, and blood vessel formation all have exciting possible uses in therapy, but can also be pathogenic when not kept under appropriate control. Misdifferentiation can lead to benign or malignant growths; uncontrolled proliferation is a cause of hypertrophy or tumorigenesis; migration to inappropriate sites may result in the integration of transplanted cells into non-target tissues; angiogenesis can be harmful if it promotes tumor growth. As we can see, like many powerful technologies, stem cells have something of a double-edged quality. These problems can be further compounded when cells have integrated into deep or difficult-to-access tissues, such as heart muscle or the brain.

Proposed uses of pluripotent stem cell-derived cell populations have particular issues as well, given the well-known propensity for both embryonic stem (ES) cells and iPS cells to trigger teratoma formation when injected subcutaneously into rodent models. iPS cells may be encumbered with additional safety issues, as the vectors used in some reprogramming methods can cause genomic instability through, for example, insertional mutagenesis. Finally, manipulation of cells of any type, such as by *ex vivo* treatment with growth factors or extended cell culture, carries risks of contamination, karyotypic instability, and changes in cellular properties and behavior as a consequence of adaptation to culture. Such contingencies must be clearly enunciated to clinical research subjects, and steps must be taken during the design of clinical studies to minimize risks and allow for the mitigation of potential adverse responses.

Despite the clear long-term safety concerns surrounding the transplantation of stem cells and their derivatives, and the lack of rigorous data on efficacy for stem cell treatments in tissues or organ systems other than the blood and immune systems, there is a rapidly growing market for treatments claiming to use stem cells to treat an extremely wide range of medical conditions, ranging from life-threatening diseases, such as amyotrophic lateral sclerosis; chronic intractable conditions, such as spinal cord injury; genetic disorders, such as Down's syndrome; disorders of unknown or poorly constrained etiology, such as autism or chronic fatigue syndrome; and quality-of-life issues, such as hair loss, facial wrinkles, and erectile dysfunction. Advertising primarily online, hundreds of clinics and companies located in jurisdictions ranging from developing economies with little history of biomedical innovation, to emerging scientific powers, to leading research nations, have subjected tens of thousands of patients to either poorly designed human medical experiments or outright fraud, some earning millions of dollars in revenue in the process.

As noted by Lysaght and Campbell, clear and scientifically sound regulatory guidelines for the testing and marketing approval of human cell and tissue products have been formulated by the United States FDA and competent authorities. That notwithstanding, calls have been made by noted ethicists, as well as by a group called the ICMS to allow for the self-regulation of interventions using autologous stem cells as a form of medical innovation, and therefore the practice of medicine, rather than as a medicinal product. Lysaght and Campbell rightly refute this view, as well as an associated proposal that "pay-for-trial" (also known as "fee-for-service") clinical research, in which the patient bears the costs of an experimental procedure, should be permitted. They point out the conundrum between calling a procedure experimental (and therefore of unknown safety and/or efficacy) and requiring patients to pay to receive it, as this inequitably shifts the entire burden of costs and risks to the paying patient, producing a dangerous ethical imbalance.

It would be beneficial to explore other, purely scientific reasons why "pay-for-trial" clinical research does not meet the basic standards of experimental design for studies involving human subjects. This has direct ethical implications as well, as it has famously been stated: "it is unethical to conduct poorly designed experiments." One obvious consequence of the patient-pays model is that it renders important aspects of clinical research design impracticable. These include randomization (as presumably paying subjects will expect to receive the active formulation rather than control), and blinding (for similar reasons). Additionally, it is well documented that the knowledge of the monetary value of a compound, including an inert placebo, has dramatic effects on its perceived effects, which could lead to the skewing of results in patient-funded clinical experiments intended to establish efficacy.

There are clear concerns regarding the social justice of such an approach as opposed to the customary scheme in which human subjects do not pay for experimental treatments. Subjects with the financial means to pay for experimental treatments will presumably have advantages in accessing such procedures, which can clearly give rise to inequitable bias in receiving effective treatments, or, paradoxically, exposure to risks in the event an experimental procedure is unsafe. In addition to the question of justice, the circularity of the logic behind the patient-pays model appears to have an inevitable link to therapeutic misconceptions. Arguments in favor of this model tend to take the form that "Patients should not be forced to wait," which carries the clear connotation of putative efficacy. Indeed, few would argue that "Patients should not be forced to wait for interventions that may be dangerous and unsafe, as well as expensive." There is also to my mind reasonable cause for concern that informed consent, in which patients are required to sign documents stating their understanding of the "experimental" nature of a procedure for which they have paid, may be perversely used for the protection of the treatment provider, rather than the patient-subject, in the sense that if an adverse reaction occurs, or a desired outcome is not achieved, they may be used to prevent legal action or other forms of recourse by patients who may not have considered the consequences of agreeing to such disclaimers.

The widespread ability of patients to participate in clinical research on a "pay-for-trial" basis may be that patients who skirted or preempted the conventional processes of recruitment, determination of eligibility, randomization, by paying for access may have other insidious effects as well. Given the inevitable defects in the design of such experiments, flawed data may enter the literature and potentially influence the standard of care toward harmful or inefficacious practices. Patients who have participated in such badly designed experiments may also be unwilling or ineligible to subsequently participate in well-designed clinical trials, which may have a potentially deleterious impact on the ability to conduct trials of adequate statistical power in "orphan" medical conditions in which patient populations are small.

I agree wholeheartedly with the authors' conclusion that adequate regulatory guidance and oversight are needed in the development of regenerative medicine, just as in other therapeutic areas, and that more thoughtful discussion of emerging ethical issues is needed as advances in fundamental and pre-clinical research fuel hopes of rapid clinical translation, and increasing numbers of first-in-human trials are initiated. I would only add that ethicists themselves will need to remain familiar with a broad range of advances in both basic and clinical research into stem cells and related fields in order for them to be able to consider and make sound recommendations regarding the potentially far-reaching implications of developments in this area of science, which simultaneously holds great promise and enormous potential for abuse.

1.3

Commentary
Regenerative Medicine and Science Literacy

Eisuke Nakazawa

Beruf is a German word that means "vocation." Edmund Husserl, a German philosopher, employed this term to describe the core concept of his ethics. In this commentary on Lysaght and Campbell's "The Ethics of Regenerative Medicine," I will examine the *Beruf* of ethicists. To this end, I will focus on the social acceptance of iPS cell research and the dimensions of relevant ethical problems. Lysaght and Campbell's discussion gives me a position from which I can address these topics. I will examine the dimensions of these ethical problems in relation to science communication. First, I will introduce contemporary examples of regenerative medical technologies, such as ES cell research and iPS cell research, and examine their ethical implications. Second, I will examine the relationship between iPS cell research and science communication. While there are various ways to achieve science communication, I will focus on biotechnology literacy as an intermediary requirement for good science communication. Finally, I will examine the mission of ethicists and conclude that the *Beruf* of ethicists working in the sciences is to be good science communicators.

1 Regenerative medicine and its ethical concerns in Japan

Much attention has been paid recently to developments in regenerative medicine. Because it appears that regenerative medicine may fulfill the human ambition to live a long healthy life, public anticipation of the fruits of this discipline has been growing steadily. In Japan, the iPS cell research conducted by Shinya Yamanaka and his team at Kyoto University is well known. In 2006, Yamanaka and his team generated mouse iPS cells, which are as pluripotent as ES cells, from adult mouse embryonic fibroblasts. Following this, in 2007, they established a technique to generate human iPS cells from adult human skin cells.[3] Yamanaka was popularly lionized all over Japan, because his

---

[3] At the same time, James Thomson at the University of Wisconsin–Madison generated human iPS cells independently.

Morton College Library Cicero, ILL

success was reported by the mass media. Whether to promote human happiness or to remain at the forefront of regenerative medicine research internationally, the Japanese government decided to promote iPS cell research after Yamanaka's successes, and has authorized for this research a relatively substantial budget, despite the prevailing dire fiscal circumstances. Therefore, the accomplishments of iPS cell research and its technical utility are matters of public concern.

The above situation has led to ethical arguments in Japan. The central issue here is the type of ethical problems that are inherent in iPS cell research. Without doubt, iPS cell studies beget fewer ethical issues than ES cell studies. To generate ES cells, researchers require zygotes or early embryos (blastocysts). iPS cells, on the other hand, are generated from adult human somatic cells, such as skin cells. Therefore, iPS cell research does not involve the moral status of human embryos.

However, this does not mean that there are no ethical problems associated with the field of iPS cell research. I think it is important to anticipate future issues, introduce legislation on tissue engineering, and thereby promote advanced, safe, and sustainable scientific research. We must insist that ethical discussions of interest should not be abstract. Of course, ethical discussions often necessitate philosophical introspection. However, many arguments are characterized by a pragmatic approach to ethical concerns. More specifically, arguments such as "How can we protect the privacy of somatic cell donors? How should we respond to incidental findings? What are the issues concerning informed consent?" are addressed in the literature on iPS ethics (Zarzeczny et al. 2009).

I endorse Lysaght and Campbell's valid statement that "much of the bioethical discussion has tended to focus narrowly around issues concerning embryonic stem cell research and, in particular, the moral status of human embryos" and wish to then "mov[e] beyond the contested philosophical issues surrounding human embryos and the meaning of life, and toward the more practical issues that arise in the translational sciences" (Lysaght and Campbell in this chapter). If ES cell research were superseded by iPS cell research, the metaphysical conflict of views on the moral status of human embryos, which nobody can settle by arbitration, would become meaningless and vanish into thin air. In this situation, Lysaght and Campbell's claim might seem trivial, because the conflict itself disappears outright. In actuality, however, that is not the case, for a couple of reasons. One of them is the technological limitation of iPS cell research. Even with progress in the field of iPS cell research, ES cell research, especially non-human ES cell research, will still be needed as a source of basic technology that provides robustness to iPS cell research. If so, it is possible that the moral status of human embryos will remain a big issue.

Another more important issue is the practical approach to ethics. I think that the most important claim in Lysaght and Campbell's discourse that we should "mov[e] beyond the contested philosophical issues surrounding human embryos" is valid not only in the area of ES cell research, but also in the field of ethics as a whole. That is, ethicists in any realm should move beyond contested philosophical issues and adopt practical approaches. Traditionally, ethicists and philosophers tend to be attracted to enigmas that have never been resolved. However, to provide practical solutions, ethicists should think about details of problems that are encountered in everyday life. This could be proposed as a part of an ethicist's ethos or creed, regardless of whether the required practical approaches pertain to a particular discipline, e.g. the field of ES cell research or iPS cell research. Lysaght and Campbell's claim is still valid, even if scholarly interests in the ES cell research develop into interests in iPS cell research.

2   Science communication and science literacy

The popular, as opposed to academic, ethical arguments about iPS cell research are not well informed, although the accomplishments of iPS cell studies and their technical utility are matters of public concern. This means that public interest in iPS cell research may not be directed appropriately. I believe this to be true for two reasons. First, it appears that a number of Japanese laypeople view with optimism the possibility of realizing the clinical potential of iPS cell research. They may assume that iPS cell research would enable the realization of science fiction-like medical technologies—for example, implantation of neural networks, eternal youth, and so on—which are currently and may always be unrealizable. Second, laypeople's interest in iPS cell research may arise from petty nationalism, supported only by an obsession for winning an imagined global competition. Although scientists and ethicists should provide laypeople with as much information as possible to help them understand the science and the issues and arrive at informed opinions, laypeople will inevitably have less information than scientists and ethicists about iPS cell research and its ethical implications. Sharing of information about the ethical implications of iPS cell research is possible only by adopting a comprehensive, panoramic view of current contexts. The lack of science communication creates mutual mistrust among scientists, ethicists, and laypeople. For instance, Lysaght and Campbell mention "stem cell tourism" and "unproven treatments." These are cases wherein science communication would play an important role. Regenerative medicine could significantly influence our society and daily lives. However, an enormous communication gap exists between laypeople and scientists. Thus, we must investigate and develop effective methods to promote mutual understanding. It will be crucial to cultivate the capabilities of laypeople to understand the basics of regenerative medicine and its significance in their lives and society.

In this sense, "biotechnology literacy," including regenerative medicine literacy, is a pressing challenge. Undoubtedly, science communication should be based not on the deficit model, but on the interactive model. The deficit model refers to "one-way communication from experts with knowledge to the public without it" (Trench 2008: 119). The interactive model or "dialogue model" engages the public in two-way communication and draws on their own information and experiences (Trench 2008). Nevertheless, even if biotechnology communication is based on an interactive model, laypeople are not likely to be able to effectively communicate with iPS cell researchers. This is because laypeople find it difficult to understand presentations made by researchers, and because researchers have still not realized the need for simple words that laypeople can understand easily. Thus, we require intermediary biotechnology communication practices and media, which can serve as a preparation for the last stage of communication in the interactive model. Biotechnology literacy will be one such form of intermediary science communication. What laypeople need to know about iPS cell research is as follows.

What are the current topics in iPS cell research? What clinical utility do they have? Do they enrich people's lives or not? What advancements do the research studies require to be of clinical utility? What are the ethical problems associated with contemporary iPS cell research? And, what problems may arise from future iPS cell research? iPS cell researchers must deliver public talks on these topics to laypeople in a way that interests them and helps them learn the issues. This is biotechnology literacy, and it can be fostered in various places. One option is to provide special lessons in elementary and middle-school education. Another option is to design liberal arts lectures for undergraduate students. Of course, science cafés or science pubs may also be a good approach to biotechnology literacy for working people.

3 Mission of the ethicists

Generally, applied ethics, including bioethics, ES cell ethics, and iPS cell ethics, is intimately involved in science communication. This changes the traditional roles of ethicists. In the past, ethicists have used their philosophical and introspective intuitions as guides. However, to think about current biotechnology and its ethical implications, ethicists require management skills, which will enable them to mediate between two parties: specialists and laypeople. These management skills also include coordination capabilities that close the divide between two groups with different background knowledge and culture. Therefore, I believe that a bioethicist simultaneously plays the role of a science communicator. I propose that, as a science communicator, the bioethicist shall listen to laypeople's opinions without relying on his or her own ethical intuition to the exclusion of public will and need; shall analyze the current status of advanced biotechnologies; and shall work toward the realization of a public-interactive science communication. This, in my opinion, is the *Beruf* of ethicists in science.

References

Lysaght, T., and Campbell, A. V. (2014). "The Ethics of Regenerative Medicine: Broadening the Scope beyond the Moral Status of Embryos," in A. Akabayashi (ed.), *The Future of Bioethics: International Dialogues*. Oxford: Oxford University Press, 5–26.

Trench, B. (2008). "Towards an Analytical Framework of Science Communication Models," in D. Cheng et al. (eds), *Communicating Science in Social Contexts: New Models, New Practices*. Dordrecht: Springer, 119–38.

Zarzeczny, A. et al. (2009). "iPS Cells: Mapping the Policy Issues," *Cell*, 139(6): 1032–7.

1.4

Commentary
Regenerative Medicine, Politics, and the High Price of Moral Constraint

Aric Bendorf and Ian Kerridge

Lysaght and Campbell provide a thoughtful overview of emerging technologies and the effects these have on the field of regenerative medicine, which they define as "a wide range of medical biotechnologies and practices, including cell-based therapies, stem cell research, gene technology, and tissue engineering" (Lysaght and Campbell in this chapter). They then go on to examine some of the problems and limitations that previous, more specific definitions of this field proposed by other authors have imposed.

The authors spend considerable time explaining some of the most recent and notable developments in the field and the historical and ethical dilemmas these developments generate. These include discussion of: unproven technologies and therapies; autologous stem cell transplants; how critically ill patients, in a desperate search for anything resembling a potential cure, can inadvertently become research subjects in unproven medical research and sponsors of research laboratories and projects; and the moral and policy implications that these issues bring to the bioethical discourse. They then conclude by stating their hopes for regenerative medicine in the future—that it may be able to evolve beyond the "contested philosophical issues surrounding human embryos and the meaning of life, and toward the more practical issues that arise in the translational sciences" (Lysaght and Campbell in this chapter).

While we agree with the paper's aim, applaud the thorough nature with which it describes the many ways that advances in regenerative medicine have been circumscribed by religious debate, and concur with their conclusion that bioethics should do more to ensure practical outcomes from the moral debate surrounding regenerative medicine, we believe that Lysaght and Campbell's discussion fails to confront a more fundamental and pernicious question—that is, *why* debate about the contested philosophical issues surrounding human embryos has constrained moral and scientific discourse underpinning regenerative medicine and, more generally, stem cell research, for so long.

We believe Lysaght and Campbell's discussion is lacking in the following key areas. First, it has tacitly assumed that the Church is a tolerant and respectful participant in the moral debate surrounding regenerative medicine.[4] Second, it ignores history and fails to take into consideration the extent to which the Church has controlled ethical discourse and hobbled scientific progress in areas with which it has disagreed. And third, we believe that Lysaght and Campbell's "hope" for a more extensive debate surrounding human embryonic stem cell research and regenerative medicine is likely to be vanquished unless bioethics recognizes that it is simply not possible for the Church to enter into meaningful debate about the creation and destruction of human embryos.

By framing the discussion of the ethics of regenerative medicine around the Church's moral judgments, Lysaght and Campbell's analysis has continued the bioethical tradition of attempting to find a pluralistic consensus amongst discordant views. This is both laudable and naïve because it mistakenly assumes that bioethical discourse occurs in an environment where all participants are equally respectful of each other's views, share common goals, are willing to compromise, and, most importantly, have equal power. The church, however, is not now, nor has it ever been, an equal or tolerant participant in moral discourse.

Prior to the Renaissance, history, philosophy, medicine, and all sciences were seen as one amalgamated subset of God's handiwork (Glick, Livesey, and Wallis 2005). Answers to questions about time, genesis, the purpose of life, natural order, illness, misfortune, natural disasters, and, especially, death were all believed to be determined by God and by faith-based cosmologies. For centuries, illiterate and fearful of factors beyond their control, the vast majority of the world's population looked to religion for answers and guidance in all areas of life. Abrahamic faith traditions provided these answers through revelation and "natural law"—establishing moral norms regarding what was pure, bad, right, wrong, good, or evil. They then amplified this power to proclaim their epistemic and moral authority supreme (Peters 1980).

Although historically swaddled in a guise of compassion and understanding, the means by which the Church has asserted its authority over these matters has, however, been neither benevolent nor benign. Its dogmatic opposition to physics, philosophy, evolutionary biology, reproductive and contraceptive practices, blood transfusions, and psychiatry make painfully clear the extent to which the church has been willing to leverage all of its power to force its will upon those who challenge it (Draper 1875; White 1900; Callahan 1970).

Despite these and countless other instances where the Church has acted malevolently against those who have threatened it, its authority has not remained uncontested. Beginning in the Renaissance, history, philosophy, science, and medicine were extracted from the Church's closely guarded dominion and began maturing into separate and independent disciplines. Copernicus, Galileo, da Vinci, Michelangelo, Lorenzo

---

[4] In this paper, our concern is with the role that Western Abrahamic faith traditions (particularly that of the Christian Churches) have played in constraining moral discourse surrounding stem cell research and regenerative medicine. Eastern faith traditions, including Buddhism, Hinduism, and Confucianism have, for the most part, not played a similar role in controlling public discourse.

de Medici, Jeremy Bentham, John Stuart Mill, Immanuel Kant, Friedrich Nietzsche, Charles Darwin, Karl Marx, Sigmund Freud, Bertrand Russell, and, more recently, Martha Nussbaum, Amartya Sen, Daniel Dennett, and Peter Singer have all challenged the moral legitimacy of faith and its accepted religious dogma. In response, however, the Church has treated many of these individuals not with tolerance, respect, and compassion, but with vengeance, abuse, ridicule, punishment, and retribution (Hooykaas 1972; Durant 1985; Larson 1997; Brooke and Cantor 1998; Blackwell 2002; Ferngren 2002).

We believe that the current status of the moral debate surrounding regenerative medicine is just one more point in a pattern of the Church's effort to restrict any ideas that threaten it. Further, we argue that this is not an issue that is peripheral to the Church— rather it lies at the very core of its base of power. We feel that the Church has so aggressively and tightly circumscribed the regenerative medicine debate because it has no other choice. While regenerative medicine raises many other moral concerns, including those raised by Lysaght and Campbell, the very possibility of regenerative medicine presupposes judgments about the moral status of the embryo and man's ability to manipulate and ultimately create life. The Church simply cannot move beyond questions of the meaning of life and the moral status of the embryo—doing so would provide a de facto validation of other moral viewpoints and would drastically undermine its own moral authority.

Recognizing the Church's historical intolerance of ideas that challenge its hegemony, why is it that, for almost 50 years, bioethics has allowed the Church, specifically the Christian religious right (Livingstone, Hart, and Noll 1999), to continue to dictate public discourse, define what is morally permissible, circumscribe scientific inquiry, and bridle scientific progress? There are a number of possible explanations. One is that despite its academic bluster, unlike the Church, bioethics has really failed to gain any traction in public discourse. A second is that bioethics has, unsurprisingly given its philosophical heritage, sought to be a voice of reason and a source of rational logic, and has been generally unwilling to critique faith traditions or even enter into the "moral domain" of the Church. Bioethics, therefore, has become a moderator and not an advocate, a conciliator and not a critic.

For bioethics to progress beyond its current seemingly intractable role of moderating debates, and transform itself into a profession or discipline that can lead, we believe that bioethics must become more critical and more political. It must advocate for logic and reason and recognize that pluralism does not demand that all arguments be treated as equally valid. Until bioethics genuinely confronts the dominance of the Church in public discourse surrounding the morality of stem cell research and regenerative medicine, progress in these fields of science will be held hostage to the Church's false and self-serving pretenses of moral equity.

What is required of bioethics to help progress regenerative medicine? We believe there are three key areas in which bioethics must adapt itself to be able to guide regenerative medicine forward. First, it must face the inevitable fact that the Church is incapable of supporting research in areas that undermine its authority. Second, bioethics must become political and assume a position of public advocacy to help educate the public with facts to counteract the insurgency of superstition and religious dogma that dominates the moral debate and determines public policy in this key area. This is not going to be achieved simply through publication of academic papers in bioethics literature. It will require sophisticated use of new social media, adoption of different non-text-based genres of communication (such as television, music, and video), specific engagement with populations that may be open to secular moral discourse (i.e. children) and greater disciplinary attention to the rhetorical construction of both moral and epistemic authority in public discourse. And third, bioethics must seek out and give voice to perspectives that are otherwise marginalized by more dominant and powerful viewpoints. Just as bioethics has been largely deaf to the concerns of the developing world and has been dominated by Western thought and Western preoccupations (Benatar, Darr, and Singer 2005), so too the bioethical discourse around regenerative medicine has been dominated by the concerns and perspectives of Abrahamic faith traditions. To counteract this, the perspectives of those who lack power must not simply be given space, but must be actively sought out and supported.

Lysaght and Campbell are right to point to the inadequacies of the moral discourse surrounding regenerative medicine. Their hope for a more rigorous and extensive discourse, however, is likely to remain unfulfilled unless bioethics confronts, head on, the root cause of its constraint.

References

Benatar, S. R., Darr, A. S., and Singer, P. A. (2005). "Global Health Challenges: The Need for an Expanded Discourse on Bioethics," *PLoS Medicine*, 2(7): e143.

Blackwell, R. J. (2002). "Galileo Galilei," in G. B. Ferngren (ed.), *Science and Religion: A Historical Introduction*. Baltimore, NJ: The Johns Hopkins University Press, 105–16.

Brooke, J. H., and Cantor, G. (1998). *Reconstructing Nature: The Engagement of Science and Religion*. Edinburgh: T and T Clark.

Callahan, D. (1970). "Contraception and Abortion: American Catholic Responses," *The Annals of the American Academy of Political and Social Science*, 387(1): 109–17.

Draper, J. W. (1875). *History of the Conflict Between Religion and Science*. New York: D. Appleton and Company.

Durant, J. (ed.). (1985). *Darwinism and Divinity: Essays on Evolution and Religious Belief*. Oxford: Blackwell.

Ferngren, G. B. (ed.). (2002). *Science and Religion: A Historical Introduction*. Baltimore, NJ: The Johns Hopkins University Press.

Glick, T., Livesey, S. J., Wallis, F. (eds). (2005). *Medieval Science, Technology, and Medicine: An Encyclopedia*. New York: Routledge.

Hooykaas, R. (1972). *Religion and the Rise of Modern Science*. Edinburgh: Scottish Academic Press.

Larson, E. (1997). *Summer for the Gods: The Scopes Trial and America's Continuing Debate over Science and Religion*. New York: Basic Books.

Livingstone, D. N., Hart, D. G., and Noll, M. A. (eds). (1999). *Evangelicals and Science in Historical Perspective*. New York: Oxford University Press.

Lysaght, T., and Campbell, A. V. (2014). "The Ethics of Regenerative Medicine: Broadening the Scope beyond the Moral Status of Embryos," in A. Akabayashi (ed.), *The Future of Bioethics: International Dialogues.* Oxford: Oxford University Press, 5–26.

Peters, E. (1980). *Heresy and Authority in Medieval Europe.* Philadelphia, PA: University of Pennsylvania Press.

White, A. D. (1900). *A History of the Warfare of Science with Theology in Christendom.* New York: D. Appleton and Company.

1.5

Response to Commentaries

Tamra Lysaght and Alastair V. Campbell

We are grateful to the authors of the three commentaries for their thoughtful responses to our paper. The response from Douglas Sipp embodies precisely the type of discussion that it is hoped that our paper will stimulate. In his commentary, Sipp rightly points out some of the issues that are raised by regenerative medicines once we step away from those concerning the moral status of human embryos. He begins by asking fundamental questions about the nature of cell-based treatments and how they differ from conventional therapeutic agents and clinical practices. If cell-based therapies are to work in the way they are expected to, then they will "functionally integrate and survive, possibly for the lifetime of the patient" (Sipp in this chapter). This expectation differs fundamentally from the pharmacodynamics and pharmacokinetics of molecular compounds, and the homogeneity and predictability of surgical techniques and medical devices. Even other biological compounds such as vaccines are not sufficiently analogous to draw parallels with the stochastic mechanisms of living cells.

As pointed out by Sipp, such considerations will be immensely important when designing clinical trials, selecting research subjects, calculating risk–benefit ratios, and providing information to patients and research participants during the consent process. Oversight of these considerations could result in the premature introduction of an intervention before it is clearly demonstrated to be safe or effective, as was demonstrated by the use of bone marrow transplantation with high-dose chemotherapy in breast cancer patients (Rettig et al. 2007). Moving promising research into clinical trials prematurely could also prove perilous as was witnessed in the first human trials of gene transfer, which resulted in the untimely death of a young American teenager and disabled an entire field of research for more than a decade (Kimmelman 2010). The need for further discussion of these issues is essential for the future of regenerative medicines.

One particular ethical issue that Sipp has raised is how the expected longevity of cell-based interventions will impact on a patient-subject's right to withdraw from research, which is a fundamental principle for all medical research. As stated in the Declaration of Helsinki, research subjects must be able "to withdraw consent to participate at any time without reprisal" (World Medical Association 2000). However, this principle is challenged by a paradigm in which the metabolic effects of a therapeutic agent are meant to be permanent and inherently so. An option that disallows novel cell treatments to be tested in humans without some type of "exit strategy" mentioned by Sipp would be neither pragmatic nor an acceptable solution for patients with few treatment options. Simply informing potential research subjects about the potential permanency and instability of cell lines also will not do. Cell-based therapies may well give cause for a reconceptualization of what it means to withdraw consent to participate in research.

Another important issue that Sipp raises is the need for bioethicists to "remain familiar with a broad range of advances in both basic and clinical research into stem cells and related fields in order for them to be able to consider and make sound recommendations" regarding the implications of emerging developments in this area of science (Sipp in this chapter). We agree wholeheartedly with the statement that bioethics scholars be kept informed about emerging developments in a broad range of scientific and clinical research, and not just the "sexy" stuff that receives the greatest media and political interest. However, we would add that the lightning-fast pace of stem cell science makes this effort nearly impossible without the scientific community itself becoming more engaged in bioethical discussion. Scientists should not place the onus of considering the many profound ethical, political, and social implications of scientific developments on bioethicists alone. Indeed, it is part of the two-way communication that Eisuke Nakazawa advocates in his commentary.

Nakazawa's commentary focuses on the need for greater communications between scientists working with iPS cells and the public. While we agree with the general principles behind Nakazawa's argument, we disagree with some of the claims made in the commentary. We dispute the claim that "iPS cell research does not involve the moral status of human embryos" and that if "ES cell research were superseded by iPS cell research, the metaphysical conflict of views on the moral status of human embryos...would become meaningless and vanish into thin air" (Nakazawa in this chapter). Nakazawa is correct in stating that, due to many technical limitations, iPS cells are unlikely to circumvent the need for ESC research. However, even if iPS cells significantly reduce the need for destructive embryo research, the metaphysical disputes over the creation and destruction of nascent human life will not disappear, particularly if these cells are differentiated into gametes and used to create human embryos (Aalto-Setälä et al. 2009). The same might be said of any reprogramming technique that is devised supposedly to avoid the moral issues concerning human embryo research.

Secondly, it is not our contention that "ethicists in any realm should move beyond contested philosophical issues and adopt practical approaches" (Nakazawa in this chapter). Rather, we argue that one can begin to appreciate and hopefully address the complexity of ethical issues that are raised by regenerative medicines once we step away from the heated debates around embryo research. We can achieve this by moving beyond the contested philosophical issues surrounding human embryos and the meaning of life, and toward the more practical issues that arise in the translational sciences. However, we do not suggest that bioethics should be *merely* pragmatic, as theoretical and normative discussion will always be required and is a necessary part of the philosophy that not only underpins the rationality of bioethics but also our pragmatic decision-making.

Nakazawa concludes that, as a science communicator, a bioethics theorist should "listen to laypeople's opinions without relying on his or her own ethical intuition to the exclusion of public will and need" and work toward "the realization of a public-interactive science communication" (Nakazawa in this chapter). We agree that as a consequence of the topics examined, bioethicists do play a de facto role of science communicators. We also believe that any profession that engages in public discourse has a responsibility to adopt an inclusive approach when considering the political, social, and ethical issues that surround scientific research and its technological applications. This means actively seeking out and engaging directly with communities that are likely to be affected most by the introduction of new technologies. However, we would add that this same argument must also apply to the scientific community.

While rejecting the "deficit model," which assumes that publics are composed of "laypersons" who are lacking in some critical scientific knowledge (Michael 1992; Wynne 1992) and that scientists simply need to disseminate more scientific and technical information in order to avoid public controversies (Lewenstein 1995), Nakazawa's commentary implicitly embraces it. Improving "biotechnology literacy" may help to improve communications between scientists and non-scientists, even though there is no convincing evidence that it improves public support for biotechnologies (Bak 2001; Sturgis, Cooper, and Fife-Schaw 2005; Sturgis, Brunton-Smith, and Fife-Schaw 2010). Yet this sounds suspiciously like a one-way communication flow from scientists to the public. For an interactive communication model to be successful, it must reject the absoluteness of scientific authority and acknowledge the opinions, beliefs, and values held by the audience (Logan 1991). For the purposes of our paper, we suggest that part of this will mean that scientists will need to communicate more directly with bioethicists and improve their own "literacy" in bioethics.

The importance of communication is also featured in the commentary of Bendorf and Kerridge. The bulk of Bendorf and Kerridge's commentary focuses narrowly on their perception of the role of "the Church" in the public debate around stem cell research and regenerative medicines, which they claim has dominated public discourse because of the challenges that this area of research brings to the Church's moral and epistemic authority. They then conclude with three recommendations for how bioethics can help to progress regenerative medicine: 1) that bioethics accept that "the Church is incapable of supporting research in areas that undermine its authority;" 2) that bioethics become political and "help educate the public with facts to counteract the insurgency of superstition and religious dogma that dominates the moral debate;" and 3) that bioethics "seek out and give voice to perspectives that are otherwise marginalized by more dominant and powerful viewpoints" (Bendorf and Kerridge in this chapter). We will address each of these three points.

The first point is flawed by Bendorf and Kerridge's monolithic and overly simplistic approach to the diversity and pluralism of Abrahamic faith traditions, which they mistakenly assume are synonymous with "the Christian Churches" that their polemic targets. Abrahamic faiths include not only Christianity but also Judaism and Islam, and neither of these religions is known to have played a significant role in the moral discourses around stem cell research. Leaders from both of these faiths have expressed support for stem cell research as well as moral objections. Thus, there is much heterogeneity both between and within the major Abrahamic faiths, which the authors would be well aware of given that Kerridge has written on the subject (Kerridge et al. 2010). As an example, the experience of the Bioethics Advisory Committee of the Singapore government (BAC) is that the Christian Churches and representatives of other faiths (including those outside the Abrahamic tradition) provide reasoned and often quite detailed commentary on issues such as the use of human embryos. The implication that they must defend their authority at all costs is certainly not evident in these submissions. In the contentious area of the use of embryonic sources for stem cells, it is true that all the Christian Churches that submitted comments on the BAC report were opposed to this proposal, but they were at pains to provide detailed documentation of their views. The other "Abrahamic faiths"—Islam and Judaism—were supportive of the use of ESCs if it was necessary for the advancement of health (See BAC 2002: Annex G).

The second point is just as worrisome. As noted in our paper, bioethics already plays a political role in providing governments and regulators with bioethical advice. However, to become a political movement, which Bendorf and Kerridge suggest, risks diminishing the ability of bioethicists to engage in reasoned and dispassionate moral discourse. The introduction of bioethics in public education curricula is laudable and entirely justifiable in the pluralistic contexts of secular societies. However, the pedagogy should be primarily about reasoning, critical thinking, and the art of argumentation, and not simply disseminating "facts" on the behalf of the scientific community as if they lack the values that we indeed attach to them. It is true that religious convictions add an element of passion to people's moral standpoints (see Campbell 2003), but this may not be entirely a bad thing, provided that those with these convictions are willing to listen to, and respect, the differing views of others. A cool and detached approach to morality is a poor motivator to moral action, and, incidentally, we note that there is considerable passion in Bendorf and Kerridge's comments, not just cool reasoning! Like Karl Popper (1945), they are not willing to tolerate the intolerant—and we support them in this view.

We agree entirely with Bendorf and Kerridge's third point that bioethics should seek out and give voice to those who are marginalized in the public debate around regenerative medicines. These voices include the women who donate their eggs and embryos to stem cell research, and the patients who seek treatments for conditions that currently are untreatable or who lack suitable treatment options (Kitzinger and Williams 2005; Lysaght, Little, and Kerridge 2011). We do not agree that broadening the debate to include a wider diversity of voices will necessarily "counteract" a discourse "dominated by the concerns and perspectives of Abrahamic faith traditions," but it may well enrich the discourse and provide everyone with a more nuanced understanding of the heterogeneity that exists between and within different communities (Bendorf and Kerridge in this chapter). To achieve this, we indeed must actively seek out and support the perspectives of those who lack the power to otherwise engage in the moral, public, and political discourses that surround regenerative medicines. To not do so, it is likely that the debates will remain as narrow and incommensurable as they have to up to now; and, like all four commentators, we hope for something better in the years ahead.

References

Aalto-Setälä, K., Conklin, B. R., and Lo, B. (2009). "Obtaining Consent for Future Research with Induced Pluripotent Cells: Opportunities and Challenges," *PLoS Biology*, 7: e42.

Bak, H. J. (2001). "Education and Public Attitudes toward Science: Implications for the 'Deficit Model' of Education and Support for Science and Technology," *Social Science Quarterly*, 82: 779–95.

Bendorf, A., and Kerridge, I. (2014). "Regenerative Medicine, Politics, and the High Price of Moral Constraint," in A. Akabayashi (ed.), *The Future of Bioethics: International Dialogues*. Oxford: Oxford University Press, 35–9.

Bioethics Advisory Committee (BAC). (2002). "Ethical, Legal and Social Issues in Human Stem Cell Research, Reproductive and Therapeutic Cloning: A Report from the Bioethics Advisory Committee Singapore," June, http://www.bioethics-singapore.org (accessed December 7, 2012).

Campbell, A. V. (2003). "Secularised Bioethics and the Passion of Religion," *New Review of Bioethics*, 1(1): 117–26.

Kerridge, I. H. et al. (2010). "Religious Perspectives on Embryo Donation and Research," *Clinical Ethics*, 5: 35–45.

Kimmelman, J. (2010). *Gene Transfer and the ethics of First-in-Human Research: Lost in Translation*. New York: Cambridge University Press.

Kitzinger, J., and Williams, C. (2005). "Forecasting Science Futures: Legitimising Hope and Calming Fears in the Embryo Stem Cell Debate," *Social Science and Medicine*, 61: 731–40.

Lewenstein, B.V. (1995). "Science and the Media," in S. Jasanoff et al. (eds), *Handbook of Science and Technology Studies*. Thousand Oaks, CA: Sage Publications, 343–60.

Logan, R. A. (1991). "Popularization and Secularization: Media Coverage of Health," in L. Wilkins and P. Patterson (eds), *Risky Business: Communicating Issues of Science, Risk, and Public Policy*. New York: Greenwood, 43–60.

Lysaght, T., Little, J. M., and Kerridge, I. H. (2011). "Marginalizing Experience: A Critical Analysis of Public Discourse Surrounding Stem Cell Research in Australia," *Journal of Bioethical Inquiry*, 8: 191–202.

Michael, M. (1992). "Lay Discourses of Science: Science-in-General, Science-in-Particular, and Self," *Science, Technology, and Human Values*, 17: 313–33.

Nakazawa, E. (2014). "Regenerative Medicine and Science Literacy," in A. Akabayashi (ed.), *The Future of Bioethics: International Dialogues*. Oxford: Oxford University Press, 31–4.

Popper, K. (1945). *The Open Society and Its Enemies*. 2 vols. London: George Routledge and Sons.

Rettig, R. A. et al. (2007). *False Hope: Bone Marrow Transplantation for Breast Cancer*. New York: Oxford University Press.

Sipp, D. (2014). "Stem Cell Clinical Research: The Biology Determines the Ethics," in A. Akabayashi (ed.), *The Future of Bioethics: International Dialogues*. Oxford: Oxford University Press, 27–30.

Sturgis, P., Brunton-Smith, I., and Fife-Schaw, C. (2010). "Public Attitudes to Genomic Science: An Experiment in Information Provision," *Public Understanding of Science*, 19: 166–80.

Sturgis, P., Cooper, H., and Fife-Schaw, C. (2005). "Attitudes to Biotechnology: Estimating the Opinions of a Better-Informed Public," *New Genetics and Society*, 14: 31–56.

World Medical Association (2000). "Declaration of Helsinki: Ethical Principles for Medical Research Involving Human Subjects," http://www.wma.net/en/30publications/10policies/b3/ (accessed December 7, 2012).

Wynne, B. (1992). "Misunderstood Misunderstanding: Social Identities and Public Uptake of Science," *Public Understanding of Science*, 1: 281–304.

2.1

Primary Topic Article
Neural Repair as a Case Study in Neuroethics

D. Gareth Jones

1 Introduction

Neuroethics emerged as a subdiscipline of bioethics, but is now regarded by many as an ethical field in its own right. Consequently, it is seen as standing over against not only bioethics but also philosophy of mind. This suggests that it is sufficiently distinct from other established disciplines to warrant its own label as proposed by Martha Farah and others (2010). The concerns of neuroethics generally centre on the increasingly effective and intrusive manner in which the tools of biomedical technology can describe, influence, and even control the brains of individuals. Consequently, its domain encompasses the influence of drugs on the brain, including their effects on memory and temperament; the various forms of neurocognitive enhancement; and the burgeoning area of neuroimaging, especially functional MRI, in basic and applied research (from economics to social policy). Further issues cover the interface between neuroscience and the law.

Extensive as are the areas covered by these topics, they pay only limited attention to neural degeneration and regeneration, a field of central interest to much of current neuroscience. Extending from the laboratory to the clinic, neural regeneration lies at the heart of the explosion within neuroscience, since it promises untold benefits for those suffering from progressive neurodegenerative conditions, such as Parkinson's disease (let alone Alzheimer's disease), and also following major loss of function resulting from strokes or trauma. The recent neuroscientific revolution is built on two developments. The first is the realization that neural plasticity is an ongoing feature of the mature brain and that neurogenesis continues in the brain well into adult life (Gurgo, Bedi, and Nurcombe 2002). The second is related, in that the adult brain contains stem cells that can, under certain circumstances, be stimulated to produce new neurons that potentially can be integrated into functioning networks in the damaged brain (Muramatsu, Ueno, and Yamashita 2009). The possibilities opened up by these expanded concepts are

* The invaluable assistance of Maja Whitaker and Mike King in every aspect of this paper is gratefully acknowledged.

immense, and have led to considerable interest in the prospects of using neural grafts and deep brain stimulation in patients with Parkinson's and other neurodegenerative diseases. More recently, considerable interest has centred on the introduction of stem cells into damaged brains with a view to their conversion into appropriate neurons to replace those lost along with their neurotransmitters and growth factors (Miller 2006).

In commenting on developments along these lines the focus of interest has been on the immediate neuroscientific challenges with their accompanying clinical applications. In responding in this manner, broader neuroethical implications have been largely overlooked, and it is on these that the current paper concentrates.

2 Reflections on the organization of the brain

A temptation in considering the brain is to view it in deceptively simple and indeed in simplistic terms. This is as much a temptation for bioethicists as for anyone else. While the details of neuroanatomical and functional organization are not of concern in this paper, what is of relevance is to underline the extraordinarily complex interconnectivity between so many of these regions and areas.

2.1 Core features of the brain: connectivity

When thinking of the way in which different parts of the brain are linked, three distinct forms of connectivity are distinguishable: anatomical, functional, and causal interactions (based on the groundbreaking work of neuroanatomists, such as Ramón y Cajal (1909), Brodmann (1909), and Swanson (2003). The foundational units described by them correspond to individual neurons, neuronal populations, and anatomically segregated brain regions. These, in turn are connected in a variety of ways: synaptic connections that link individual neurons at the microscopic level; networks connecting neuronal populations at the intermediate level; and brain regions linked by fibre pathways at the macroscopic level. Each of these levels has to be understood in its own terms, and all point in the same direction—that no part of the brain can be isolated from numerous related parts, in terms of contact between individual neurons, fibres of neuronal processes and columns connecting functionally related neural areas, and inter-regional pathways connecting brain regions. An appreciation of these interconnections demonstrates that it is not possible to completely isolate one brain area from a number of others. For instance, the primary motor cortex also receives information related to visual cues, sensation, coordination, speech, and emotions. This results from links between its association area and those dealing with auditory, touch, and visual information.

2.2 Core features of the brain: plasticity

The second core feature of the brain is its plasticity. The developmental period is characterized by an initial overproduction of neurons, when there is massive competition between them, with only 50 per cent surviving into adulthood (Buss, Sun, and Oppenheim 2006; Stiles and Jernigan 2010). The fascinating aspect of this phenomenon is that it is the external environment that plays a crucial role in determining which synaptic connections between neurons persist and, therefore, which neurons survive.

External inputs have an extensive influence on the developing brain, interacting with internal drivers to mould the end product that is the adult brain, and hence the adult individual. It is because of this close interrelationship between the developing brain and extrinsic factors that normal development can readily be disrupted (Neville and Bavelier 2002; Markham and Greenough 2004). Consequently, numerous influences during development can have devastating consequences for a child's subsequent intelligence and behaviour. The converse also holds: a stimulating environment can increase the complexity of neural organization, in turn altering many facets of the behavioural repertoire of the growing individual. What we are as people emerges from this ongoing dialogue between the neural and genetic material we inherit, the worlds we occupy, and the worlds we ourselves construct (Curley et al. 2011; Stiles 2011).

Many examples of neuroplasticity, sometimes colloquially referred to as 'rewiring the brain', are encountered in adult life. These include: playing the piano (Lappe et al. 2011), juggling (Voelcker-Rehage and Willimczik 2006), basketball (Park et al. 2009), ballet (Hanggi et al. 2010), badminton (Jin et al. 2010), studying mathematics (Aydin et al. 2007) and phonetics (Golestani, Price, and Scott 2011), driving a taxi in London (Maguire, Woollett, and Spiers 2006), and even long-term romantic love (Acevedo et al. 2012). A fascinating potential effect of the neuroplasticity may arise from our increasing dependence upon Google and other search engines (Carr 2008). By allowing us to offload the memorizing of details, web search engines like Google could facilitate the development of higher cognitive functioning (Bohannon 2011).

The characteristic feature of these studies is that in most of them the rewiring is the result of a repetitive activity. Hence, care has to be exercised in generalizing from them to all neural functioning to suggest that rewiring is achieved far more readily than may be the case. Nevertheless, they demonstrate the validity of the assertion that neural rewiring does occur, and may be relatively common in normal human life. It is unfortunate that terms such as 'rewiring the brain' can lend the phenomenon an air of danger suggesting that it should *in itself* be a matter of concern. The kind of scaremongering that conflates the descriptive and the normative is exemplified by Wolf's unhelpful claim that exposure to pornography rewires men's brains (Wolf 2011).

While one should not conclude that rewiring is more extensive than is the case, it is a pertinent reminder that the rationale for introducing neural grafts into the brain (section 4) emanates from the brain's inherent plasticity. However, by the same token any unwanted subsidiary effects are also due to this same phenomenon.

2.3 Core features of the brain: neurogenesis in the adult brain

The brain's plasticity is the first stepping stone. The second is the flip side of plasticity, ongoing neurogenesis after the early developmental period. This phenomenon carries with it the message that, when neurons are damaged in the post-developmental brain, they can potentially be replaced by new ones.

It appears that some neurons are produced throughout the entire life of an individual. However, this is probably a selective process, applying to certain neuronal populations in the dentate gyrus of the hippocampus and olfactory bulb (Conover and Notti 2008). In these areas the newborn neurons appear to replace dying ones, and become integrated into normal neural networks. The production of new neurons in the adult dentate gyrus is regulated by physiological cues such as stress, suggesting that neurogenesis is functionally significant (Gould and Tanapat 1999). Additionally, degenerating neurons may to some extent be replaced by newly generated ones (Kee, Preston, and Wojtowicz 2001).

In the neocortex, there is a low level of neurogenesis, although the newly generated neuron-like cells survive only for short periods, and may not differentiate into fully functional neurons (Cameron and Dayer 2008).

In short, the brain is characterized by remarkably dynamic features, stemming from its complex circuitry and connectedness at each descriptive level, its ongoing synaptic plasticity, and even the ongoing production of neurons at selected sites and under certain conditions. Consequently, efforts to rectify pathological changes and re-establish failed or degenerating pathways and connections take place against a background constantly being moulded by internal and external forces.

3 Parkinson's disease: a model neurodegenerative disorder

Of all the neurodegenerative conditions that might eventually benefit from neural grafting, the one on which most attention has been focused is Parkinson's disease (PD). This is because of the discreteness of the degeneration within the brain. All the symptoms of Parkinson's disease result from damage to the basal ganglia, the damage being to one or more of their constituent regions (Obeso et al. 2008). The neurons that are destroyed are principally in the substantia nigra, and are important in the control of movement. Since these neurons function by releasing one particular neurotransmitter, dopamine, their destruction in Parkinson's disease leads to a loss of dopamine and consequent inability for this part of the brain to carry out its normal motor functions.

Early in the course of the disease a dramatic restoration of neurological function occurs in response to the dopamine precursor, levodopa (L-DOPA), and to dopamine-receptor agonists. However, with the progression of the disease, the response to L-DOPA and other drugs is often diminished, possibly because of the continued loss of dopaminergic nerve terminals and the necessary receptors. To make matters worse, the dopaminergic drugs also have side effects, such as *dyskinesias* (purposeless, involuntary movements) and *hallucinations*. When these occur they limit the usefulness of the drug regimes. The loss of response to L-DOPA is shown by the appearance of an 'on–off' phenomenon, in which periods of continual immobility or 'freezing spells' ('off') alternate with excessive abnormal movements ('on').

The straightforwardness of this account is misleading, since there is also a host of non-motor symptoms (Poewe 2008; Chaudhuri and Schapira 2009; Park and Stacy 2009; Chaudhuri et al. 2011). These occur in over 90 per cent of patients. In general, non-motor symptoms correlate with advancing disease but others, including sleep disorder and depression, occur before overt motor symptoms present themselves (Chaudhuri and Schapira 2009). Of considerable relevance to this present paper is neuropsychiatric dysfunction. Depression is common, with loss of initiative and assertiveness, while anhedonia (inability to experience pleasure from activities usually found enjoyable) and anxiety are common. Also encountered are cognitive dysfunction, psychotic episodes, and dementia.

The devastating nature and refractory quality of these clinical symptoms have led to numerous efforts at overcoming them. These include neural grafting and direct electrical stimulation of brain regions. The intrusive nature of these procedures raises ethical queries that are accentuated by the interconnectedness, complexity, and plasticity of the adult brain. All too often ethical assessments ignore these neural features, and thereby overlook a range of pertinent considerations that are significant for neuroethics.

4 Transplantation studies in PD

4.1 Adrenal medulla transplantation

The first foray into transplantation to alleviate the symptoms of PD took place in the mid 1980s and involved the use of adrenal chromaffin cells from the patients' own adrenal glands. The procedure was initially carried out on four patients with advanced PD in two separate studies in Scandinavia (Backlund et al. 1985; Lindvall et al. 1987). Overall the results were disappointing.

These first clinical trials were initiated in the absence of any convincing data to suggest that adrenal grafting was likely to be either safe or efficacious in human patients. The sparse evidence that did exist at the time was from a small number of studies in rodents (Freed et al. 1981; Freed et al. 1983; Herrera-Marschitz et al. 1984; Strömberg et al. 1984). They failed to answer many of the most fundamental scientific questions regarding neural grafting, including: the amount of tissue required, whether the grafts should be placed in one or both hemispheres, the optimal site for graft placement, or what factors are important for long-term graft survival. There had been no successful grafting in non-human primates (Sladek and Shoulson 1988). In fact, shortly *after* grafting commenced in human patients, a report was published on adrenal transplantation in the rhesus monkey, in which graft survival was extremely poor (Morihisa et al. 1984).

One of the more controversial trials was carried out on two patients in Mexico by Madrazo, Drucker-Colín, and colleagues (1987). Both patients appeared to exhibit substantial improvements following adrenal grafts, in complete contrast to those reported in earlier studies (Backlund et al. 1985; Lindvall et al. 1987). They were so dramatic that questions were raised over their authenticity, and no one was able to replicate the findings. However, Madrazo's study created a surge of enthusiasm for adrenal medullary grafting in many countries (Lieberman 1987; Sullivan 1987). At best, the results were only of moderate benefit for some patients, while the trauma of the surgery led to a mortality rate of up to 20 per cent (Goetz et al. 1989; Porena et al. 1996). There was no evidence of reinnervation of the motor region (Dohan et al. 1988; Peterson, Price, and Small 1989; Forno and Langston 1991).

This early foray into neural grafting was far from a good illustration of ethical practice and was unlikely to yield substantial data of benefit to PD patients or to developmental neuroscience. It ignored basic principles of neural organization as well as basic ethical considerations, such as the need for scepticism, the importance of sound animal research, and insistence on adequately powered studies and peer-reviewed publications when human studies are undertaken.

4.2 Initial neural grafting

The general failure of adrenal medulla grafting prompted a move to the use of neural tissue obtained from aborted human fetuses. Despite the ethical constraints associated with this approach (Jones 1991), convincing pre-clinical studies suggested that grafting of fetal neural tissue was a very promising treatment for PD (for a review, see Bingaman and Bakay 2000).

The earliest results of fetal neural grafting in PD appeared in the literature in 1988. These reports provided few details (Hitchcock et al. 1988; Madrazo et al. 1988) and as such are difficult to assess. However, they were characterized by their optimism. Beneficial effects were reported to occur within days of surgery, and on both sides of the body, even though this timeline is too quick and the grafts were placed unilaterally. These findings contradicted what was expected from the results of experimental animal work.

Soon after publication of these early findings an insightful overview of the issues was produced by Sladek and Shoulson (1988). They pointed to a lack of animal studies; uncertainty about the placing of grafts; a low 10–20 per cent survival rate of grafted neurons; the possibility of tumour formation; the need for controlled clinical trials to clarify a host of technical matters; and unpacking of ethical considerations.

These points were to prove exceptionally insightful for all subsequent studies. However, were they taken seriously? A search of the *2011 Science Citation Index* through the *ISI Web of Science* revealed that, while the 1988 article by Sladek and Shoulson (1988) has been cited 68 times by other authors, the vast majority simply referred to it in passing. In other words, the criteria they had set forth were not followed up. Even at this early stage in the development of neural grafting, the excitement and prospects it held out overshadowed any serious ethical analysis of potential scientific and clinical pitfalls.

4.3 The next few years

The first detailed report of fetal neural grafting in humans appeared in 1989 (Lindvall et al. 1989). The backdrop was the acute need for new therapeutic approaches in PD; encouraging results with fetal grafting in rodents and non-human primates over a ten-year period; and the availability of provisional ethical guidelines for the use of human fetal material for grafting purposes. Two patients with advanced PD received grafts with no major complications. The results were somewhat disappointing, but the authors contended that the small positive effects provided a rationale for pursuing fetal neural grafting.

In 1992 three studies appeared in the same issue of *The New England Journal of Medicine*. Two of the studies were in patients with idiopathic PD (Freed et al. 1992; Spencer et al. 1992), while the third was in two young adults with severe MPTP-induced Parkinsonism (Widner et al. 1992). The methodology varied between, and even within, these studies, making generalizations and comparisons difficult. The greatest benefits were seen in the MPTP-induced Parkinsonian patients. In the accompanying editorial, Fahn (1992) concluded that, while the procedure remains experimental, the results justify the effort and cost of such a complex procedure. In his view the studies should spur optimism.

There is tension here between a justifiably critical assessment of the limitations of the studies, and the optimistic conclusion that work should continue. Balancing legitimate scientific scepticism, the desire to find a better means of treatment for patients now and in the future, and the welfare of current patients subject to experimental procedures, is a delicate act. The literature of the time showed no evidence of grappling with ethical constraints. The paradigm was one of relative hubris—neural grafts can overcome the devastation wrought by Parkinson's disease, even though the causal factors remained unclear.

4.4 Overview of clinical trials to the present day

Further clinical trials followed (Hagell and Brundin 2001; Bjorklund et al. 2003), and the general consensus up to the year 2001 was positive, though not unreservedly so. There was evidence that human fetal neurons survive and function in the brains of patients with PD for up to six years in some patients (Wenning et al. 1997). Post mortem results demonstrated good survival and integration of grafted neurons into the host brain (Kordower et al. 1995; Hagell and Brundin 2001). There was sustained symptomatic improvement in a majority of the grafted patients, allowing a reduction in L-DOPA treatment (Clarkson 2001) while in the most successful cases it was possible to withdraw L-DOPA treatment altogether (Olanow, Freeman, and Kordower 1997). On the negative side, functional recovery in fetal neural trials was never more than partial. However, there was general consensus that fetal neural transplantation was worth pursuing as a therapeutic option for PD. Further clinical trials were recommended.

A small number of double-blind placebo-controlled trials were then carried out (Freed et al. 2001; Olanow et al. 2003). The control subjects were PD patients who received sham operations but no neural grafts. These studies revealed a clear clinical improvement following grafting in patients under the age of 60, but far less in older patients. In addition, some of the more recent trials revealed that the treatment is associated with side effects (dyskinesias) and in some cases morbidity due to subdural hemorrhages (Freed et al. 2001; Hauser et al. 2002; Olanow et al. 2003; Freeman et al. 2003). The Network of European CNS Transplantation and Restoration (NECTAR) raised concerns over one of these studies, including the use of sham neurosurgical procedures (Nikkhah 2001). Sham surgery has also come in for criticism on ethical grounds (Macklin 1999; Polgar and Ng 2005). More recently, evidence has emerged that, over a 10–16-year period, the underlying cause of PD may destroy the grafts over time (Kordower et al. 2008; Li et al. 2008; Mendez et al. 2008).

As those involved in this research look at the current state of play, it is generally conceded that a number of highly significant technical issues remain to be addressed before trials should continue (Lindvall and Bjorklund 2004; Winkler, Kirik, and Bjorklund 2005; Brundin, Barker, and Parmar 2010). In addition, the need for further animal studies to investigate the mechanisms underlying side effects continues. These suggestions are hauntingly reminiscent of similar comments over the past 20 or more years. Despite the uncertainties a European multi-centre trial called Transeuro has recently begun

(Holden 2009; Allan, Petit, and Brundin 2010) with the aim of clarifying some of the outstanding scientific and clinical issues.

5 Relevance of grafting studies for neuroethics

What sustains and energizes a field such as this one? What is the rationale behind the ongoing commitment by scientists and clinicians to an approach that, whatever its ulti-mate benefits turn out to be, continues to be ambiguous? Any answer brings us face-to-face with a host of social and ethical imperatives.

5.1 A paradigm of optimism

One of the dominant messages to emerge is the optimism of most reports. The gen-eral consensus appeared to be that there remained numerous ways of improving the then current techniques of neural grafting, and hence clinical trials were warranted. However, it is unclear to what extent this optimism stemmed from a basic belief in the worthwhile nature of this approach rather than from an objective assessment of the data.

It has emerged that optimism drives an experimental approach for year after year on the grounds that convincing data and a satisfactory approach will be found. Herein lies hope, both for patients and researchers. On the surface this is an eminently ethical road to pursue, and yet it raises the question of what criteria will be used to determine the length of time a field can be pursued as a worthwhile endeavour in the absence of con-vincing clinical results. At some point the question arises: are vulnerable patients being exploited?

Optimism of this ilk is repeatedly found in many of the conditions that crop up in neuroethical discussion where it serves as a major driver of expectations and hopes. Repeatedly the optimism is not tempered by realistic assessment of the state of the clini-cal science. Consequently, the ethical debate may be diverted into highly speculative areas to the detriment of far more pressing ethical issues. This has been brought out by a number of commentators, even if not within the specific domain of neuroethics (Jones 2006; King, Whitaker, and Jones 2011; Lysaght and Campbell 2013).

5.2 Clinical equipoise

The search for better brains, or even as a means of controlling an individual's inad-equately functioning motor system, is a powerful one. This in turn has extensive ethical repercussions that, while relevant in a condition like Parkinson's disease, are far more pressing when discussing the many possibilities of, say, cognitive enhancement.

The Parkinson's example demonstrates the uncertainty of the boundary between therapeutic and experimental studies. However, this boundary is rarely invoked when considering ways of blocking or dampening traumatic memories, removing traces of guilt, reducing anxiety, or improving problem-solving abilities. The underlying assump-tion appears to be that any or all of these will one day be readily accomplished with few negative side effects and with few teething problems. Neither is much thought given to controlled trials, or possible effects resulting from administering what turn out to be excessive levels of drugs (such as excessive dopamine agonists in Parkinson's disease that convert moderate patients into obsessive gamblers (Dodd et al. 2005)).

Ethical attention is usually directed onto concerns raised by the issue at hand, such as memory enhancement or guilt removal. However, there is a preliminary stage of ethical analysis and this is how we arrive at the expected modification. The complexity and interconnectedness of brain circuits and regions make it highly unlikely that the intended effect will be the only one achieved. Even if in the long term this turns out to be the case, wrong turns and unwanted effects will undoubtedly characterize the intervening experimental stages.

The history of neural grafting raises the question of the requirements necessary to ethically justify surgery of this nature. A research proposal is unethical if it lacks scientific validity, since participants may be inconvenienced or put at risk for no clear benefit (Campbell, Gillett, and Jones 2005). Every research proposal must be subjected to stringent scientific assessment to ensure the presence of a useful and valid hypothesis and to ensure that the research design will yield the desired result.

Neural grafting research is therapeutic, since these patients have a serious debilitating condition and are expecting to benefit from the procedures undertaken on them. Clinical equipoise requires that in therapeutic trials patients might reasonably expect an improvement in their condition roughly equivalent to that of standard treatment. In practice patients may expect more than this, especially those whose conditions are especially difficult and whose hopes are high. Managing these expectations when gaining consent is an important consideration for any experimental work with patients. As well as these considerations, the effects of the treatment must be capable of being isolated statistically and evaluated in a scientifically rigorous way, for example by comparing the new treatment (e.g. grafting) with conventional treatment (e.g. drug regime alone in this case).

In addition there is also the expectation that the procedure will contribute towards the benefit of patients in the future. This entails previous experimental knowledge sufficient to justify the approach, a sufficient number of patients to enable stringent assessment of the outcome, and peer review of the study.

5.3 The place of controls

Controlled neural grafting trials were initiated in 2001 (Freed et al. 2001). Earlier studies were unblinded, uncontrolled, the number of patients was very small, and surgical approaches varied considerably between studies. This has made it extremely difficult to compare the results of grafting procedures in different groups of patients, a situation with serious ethical implications let alone scientific ones. If patients have been placed at unnecessary risk and have been subjected to procedures with limited prospects of beneficial effects, the balance between beneficence and maleficence has wrongfully tipped towards the latter.

The main argument in favour of randomized controlled trials is that they constitute the only way to exclude the possibility that clinical improvements are due to a placebo effect (Freeman et al. 1999). On the other hand, patients should not be exposed to the risks associated with sham surgery when they are not expected to benefit from it (Macklin 1999). For Dekkers and Boer (2001) sham surgery is not needed since the question of the clinical benefits of neural grafting can be answered by other means, while sham surgery itself does not amount to a true placebo.

Once again, the intricacies of brain-invasive procedures shine through. Even the legitimate desire to employ adequate controls is proving problematic. While these concerns do not amount to an adequate reason for desisting with work of this nature, they demonstrate with startling clarity the problems inherent in conducting this type of work in an ethically appropriate fashion. The issues raised here are relevant to all other forms of neural experimentation, and need to be seriously considered as part of any ethical assessments undertaken as part of these burgeoning neuroethical debates.

6 Deep brain stimulation in Parkinson's disease

One alternative to grafting is the use of deep brain stimulation (DBS). In DBS, electrical signals generated in a subcutaneously placed unit are sent to electrodes implanted in the motor regions of the brain. The aim of these is to stimulate the function of the motor regions detrimentally affected by the loss of the dopamine producing neurons in PD. It is used when routine treatments have become ineffective, although care has to be exercised since it may have negative side effects including personality changes (Glannon 2009). Worldwide more than 80,000 patients have been provided with these implants.

DBS is also cautiously used as an experimental treatment for intractable depression, obsessive compulsive disorder, and Tourette syndrome (Rabins et al. 2009). Additionally, it is sometimes used to treat psychiatric disorders, as well as forms of cluster headaches, epilepsy, and disorders of consciousness like the minimal conscious state (see Synofzik and Schlaepfer 2008; Clausen 2010).

The experimental treatment of patients includes exploring new implantation sites and these have a good scientific rationale (Greenberg, Rauch, and Haber 2009; Rabins et al. 2009). Commendably, this research is proceeding very cautiously with stringent patient selection criteria, and occurs best under the leadership of specialist interdisciplinary teams (Greenberg, personal communication, 7 September 2011).

When DBS is used in PD, its aim is to alleviate the motor symptoms that, by the stage at which DBS is employed, are debilitating. However, the positive effects of DBS in controlling these symptoms may be accompanied by a range of transient and treatable neuropsychiatric symptoms including depression and apathy (Voon et al. 2006). If side effects of this nature are minor, the alleviation of the crippling motor deficiencies will likely be welcomed by most patients. The underlying assumption is that there are no ethically objectionable effects on the patients' identity. Inevitably, the removal of a debilitating neurological condition like Parkinson's disease can itself affect self-identity; however, where the effects are perceived by the patient to be a restoration of their 'usual self', they will not be of great ethical concern since the change is strictly therapeutic.

Nevertheless, follow-up studies have looked in detail at side effects. One strand of investigations has shown that there are a few relatively minor or manageable psychiatric side effects. These include meta-analyses (Voon et al. 2006), randomized, controlled, multi-centre studies (Witt et al. 2008), and large studies (Funkiewiez 2001). In contrast, case studies have unearthed more troubling results. These include pathological crying (Okun et al. 2004; Wojtecki et al. 2007), mirthful laughter (Krack et al. 2001), and mania with psychotic or hypersexual symptoms (Romito et al. 2002; Raucher-Chéné et al. 2008). There have been a number of reports of dementia (however, this is also a symptom of PD itself), mania, transient hypomanic state, and long-term apathy. Affective and psychiatric side effects have been reported in up to a quarter of DBS patients, with increased suicide rates also being reported (Clausen 2010). There was one case where the patient was not aware of his hypomanic state and developed criminal behaviour (Mandat, Hurwitz, and Honey 2006).

However, these various side effects may diminish spontaneously over time or can often be resolved either by altering the target of DBS or through pairing DBS with other treatment. These side effects, while uncommon, remind us that few treatments are without any side effects, and these have to be taken into account in any ethical assessment of interventions into the brain.

6.1 Scientific precision of DBS

DBS provides an instructive counterpoint to neural grafting in that it is directed far more precisely at well-defined neural targets within the basal ganglia (Ponce and Lozano 2010; Franzini et al. 2011). This precision provides considerable assurance that the areas being targeted are ones that are malfunctioning in PD and giving rise to the symptoms being experienced by individual patients. This increasing clinical specificity is a major positive ethically.

DBS appears to be effective in reducing motor fluctuations and dyskinesias. Moreover multi-centre control trials suggest that DBS is more effective than the best available medical therapy in improving motor function and quality of life, and in reducing dyskinesias (Weaver et al. 2009). It is most effective in those who respond well to L-DOPA, but for whom medication-related complications make L-DOPA therapy no longer acceptable. DBS offers relief similar to L-DOPA but without the side effects.

It is likely that DBS produces its clinical benefit by disrupting the pathological activity in the neural circuitry linking the basal ganglia and motor cortex. However, the precise mechanism by which DBS acts on the brain to alleviate symptoms is not conclusively understood. There is increasing evidence that the effects of DBS are complex, and that it produces long-term changes in the brain, altering excitability and plasticity (Prescott et al. 2009), and driving neurogenesis (Toda et al. 2008). These, as pointed out previously, are fundamental neural processes, and if DBS does indeed influence them, some of its effects in all probability are widespread and lasting.

In spite of these encouraging outcomes, there can be complications, including massive brain hemorrhage, permanent or transient neurological deficits, postoperative seizures, infection, and hardware complications (Franzini et al. 2011).

6.2 Ethical responses: authenticity and alienation

The usual range of research ethics issues are overshadowed by more specific ones relating to DBS-induced changes in mood and behaviour (Duggan et al. 2009; Clausen 2010), as well as notions of alienation and authenticity (Kraemer forthcoming). While for some patients treatment with DBS cured the feeling of alienation that living with PD had brought about ('Now that I am better I feel like myself again'), for others the treatment brought a feeling of alienation even though it cured the motor symptoms ('I don't recognize myself now that I don't suffer from PD ...I feel like a machine'). For the latter group, the loss of what was an important goal, namely, striving to fight the symptoms of PD, as well as altered body image, are key factors in such responses.

To some degree personal identity is altered by many kinds of surgery, e.g. limb amputation, mastectomy, hysterectomy, and prostate surgery. Our identity is in many ways tied to our bodily function and capabilities. DBS is similar to these other surgeries, in that it can have profound implications for physical functioning of the patient's body. However, it may differ in that it can cause specific alterations to components of one's fundamental sense of self by affecting directly elements of the psyche that reside in the brain (memory, emotion, cognition) (Lipsman, Zener, and Bernstein 2009). For some, these effects of DBS and other neurosurgical interventions pose deep problems because identity (in a psychological and narrative sense) is affected. However, the depth of the problem varies according to how dynamic a view of psychological and narrative identity is permitted. DBS-induced changes may change identity from its desired stasis and therefore be regarded as problematic, or it may represent one of the dynamic changes that identity undergoes during our varied life courses.

Other views claim that identity is constituted only in part by one's psychological attributes and characteristics, but more through one's negotiated relations with others (Baylis forthcoming). According to this relational view, identity is constituted by who we are in ourselves but also who others will let us be. Accordingly, alterations to psychological and physical characteristics are only part of what matters, and it is how these integrate with the responses of others to perceived changes in identity that ultimately determines identity. From this point of view alterations in psychological characteristics from DBS need not necessarily be a problem unless they undermine the ability of the individual to meaningfully participate in the relations that drive identity.

Providing dramatic side effects are avoided, the concerns relating to identity that arise from DBS in the majority of patients are in large part similar to those that arise in the alleviation of any major illness. Crucially however, the effects of DBS can be altered significantly by altering target sites for stimulation, and unlike neural grafting the possibility of discontinuing the treatment and its effects is feasible (possible lasting effects due to plastic alterations of the brain notwithstanding). Treatment must take these concerns into account and proceed with caution and sensitivity to the views of the patient, especially whether they are aware of potential identity-concerning implications of the treatment prior to giving consent.

7 Neural grafting, DBS, and neuroethics

Future vistas lead to possibilities closely related to those envisaged by proponents of neurocognitive enhancement. This may not be the intention, but as the inherent plasticity of the brain is exploited, as memories and moods are modified and even improved by changes to neurotransmitter levels, and as neural implants and genetic manipulation are increasingly utilized to remedy neural deficiencies, will changes to our brains alter how we view ourselves and are seen by others? None of these prospects would be on the horizon were it not for the latent neuroregenerative properties of the human brain. But how easy is it going to be to optimize these properties and utilize them in ways that will enhance human neural functioning in the desired directions?

In attempting to answer this question, I have analysed two treatment approaches to PD. Neither neural grafting nor DBS has grandiose objectives; they are simply approaches to the treatment of PD even though both exist on the border between therapy and experiment. Neither can be classed as an enhancement and those involved in applying them would not wish them to be seen in such terms. Surprisingly perhaps, the development of each of them has raised a raft of clinical and ethical challenges. The contention of this paper is that these challenges are common to all the innovations that constitute the core of neuroethical debate.

By taking a neurodegenerative disease where the neuronal population lost is accurately known and where it is definitively known which neurons or their neurotransmitter are to be replaced, one has as straightforward a model system as one is likely to encounter. And yet there are potential problems, consideration of which yields three salutary messages that deserve serious assessment by neuroethicists.

The *first* highlights the interconnectivity of the regions and functional areas within the brain, and consequently the non-modular nature of the brain's organization. This is brought out by the experience of DBS that shows very clearly that this means of alleviating symptoms of motor system dysfunction may have implications for other facets of the individual's neural responses, including their identity, while other psychiatric repercussions are sometimes evident. The message for neuroethical consideration is that attempts to alter specific brain characteristics, whether memory, intelligence, or cognitive ability are likely to have unanticipated effects on personality characteristics, authenticity, and self-awareness. These possibilities may prove to be counter-indications to proceeding with some forms of, say, cognitive enhancement.

A *second* issue of note emerged with the experience gained by neural grafting, with its prolonged experimental period. This is a timely reminder that what appear to be straightforward intrusions into the brain (surgical or pharmacological) will probably turn out to be far from straightforward in practice. Neuroethical debate has tended to assume that the only discussion that needs to be held is whether the project is worthwhile. Its scientific and clinical feasibility has played little, if any, part in the debate. Neural grafting points to the pitfalls of this approach. The path from concept to application may well be tortuous and strewn with ethical questions. Neuroethics needs to pay far more attention than heretofore to the issues inherent within this path.

A *third* issue is that of the adult brain's plasticity and ongoing neurogenesis. Attempts to modify the brain have to be seen within this context, and not that of a supposedly status quo structure. The brain is constantly responding to internal and external changes, so that intrusions may have surprising effects that cannot be precisely determined in advance. Are our forays into the brain based on a misleading mechanistic model of the brain? Alongside this query we need to ask whether expectations are based on an assumption that the microstructure of the brain can be remodelled as if it was in its developmental stages. This is an area ripe for neuroethical considerations, since if this is overlooked we may find that we are indulging in misleading hyperbole. Of one thing we can be certain: intrusions into the brain are not on a par with intrusions into any other organs.

Neuroethics has a great deal to learn from the matters raised by therapeutic endeavours in treating PD. Far more attention should be given to what at first glance may appear to be nothing more than forays into clinical ethics. Their relevance for neuroethics is considerable.

References

Acevedo, B. P. et al. (2012). 'Neural Correlates of Long-Term Intense Romantic Love', *Social Cognitive and Affective Neuroscience*, 7(2): 145–59.

Allan, L. E., Petit, G. H., and Brundin, P. (2010). 'Cell Transplantation in Parkinson's Disease: Problems and Perspectives', *Current Opinion in Neurology*, 23(4): 426–32.

Aydin, K. et al. (2007). 'Increased Gray Matter Density in the Parietal Cortex of Mathematicians: A Voxel-Based Morphometry Study', *American Journal of Neuroradiology*, 28(10): 1859–64.

Backlund, E. O. et al. (1985). 'Transplantation of Adrenal Medullary Tissue to Striatum in Parkinsonism: First Clinical Trials', *Journal of Neurosurgery*, 62(2): 169–73.

Baylis, F. (Forthcoming). '"I am who I am": On the Perceived Threats to Personal Identity from Deep Brain Stimulation', *Neuroethics*, Advance online publication, 13 September 2011. DOI: 10.1007/s12152-011-9137-1.

Bingaman, K. D. and Bakay, R. A. (2000). 'The Primate Model of Parkinson's Disease: Its Usefulness, Limitations, and Importance in Directing Future Studies', *Progress in Brain Research*, 127: 267–97.

Bjorklund, A. et al. (2003). 'Neural Transplantation for the Treatment of Parkinson's Disease', *Lancet Neurology*, 2(7): 437–45.

Bohannon, J. (2011). 'Searching for the Google Effect on People's Memory', *Science*, 333(6040): 277.

Brodmann, K. (1909). *Vergleichende Lokalisationslehre de Großhirnrinde in ihren Prinzipien dargestellt auf Grund des Zellenbaues*. Leipzig: Johann Ambrosius Barth.

Brundin, P., Barker, R. A., and Parmar, M. (2010). 'Neural Grafting in Parkinson's Disease Problems and Possibilities', *Progress in Brain Research*, 184: 265–94.

Buss, R. R., Sun, W., and Oppenheim, R. W. (2006). 'Adaptive Roles of Programmed Cell Death during Nervous System Development', *Annual Review of Neuroscience*, 29: 1–35.

Cameron, H. A. and Dayer, A. G. (2008). 'New Interneurons in the Adult Neocortex: Small, Sparse, but Significant?' *Biological Psychiatry*, 63(7): 650–5.

Campbell, A. V., G. Gillett, and D. G. Jones. (2005). *Medical Ethics*. Melbourne: Oxford University Press.

Carr, N. (2008). 'Is Google Making Us Stupid? *The Atlantic*, July–August, http://www.theatlantic.com/magazine/archive/2008/07/is-google-making-us-stupid/6868/ (accessed 23 September 2011).

Chaudhuri, K. et al. (2011). 'Parkinson's Disease: The Non-Motor Issues', *Parkinsonism and Related Disorders*, 17(10): 717–23.

Chaudhuri, K. and Schapira, A. H. V. (2009). 'Non-Motor Symptoms of Parkinson's Disease: Dopaminergic Pathophysiology and Treatment', *The Lancet Neurology*, 8(5): 464–74.

Clarkson, E. D. (2001). 'Fetal Tissue Transplantation for Patients with Parkinson's Disease: A Database of Published Clinical Results', *Drugs and Aging*, 18(10): 773–85.

Clausen, J. (2010). 'Ethical Brain Stimulation: Neuroethics of Deep Brain Stimulation in Research and Clinical Practice', *The European Journal of Neuroscience*, 32(7): 1152–62.

Conover, J. C., and Notti, R. Q. (2008). 'The Neural Stem Cell Niche', *Cell and Tissue Research*, 331(1): 211–24.

Curley, J. P. et al. (2011). 'Social Influences on Neurobiology and Behavior: Epigenetic Effects during Development', *Psychoneuroendocrinology*, 36(3): 352–71.

Dekkers, W., and Boer, G. (2001). 'Sham Neurosurgery in Patients with Parkinson's Disease: Is It Morally Acceptable?' *Journal of Medical Ethics*, 27(3): 151–6.

Dodd, M. L. et al. (2005). 'Pathological Gambling Caused by Drugs Used to Treat Parkinson Disease', *Archives of Neurology*, 62(9): 1377–81.

Dohan, P. C. et al. (1988). 'Autopsy Findings in a Parkinson's Disease Patient Treated with Adrenal Medullary to Caudate Transplant', *Society of Neuroscience Abstracts*, 1: 8.

Duggan, P. S. et al. (2009). 'Unintended Changes in Cognition, Mood, and Behavior Arising from Cell-Based Interventions for Neurological Conditions: Ethical Challenges', *American Journal of Bioethics*, 9(5): 31–6.

Fahn, S. (1992). 'Fetal-Tissue Transplants in Parkinson's Disease', *The New England Journal of Medicine*, 327(22): 1589–90.

Farah, M. J. (ed.). (2010). *Neuroethics: An Introduction with Readings*. Cambridge, MA: MIT Press.

Forno, L. S. and J. W. Langston. (1991). 'Unfavorable Outcome of Adrenal Medullary Transplant for Parkinson's Disease', *Acta Neuropathologica*, 81(6): 691–4.

Franzini, A. et al. (2011). 'Deep Brain Stimulation for Movement Disorders: Considerations on 276 Consecutive Patients', *Journal of Neural Transmission*, 118: 1497–510.

Freed, C. R. et al. (1992). 'Survival of Implanted Fetal Dopamine Cells and Neurologic Improvement 12 to 46 Months after Transplantation for Parkinson's Disease', *The New England Journal of Medicine*, 327(22): 1549–55.

Freed, C. R. et al. (2001). 'Transplantation of Embryonic Dopamine Neurons for Severe Parkinson's Disease', *The New England Journal of Medicine*, 344(10): 710–19.

Freed, W. et al. (1981). 'Transplanted Adrenal Chromaffin Cells in Rat Brain Reduce Lesion-Induced Rotational Behaviour', *Nature*, 292(5821): 351–2.

Freed, W. J. et al. (1983). 'Catecholamine Content of Intracerebral Adrenal Medulla Grafts', *Brain Research*, 269(1): 184–9.

Freeman, T. B. et al. (1999). 'Use of Placebo Surgery in Controlled Trials of a Cellular-Based Therapy for Parkinson's Disease', *The New England Journal of Medicine*, 341(13): 988–92.

Freeman, T. B. et al. (2003). 'Surgical Placebo Controlled Trial of Human Fetal Nigral Transplantation in Parkinson's Disease (PD)', Program No. 656.3, Neuroscience 2003 Abstracts. Washington, DC: Society for Neuroscience.

Funkiewiez, A. (2001). 'Behavioral and Mood Changes Associated with Bilateral Stimulation of the Subthalamic Nucleus: A Consecutive Series of 98 Parkinsonian Patients', *Neurology*, 56(suppl 3): A274.

Glannon, W. (2009). 'Stimulating Brains, Altering Minds', *Journal of Medical Ethics*, 35(5): 289–392.

Goetz, C. G. et al. (1989). 'Multicenter Study of Autologous Adrenal Medullary Transplantation to the Corpus Striatum in Patients with Advanced Parkinson's Disease', *The New England Journal of Medicine*, 320(6): 337–41.

Golestani, N., Price, C. J., and Scott, S. K. (2011). 'Born with an Ear for Dialects? Structural Plasticity in the Expert Phonetician Brain', *The Journal of Neuroscience*, 31(11): 4213–20.

Gould, E., and Tanapat, P. (1999). 'Stress and Hippocampal Neurogenesis', *Biological Psychiatry*, 46(11): 1472–9.

Greenberg, B. D., Rauch, S. L., and Haber, S. N. (2009). 'Invasive Circuitry-Based Neurotherapeutics: Stereotactic Ablation and Deep Brain Stimulation for OCD', *Neuropsychopharmacology*, 35(1): 317–36.

Gurgo, R. D., Bedi, K. S., and Nurcombe, V. (2002). 'Current Concepts in Central Nervous System Regeneration', *Journal of Clinical Neuroscience*, 9(6): 613–17.

Hagell, P., and Brundin, P. (2001). 'Cell Survival and Clinical Outcome Following Intrastriatal Transplantation in Parkinson Disease', *Journal of Neuropathology and Experimental Neurology*, 60(8): 741–52.

Hanggi, J., S. et al. (2010). 'Structural Neuroplasticity in the Sensorimotor Network of Professional Female Ballet Dancers', *Human Brain Mapping*, 31(8): 1196–206.

Hauser, R. A. et al. (2002). 'Bilateral Human Fetal Striatal Transplantation in Huntington's Disease', *Neurology*, 58(5): 687–95.

Herrera-Marschitz, M., et al. (1984). 'Adrenal Medullary Implants in the Dopamine-Denervated Rat Striatum. II. Acute Behavior as a Function of Graft Amount and Location and Its Modulation by Neuroleptics', *Brain Research*, 297(1): 53–61.

Hitchcock, E. R. et al. (1988). 'Embryos and Parkinson's Disease', *Lancet*, 1(8597): 1274.

Holden, C. (2009). 'Fetal Cells Again?' *Science*, 326(5951): 358–9.

Jin, H. et al. (2010). 'Athletic Training in Badminton Players Modulates the Early C1 Component of Visual Evoked Potentials: A Preliminary Investigation', *International Journal of Psychophysiology*, 78(3): 308–14.

Jones, D. G. (1991). 'Fetal Neural Transplantation: Placing the Ethical Debate within the Context of Society's Use of Human Material', *Bioethics*, 5(1): 23–43.

Jones, D. G. (2006). 'Enhancement: Are Ethicists Excessively Influenced by Baseless Speculations?' *Medical Humanities*, 32: 77–81.

Kee, N. J., Preston, E., and Wojtowicz, J. M. (2001). 'Enhanced Neurogenesis after Transient Global Ischemia in the Dentate Gyrus of the Rat', *Experimental Brain Research*, 136(3): 313–20.

King, M., Whitaker, M., and Jones, D. G. (2011). 'Speculative Ethics: Valid Enterprise or Tragic Cul-De-Sac?' in A. Rudnick (ed.), *Bioethics in the 21st century*. Rijeka: InTech, 139–58.

Kordower, J. H. et al. (1995). 'Neuropathological Evidence of Graft Survival and Striatal Reinnervation after the Transplantation of Fetal Mesencephalic Tissue in a Patient with Parkinson's Disease', *The New England Journal of Medicine*, 332(17): 1118–24.

Kordower, J. H. et al. (2008). 'Lewy Body-Like Pathology in Long-Term Embryonic Nigral Transplants in Parkinson's Disease', *Nature Medicine*, 14: 504–6.

Krack, P. et al. (2001). 'Mirthful Laughter Induced by Subthalamic Nucleus Stimulation', *Movement Disorders*, 16(5): 867–75.

Kraemer, F. (Forthcoming). 'Me, Myself, and My Brain Implant: Deep Brain Stimulation Raises Questions of Personal Authenticity and Alienation', *Neuroethics*, Advance online publication, 12 May 2011. DOI: 10.1007/s12152-011-9115-7.

Lappe, C. et al. (2011). 'Cortical Plasticity Induced by Short-Term Multimodal Musical Rhythm Training', *PLoS One*, 6(6): e21493.

Li, J.Y. et al. (2008). 'Lewy Bodies in Grafted Neurons in Subjects with Parkinson's Disease Suggest Host-to-Graft Disease Propagation', *Nature Medicine*, 14: 501–3.

Lieberman, A. (1987). 'Adrenal Grafts for Parkinson's Disease', *The New England Journal of Medicine*, 317(17): 1092.

Lindvall, O., and Bjorklund, A. (2004). 'Cell Therapy in Parkinson's Disease', *NeuroRx*, 1(4): 382–93.

Lindvall, O. et al. (1987). 'Transplantation in Parkinson's Disease: Two Cases of Adrenal Medullary Grafts to the Putamen', *Annals of Neurology*, 22(4): 457–68.

Lindvall, O. et al. (1989). 'Human Fetal Dopamine Neurons Grafted into the Striatum in Two Patients with Severe Parkinson's Disease: A Detailed Account of Methodology and a 6 Month Follow-Up', *Archives of Neurology*, 46: 615–31.

Lipsman, N., Zener, R., and Bernstein, M. (2009). 'Personal Identity, Enhancement, and Neurosurgery: A Qualitative Study in Applied Neuroethics', *Bioethics*, 23(6): 375–83.

Lysaght, T., and Campbell, A.V. (2014). 'The Ethics of Regenerative Medicine: Broadening the Scope beyond the Moral Status of Embryos', in A. Akabayashi (ed.), *The Future of Bioethics: International Dialogues*. Oxford: Oxford University Press, 5–26.

Macklin, R. (1999). 'The Ethical Problems with Sham Surgery in Clinical Research', *The New England Journal of Medicine*, 341(13): 992–6.

Madrazo, I. et al. (1987). 'Open Microsurgical Autograft of Adrenal Medulla to the Right Caudate Nucleus in Two Patients with Intractable Parkinson's Disease', *The New England Journal of Medicine*, 316(14): 831–4.

Madrazo, I. et al. (1988). 'Transplantation of Fetal Substantia Nigra and Adrenal Medulla to the Caudate Nucleus in Two Patients with Parkinson's Disease', *The New England Journal of Medicine*, 318: 51.

Maguire, E. A., Woollett, K., and Spiers, H. J. (2006). 'London Taxi Drivers and Bus Drivers: A Structural MRI and Neuropsychological Analysis', *Hippocampus*, 16(12): 1091–101.

Mandat, T., Hurwitz, T., and Honey, C. (2006). 'Hypomania as an Adverse Effect of Subthalamic Nucleus Stimulation: Report of Two Cases', *Acta Neurochirurgica*, 148(8): 895–8.

Markham, J. A., and Greenough, W. T. (2004). 'Experience-Driven Brain Plasticity: Beyond the Synapse', *Neuron Glia Biology*, 1(4): 351–63.

Mendez, I. et al. (2008). 'Dopamine Neurons Implanted into People with Parkinson's Disease Survive without Pathology for 14 Years', *Nature Medicine*, 14: 507–9.

Miller, R. H. (2006). 'The Promise of Stem Cells for Neural Repair', *Brain Research*, 1091(1): 258–64.

Morihisa, J. M. et al. (1984). 'Adrenal Medulla Grafts Survive and Exhibit Catecholamine-Specific Fluorescence in the Primate Brain', *Experimental Neurology*, 84(3): 643–53.

Muramatsu, R., Ueno, M., and Yamashita, T. (2009). 'Intrinsic Regenerative Mechanisms of Central Nervous System Neurons', *Bioscience Trends*, 3(5): 179–83.

Neville, H. and Bavelier, D. (2002). 'Human Brain Plasticity: Evidence from Sensory Deprivation and Altered Language Experience', *Progress in Brain Research*, 138: 177–88.

Nikkhah, G. (2001). 'Neural Transplantation Therapy for Parkinson's Disease: Potential and Pitfalls', *Brain Research Bulletin*, 56(6): 509.

Obeso, J. A. et al. (2008). 'Functional Organization of the Basal Ganglia: Therapeutic Implications for Parkinson's Disease', *Movement Disorders*, 23(Suppl 3): S548–59.

Okun, M. et al. (2004). 'Pseudobulbar Crying Induced by Stimulation in the Region of the Subthalamic Nucleus', *Journal of Neurology, Neurosurgery and Psychiatry*, 75(6): 921.

Olanow, C. W., Freeman, T. B., and Kordower, J. H. (1997). 'Neural Transplantation as a Therapy for Parkinson's Disease', *Advances in Neurology*, 74: 249–69.

Olanow, C. W. et al. (2003). 'A Double-Blind Controlled Trial of Bilateral Fetal Nigral Transplantation in Parkinson's Disease', *Annals of Neurology*, 54(3): 403–14.

Park, A. and Stacy, M. (2009). 'Non-Motor Symptoms in Parkinson's Disease', *Journal of Neurology*, 256: 293–8.

Park, I. S. et al. (2009). 'Experience-Dependent Plasticity of Cerebellar Vermis in Basketball Players', *Cerebellum*, 8(3): 334–9.

Peterson, D. I., Price, M. L., and Small, C. S. (1989). 'Autopsy Findings in a Patient Who Had an Adrenal-to-Brain Transplant for Parkinson's Disease', *Neurology*, 39(2 Pt 1): 235–8.

Poewe, W. (2008). 'Non Motor Symptoms in Parkinson's Disease', *European Journal of Neurology*, 15: 14–20.

Polgar, S. and Ng, J. (2005). 'Ethics, Methodology, and the Use of Placebo Controls in Surgical Trials', *Brain Research Bulletin*, 67(4): 290–7.

Ponce, F. A. and Lozano, A. M. (2010). 'Deep Brain Stimulation State of the Art and Novel Stimulation Targets', *Progress in Brain Research*, 184: 311–24.

Porena, M. et al. (1996). 'Autologous Adrenal Medullary Transplant in Parkinson's Disease: Critical Review of Our Results in 13 Patients', *Neurourology and Urodynamics*, 15(3): 195–201.

Prescott, I. A. et al. (2009). 'Levodopa Enhances Synaptic Plasticity in the Substantia Nigra Pars Reticulata of Parkinson's Disease Patients', *Brain*, 132(Pt 2): 309–18.

Rabins, P. et al. (2009). 'Scientific and Ethical Issues Related to Deep Brain Stimulation for Disorders of Mood, Behavior, and Thought', *Archives of General Psychiatry*, 66(9): 931.

Ramón y Cajal, S. (1909). *Histologie du systeme nerveux de l'homme et des vertebres*. Paris: Maloine.

Raucher-Chéné, D. et al. (2008). 'Manic Episode with Psychotic Symptoms in a Patient with Parkinson's Disease Treated by Subthalamic Nucleus Stimulation: Improvement on Switching the Target', *Journal of the Neurological Sciences*, 273(1–2): 116–17.

Romito, L. M. et al. (2002). 'Transient Mania with Hypersexuality after Surgery for High Frequency Stimulation of the Subthalamic Nucleus in Parkinson's Disease', *Movement Disorders*, 17(6): 1371–4.

Sladek, J. R., Jr. and Shoulson, I. (1988). 'Neural Transplantation: A Call for Patience Rather than Patients', *Science*, 240(4858): 1386–8.

Spencer, D. D. et al. (1992). 'Unilateral Transplantation of Human Fetal Mesencephalic Tissue into the Caudate Nucleus of Patients with Parkinson's Disease', *The New England Journal of Medicine*, 327(22): 1541–8.

Stiles, J. (2011). 'Brain Development and the Nature Versus Nurture Debate', *Progress in Brain Research*, 189: 3–22.

Stiles, J. and Jernigan, T. L. (2010). 'The Basics of Brain Development', *Neuropsychology Review*, 20(4): 327–48.

Strömberg, I. et al. (1984). 'Adrenal Medullary Implants in the Dopamine-Denervated Rat Striatum. I. Acute Catecholamine Levels in Grafts and Host Caudate as Determined by HPLC-Electrochemistry and Fluorescence Histochemical Image Analysis', *Brain Research*, 297(1): 41–51.

Sullivan, W. (1987). 'Mexican Procedure For Parkinson's Will Be Used By Surgeons Here', *New York Times*, 15 April.

Swanson, L. W. (2003). *Brain Architecture: Understanding the Basic Plan*. Oxford: Oxford University Press.

Synofzik, M. and Schlaepfer, T. E. (2008). 'Stimulating Personality: Ethical Criteria for Deep Brain Stimulation in Psychiatric Patients and for Enhancement Purposes', *Biotechnology Journal*, 3(12): 1511–20.

Toda, H. et al. (2008). 'The Regulation of Adult Rodent Hippocampal Neurogenesis by Deep Brain Stimulation', *Journal of Neurosurgery*, 108(1): 132–8.

Voelcker-Rehage, C., and Willimczik, K. (2006). 'Motor Plasticity in a Juggling Task in Older Adults: A Developmental Study', *Age and Ageing*, 35(4): 422–7.

Voon, V. et al. (2006). 'Deep Brain Stimulation: Neuropsychological and Neuropsychiatric Issues', *Movement Disorders*, 21(Suppl 14): S305–27.

Weaver, F. M. et al. (2009). 'Bilateral Deep Brain Stimulation vs Best Medical Therapy for Patients with Advanced Parkinson Disease: A Randomized Controlled Trial', *JAMA*, 301(1): 63–73.

Wenning, G. K. et al. (1997). 'Short- and Long-Term Survival and Function of Unilateral Intrastriatal Dopaminergic Grafts in Parkinson's Disease', *Annals of Neurology*, 42: 95–107.

Widner, H. et al. (1992). 'Bilateral Fetal Mesencephalic Grafting in Two Patients with Parkinsonism Induced by 1-Methyl-4-Phenyl-1,2,3,6-Tetrahydropyridine (MPTP)', *The New England Journal of Medicine*, 327(22): 1556–63.

Winkler, C., Kirik, D., and Bjorklund, A. (2005). 'Cell Transplantation in Parkinson's Disease: How Can We Make It Work?' *Trends in Neurosciences*, 28(2): 86–92.

Witt, K. et al. (2008). 'Neuropsychological and Psychiatric Changes after Deep Brain Stimulation for Parkinson's Disease: A Randomised, Multicentre Study', *The Lancet Neurology*, 7(7): 605–14.

Wojtecki, L. et al. (2007). 'Pathological Crying Induced by Deep Brain Stimulation', *Movement Disorders*, 22(9): 1314–16.

Wolf, N. (2011). 'Is Pornography Driving Men Crazy?' *Global Public Square, CNN World*, 30 June, http://globalpublicsquare.blogs.cnn.com/2011/06/30/is-pornography-driving-men-crazy/ (accessed 26 August 2011).

2.2

Commentary
Some Issues in Neuroethics

Jing Bai and Renzong Qiu

In his paper 'Neural Repair as a Case Study in Neuroethics', Professor Gareth Jones took Parkinson's disease as a case study to overview the progress of transplantation studies, grafting studies, and DBS, as well as neuroethical issues. In what follows we would like to argue for the importance of clinical trials in therapeutic brain interventions of these kinds, and to provide some information on neuroethics in China, as well as the Chinese perspective on it.

Clinical trials in neural repair

As Professor Jones rightly pointed out, the human brain is an organ with fascinating complexity, interconnectivity, and plasticity. It is also a central and vital organ in the human body, and in the relationship between the human body and its environment. It follows from this that we have to be very prudent, careful, and stringent in the risk–benefit assessment of any such intervention. When making therapeutic interventions involving the brain, clinical trials are of crucial importance, no matter whether the intervention is pharmacological, surgical, or DBS.

One reason why we must stress the importance of clinical trials is that in mainland China physicians and investigators have, on many occasions, deliberately characterized clinical trials as medical care, thereby avoiding ethical review and a formal informed consent process. In China, and perhaps also in other parts of the world, transplantation of fetal brain tissues to treat Parkinson's disease, psychosurgery for detoxification, or currently fashionable stem cell therapy are provided to patients as routine clinical services by health-care institutions and doctors for various reasons (including financial). These institutions are often reluctant to conduct clinical trials to prove the safety and effectiveness of the therapeutic intervention they recommend, providing various reasons or excuses for avoiding or bypassing clinical trials.

One reason given for avoiding clinical trials is that only patients know what is effective or not. Medical history has taught us, however, that patients' responses as well as physicians' responses are subjective; and whilst they offer important and useful clues, they by no means provide conclusive evidence of the safety and efficacy of the drug or other therapeutic method.

The other reason given for avoiding randomized controlled trials (RCTs) is that they harm patients. However, before embarking on clinical trials any new therapeutic intervention is at clinical equipoise with the existing method. That is, even though some doctors may favor this new intervention, the medical community as a whole has not accepted it, and persuasive data to prove its safety and effectiveness are still lacking. In this situation, the new intervention, if it became a routine clinical service, might harm the patients more than the existing intervention or even placebo. The purpose of clinical trials is to break the equipoise by proving which intervention is safer, or more efficacious: the intervention in the experimental arm or the control arm. Overall, RCTs will bring great benefits to patients and society at large. The possible harms of RCTs can be minimized through conscientious and careful efforts.

In what follows we shall elucidate our points with some examples.

CASE 1: **Treating Parkinson's disease with fetal tissue transplantation**
According to Erika Check (2003a; 2003b), before the results of clinical trials were reported, the effectiveness of treating PD with fetal tissue transplantation had been affirmed in many clinical case reports. However, a number of clinical trials conducted around 2003 refuted the claim that such transplantation is effective. On 29 August 2003, the journal *Nature* reported clinical trials conducted at Mount Sinai School of Medicine in New York that failed to show any benefit for the patients. An earlier n-ical trial at the University of Colorado also found it to be of no benefit for patients. 'This demonstrates that scientists often pretend to proceed with human experiments on the basis of scientific evidence when, in fact, they are deluding themselves, their patients and families, and the public with unsubstantiated "promising" claims' (Check 2003b).

CASE 2: **Detoxification by psychosurgery**
A number of years ago, many hospitals in China developed a treatment in which drug addiction was treated with psychosurgery. The rationale was that there is a reward system for drug use in the brain located in the accumbens septi, and that excision of a specific part of the accumbens septi cured the addiction—and the psychological addiction in particular would be removed too. Altogether 738 drug users underwent the operation in more than 20 hospitals all over China. But the precise part of accumbens septi that was removed was different in different hospitals. At an expert workshop in Xian under the sponsorship of the Ministry of Health (MOH) on 2–3 March 2005, six hospitals reported their findings with different parts of the accumbens septi removed. All hospitals claimed that the effectiveness rate was almost 85 per cent. The bioethicists who attended the meeting commented: If each of you is correct individually, then all of you are wrong in sum, because each of you only removed one part; the other five parts remain intact. The workshop ended with the MOH's announcement that the surgery as a routine practice was prohibited.

CASE 3: **Antiretroviral treatment as HIV prevention**

The importance of clinical trials has been explicitly demonstrated in recent trials in HIV treatment and prevention. For many years, physicians and public health experts believed on the basis of their experience that antiretroviral treatment (ARV) plays a role in HIV prevention. However, these experiences do not constitute conclusive evidence of the effectiveness of ARV in preventing HIV. According to Jon Cohen, such evidence was, however, provided by the HIV Prevention Trials Network study known as HPTN 052. This study showed that 'ARVs reduced the risk of heterosexual transmission by 96 per cent' (Cohen 2011: 1628). James D. Shelton has remarked that '[t]he HPTN 052 randomized study confirmed earlier experiences that, if the HIV-positive partner in a discordant couple took ARVs, transmission to the HIV-negative partner was virtually eliminated' (Shelton 2011: 1646). As a result of this study, ARVs are now seen as providing a breakthrough for HIV prevention. 'Indeed, the Executive Director of UNAIDS Michel Sidebe described it as "game changing"' (Shelton 2011: 1646).

CASE 4: **'Stem cell therapy'**

It is estimated that there may be 400 hospitals which provide unregulated and unproven so-called 'stem cell therapy'. Some of these exploit desperate patients through misleading and exaggerated advertisements, invalid, or even no informed consent procedure, and overcharging of medical costs. Many foreigners went to mainland China as medical tourists to seek such therapy.

Recently the Ethics Committee of MOH developed the 'Ethical Guidelines on Clinical Trials and Applications of Human Adult Stem Cells', which emphasize the distinction between pre-clinical research, clinical trials, and clinical practices.

The Guidelines emphasize that pre-clinical (laboratory and animal) research must precede clinical trials, and that clinical trials are a necessary condition for clinical application. Adult stem cells are permitted to be translated into clinical applications only after sufficient evidence of safety and efficacy have been obtained during the two steps of scientific research (pre-clinical research and clinical trials), the results have been evaluated scientifically and ethically, and the application has been approved by health administration. Those adult stem cells which are not specially processed *in vitro*, such as hemopoietic stem cells and cartilage cells, and which are routinely used to treat diseases of the blood system, corneal injuries, or cartilage injuries, are exempted from the Guidelines.

The Guidelines also stipulate the conditions under which innovative therapy or experimental treatment with adult stem cells can be permitted. The main situation in which such treatment is permitted is for patients with untreatable and fatal diseases who insistently request treatment with adult stem cells. Even in this situation the patients selected for innovative treatment should be those whose cancer is either at a late stage or untreatable, or those with debilitating and fatal diseases. Both clinical trials and experimental treatment require ethical review and informed consent.

In our opinion the distinction and connection between pre-clinical research, clinical trials, and clinical applications are valid and important for therapeutic brain intervention (Qiu and Zhai 2011).

The Chinese perspectives on 'clinical trials' in neural repair

On 15 October 2011 the First National Conference on Neuroethics was held in Wuhan, Central China. The issues reported and discussed include:

Ethical issues in pharmacological brain interventions;
Ethical issues in surgical brain interventions;
Ethical issues in brain–machine interface;
Ethical issues in neuroimaging;
The distinction between treatment and enhancement; and
The neural basis of human morality; etc.

In China, as well as around the world, the nature of the relationship between neural activities and cognitive activities is viewed as a fundamental philosophical issue between matter and consciousness. It is not for neuroethics to deal with this issue. It can be classified as a philosophical (not merely ethical) issue. Neuroethics should focus on normative issues in neurosciences, that is on the question of what ought to be done (the substantial ethical issues), and on how (the procedural ethical issues). Such a neuroethics perspective can then be applied to the innovation, research, development, and application of neurosciences. So we had better distinguish between neurophilosophy and neuroethics.

References

Check, E. (2003a). 'Parkinson's Transplant Therapy Faces Setback', *Nature*, 472: 987. http://www.nature.com/news/1998/030825/full/news030825-4.html (accessed 6 December 2012).

Check, E. (2003b). 'Parkinson's Fetal Tissue Transplant Experiment Fails', *Nature*, published online, 28 August 2003, http://www.ahrp.org/infomail/03/08/29.php (accessed 6 December 2012).

Cohen, J. (2011). 'HIV Treatment as Prevention', *Science*, 334(6063): 1628.

Qiu, R. Z. and Zhai, X. M. (2011). 'Stem Cell Research and Its Clinical Application in China: Interactions between Science, Ethics, and Society,' in *Bioethics and the Global Politics of Stem Cell Science: Medical Applications in a Pluralistic World*, edited by Alastair Campbell and Benjamin Capps, Imperial College Press, UK and World Scientific Publishing Co.

Shelton J. D. (2011). 'ARVs as HIV Prevention: A Tough Road to Wide Impact', *Science*, 334: 1646.

2.3

Commentary

Public Participation as a Potential Counter Strategy against Unethical Optimism

Taichi Isobe, Nozomi Mizushima, and Osamu Sakura[1]

Issues raised in the primary topic article

In the present commentary, we begin by organizing Jones's contentions. We then introduce the perspectives of public participation in specialized areas and upstream engagement, previously emphasized in the field of STS (science, technology, and society study), and propose a counter strategy against unethical 'optimism.'

Jones criticizes clinical studies in Parkinson's disease, arguing that experiments carried out on nerve grafting and nerve regeneration have continued for more than 20 years without proper evaluation and have produced little in the way of significant results. He further states that this can no longer be ethically ignored, as it has brought hardly any benefits to patients with Parkinson's disease or to the development of the neuroscience field. In 1988, in the earliest stages of nerve grafting, studies were being performed in human subjects before results from animal experiments had sufficiently accumulated. Bias was observed in the research procedure. For example, evaluation of nerve graft outcomes was performed immediately after transplantation. These initial evaluations yielded optimistic results; however, nerve graft outcomes were never evaluated at later time points post surgery. According to Jones, such optimism was the cause of the observed bias. Ethical warnings concerning nerve graft experiments had already been voiced by Sladek and Shoulson (1988) (cited in the primary topic article). Unfortunately, few researchers took their suggestions seriously, and the experimental protocols and ethical standards they proposed were not followed in subsequent studies related to nerve grafting and nerve regeneration. Optimism had thus concealed the potential risks associated with these procedures. Recently, ethical issues with experiments focused on nerve grafting and nerve regeneration are being raised once again; however, these issues are a mere repetition of what had been suggested more than 20 years ago.

---

[1] Authors are listed in alphabetical order; all authors contributed equally.

Jones goes on to discuss DBS as a treatment alternative for Parkinson's disease. The therapeutic efficacy of DBS has been confirmed, with only a few safety concerns. Therefore, the therapy will likely be accepted by many patients if side effects are not severe. However, one inherent problem to consider is that the precise mechanisms of how the brain undergoes transformation are not completely understood. The effects of DBS are complicated, and indications highlighting the long-term changes that occur in the brain have begun to emerge (i.e. problems associated with the loss of authenticity and a sense of alienation in patients have been reported). Jones emphasizes that issues associated with DBS treatment must be considered and consent obtained prior to treatment.

We believe that Jones's discussion on nerve grafting and regenerative medicine and his analysis of the ethical problems associated with experimental and clinical studies related to Parkinson's disease are important. Jones points out that clinical studies on nerve grafting and regeneration place an enormous burden on test subjects. In addition, controlling the experimental conditions and increasing the chances of benefiting the patients are important from an ethical perspective. In neuroethics, the risks and benefits related to the emergence of a new treatment method often become points of contention.

Jones debates his contentions from the viewpoint of researchers and physicians to guarantee scientific validity and increase the rigor of research protocols. The issues raised are of course important, and Jones's proposals are effective. However, we believe that the solutions to these issues cannot be achieved by these proposals alone. In fact, Jones suggests that research 'optimism' leads to a variety of ethical problems, which cannot be resolved simply by guaranteeing scientific validity or strengthening research protocols. This is precisely why, as Jones criticizes, various ethical problems similar to those posed 20 years ago continue to surface. We propose the participation of non-experts as a possible solution against 'optimism' among researchers and physicians. Case studies and practical examples of public participation in scientific research and development are accumulating in the field of STS. In the present commentary, we highlight three representative examples of participatory research to complement the topic article.

Public participation: its power and effectiveness

The issue of public participation in science and technology stems back to the 1970s. At the time, there was a growing awareness of trans-scientific problems, that is, problems that could not be solved without science but could not be solved by science alone (Weinberg 1972). Examples of failures in science and technology based on the uncertainty of science (e.g. nuclear power generation and mad cow disease), in addition to those involving the clash of social interests or values (e.g. genetically modified foods and the clash of religion and science), have been frequent. Rather than experts governing science and technology alone, the active participation of citizens with viewpoints and standards of which experts are poorly aware is required in science and technology (Kasemir et al. 2003; Creighton 2005; Einsiedel 2008). What we refer to as 'viewpoints and standards of which experts are poorly aware' may be an event at the scientific level or an event based on a citizen's experiences which differ completely from an expert's viewpoint (i.e. a non-scientific event). Therefore, 'public participation in science and technology' does not necessarily refer to citizens who lack the expert knowledge in a relevant field or who work in a research laboratory or clinical setting together with scientists and/or physicians. There are, however, examples of non-experts who understand and who have acquired expert knowledge, and can thus participate in the development process of science and technology. In general, the expected role of non-experts involves introducing a variety of social contexts and norms to the governance of science and technology, which cannot be handled by experts alone. We present three case studies below which are related to public participation in the field of medicine. In one example, the local knowledge of a non-expert was far more effective than the framework or viewpoint of the expert. Finally, from the case studies presented below, we explore measures to curb the 'optimism' which was criticized by Jones in the topic article.

The first case concerns AIDS research (Epstein 1995; Epstein 1996). The most striking aspect of AIDS research in the United States is that a variety of actors were involved in establishing reliable scientific knowledge. Epstein (1996) emphasized that AIDS research was not a political activity influenced by social movement, but rather an accumulation of reliable scientific knowledge in a variety of forms, which allowed activists and patient groups to participate in establishing scientific knowledge. Such activists and patient groups brought about changes in the conscious implementation of biomedical research and therapeutic techniques. This stands against the general notion that science is an independent activity with high barriers to public participation. Epstein (1996: 338) carried out his analysis by focusing on the fact that 'activists [who were] involved in treatment' intervened in the design, methods, and interpretation of clinical trials aimed at measuring the safety and efficacy of AIDS drugs. In AIDS research, there was cooperative discussion between activists and patient groups while selecting methods to test drug efficacy and for the selection of terms to denote diseases. In the early 1980s, 'gay-related immunodeficiency disease' (GRID) was a commonly used term. However, the term was changed to AIDS given the pressure and demands by the American Homosexual Association. In addition, AIDS patients in the mid 1980s who had been participating in a clinical trial for AZT (a drug that was thought to suppress the disease) acquired a voice and thus contributed to and influenced experimental progress (Bucchi & Neresini 2008). Such patients argued that it was possible to distinguish between the placebo and therapeutic agent. As a result, the Food and Drug Administration (FDA) of the United States accepted these arguments as valid and allocated a larger budget to advance more rigorous clinical trials in a shorter period of time. Another example was the clinical trial of the aerosol pentamidine (aerosol nebulizer), which was used for pneumocystis pneumonia, a disease associated with AIDS (Bucchi & Neresini 2008). This became the first example in which a group of activists carried out a clinical trial (that scientists had refused to conduct) with human subjects. As a result, the use of pentamidine was approved by the FDA in 1989 and commercialization was achieved from data collected through community-based participatory experimentation. This case demonstrates that citizens, who might normally be seen as amateurs and who have understood the content and methods of biomedical research, have played a meaningful role in establishing scientific knowledge in AIDS research.

The second case concerns research on muscular dystrophy (Callon and Rabeharisoa 2003). An organization known as the French Muscular Dystrophy Association (AFM), which was established by patients with muscular dystrophy and their families, has played an important role in muscular dystrophy research. In the 1950s, the medical and scientific fields showed no interest in muscular dystrophy. Moreover, social interest was low. However, the AFM actively carried out activities to improve these conditions. At the time of the AFM's establishment in 1958, muscular dystrophy was regarded as a rare disease. The likelihood of obtaining rewarding results by those who conducted research on the disease was too low for any expert to specialize in muscular dystrophy. By promoting clinical data collection, conducting patient surveys, and establishing a gene bank, the AFM accumulated the scientific and empirical knowledge which had been lacking in this field. As a result, muscular dystrophy gained social interest and became entrenched in the awareness of experts as an appropriate subject matter worthy of scientific pursuit (Bucchi & Neresini 2008). The AFM not only improved social recognition of muscular dystrophy, but also changed the awareness of experts. Furthermore, the AFM advocacy brought about important results in the field and helped redefine the research direction of experts, further promoting the creation of new research directions and research structures (Bucchi & Neresini 2008). For example, Genethon, an organization established by the AFM in 1990, studies gene rearrangements associated with muscular dystrophy and conducts research on issues previously considered impossible to explore by public and private research organizations (Callon and Rabeharisoa 2003). This case demonstrates that for a disease like muscular dystrophy—one not previously recognized as a subject of scientific study and with poor social recognition—an organization established by patients and families determined the direction of scientific research and also changed the social status of the disease.

The third case concerns the 'Cumbrian sheep farmers' (Wynne 1996). They live in the Lake District of northern England where the farmers suffered due to radioactive contamination in their sheep and upland pastures from the 1986 Chernobyl nuclear power plant accident. The purchase and sale of sheep became regulated, prompting farmers to seek advice from experts on radioactive substances. Although the advice was scientifically valid, their advice did not take into account the uniqueness of each situation, difference among soils, and further ignored farmers' knowledge about the characteristics of the behavior and ecology of sheep. The farmers began to implement scientific activities in their farming work (e.g. monitoring, sampling, and field analysis). During this process, farmers came to realize the scientific discrepancies that exist when acquiring scientific knowledge; that is, the farmers came to understand the uncertainty inherent to science. In one example, a sheep farmer performed radioactivity measurements on 500 sheep, showing that 13–14 had measurements which exceeded normal values. However, examination by an inspector revealed that only three sheep had measurements above normal values. The farmer argued that this difference came from the expert's poor understanding of sheep (i.e. sheep jump slightly when they move). While conducting such measurements, accurate values cannot be obtained unless the Geiger counter is fixed to the sheep's backside. From case studies relating to exchanges between scientists and sheep farmers over radioactive substances in the Cumbria region, Wynne (1996) concluded that the scientific viewpoint, just like other viewpoints, is rooted in society, and is conditional and imbued with values. By terminating the practice of restricting discussion groups to a very limited number of scientific experts and by recognizing as proper the critical discussion of scientific knowledge by a new and socially extended discussion group, the social definitions established by such a group can be incorporated when the relevant scientific expertise is utilized. Tateishi (2011) emphasizes that the arguments and assertions made by the sheep farmer, while different from that of the scientist, are equally rational. Therefore, in science, which behaves as if it were value neutral, the institutional forms and values are biased. From the viewpoint of a non-expert group such as the sheep farmers, who had on-the-spot knowledge, a different rationality was formed (Tateishi 2011).

Concluding remarks

In this commentary, we provided an overview of three case studies (i.e., AIDS, muscular dystrophy research, and the shepherds of Cumbria) as examples of public participation in science and technology. The participation of non-experts in an expert field has the potential to break biases and restricted perspectives. With respect to nerve grafting and nerve regeneration, Jones proposes to change the decision-making process by introducing non-expert engagement. We believe that an important factor which gives rise to ethical problems in clinical research is that evaluations and decisions are commonly carried out within a closed expert community. For example, it is not sufficient to listen to the opinions of test subjects and patients regarding 'regeneration.' Jones pointed out that some patients who had received DBS treatment construed changes in 'self' in a negative manner. Accordingly, it is necessary to survey patient opinions, and reflect them in the development of therapies and research objectives. Likewise, it is necessary to fully understand the opinions of patients and their families prior to initiating such studies. For example, the Japan Spinal Cord Foundation (http://www.jscf.org/jscf/), an incorporated non-profit organization, is advancing technical evaluations and guidelines in collaboration with researchers in neuroscience and regenerative medicine. Both researchers and patients will benefit by making use of this sort of network. Be it nerve regeneration or DBS, changing the patient's 'self' as a result of treatment is clearly possible. Therefore, thinking of the test subject or patient as the only agent of consent is an inadequate assumption in neuroscience.

The three case studies highlighted here indicate that the perspectives of the public parties involved may lead to new research directions. We believe that by designing experiments and treatments in a way that actively incorporates the perspectives and awareness of patients—different from those of expert groups in terms of view and understanding—experiments and clinical work based on 'optimism,' so criticized by Jones, will be deterred. Furthermore, this proposal will apply not only to nerve grafting and regeneration, but to other cutting-edge medical fields as well, as treatments and basic experiments are not only for physicians and researchers to monopolize.

References

Bucchi, M. and Neresini, F. (2008). 'Science and public participation,' in E. Hackett et al. (eds), The Handbook of Science and Technology Studies. Cambridge: MIT Press, 449–72.

Callon, M. and Rabeharisoa, V. (2003). 'Research 'in the Wild' and the Shaping of New Social Identities,' Technology in Society, 25: 193–204.

Creighton, L. J. (2005). The Public Participation Handbook: Making Better Decisions through Citizen Involvement. San Francisco, CA: Jossey-Bass.

Einsiedel, F. E. (2008). 'Public Participation and Dialogue,' in M. Bucchi and B. Trench (eds), Handbook of Public Communication of Science and Technology. Abingdon: Routledge, 173–84.

Epstein, S. (1995). 'The Construction of Lay Expertise: AIDS Activism and the Forging of Credibility in the Reform of Clinical Trials,' Science, Technology, and Human Values, 20(4): 408–37.

Epstein, S. (1996). Impure Science: AIDS, Activism, and the Politics of Knowledge. Berkeley, CA: University of California Press.

Kasemir, B. et al. (2003). Public Participation in Sustainability Science: A Handbook. Cambridge: Cambridge University Press.

Sladek, J. R., Jr. and Shoulson, I. (1988). 'Neural Transplantation: A Call for Patience Rather than Patients', Science, 240(4858): 1386–8.

Tateishi, Y. (2011). 'Translator's Comments: Brian Wynne's Sociology of Science,' Shisô (Thought), no. 1046: 64–70.

Weinberg, M. A. (1972). 'Science and Trans-Science,' Minerva, 10(2): 209–22.

Wynne, B. (1996). 'Misunderstood Misunderstandings: Social Identities and Public Uptake of Science,' in A. Irwin and B. Wynne (eds), Misunderstanding Science? The Public Reconstruction of Science and Technology. Cambridge: Cambridge University Press, 19–46.

2.4

Commentary
Three Problems with Treatments for Parkinson's Disease

Yukihiro Nobuhara

Citing the interconnectedness of brain regions, neural plasticity, and neural development as the three central characteristics of the brain, Gareth Jones discusses ethical issues regarding cell grafting and deep brain stimulation, two representative treatments for Parkinson's disease. While he presents many interesting arguments, I would like to comment on three of them in particular.

The problem of optimism without scientific evidence

In general, a treatment performed on a patient suffering from a disease must be shown scientifically to have an effect on curing the disease without any serious side effects. Otherwise, an ethical problem arises. Yet, in grafting treatment for Parkinson's disease, various attempts are made at grafting despite a lack of scientific validation. Jones identifies a major ethical issue here.

According to Jones, grafting treatments for Parkinson's disease are performed despite a lack of scientific evidence for their success because significant room for improvement remains for treatment methods. There is a general consensus that attempting grafting is clinically justified, but Jones points out that performing treatments based on optimism without scientific evidence carries the danger of patients being used as tools of experimentation: an ethically problematic scenario. Furthermore, suppressing such optimistic arguments with realistic evaluations of treatment efficacy is difficult. Jones and other ethicists note that because of this, ethical arguments tend to avoid the pressing problems created by optimism and turn instead to extremely speculative problems (5.1).

Certainly, as Jones argues, optimism without scientific evidence, and experimental treatments based on it, should be avoided. But a fundamental solution to the problems surrounding optimism cannot be reached simply by rejecting optimism on rational or ethical grounds. Jones himself concedes that this sort of optimistic thinking will not disappear, even if exposed to realistic evaluation. Even without scientific evidence, the expectation that a superior treatment option will become available some day represents an important hope for both patients and researchers.

Patients cannot help but seek some kind of treatment for severe illnesses like Parkinson's disease. They hold on to faint hope even in the absence of scientific evidence of the treatment's efficacy, even if the treatment has no hope of being effective when considered rationally. Physicians also want to accommodate patients' hopes, even if it means trying treatments with unclear effects. This kind of psychological state may be irrational, but when facing a severe illness it may be the natural response of human nature.

Of course, even if natural, such situations should be avoided. Physicians in particular should not attempt treatments with uncertain results, even if the patient desires it. However, if physicians do not attempt such therapies, even more serious problems might arise. Patients may think that the physician has given up on them, and turn to pseudoscientific treatments as a last hope. These treatments may not simply fail to have an effect, but could also have serious side effects.

Given such dangers, we should avoid situations in which patients demand treatments based on optimism rather than scientific evidence and in which physicians give in. This does not mean abandoning patients to despair; instead, it should prompt physicians to find other ways to save patients, from a perspective other than treatment. For example, we must help patients rethink the meaning of their lives and fundamentally question what it means to live. This may not be the job of physicians or even of neuroethicists, but it perhaps represents a task for ethics.

The need for a deep understanding of identity

Jones specifically discusses issues of identity as they relate to Parkinson's treatments involving deep brain stimulation (6.2). Identity issues can occur following physical operations such as quadruple amputations and hysterectomies, but severe identity issues arise in therapies that directly involve cognitive ability, like those for Parkinson's disease. Jones makes the interesting observation that the severity of these problems changes depending on how dynamic one perceives narrative identity to be. For those who reject such a dynamic nature, the psychological problems caused by deep brain stimulation may lead to a loss of identity. Those who instead accept a more dynamic view are able to adjust while maintaining their identity. In other words, the change becomes just one of the many that the self experiences on the path of life.

This is indeed an important observation. Personal identity has long been debated among philosophers, and there is no sign of agreement about it; thus it may be impossible to ever reach a fundamental consensus. Conversely, this means that there may be flexibility and arbitrariness in personal identity. It appears that there is quite a lot of flexibility with narrative identity in particular. When an individual experiences a major change in memory or personality, whether they perceive themselves as the same person or not depends on whether they can maintain a consistent narrative of the self through that change. Even where two people experience the same sort of memory or personality change, the capacity of each to maintain a consistent narrative may differ.

If that is the case, then it is important for patients who undergo treatments that may threaten their identity, such as those for Parkinson's disease, to have a deep understanding of their own identities. What is self-identity? What, in particular, is narrative identity? How much leeway does it allow? What constitutes a consistent self-narrative? How can one weave such a narrative? In order to accommodate changes that may arise from treatments, it is important that patients form a deep understanding of these issues before, or even after, treatment.

At first glance, it may appear best to adopt the perspective that one's identity be maintained at all costs, but this is not necessarily the case. This stance may be desirable in many cases because it lessens shock, but in some cases, it may be preferable to make a break with the past self and be reborn as a new person. Decisions regarding which approach to adopt should consider this possibility.

Jones also incorporates Baylis's theory of relations, and argues that identity is not just a psychological characteristic, but also includes interpersonal relations. Based on this argument, even if deep brain stimulation causes major changes in psychological characteristics, it is not necessarily a serious problem as long as it does not result in the patient severing relationships. Therefore, identity maintenance is possible by continuing personal relationships.

This is an adequately persuasive argument. Relationships are constitutively involved in identity, and aspects of these relationships are particularly important for narrative identity. How one relates to, evaluates, and is evaluated by other people constitutes an important, indispensible component—perhaps the most central component—of constructing a consistent narrative of the self. Therefore, when a major change in the patient's psychological characteristics occurs as a result of Parkinson's treatment, it is very difficult for the patient to form a consistent narrative of the self spanning treatment if people around the patient fail to regard them as the same person, and consequently interact with them in different ways, even if the patient perceives themselves as the same person as before.

Narrative self-identity is not just a matter of how the person concerned understands it, but also of how people around the patient view it. Consequently, both the patient and those around them need to deepen their understanding of identity.

Negative effects of the mechanistic brain model

Toward the end of his article, Jones points out that neurological interventions could cause unanticipated deleterious effects based on the mechanistic brain model, which tends to invite misunderstanding. There is close interaction between brain regions, and even the adult brain has plasticity. The brain is constantly changing in a holistic way in response to internal and external changes. As a result, there is a high likelihood that interventions in just a small part of the brain could have an impact throughout the entire brain. It is important not to lose sight of this point, especially if one adopts the atomistic and mechanistic view that the brain is composed of independent modules such that the impact of an intervention in one module will remain in that module, since those who take this view risk failing to account for the global effects caused by interventions in the brain.

This observation is extremely important. Viewing the brain as a machine composed of parts independent from one another might be a major mistake. A holistic view of the brain as composed of parts that interact closely with one another, and together perform numerous functions, may be closer to the truth. If so, function-specific interventions in the brain (those that aim to improve or strengthen a specific cognitive function while not affecting any others) are nearly impossible, regardless of whether the intervention is pharmacological or surgical.

The localization theory of cognitive function remains dominant. According to this theory, each cognitive function exists in a specific region of the brain and manifests as neural activity in that specific region. Attempts to use imaging technology such as fMRI to identify neural correlates of individual cognitive functions are especially attractive to localization theorists. For example, fMRI has been used to measure brain activity at the time a study participant tells a lie in an attempt to identify the brain regions involved in lying. These studies have shown that the brain regions involved in lying are spread throughout the brain rather than limited to a specific region, but this is interpreted to mean that lying is a composite cognitive function with each component function localized to a specific brain region, allowing localization theory to be maintained.

There are several serious problems with the localization theory of function, and I would like to point out two of them here. First, there is an influential idea that what we call 'cognitive function' exists to make our own actions comprehensible within our folk psychology. Comprehension here includes comprehension of causality that does not conform to rationality, such as the interpretation of irrational actions caused by emotion; but it mainly refers to rational understanding. In the localization theory of function, the functions of brain regions are assumed to be mechanistic functions in the machine known as the brain, i.e. causal-nomological functions. If so, the rational cognitive functions in folk psychology cannot be the functions of certain brain regions. They would have to be realized holistically by the total activity of a wide range of brain regions, along with various other cognitive functions.

Yet, even if the rational cognitive functions supposed by folk psychology are not realized by specific brain regions, there is still the possibility that each region of the brain is responsible for a specific function. Such specific functions are not those of folk psychology, but functions identified by the causal role each region of the brain plays. The localization theory of function may be correct in the sense that brain regions each fulfil specific causal functions. However, this does not mean that regions of the brain perform their roles independently. There is close interaction between each region of the brain, and brain regions perform functions through that interaction. That is, the functions of brain regions are interdependent.

The modularity model of the brain, by presenting the image that brain regions perform specific functions on their own, tends to invite misunderstanding. Even when conceptualizing the brain as composed of modules, it is important to note that each module is dependent on others and specific functions are not performed by single modules. Interventions in one module affect not only the functioning of that module, but also the functions of many others. It is impossible, or at least extremely difficult, to freely manipulate the function of a single brain region.

This does not, of course, mean that it is impossible to treat illnesses using interventions such as deep brain stimulation. Such interventions certainly have the potential to bring about therapeutic effects. Yet, when a specific intervention is performed to eliminate a specific symptom, it is always necessary to be aware of the possibility of other effects. The treatment can be considered successful if these effects are not very serious; but if serious, the treatment cannot be deemed successful even if the problematic symptom is eliminated. The brain works in a holistic manner. Consequently, atomistic brain manipulation is impossible. Thus, when conducting neurological interventions, it is important to understand correctly the holistic nature of the brain.

2.5

Response to Commentaries
The Optimism of Misguided Ventures in Repairing the Brain

D. Gareth Jones

Introduction

The aim of my paper 'Neural Repair as a Case Study in Neuroethics' was to draw attention to the immense challenges encountered by scientists and clinicians in overcoming degenerative changes in the brains of adults. However, I also argued that it is not sufficient to dwell exclusively on these challenges, since they in turn introduce a host of equally problematic ethical ones. The point to which I wished to draw attention is that the neural and ethical challenges are intertwined. If it were not for the inherent complexity of brain organization, any ethical challenges would be far less compelling. If there were relatively straightforward ways of overcoming the degeneration and its clinical effects, clinical trials would also be straightforward and accompanying ethical issues would be minimal. But this is not the case, even with such a well-known condition as PD that, in neurological terms, presents as a relatively simple model of neurodegeneration confined as it is to the loss of one population of neurons in one brain region. Nevertheless, the consequences of this loss spread beyond the motor system.

As I demonstrated in the paper, attempts at using grafts to serve as a source of replacement neurons over a period of 20 years have proved depressingly unproductive. While the results have not been universally negative, and while there have been successes, the trials have largely been experimental in nature. They have failed to break through into self-evidently therapeutic territory. Perhaps this should not have been surprising, since there were indications from early on that the experimental demands would prove formidable (Sladek and Shoulson 1988). And yet little was made of these indications, largely, I argued, on account of the inbuilt optimism of both scientists and clinicians. The conceptual environment was that, given further studies and adjusted experimental protocols along with longer-term follow-up, problems could be overcome. All these possibilities were reasonable, and yet the experimentation—because that is what it became—was being conducted on human patients. In my view 'the optimism [was] not tempered by realistic assessment of the state of the clinical science' (Jones in this chapter). There was nothing flagrantly unethical in this, but the inherent optimism of the scientific method had taken over, possibly to the detriment of the welfare of human patients suffering from a debilitating neurological condition. This has ethical consequences that all too readily go unrecognized.

It is striking that in the early days of neural grafting there was vigorous ethical debate about the use of neural tissue from aborted fetuses (Jones 1991), stemming from concerns about abortion and the ends to which aborted fetuses were being put. Legitimate as that debate may have been, it centred on a well-recognized topic of ethical concern. By contrast, debate over the ethical issues arising from ongoing experimental treatment on vulnerable patients has proved elusive, with attention confined to progress being made within the clinical arena.

The nature of optimism

The paradigm of optimism touched on in my paper referred to the scientifically driven optimism of the researchers and their associates. It stemmed as I have argued from the manner in which the science was conducted. Too little attention was paid to experimental issues that could have been foreseen but were only recognized during ongoing studies. Coupled with this was an attitude that even minor advances justified further exploration and hence further studies. The optimism of the clinicians was closely linked to their reading of the state of the science and this undoubtedly played a role in encouraging patients and their families to undergo these procedures. The critical aspect of this form of optimism is that it emanates from the health professionals and therefore is controlled by limits they themselves set.

The same cannot be said of some other procedures, such as so-called stem cell therapy, to which Jing Bai draws our attention, and in which the mythology surrounding 'stem cells' has taken on a life of its own (Bai in this chapter). There are instances galore of claims that transfusions of autologous stem cells are capable of treating a panoply of diseases and injuries, ranging from blindness to cerebral palsy, and brain injury to multiple sclerosis (Barclay 2009; Kiatpongsan and Sipp 2009).[2] The thrust of such claims is that they are available now in countries such as China, and there is no need to wait until the treatments become available in countries like the US and UK. The claims are accompanied by illustrations of people whose ailments have been rectified and who are advocates for the work of the clinic in question. In scientific terms the expectations are unrealistic since the claims are based on adult stem cells, such as mesenchymal stem cells, having the capability of overcoming conditions from arthritis and skeletal injuries to inflammatory diseases like Crohn's disease and asthma, and even including multiple sclerosis. In this instance, the optimism displayed by patients and their families stands in stark contrast to the far more cautious prospects held out by medical researchers.

---

[2] See, for example, http://stemcellschina.com, http://stemcelltreatment.co.nz, and http://www.cells4health.com.

The ethical issues raised in the two domains differ substantially. I have referred to the one as scientifically driven optimism, whereas the other far more commonly encountered variety is scientifically uninformed and indeed may fly in the face of scientific evidence (Barclay 2009). The unrealistic expectations of the latter are of a different variety from those of the former. Medico-scientific research is a gradual process, in which successes and failures contribute to building up a picture of treatment options. The anticipated potential of a particular approach may not be realized, and that approach may have to be discontinued. Hypotheses may be overthrown and cherished ideas overturned. By contrast, what I am describing as scientifically uninformed approaches do not abide by any such constraints. Hence, the claims that benefits are immediately available even when clinical trials from medical researchers suggest the results are no more than preliminary and experimental in nature. By denying the place and necessity of clinical trials, the gap between the experimental and clinical practice has been dangerously obliterated.

From this it follows that medical researchers need to take into account the effects of their scientifically driven optimism when the subjects of their research are human patients. This is the 'hopeful principle' that has been so well critiqued by Holm and Takala (2007). Acknowledgement of the problems inherent in this may restrict some of their scientific ventures but it is necessary if they are to take seriously ethical values such as beneficence and nonmaleficence. It is also important that they do not provide those running unregulated clinics with optimistically framed preliminary data on which to base their dubious claims.

Consequently, it is incumbent upon medical researchers to temper the hype with which they report results and possible breakthroughs. This is an extension of what was discussed in my paper, although it has not characterized the PD work. The realm of stem cells, however, has been different, particularly over claims and counterclaims regarding the relative efficacy of embryonic and adult stem cells (see, for example, Smith, Neaves, and Teitelbaum 2006; Prentice and Tarne 2007). This is well brought out by Jing Bai in her commentary on the profusion of unregulated stem cell clinics in China (Bai in this chapter).

Hype and uncontrolled claims have emerged on too many occasions when scientists have been vigorous advocates of the potential medical benefits of embryonic stem cell research (Witherspoon Council on Ethics and the Integrity of Science 2012). This has generally been a feature of political debate over whether there should be legislative support for, as well as financial support of, various forms of research utilizing human embryos. Public sympathy for such research is greatly accentuated by claims of imminent medical breakthroughs, including prospective benefits in the treatment of neurodegenerative diseases, such as PD. The contrary case has been put by opponents of embryo research and the derivation of embryonic stem cells, with their exaggeration of the therapeutic benefits of adult stem cell research (Prentice 2005). In battles in which one category of hype is pitted against an opposing category, the nuances of scientific niceties tend to disappear even for medical researchers.

The problems encountered with neural grafting do not appear to have informed the debate, even though they are highly relevant in the face of the challenges inherent in establishing new functional synaptic connections in a disorganized cellular environment (Snyder, Daley, and Goodell 2004). It is at this point that the well-publicized optimism of clinicians raises the expectations and hopes of the general public to unrealistic heights. This may well be an illustration of what Hofmann (2009) terms 'the appeal to novelty'—belief in the new, especially belief in the potential of technology.

These comments highlight the dialectic between physician and patient. Yukihiro Nobuhara reminds us that physicians 'want to accommodate patient hopes, even if it means trying treatments with unclear effects' (Nobuhara in this chapter). If this does not happen, the conclusion reached by patients may well be that the physician has given up on them, thereby tempting them to move in the direction of pseudoscientific treatments as a final resort. It is here that ethical reflection becomes so important. What are the options? One route is to abandon patients to despair (nothing more can be done medically). A second way forward is to provide an alternative treatment that promises some (even limited) respite for patients but is in keeping with well-established scientific and clinical principles. A third route is to provide patients with an alternative (non-technological) perspective that helps them cope with the inevitable limitations of their existence, even in the face of increasing debility.

These three routes represent a continuum from a narrowly research-focused and biomedical stance to one in which the limits of biomedical intervention are accepted but can be viewed through a much broader holistic lens. The second and third routes have a perspective of hope, even if not a superficial form of optimism (of a cure around the corner or of substantial immediate improvement), and these two are firmly embedded in realistic assessment of clinical reality. This is of particular importance for neuroethics, where the clinico-scientific challenges are paramount and where the organ diseased or injured has such a major part to play in self-identity and in making us the sort of people we are. By contrast the first route requires careful handling, since if too narrowly focused it could lead to despair on the part of patients. This is not inevitable, but to avoid this pitfall some elements of the other routes are essential. This is an ethical obligation for clinicians if patients are to be treated in a beneficent manner.

Therapeutic misconception

Jing Bai helpfully points out the hazard of confusing clinical trials with medical care, as a means of avoiding ethical review and informed consent (Bai in this chapter). While care is needed before assigning dubious motives to clinicians, this does not apply when clinics function by offering services that have not been peer reviewed and when no attempt has been made to publish results of the outcomes of ongoing treatment (Lau et al. 2008; Kiatpongsan and Sipp 2009). In such cases there is a startling disconnect between the paucity of serious research and the profligacy of treatments offered in the clinic.

A counterargument by clinics mentioned by Jing Bai is that the ultimate test is the effect on patients, in the sense that only they know what is effective for them. While patients' responses constitute an important ingredient in determining what does or does not work, by itself it can be seriously misleading. This is because in the absence of a means of following up patients we lack an objective assessment of their ongoing condition. This, of course, gets us back to clinical trials, and to the other counterargument that randomized controlled trials would harm patients. As Jing Bai reminds us, the purpose of clinical trials is to break the equipoise by showing what is safe and efficacious in both arms—experimental and control.

Taking this further, Jing Bai refers not only to neural grafting in PD, but also detoxification by psychosurgery, antiretrovirus treatment in HIV prevention (where the positive contribution of clinical trials is very usefully brought out), and stem cell therapy. It is in this last area that, as discussed in the previous section on 'The nature of optimism', exaggeration and hype reach new heights, and where the threat of deceiving gullible and emotionally vulnerable patients is immense.

While the clinics covered by the neural grafting experiments described in my paper do not fall into this category, the unethical excesses characteristic of highly dubious clinics feed off responsible experimentation unless enormous care is taken to distinguish adequately between pre-clinical research, clinical trials, and clinical practices (as pointed out by Jing Bai). Using the criteria outlined in Jing Bai's commentary, the initial adrenal medulla grafts would be condemned, although the initial neural grafts would be acceptable. Ethical unacceptability became evident with the continued lack of success in restoring adequate functioning in patients. As stated previously, the scientific method demands openness to discontinuation of experiments and a willingness to forgo what once appeared to be promising avenues of research and therapy.

Public participation

Taichi Isobe and co-workers in their commentary propose that non-experts participate in decision-making, thereby serving as a bulwark against the optimism of researchers and physicians (Isobe, Mizushima, and Sakura in this chapter). They have in mind non-experts who have sufficient understanding and expert knowledge of the area in question. The first case they raise is that of AIDS research involving activists and patient groups. Their second case concerning muscular dystrophy involved patients raising the awareness of researchers by promoting data collection, conducting patient surveys, and establishing a gene bank. The third case of the Cumbrian sheep farmers illustrated how farmers were able to complement the approach of scientists by integrating their knowledge of local conditions into scientific analysis. Against this background Isobe and co-workers argue that in research on conditions such as PD, patient opinion should be surveyed and reflected in the development of therapies. They refer to patients' reactions to changes in self-identity and self-image in DBS.

I have sympathy with their conclusion that the test subject should not simply be regarded as an agent of consent. However, each of the case studies they employ has a distinctive characteristic, namely that the patients concerned have some specific knowledge or perspective to bring to the research, knowledge unavailable to the researchers themselves. This illustrates the mutuality of the enterprise that, they contend (and I agree), should be utilized to the full. However, I remain to be convinced that this approach has as much to contribute in the neural regeneration area, where relevant patient feedback (regarding research imperatives) is far more limited.

I also consider it would be disingenuous to apply this model to the stem cell area where patients are not contributing data or perspective to the treatment carried out in expensive unregulated clinics. There is no research in these instances, only 'assured' treatment. In no sense can the patients be regarded as active participants in ongoing research.

Neural complexity

The problems resulting from uncontrolled hype are found in all areas of biomedicine. However, a thesis in my paper was that it is far more serious in the brain than probably in relation to any other organ system of the body. This stems from the complex organization of the brain, and the nature of the neural interactions within the brain. Nobuhara picks up on the comments I made about these interactions and therefore the limitations of viewing the brain as a series of independent modules (Nobuhara in this chapter). He helpfully reminds us that acceptance of the localization theory of brain function does not lead to the conclusion that brain regions perform their roles independently. General as these comments are, they are highly relevant to our approach to both neural grafting and DBS in attempting to alleviate the worst effects of PD.

This is well brought out by Nobuhara's comments on the flexibility and arbitrariness of human identity. This leads him to stress that patients about to undergo invasive treatments for PD need to form a deep understanding of their own self-identity, since this may be altered by treatment. Identity maintenance may be made possible by the continuation of personal relationships. These considerations immediately take us beyond the narrow focus of medical research, although they in no way invalidate it. But they clearly underscore the necessity of taking account of detailed patient feedback. Even more important, they point to the priority to be accorded long-term follow-up of patients and rigorous peer-reviewed clinical trials. These are of even greater importance in research centred on the brain than in any other area.

What is neuroethics?

Jing Bai has written that 'Neuroethics should focus on normative issues in neurosciences, that is on the question of what ought to be done (the substantial ethical issues), and on how (the procedural ethical issues)' (Bai in this chapter). In this she contrasts neuroethics from neurophilosophy. More specifically she lists the issues discussed at the First National Conference on Neuroethics in China in 2011. These include ethical issues in pharmacological and surgical brain interventions, neuroimaging, and brain–machine interfaces. While I agree with these emphases, the additional point I wish to make is that priority should be given to topics of immediate relevance. While highly speculative scenarios may prove intellectually stimulating (King, Whitaker, and Jones 2011), my paper and these responses have attempted to demonstrate the urgency with which we should approach research-based clinical issues. It is only as these issues are tackled that we begin to appreciate the close interplay of science and ethics. Long-term projects like those of neural grafting, and more recently DBS, in Parkinsonian patients would benefit from active ethical reflection on their character and future directions. The more neuroethics is seen as an integral part of clinical research projects the more valuable it will be.

It has also become evident that the boundary between neuroethics and clinical ethics is far from impregnable. Additionally, while neuroethics is gaining an increasingly well-established place alongside the central core of bioethics, it would be unhelpful to regard it as independent of bioethics. The question of whether neuroethics should be accorded an independent status remains a matter of contention, although, as I believe these responses and my paper have shown, a great deal will be lost if the separation is too great. There is room for fruitful interchange between the two, as there is with the science underlying ethical debate.

References

Bai, J. and Qui, R. (2014). 'Some Issues in Neuroethics', in A. Akabayashi (ed.), *The Future of Bioethics: International Dialogues*. Oxford: Oxford University Press, 65–8.

Barclay, E. (2009). 'Stem-Cell Experts Raise Concerns about Medical Tourism', *Lancet*, 373(9667): 883–4.

Hofmann, B. (2009). 'Fallacies in the Arguments for New Technology: The Case of Proton Therapy', *Journal of Medical Ethics*, 35(11): 684–7.

Holm, S. and Takala, T. (2007). 'High Hopes and Automatic Escalators: A Critique of Some New Arguments in Bioethics', *Journal of Medical Ethics*, 33(1): 1–4.

Isobe, T., Mizushima, N., and Sakura, O. (2014). 'Public Participation as a Potential Counter Strategy against Unethical Opinion', in A. Akabayashi (ed.), *The Future of Bioethics: International Dialogues*. Oxford: Oxford University Press, 65–74.

Jones, D. G. (1991). 'Fetal Neural Transplantation: Placing the Ethical Debate within the Context of Society's Use of Human Material', *Bioethics*, 5(1): 23–43.

Jones, D. G. (2014). 'Neural Repair as a Case Study in Neuroethics', in A. Akabayashi (ed.), *The Future of Bioethics: International Dialogues*. Oxford: Oxford University Press, 46–64.

Kiatpongsan, S., and Sipp, D. (2009). 'Monitoring and Regulating Offshore Stem Cell Clinics', *Science*, 323(5921): 1564–5.

King, M., Whitaker, M., and Jones, D. G. (2011). 'Speculative Ethics: Valid Enterprise or Tragic Cul-De-Sac?' in A. Rudnick (ed.), *Bioethics in the 21st Century*. Rijeka: InTech, 139–58.

Lau, D. et al. (2008). 'Stem Cell Clinics Online: The Direct-to-Consumer Portrayal of Stem Cell Medicine', *Cell Stem Cell*, 3(6): 591–4.

Nobuhara, Y. (2014). 'Three Problems with Treatments for Parkinson's Disease: Comments on Gareth Jones "Neural Repair as a Case Study in Neuroethics"', in A. Akabayashi (ed.), *The Future of Bioethics: International Dialogues*. Oxford: Oxford University Press, 75–9.

Prentice, D. A. (2005). 'Live Patients and Dead Mice', *Christianity Today*, 49(10): 71.

Prentice, D. A. and Tarne, G. (2007). 'Treating Diseases with Adult Stem Cells', *Science*, 315(5810): 328.

Sladek, J. R., Jr. and Shoulson, I. (1988). 'Neural Transplantation: A Call for Patience Rather than Patients', *Science*, 240(4858): 1386–8.

Smith, S., Neaves, W., and Teitelbaum, S. (2006). 'Adult Stem Cell Treatments for Diseases?' *Science*, 313(5786): 439.

Snyder, E. Y., Daley, G. Q., and Goodell, M. (2004). 'Taking Stock and Planning for the Next Decade: Realistic Prospects for Stem Cell Therapies for the Nervous System', *Journal of Neuroscience Research*, 76(2): 157–68.

Witherspoon Council on Ethics and the Integrity of Science. (2012). 'The Stem Cell Debates: Lessons for Science and Politics', *The New Atlantis*, Winter: 9–60.

SECTION B

Enhancement

3.1

Primary Topic Article
Autonomy and the Ethics of Biological Behaviour Modification

Julian Savulescu, Thomas Douglas, and Ingmar Persson

Much disease and disability are the result of lifestyle behaviours. For example, the contribution of imprudence in the form of smoking, poor diet, sedentary lifestyle, and drug and alcohol abuse to ill health is now well established. More importantly, some of the greatest challenges facing humanity as a whole—climate change, terrorism, global poverty, depletion of resources, abuse of children, overpopulation—are the result of human behaviour. In this chapter, we will explore the possibility of using advances in the cognitive sciences to develop strategies to intentionally manipulate human motivation and behaviour. While our arguments apply also to improving prudential motivation and behaviour in relation to health, we will focus on the more controversial instance: the deliberate targeted use of biomedicine to improve moral motivation and behaviour. We do this because the challenge of improving human morality is arguably the most important issue facing humankind (Persson and Savulescu 2012b). We will ask whether using the knowledge from the biological and cognitive sciences to influence motivation and behaviour erodes autonomy and, if so, whether this makes it wrong.[1]

1 Cognitive science and behaviour modification

One of the emerging subdisciplines of the cognitive sciences is the cognitive science of motivation and behaviour. Advanced techniques in neuroscience, such as functional magnetic resonance imaging, together with sophisticated pharmacological, psychological, and economic experiments have begun to shed light on the subtle neural and psychological bases of motivation and behaviour. Perhaps the most controversial area of such research is investigating those features of psychology which are characteristic of our humanity: rationality and morality. Though the main controversies surrounding this research have focused on what it tells us about the nature of rationality and morality,

---

[1] This chapter is based on the article forthcoming in the *Monist*.

there is another, more neglected way in which progress in the cognitive sciences may have even more morally significant implications: it may yield new means of *modifying* morally significant aspects of motivation and behaviour (henceforth, 'moral motivation and behaviour'). In this chapter, we will explore not what neuroscience tells us about the nature of rationality and morality, but rather how ethics could justify the use of radical advances in the neurosciences for the purposes of modifying moral motivation and behaviour.

Behavioural manipulation, or 'mind control' as it is often loosely put, has a bad name. Crude forms of mind control, such as brainwashing or torture, have been around for millennia. Electrical brain implants were in the past used to 'treat' homosexuality, while radical psychosurgery was used to control aggression (Greely 2008). Such forms of mind control were either used in the service of misguided goals or were performed without adequate protections for those subjected to them. However, safe and allegedly ethical means of influencing motivation and behaviour are being employed or advocated. For example, psychological research is affording strategies to influence behaviour by manipulating unconscious stimuli (Kiesel et al. 2006). One prominently discussed technique is the 'nudge' strategy, which harnesses knowledge about cognitive biases that may influence voluntary choice (Thaler and Sunstein 2008). To date, nudges have largely been advocated as means to improve health (see, for example, Charkrabortty 2008), but they can also be used to influence moral behaviour. For example opt-out systems for organ donation take advantage of a form of status quo bias to encourage registration for post-death organ donation.

'Nudging' is an example of a scientifically informed *institutional* strategy that can be used to alter moral motivation and behaviour. Some have raised autonomy-based concerns about nudge techniques (see, for example, Bovens 2008). But in this article we will focus on what many find more concerning: techniques to alter moral motivation and behaviour that operate by directly manipulating our *biology*, not our social environment.

A number of commonly employed antidepressants and antihypertensives (Terbeck et al. under review) affect moral behaviour as a side effect. Indeed, a number of drugs are already prescribed specifically for their behaviour-altering effects, some of which are morally significant: the anti-alcohol-abuse drug disulfuram, the weight-loss drug orlistat, and anti-libidinal agents sometimes used to reduce sexual reoffending. Neuropsychology is beginning to provide more robust evidence for biological correlates of morally relevant traits such as aggression, trust, and empathy. For example, Ramachandran and colleagues have begun to identify neural loci of empathic responses in humans and animals (Ramachandran and Oberman 2006). This research may lead to pharmacological interventions to alter empathy, cooperation, and trust (e.g. De Dreu et al. 2011). Indeed, our own empirical research has already shown that propranolol can reduce implicit racial bias (Terbeck et al. 2012) and produce less utilitarian judgement (Terbeck et al. under review).

Other possible techniques for biologically influencing choices include transcranial magnetic stimulation, deep brain stimulation, transcranial direct current stimulation, and optogenetics, offering the prospect of profound manipulation using genetic manipulation and targeted optic stimulation of precise areas of the brain. These technologies can directly modify behaviours, perhaps including addictive behaviour (Carter, Hall, and Nutt 2009). Indeed, transcranial magnetic stimulation can affect behaviour without subjects' awareness (Brasil-Neto et al. 1992).

1.1 The prospect of moral bioenhancement

Could such cognitive science be used to biologically improve decisions about good and bad, or right and wrong? Could it be used to biologically reduce weakness of will? At present there is no one drug or other biological manipulation that improves moral behaviour in all people in all circumstances. However, there are reasons to believe that manipulation of biology could be used to influence moral behaviour.

As discussed, hormonal manipulation to reduce libido in sexual offenders such as paedophiles is a crude form of moral enhancement. Improving impulse control with Ritalin and Adderall in children with attention deficit disorder reduces imprudent and immoral behaviour, such as violence against others, and may also, in some cases, be an example of crude moral bioenhancement.

The possibility also exists of moral bioenhancement amongst the general population. A number of studies have shown clear effects on moral behaviour through the hormone and neurotransmitter oxytocin. Oxytocin is known to play a key role in birth and breastfeeding. Higher levels of the hormone have been linked to maternal care, pair bonding, and other pro-social attitudes, such as trust, sympathy, and generosity (Insel and Fernald 2004).

Oxytocin levels vary and can be increased through certain external stimuli, such as sex and physical contact. They can also be elevated by a simple nasal spray, which is the delivery method of many of the experiments measuring its effects. In addition, several commonly used drugs are also thought to affect the release or metabolism of oxytocin. Over 100 million women worldwide use the conbined oral contraceptive pill. An estimated 300 million people worldwide suffer from asthma, for which one of the most effective treatments is glucocorticoids.

Both these are associated with an effect on oxytocin levels, with the contraceptive pill associated with elevated baseline oxytocin levels and an increase in oxytocin secretion (Silber et al. 1987; Stock, Karlsson, and von Schoultz 1994), and glucocorticoids are thought to modulate both the release of oxytocin and the expression of oxytocin receptors in some parts of the brain (Link, Dayanithi, and Gratzl 1993; Liberzon and Young 1997).

The effects of increased levels of oxytocin have been shown to be significant. For example, Kosfeld and collaborators investigated the relationship between oxytocin and trust in a simple game of cooperation (Kosfeld et al. 2005). In the experiment, subjects were randomized and given a spray containing either a placebo or oxytocin. They were allocated into pairs consisting of an investor and a trustee. The investor was given a sum of money and allowed to choose how much to pass to the trustee, who would receive three times the investor's amount. The trustee then had to decide how much to return to the investor. The investor's initial decision indicated the level of trust, and the trustee's return was an indication of trustworthiness and gratitude. The greater the initial payment chosen by the investor, the better the potential return for both players—but this could only be realized by the investor if the trustee responded accordingly—if they were trustworthy. The study showed that investors who had received oxytocin instead of the placebo exhibited significantly more trusting behaviour. Oxytocin has also been shown to facilitate increased cooperation in a number of other coordination problems (see, for example, Declerck, Boone, and Kiyonari 2010).

However, oxytocin's effects are complicated. Other research has shown that the pro-cooperation effects of oxytocin may be restricted to others perceived as members of the same group (De Dreu et al. 2010; De Dreu et al. 2011). Indeed, it may even reduce cooperation with out-group members (De Dreu et al. 2010).

Another neurotransmitter implicated in moral behaviour is serotonin. Again, serotonin is naturally occurring, varying according to external stimuli, which is involved in mood regulation. It can also be affected by selective serotonin reuptake inhibitors (SSRIs), which are commonly prescribed for depression, anxiety, and obsessive compulsive disorder. In 2003, in the UK alone, 19 million prescriptions for SSRIs were issued. SSRIs slow the reabsorption of serotonin, thereby making more of it available to stimulate receptors. But SSRIs have a side effect: they seem to make subjects more fair-minded and willing to cooperate. Tse and Bond (2002) measured its effects by observing subjects given the SSRI citalopram as they played the 'Dictator' game. In this game, some subjects are assigned the roles of dictator and are given a sum of money to divide between themselves and another participant. Tse and Bond found that subjects who had ingested citalopram made the division more equally than the control group. Conversely, studies have shown that depletion of a precursor of serotonin (tryptophan), which would in turn lead to reduced levels of serotonin, leads to lower rates of cooperation in the 'Prisoner's dilemma' game (Wood et al. 2006). Crockett and colleagues (2008) found that lowered levels of tryptophan led to a greater propensity in subjects to reject offers perceived as unfair, relative to controls. This suggests that SSRIs, by increasing serotonin levels, affect subjects' assessment of what counts as (unacceptably) unfair, possibly leaving them more vulnerable to exploitation.

2 The ethics of moral bioenhancement

While the technology to biologically influence moral motivation and behaviour is still in its infancy, or even pre-embryonic stages, it seems likely that science will afford ever more powerful interventions. Douglas (2008) has argued that it might be permissible for individuals to use these interventions to bring about more moral motivation and behaviour in themselves, though he also raises concerns about the possible misuse of technology: concerns which may militate against seeking to develop them. By contrast, Persson and Savulescu have argued that the development of these technologies should be prioritized and aggressively pursued, such is the need for moral enhancement (Savulescu and Persson 2008; Persson and Savulescu 2011; Savulescu and Persson 2011; Persson and Savulescu 2012a; Persson and Savulescu 2012b; Persson and Savulescu 2013).

One objection that is frequently raised against mind control and behavioural manipulation, even for a person's own benefit but especially when it is for the purposes of promoting more moral behaviour, is that it would compromise our freedom and autonomy.

It is this objection that we wish to spell out and address in this paper. First, however, we should offer some thoughts on the likely nature of moral bioenhancement.

3 The nature of moral bioenhancement

A moral enhancement is, we will assume, an intervention that makes it more likely that you will act morally, in some future period, than would have been the case if it were not used. One acts morally when one does the right thing, and for the right reason(s). In many circumstances there would be disagreement about what actions, and reasons for acting, are right. What constitutes moral enhancement will depend on what accounts of right action and right motivation are correct.

What constitutes right action is contested. Kantians, utilitarians, virtue theorists, deontologists, and religious ethicists may all disagree on what the right action is. There is also significant disagreement about what sorts of motivations are the right ones to have and act on. Kant famously claimed that to act in a way that has true moral worth—rather than merely conforming to morality—one must act from the motive of duty (Kant 1964). This view has sometimes been taken to imply that the right motive for action is *moral reasoning*. One must reason about what duty requires and then act accordingly. But others would allow that emotions such as sympathy can produce genuinely moral action (Mill 1979; Arpaly 2003), and some would question whether moral reasoning is even capable of producing action with the support of emotions or desires that are external to reasoning itself (Hume 1978).

But despite this significant disagreement, there are areas of agreement. For example, almost every ethical theory says it is wrong to kill an innocent person in non-extra-ordinary circumstances. And on any plausible ethical theory, certain capacities will be necessary to act for the right reasons. For example, right motivation surely requires the capacity to act for the sake of others, or for morality itself, rather than in self-interest. This requires that one can conceptualize and be motivated by morality or the interests of others.

3.1 Self-sacrifice and altruism

It is characteristic of morality, as opposed to prudence or self-interest, that it requires the sacrifice of one's own interests for the sake of others, or at least for the sake of some moral code. It is a prerequisite of moral action that one should sacrifice/constrain one's own self-interest for the sake of others or of morality.

For example, proponents of most moral theories could accept a principle of easy rescue stating that, when (i) the harm to A of F'ing is small, (ii) the benefit to another/others, B, is great, and (iii) there is no harm to third parties, then A should F. Even this undemanding and relatively uncontroversial principle requires some minor sacrifices of self-interest.

Perhaps, some might argue, there is no duty of easy rescue. But any morality requires that we do not kill innocent persons, or at very least, innocent in-group members for no good reason. In some cases, it will be against our interests to refrain from killing someone. Perhaps it is frequently so. A controlling spouse, a demanding boss, a person who blocks your chances of advancement. In all these cases, morality requires that you set aside your interests and not kill.

Thus, a willingness to sacrifice one's own interests is required by even undemanding moralities. Yet it is something which, like all human characteristics, varies from person to person. Some will be less inclined to make sacrifices, or less often or of very small magnitude.

Various factors predictably increase self-sacrifice. For example, if one derives pleasure from self-sacrifice, this will increase willingness to sacrifice one's interests. The praise or esteem of others increases self-sacrifice. Rituals, dances, induction ceremonies, etc. have all been used to increase self-sacrifice of members of groups. In the future, it will become possible to not only manipulate the situational and social determinants of self-sacrifice, but also the biological determinants.

This can be seen by comparing the sexes. It is plausible to think that in general women have a greater capacity for self-sacrifice than men. Baron-Cohen (2003) argues that women have a greater capacity for empathy than men. If men could be made more like typical women with respect to empathy, this might increase their willingness to sacrifice their own interests for the sake of others, at least in some circumstances. This could qualify as a moral enhancement on almost any widely accepted account of morality.

Of course, the acquisition of any single trait which contributes to more moral behaviour can be used for immoral purposes. For example, greater willingness to self-sacrifice will not always qualify as a moral enhancement. Some Nazis described having to overcome their revulsion at killing Jews for the sake of others (future generations of Aryan Germans). Heinrich Himmler reportedly told his masseur that 'It is the curse of greatness that it must step over dead bodies to create new life. Yet we must…cleanse the soil or it will never bear fruit. It will be a great burden for me to bear' (Kersten 1956: 120). Himmler would not have been morally enhanced by an intervention that made him even more willing to kill Jews for the sake of future Germans, for he accepted a mistaken view according to which Jews were not persons, and their interests should be attached no weight. But for those whose descriptive and moral views are less mistaken, increasing the willingness to sacrifice one's own interests may result in a stronger disposition to act morally.

3.2 Violence and aggression

The opposite of promoting another's interests is damaging another's interests. Since harming others is often immoral, traits which increase harmful behaviour tend thereby to increase immoral behaviour. The reduction in these tendencies would thus often qualify as a moral enhancement. An obvious example is the treatment of psychopathy. But more common are personality disorders.[2] Especially dangerous amongst these is antisocial personality disorder (75 per cent of prison inmates have this) and borderline personality disorder.

Personality disorder affects 5–10 per cent of the population, placing heavy demands on psychiatric, social, and forensic services (NIMHE 2003): 64 per cent of male and

---

[2] Thanks to Hannah Pickard for contributing details on personality disorder.

50 per cent of female offenders have personality disorder (NOMS 2011). Traits associated with many personality disorders include criminal behaviour, addiction, self-harm, violence, selfishness, recklessness, impulsivity, lack of empathy and remorse, poor anger management, and willingness to exploit others. Personality disorder has an inherently moral component: traits are moral failings that harm self and others (Charland 2004; Pickard 2009; Pickard 2011).

Alongside genetic predisposition (Lang and Vernon 2001), the strongest predictor of personality disorder is early-environment psychosocial adversity. Personality disorder is associated with parental psychopathology, institutional care, sexual, emotional, and physical abuse (Paris 2001). The chaotic/violent behaviour and emotional instability diagnostic of personality disorder mirrors early environment. Patients with personality disorder did not have the opportunity to learn moral skills.

There is increasing evidence that personality disorder can be treated pharmacologically and psychologically. Antidepressants are recommended for depressive symptoms and impulsivity (NIMHE 2003); sedatives for short-term crises (NICE 2009). There are specific psychological therapies: cognitive-behavioural therapy (Davison 2008), dialectical behavioural therapy (Linehan and Dimeff 2001), and STEPPS (Blum et al. 2008); mentalization-based therapy (Fonagy et al. 2004); and therapeutic communities (Lees, Manning, and Rawlings 1999). These develop theory of mind skills and self-control as well as promoting personal and social responsibility (Pickard 2011). Psychiatric interventions are acting as moral enhancers (Pearce and Pickard 2009).

In addition to treating personality disorder, it may be possible to reduce aggression by modifying more subtle psychological factors. Baron-Cohen notes that empathy can act as a 'brake on aggression' (2003: 35). Thus, we should expect that a lesser male capacity for empathy could go with the greater display of male aggression, which is borne out by the statistics of crimes such as murder (see, e.g., Baron-Cohen 2003: 36). If women do have a lower tendency to harm others overall, it seems that in principle we could make men more moral by biomedical methods by making them more like women, or rather, more like the men who are more like women in respect of empathy and aggression.

3.3 Racial and sexual bias

It would be fairly uncontroversial that freedom from certain biases—such as racial and sexual bias—is conducive to acting morally in many contexts. Such biases are frequently impediments both to right motivation and to right action. Though there is disagreement about precisely what motives are the right motives for action, it would be widely accepted that these motives should be free from racial and sexual bias. Biased reasoning and conative states driven by biases are *not* the right motives for action. Similarly, while there is considerable disagreement about right action, it would be widely accepted that sexually and racially discriminatory conduct is often wrong.

It is tempting to think that racism and sexism are, at least in Western societies, largely a thing of the past. But the evidence suggests not. Though racial bias is notoriously difficult to measure, most research suggests that, though it has declined since 1960, it remains present. Regression analyses typically find that black US men earn less than their white counterparts even after correction for alternative explanatory factors such as educational attainment and age (Darity, Guilkey, and Winfrey 1996; Rodgers and Spriggs 1996;

Gottschalk 1997). Darity and Mason (1998: 71) estimate that in 1980 and 1990 black men in the United States were paid 12–15 per cent less than white men as a result of racial discrimination. Additionally, black males with darker skin appear to fare worse in the labour market than black males with lighter skin, again, after correction for other explanatory variables (Ransford 1970; Keith and Herring 1991; Johnson, Bienenstock, and Stoloff 1995). Further direct evidence of bias comes from court proceedings (successful suits for racial discrimination remain frequent) and audits, in which pairs of actors who differ in race but are trained to perform equally well at interview apply for the same position with matched curricula vitae. A series of such audits in the United States found that black male actors were three times more likely to be turned down for a job than white male actors (Fix, Galster, and Struyk 1993: 79–81). Similar evidence is available for sexual bias (Neumark, Bank, and Van Nort 1996). In one interesting study, Goldin and Rouse (2000) found that where symphony orchestras move from auditioning candidates in the view of auditioners to 'blind' auditions, the average likelihood of women being selected increases by 50 per cent.

Tendencies to favour the members of a particular sex or racial group may not always qualify as biases, since in some cases the preference may be morally permissible. For example, most of us would find it permissible for a person to favour members of a particular sex or race when considering who to invite on a date, or who to accept for the roles of Othello or Desdemona in a play. But in many cases, racial and sexual preferences do amount to biases.

There is an emerging understanding of the biological bases of racial bias. Several neuroimaging studies have suggested that activation of the amygdala—part of the brain that has been implicated in emotion—may underpin this bias. Lieberman and collaborators found that both black and white subjects exhibited greater amygdala activation on functional magnetic resonance imaging when presented with photos of black Americans as compared to photos of white Americans (Lieberman et al. 2005). Other studies have identified a correlation between these amygdala responses and implicit racial attitudes revealed by psychological tests (Phelps et al. 2000; Amodio 2008). These findings are consistent with the view that negative implicit evaluative reactions to certain racial groups are mediated by differences in amygdala activity, plausibly due to the amygdala's role in emotion. There is some further support for this hypothesis. For example, the only persons known to lack a consistent tendency to discriminate on the basis of race are the victims of Williams syndrome, a rare chromosomal abnormality associated with reduced fear in social situations (Santos, Meyer-Lindenberg, and Deruelle 2010). This suggests a possible role for the emotion of fear in mediating racial bias.

Though this research is very far from yielding biological interventions capable of selectively and reliably attenuating racial bias, one might expect that further scientific progress will ultimately lead to the development of such techniques. At least, it would be bold to rule this out. These techniques might well constitute moral enhancements, at least in some individuals and circumstances.

3.4 Other morally relevant traits

There are other traits which are conducive to acting morally in many circumstances. Willingness to cooperate with other people is one. As we have seen, SSRIs increase willingness to cooperate (though they may have other undesirable moral effects). Another trait is impulse control. If one cannot withstand temptation and delay gratification, one will be less likely to sacrifice one's own interests for the interests of others or a moral code. Drugs which increase impulse control thus contribute to more moral behaviour. Ritalin, Adderall, and other drugs improve impulse control in children with attention deficit disorder, indeed reducing violence and antisocial behaviour.

Of course, modification of these traits could be done for nefarious purposes, making someone, for example, a more effective criminal. Moreover, even when done with good intentions, attempts at moral bioenhancement might misfire. It is easy to imagine circumstances in which an isolated enhancement of any single one of the traits we have suggested would produce moral disenhancement rather than enhancement—recall the case of Himmler above—though this risk might be mitigated by enhancing a combination of traits. Similarly, in some people, enhancing one or more of the traits we have discussed might fail to produce moral enhancement because that individual already possesses the trait(s) in question to an optimal (or supra-optimal) degree: it is possible to be too self-sacrificing from the point of morality, so enhancing those the willingness to self-sacrifice of those who already possess this trait to a high degree might lead to moral deterioration. Our point is merely that, in many people, enhancing one or more of the traits we have discussed would, in many circumstances, result in that individual being more likely to act morally than would otherwise have been the case.

4 Moral bioenhancement and freedom

We now turn to consider an objection to moral bioenhancement raised recently by John Harris. Harris traces the objection to Milton (Harris 2011: 103):

Famously, in Book III of *Paradise Lost* Milton reports God saying to his 'Only begotten Son' that if man is perverted by the 'false guile' of Satan he has only himself to blame:
> whose fault?
> Whose but his own? Ingrate, he had of me
> All he could have; I made him just and right,
> Sufficient to have stood, though free to fall. (requoted from Milton ([1667] 2000): lines 96ff.)

It is not immediately clear that there is anything in this passage that should concern a proponent of moral bioenhancement. If we read the claim that humans are 'sufficient to have stood' as implying that there is no *need* for moral enhancement—that humans already have sufficiently moral motives and behaviour—then it will look clearly false. It will also look inconsistent with Harris's own admission that we often succumb to temptation (Harris 2011: 103–4), and often have purposes other than, and in conflict with, moral goals (Harris 2011: 104). If, on the other hand, it is understood as holding merely that humans have the *capacity* for sufficiently moral motives and behaviour (henceforth, the capacity to be moral), then it seems quite consistent with the thought that moral bioenhancement would be morally permissible and indeed desirable. We could undergo moral bioenhancements that further enhanced this capacity, or that disposed us to exercise it more effectively.

Why, then, does Harris appeal to Milton? Harris explains:

God was, of course, speaking of the fall from Grace when congratulating herself on making man 'sufficient to have stood though free to fall'; she was underlining the sort of existential freedom…which allows us the exhilaration and joy of choosing (and changing at will) our own path through life. And while we are free to allow others to do this for us and to be tempted and to fall, or be bullied, persuaded, or cajoled into falling, we have the wherewithal to stand if we choose. So that when Milton has God say mankind 'had of me all he could have', he is pointing out that while his God could have made falling impossible for us, even God could not have done so and left us free. Autonomy surely requires not only the possibility of falling but the freedom to choose to fall, and that same autonomy gives us self-sufficiency; 'sufficient to have stood though free to fall'. (Harris 2011: 103)

And then,

part of Milton's insight is the crucial role of personal liberty and autonomy: that sufficiency to stand is worthless, literally morally bankrupt, without freedom to fall.…[M]y own view is that I, like so many others, would not wish to sacrifice freedom for survival. I might of course lack the courage to make that choice when and if the time comes. I hope however that I would, and I believe, on grounds that have more eloquently been so often stated by lovers of freedom throughout history, that freedom is certainly as precious, perhaps more precious than life. (Harris 2011: 110–11)

Moral enhancement thus, according to Harris, is wrong because it restricts the freedom to do wrong and thereby reduces personal autonomy.

Harris's argument has a theological parallel in the free will defence of theism. The argument from evil holds that there can be no omnipotent, omniscient, and benevolent God, since that God would not allow evildoing to occur. The free will defence maintains, in reply, that evildoing is a consequence of our possessing the freedom to do evil, which is, all things considered, good. Though the freedom to do evil possesses the great instrumental disvalue of allowing evildoing, it also possesses some other, greater value. Thus, God rightly bestowed on us the freedom to do evil despite the risk of wrongdoing that this created.

Similarly, Harris would say, we would be right to retain our freedom to act immorally by declining moral bioenhancement, despite the risk of wrongdoing that this entails. His argument implies both that moral enhancement would deprive us of our freedom to act immorally, and that the disvalue of this loss of freedom would exceed any value associated with a reduction in the rate of wrongdoing. In what follows we respond to these claims.

4.1 Must moral bioenhancement restrict the freedom to act immorally?

Moral bioenhancement, and biological behaviour manipulation more generally, need not restrict freedom. It could simply make us more like the most morally virtuous individuals already among us. To see this, suppose that women are, in at least some circumstances, more disposed to act morally than men because their greater empathy leads them to make greater personal sacrifices in certain circumstances where self-sacrifice is what is required. Then men might be morally enhanced by being made more like women in their capacity for empathy. Plainly, this would not make the men less free to do wrong. For women are not less free to act immorally than men. And certainly they are not barred from acting wrongly by their greater empathy.

This result holds regardless of whether human action is determined. Suppose, first, that our behaviour is fully determined but that our freedom is compatible with it being fully determined whether or not we shall do what we take to be good. In this case, effective moral bioenhancement will not reduce our freedom; it will simply bring about circumstances where we are more often, or always, determined to do what we take to be good. The actions would be those of someone today who is morally perfect.

However, if we are free only because, by nature, we are not fully determined to do what we take to be good, then moral bioenhancement can never be fully effective because its effectiveness is limited by our indeterministic freedom. So, irrespective of whether determinism or indeterminism reigns in the realm of human action, moral bioenhancement will not curtail our freedom.

Some critics of moral bioenhancement seem to think that we risk becoming automatons who do not act for reasons. Harris writes that moral bioenhancement will 'make the freedom to do immoral things impossible, rather than simply making the doing of them wrong and giving us moral, legal, and prudential reasons to refrain' (2011: 105). However, the morally bioenhanced could still act for the same reasons as un-enhanced humans who act morally. The sense in which it is 'impossible' for morally bioenhanced people to do what they regard as immoral will be the same as it is already for the virtuous person: it is psychologically or motivationally out of the question. People who are morally good and always try to do what they regard as right are not necessarily less free than those who sometimes fail to do so.

To take a final parallel, consider someone who reads a good novel. Such a person might be brought to vividly imagine what it is like to be another person to a much finer and deeper degree. As a result, he empathizes with that character and develops sympathy for him. Such a moral enhancement does not rob freedom. If anything, it facilitates richer imagination of what life is like and its alternatives. If a pill were to do the same thing, it would be no different, regarding its effects on freedom, to a novel. If a pill were to make people more open to the experiences and lives of others, this would no less erode freedom than reading Tolstoy. Consider the following example.

4.2 Beggar in the street

Sarah is a lawyer at a London firm. She is asked to take on an extra hour per week on pro bono work, but prefers to spend the time relaxing with friends in a bar. Sarah takes a drug which makes her more interested in the suffering of others, more empathetic, more capable of vividly imagining what it would be like to be in another person's shoes. The drug is like a pair of moral spectacles, clarifying her vision of other people's experiences. She sees pro bono clients not as an extra hour of her time spent working, but as people caught in a complex legal system, confused, stigmatized, and lacking the funds to pay for justice. She sees how their lives will go with her expert help and how they will go without it. She decides to give up her time for the clients.

In this case, Sarah retains the same deliberation and judgement. Sarah acts for reasons, in the same way that anyone does. She has simply viewed the original circumstances in a different way. Sarah's giving of her time was not unfree; it was virtuous. Imagine that

Sarah, when she took the drug, always behaved in the morally correct way. She would not be unfree. She would be the most virtuous person.

Consider now James. James is a district court judge in a multi-ethnic area. He was brought up in a racist environment and is aware that emotional responses introduced during his childhood still have a biasing influence on his moral and legal thinking. For example, they make him more inclined to counsel jurors in a way that suggests a guilty verdict, or to recommend harsher sentencing, when the defendant is African-American. James recognizes this and dislikes it. A drug is available that would help to reduce his aversion to African-Americans, thus mitigating his bias. It would help him to do the right thing. And, since it would remove one inappropriate motive—racial aversion—it would help him to do it for the right reasons.

Taking this drug might plausibly be said to increase rather than decrease James's freedom. For the aversive reaction that it attenuates might itself be thought to be a constraint on his freedom. Suppose we draw a distinction between the true or authentic self, and the brute self. An agent acts freely, let us say, when her true self determines what she does. If James's racial aversion is part of his brute self—which seems plausible—then the drug helps to free his true self from brute constraints. It helps to enhance his freedom.

It may be that as our understanding develops, moral bioenhancement will be most effective in children during their early development. Perhaps by giving them drugs or other biological manipulation we will be able to increase their ability to more easily learn to behave morally, just as cognitive enhancement may enable them one day to learn to study more easily and effectively. Moral bioenhancement will of course rest on a conventional moral education: children would still need to be taught correct values, and the importance of acting on values, etc., just as cognitive enhancers do not work without education and study. But the moral bioenhancement may allow the education we routinely give our children to be more effective.

For example, most parents would aim to encourage children to recognize suffering in other people, and to respond by trying to ameliorate it. Some would argue that engineering this biologically would restrict the child's open future. But we do this all the time through education, stories, literature, and punishment and we do not believe it to restrict the freedom to act immorally. Why should it make a difference if we should we do this biologically?

It might be objected that we have painted an unwarrantedly rosy picture of the likely nature of moral bioenhancement. Such enhancements might be unlikely to take the form of drugs that enhance empathy or imagination, reduce unwanted racial aversion, or aid childhood moral development. More likely, it might be thought, they would simply remove the option of acting immorally. For example, neurofeedback might be used to condition irresistible disgust reactions at the thought of harming others. Such interventions surely would restrict the freedom to act immorally. But would they thereby diminish our *autonomy*? And if so, would this render them morally unjustified, all things considered?

4.3 *Perfect mind control: phone hacking*

It is 2100. The mobile phone evolved into a brain–computer interface allowing a wide range of communications under direct mind control. One could communicate just by thinking and directing one's thoughts to a target person or artificial intelligence. The iPhone 10EEE was so useful and successful that every parent implanted one into the earlobe of their children, like an earring. People without the iPhone 10EEE came to be seen as disabled because they could not communicate sufficiently. They were the deaf and blind of their generation. Governments soon implanted these cheap devices into all newborns as a way of enabling their lives and securing their human rights.

Technology progresses relentlessly and exponentially in other directions. It becomes possible to evaluate and intervene in human intention by hacking into the iPhone 10EEE communications network. A small government spin-off perfects MT, or moral technology. It can pick up intentions to perform grossly immoral actions and intervene to change these. Traditional government realizes the potential and implements MT.

MT is only designed to prevent gross immorality. It only intervenes in human action to prevent great harm, injustice, or other deeply immoral behaviour from occurring. For example, murder of innocent people no longer occurs. As soon as a person forms the intention to murder, and it becomes inevitable that this person would, without intervention, act to kill, MT would intervene. The would-be murderer would 'change his mind'. MT does not intervene in trivial immoral acts, like minor instances of lying or cheating. Only when a threshold insult to some sentient being's interests is crossed is MT deployed.

Humans are still free to act morally, since if they choose to do so, MT does not intervene. They are only unfree to do grossly immoral acts, such as killing or raping. This is seen as preferable to physical incarceration, which physically restricts the freedom to be immoral. It is seen as preferable that would-be murderers change their minds, rather than that an innocent person is killed and then the murderer incarcerated for life. A would-be murderer never knows that her intentions have been changed by an authority outside herself. It seems to her that she has 'changed her mind'—she experiences a life of complete freedom, though she has not been free. And no one is ever wrongfully killed.

There had been quite a bit of controversy over what should be classified as 'grossly immoral action' which should be within the purview of MT. Should cheating in exams be extinguished? Marital infidelity? The cognitively and morally enhanced government decides that only those acts which would have resulted in imprisonment of a person should be modified. Thus prisons are abolished.

It is this kind of world which objectors to moral enhancement such as Harris fear. Human beings are no longer 'free to fall' or at least not free to fall a long way. It might be wondered what is so bad with such a world after all. It is true that people are in one way less free in the world with MT. But plausibly everyone is much better off for the absence of evil. There is no physical incarceration or great harm wrought by one human being on another.

We return to the question of whether restricting the freedom to do wrong might be morally justified, all things considered, in section 4.6 below. However, for the moment, we focus on the more limited question of whether it would reduce *autonomy*. Plausibly, the reason for caring about the freedom to do wrong is that we have reason to protect our autonomy—roughly speaking, our control over our lives. If a restriction on our freedom to do wrong would thereby restrict our autonomy, it might be of moral concern. But if it would not, it is not clear that it should trouble us.

Though MT does compromise the freedom to do wrong, there are at least two circumstances in which it might be thought not to compromise autonomy or self-government. One of these circumstances is where the immoral action prevented by MT would have been the result of an inauthentic or irrational desire. The other is where a person had voluntarily chosen to be connected to MT as a form of precommitment contract. The case in which autonomy could most plausibly be said to have been preserved is where both of these circumstances obtain: where an individual forms a precommitment contract to prevent himself from acting on an irrational (or inauthentic) desire. The paradigm example of such a case is Ulysses and the Sirens.

4.4 Ulysses and the Sirens

The story of Ulysses and the Sirens provides an example of what can be called an obstructive desire. Ulysses was to pass 'the Island of the Sirens, whose beautiful voices enchanted all who sailed near. [They] ... had girls' faces but birds' feet and feathers ... [and] sat and sang in a meadow among the heaped bones of sailors they had drawn to their death,' so irresistible was their song. Ulysses desired to hear this unusual song,' but at the same time wanted to avoid the usual fate of sailors who succumbed to this desire. So he plugged his men's ears with beeswax and instructed them to bind him to the mast of his ship. He told them: '[I]f I beg you to release me, you must tighten and add to my bonds.' As he passed the island, 'the Sirens sang so sweetly, promising him foreknowledge of all future happenings on earth'. Ulysses shouted to his men to release him. However, his men obeyed his previous orders and only lashed him tighter. They passed safely (Graves 1960: Vol. 2, 361).[3]

Before sailing to the Island of the Sirens, Ulysses made a considered evaluation of what was best for him. Thinking clearly, with all the facts before him, he formed a plan which would enable him to both hear the song of the Sirens and live. His order that he should remain shackled was an expression of his autonomy.

Moreover, his order prevented him from acting on an irrational desire. In the grip of the Sirens' song, Ulysses's strongest desire was that his men release him. At the time, this may have been his only desire. But it was an irrational desire. The song of the Sirens was irresistible. It is plausible to assume that this song so preoccupied those who heard it that they could think of nothing else. It consumed the listener's attention and so prevented vivid imagination of other alternatives. The desire to move closer to the Sirens was irrational because it was not the result of vivid imagination of all alternatives and because it prevented the satisfaction of a rational desire (to hear the Sirens' song and stay alive). There are thus two reasons why Ulysses's precommitment did not restrict his autonomy: because it was itself the result of an autonomous choice, and because the desires it frustrates were irrational and thus, plausibly, impediments to autonomy.[4]

---

[3] All quotations in this paragraph are from this work.

[4] The notion that some desires can frustrate the expression of our autonomy is also described by Young (1986, especially pp. 9, 14, 50, 56), Frankfurt (1989, especially pp. 68–71), and Watson (1989, especially pp. 109–10, 117). The last two writers use the term freedom rather than autonomy. Feinberg (1973) gives a detailed list of the kinds of states which can interfere with autonomy.

Where an individual voluntarily connects to MT to prevent acting on an irrational desire, MT achieves the same thing as wax and lashings in Ulysses's case.

4.5 *Rationalist autonomy*

We have suggested that MT may not compromise autonomy where it is a precommitment contract or where the desire to do wrong is, or is based on, an irrational or inauthentic desire. But thus far we have defended this suggestion only by offering a case designed to pump intuitions. In this section, we seek to give some theoretical backing to our suggestion. To do this, it is necessary to say something more about the nature of autonomy.

Autonomy is not mere choice by a competent agent. The word 'autonomy' comes from the Greek: *autos* (self) and *nomos* (rule or law) (Dworkin 1988: 12). Autonomy is self-government or self-determination. Being autonomous involves freely and actively making one's own evaluative choices about how one's life should go. But autonomous choice is not merely intentional. What distinguishes autonomous choice from mere choice is that it is evaluative, employing a person's normative capacities. It is based on full (or at least as full as possible) appreciation of the nature of the options on offer, and so requires both information and rational deliberation to form rational beliefs. One of us has elsewhere called this a rational choice and defended a rationalist account of autonomy. It could be called a Kantian account.

P rationally desires some state of affairs, that q, if and only if P desires that q while in possession of all relevant, available information, without making relevant errors of logic and while vividly imagining what each alternative course of action and resulting state of affairs would be like.

Arguably, one necessary condition for a choice to be autonomous is that it be based on or satisfy a rational desire. If choosing to do immoral things would be based on an irrational desire, then preventing a person from so acting would not constrain the person's autonomy (Savulescu 1994).

The paradigm of a person P autonomously choosing between A and B is that, having appreciated the nature of A and B, this P judges that one is better than the other. Why is appreciation of the nature of A and B important? It will not do, when imagining what A is like, to imagine some state of affairs which is more like B, or some other state of affairs. If this person were to choose A under these circumstances, what P would really want is B, or something else entirely.

To appreciate A and B as they are, this person must know what each is like. She needs relevant, available information. For example, in considering whether to go on some diet, a person needs to know what all its effects will be, on weight, health, her financial and temporal assets.

In processing information, it is important not to make any errors of logic. Logic enables us to transfer information and belief into the widest web of rational belief. Steve Jobs, the Apple pioneer who died recently of pancreatic cancer, was initially diagnosed with a neuroendocrine cancer and it is rumoured that this was possibly treatable. However, Jobs allegedly elected complementary/alternative medicine and delayed definitive surgical treatment for nine months, by which time the cancer had metastasized (Smith 2011). Assuming these rumours to be true for the purposes of argument, if Jobs had had access to accurate information, his choice may have been explained by a failure of logic, resulting in irrational beliefs. Suppose that a person is provided with information and reasons in the following way.

(1)   There is a chance surgery will have serious adverse effects. (True)
(2)   Alternative medicine has no risk of serious adverse effects. (True)

Therefore, if I want to best survive my cancer, then I should have alternative medicine. (False)

All that can be concluded from (1) and (2) is that if I want the treatment with fewer side effects, then I should choose alternative medicine. These premises say nothing about the effectiveness of surgery or alternative therapy.

Logic is important so that a person can utilize available facts properly. False beliefs which arise from correctable errors of logic corrupt a person's appreciation of the nature of the options, and so reduce the autonomy of his choice.

Importantly, autonomous choice also requires 'vivid imagination' of the alternatives if one is to appreciate fully their nature as options. Here is an argument to that effect.

The concept of choice entails that at least two alternatives are available. But it is necessary to distinguish between subjectively and objectively available alternatives. Two objective alternatives may exist with only one subjective alternative.

Consider the following example, after Locke.[5] A person in a room is led to believe that the room is locked, when in fact one door is open. This person has two objective alternatives (leave or stay) but only one subjective alternative (stay).

It is only after a person has presented herself with subjective alternatives that she can choose the one which she judges is best. One's choice cannot be fully self-determining if one believes that the path one sets upon is the only path available. As far as demonstrating that a choice is autonomous, it is not enough to show that objective choices exist. There must be some evidence that subjective choice exists.[6]

In order to be self-determining, then, it is necessary to present at least two alternatives to oneself. However, being autonomous requires more than this. Imagine that P wants to do A. P believes that he could also do B. However, it is A that P wants to do, and P does not think about B. In one sense, it can be said that P has chosen to do A, but is doing A an expression of P's self-determination? Self-determination is an active process of actually determining the path of one's life. In order to judge what is best for himself, P must think and imagine what it would be like for him if A and B obtained, and what the consequences, at least in the short term, of each of these would be for him. Thus, not only must P know what A and B are like, but he must also imagine what A and B would be like for him. This is vivid imagination.

One's rational objects need not be egoistic. One can autonomously care about morality and moral ends. But to be autonomous, these must have been rationally evaluated.

---

[5] In Locke's case, the person believes the door is open when in fact it is locked (Locke 1924: Book II, Chapter XXI, Sec. 10).

[6] Kahneman and Varey note: 'A basic tenet of psychological analysis is that the contents of subjective experience are coded and interpreted representations of objects and events. An objective description of stimuli is not adequate to predict experience because coding and interpretation can cause identical physical stimuli to be treated as different and different ones to be treated as identical' (Kahneman and Varey 1991: 141).

It is true that irrationality, spontaneity, and impulsivity can be a part of an autonomous life, but only if rationally endorsed at some time, at some higher level. A completely irrational unreflective life is not an autonomous life, even if it is wholeheartedly endorsed, on this Kantian account.

What compromises autonomy? On a full-blooded rationalist account, many things will compromise autonomy: relevant false beliefs, invalid or incomplete logic, lack of vivid imagination. The choice to do wrong may often be irrational for one or more of these reasons. Where this is the case, it would not, on the rationalist account, compromise the agent's autonomy. It may be preferable to correct false or irrational belief, errors of logic, and facilitate imagination. But this may not be possible or practicable. In these cases, employment of MT, even in cases of competent adults who have not consented to its use, may not offend autonomy and may actually open the door to a more autonomous life preventing incarceration and so promoting a wider range of options.

4.6 The value of the freedom to fall

The objector to moral enhancement by means of MT might respond: 'It is fine to allow voluntary use of MT to prevent oneself from acting in immoral and non-autonomous ways. But it is not fine to coerce people to adopt MT. Indeed, this is problematic even where the behaviour that MT prevents would be non-autonomous. For the act of forcing MT on someone against their will or without their consent is itself an infringement of autonomy. We should not restrict others' autonomy, even where doing so will in the long run increase their autonomy. Thus, for example, it would be wrong to use MT on a child who cannot consent to it, or to use it on a competent adult who refuses consent. Moreover, MT would almost certainly have to be used in this way. Criminals would be unlikely to voluntarily request MT so that, in order to eradicate crime, it would need to be involuntarily employed.'

But would it be wrong to infringe the autonomy of a child or adult to prevent grossly immoral action? Autonomy is only one value. We would be negligent if we did not physically restrain a child we knew to be about to commit murder. We work very hard to develop moral education for children, aimed at shaping their desires. MT would only remove the most harmful desires, leaving the child free to develop without the taint of having commited murder or other serious harm that would be a burden for the rest of his life, and MT would achieve this without imprisonment.

The criminal justice system also restrains autonomy in many, varied, and serious ways, largely in order to prevent grossly immoral action. And these restraints on autonomy are widely thought to be justified.

It might be objected that there is a difference between restricting someone's autonomy externally (say through incarceration) and restricting someone's autonomy internally (as with MT). Incarceration impedes autonomy by limiting our freedom of movement. But MT directly changes our bodily (brain) and mental states. Arguably, we have a stronger claim to bodily and mental non-interference than we do to freedom of movement. Thus, MT might seem to be a more serious restriction on autonomy than incarceration.

However, even if the distinction between internal and external restrictions has moral significance, it is not clear that this objection can be sustained, since incarceration and other putatively justified restrictions on autonomy designed to prevent gross immorality *do* in fact cause internal changes. A person's brain and mind are not unaffected by being imprisoned for 20 years, say.

Moreover, even if MT *is* a more serious restriction on autonomy than widely accepted restraints currently imposed by the criminal justice system, it may still be justified. For those existing restraints have proven rather poor at preventing gross immorality. Crime remains prevalent. MT, as we described it, would be much more effective at preventing gross immorality than is, say, incarceration. So it might be justified even if it constitutes a more serious restriction on autonomy.

In the world of MT, serious crime would be non-existent. There would be great benefits to society in general, but MT would also be of great benefit to potential criminals: they would no longer risk losing their freedom by imprisonment or capital punishment by committing serious crime. In the absence of effective moral enhancements that do not restrict autonomy, the loss of freedom in one domain of our lives, to commit evil deeds, would surely be worth the benefits. We would be otherwise free. Even in those cases in which MT does undermine autonomy, the value of human well-being and respect for the most basic rights of others plausibly outweighs the value of autonomy.

Of course, there might be other objections to MT. It could be argued, for example, that MT would be too prone to misuse, or that its acceptance would be the beginning of a slippery slope to unjustified restrictions on mental autonomy. Our point is that the very use of MT would not always constitute an unjustified restriction on autonomy. In some cases its use would not restrict autonomy at all. And in others, it would restrict autonomy, but justifiably.

5 Conclusion

Moral bioenhancement (or its opposite) may already be occurring in small ways when drugs like SSRIs are taken for psychiatric indications. However, there has been no strategic programme to use knowledge from the science of morality to deliberately and effectively improve moral motivation and behaviour through biological means. But such enhancement seems possible and, in many ways, desirable.

In this chapter, we have addressed the objection that moral bioenhancement is wrong because it would compromise the freedom to act immorally and thereby undermine personal autonomy. We have argued that moral bioenhancements need not restrict freedom, and that where they do they may, as with Ulysses, nevertheless preserve personal autonomy. Moral bioenhancements which work by enhancing capacities for empathy or imagination, by removing xenophobic aversions, or by aiding childhood moral development do not diminish autonomy. They may enhance it.

There might be instances of biological intervention to produce moral action that do control the moral agent, subjugating that person to the will of another, thus diminishing her autonomy. But such interventions might nevertheless be justified by the benefits that they produce, as are certain existing crime-prevention measures. Even if they do reduce freedom and autonomy, the value of behavioural control may outweigh this loss.

Note that, although we have focused on the case of *biological* interventions to enhance moral motivation and behaviour, our arguments also have implications for other varieties of moral enhancement—varieties that are perhaps more likely to be widely adopted. The cognitive sciences have already given rise to social-institutional reforms capable of altering human moral behaviour, for example, nudge techniques. One objection that has sometimes been raised to the use of these techniques is that they restrict autonomy. Though a full discussion of these objections lies beyond the scope of this article, we believe that our discussion of moral bioenhancement suggests reasons to doubt that the objections will count decisively against using nudge techniques, at least when the aim is to prevent gross immorality.

References

Amodio, D. M. (2008). 'The Social Neuroscience of Intergroup Relations', *European Review of Social Psychology*, 19(1): 1–54.

Arpaly, N. (2003). *Unprincipled Virtue: An Inquiry into Moral Agency*. New York: Oxford University Press.

Baron-Cohen, S. (2003). *The Essential Difference: Male and Female Brains and the Truth about Autism*. New York: Basic Books.

Blum, N. et al. (2008). 'Systems Training for Emotional Predictability and Problem Solving (STEPPS) for Outpatients with Borderline Personality Disorder: A Randomized Controlled Trial and 1-Year Follow-Up', *American Journal of Psychiatry*, 165:468–78.

Bovens, L. (2008). 'The Ethics of Nudge', in T. Grüne-Yanoff and S. O. Hansson (eds), *Preference Change: Approaches from Philosophy, Economics, and Psychology*. Berlin: Springer, 207–20.

Brasil-Neto, J. P. et al. (1992). 'Focal Transcranial Magnetic Stimulation and Response Bias in a Forced-Choice Task', *Journal of Neurology, Neurosurgery, and Psychiatry*, 55:964–6.

Carter, A., Hall, W., and Nutt, D. (2009). 'The Treatment of Addiction', in A. Carter, B. Capps, and W. Hall (eds), *Addiction Neurobiology: Ethical and Social Implications*. Luxemburg: Office for Official Publications of the European Communities, 53–68.

Charkrabortty, A. (2008). 'From Obama to Cameron: Why Do So Many Politicians Want a Piece of Richard Thaler?' *The Guardian*, 8 July.

Charland, L. (2004). 'Moral Treatment and the Personality Disorders', in J. Radden (ed), *The Philosophy of Psychiatry: A Companion*. Oxford: Oxford University Press, 64–77.

Crockett, M. J. et al. (2008). 'Serotonin Modulates Behavioral Reactions to Unfairness', *Science*, 320:1739.

Darity, W. A., Jr., Guilkey, D. K., and Winfrey, W. (1996). 'Explaining Differences in Economic Performance among Racial and Ethnic Groups in the USA: The Data Examined', *American Journal of Economics and Sociology*, 55(4): 411–25.

Darity, W. A., Jr., and Mason, P. L. (1998). 'Evidence on Discrimination in Employment: Codes of Color, Codes of Gender', *Journal of Economic Perspectives*, 12(2): 63–90.

Davison, K. (2008). *Cognitive Therapy for Personality Disorder*. 2nd edition. London: Routledge.

De Dreu, C. K. W. et al. (2010). 'Neuropeptide Oxytocin Regulates Parochial Altruism in Intergroup Conflicts among Humans', *Science*, 328:1408–11.

De Dreu, C. K. W. et al. (2011). 'Oxytocin Promotes Human Ethnocentrism', *Proceedings of the National Academy of Sciences*, 108(4): 1262–6.

Declerck, C. H., Boone, C., and Kiyonari, T. (2010). 'Oxytocin and Cooperation under Conditions of Uncertainty: The Modulating Role of Incentives and Social Information', *Hormones and Behavior*, 57(3): 368–74.

Douglas, T. (2008). 'Moral Enhancement', *Journal of Applied Philosophy*, 25(3): 228–45.

Dworkin, G. (1988). *The Theory and Practice of Autonomy*. Cambridge: Cambridge University Press.

Feinberg, J. (1973). *Social Philosophy*. Englewood Cliffs, NJ: Prentice-Hall.

Fix, M., Galster, G. C., and Struyk, R. J. (1993). 'An Overview of Auditing for Discrimination', in M. Fix and R. J. Struyk (eds), *Clear and Convincing Evidence: Measurement of Discrimination in America*. Washington, DC: Urban Institute Press, 1–68.

Fonagy, P. et al. (2004). *Affect Regulation, Mentalization, and the Development of the Self*. London: Karnac.

Frankfurt, H. (1989). 'Freedom of the Will and the Concept of a Person', in J. Christman (ed), *The Inner Citadel: Essays on Individual Autonomy*. New York: Oxford University Press, 63–76.

Goldin, C., and Rouse, C. (2000). 'Orchestrating Impartiality: The Impact of "Blind" Auditions on Female Musicians', *American Economic Review*, 90(4): 715–41.

Gottschalk, P. (1997). 'Inequality, Income Growth, and Mobility: The Basic Facts', *Journal of Economic Perspectives*, 11(2): 21–40.

Graves, R. (1960). *The Greek Myths*. Volume 2. London: Penguin.

Greely, H. T. (2008). 'Neuroscience and Criminal Justice: Not Responsibility but Treatment', *Kansas Law Review*, 56(5): 1103–38.

Harris, J. (2011). 'Moral Enhancement and Freedom', *Bioethics*, 25: 102–11.

Hume, D. (1978). *A Treatise of Human Nature*. 2nd edition. Edited by L. A. Selby-Bigge. Oxford: Clarendon Press.

Insel, T. R., and Fernald, R. D. (2004). 'How the Brain Processes Social Information: Searching for the Social Brain', *Annual Review of Neuroscience*, 27: 697–722.

Johnson, J. H., Bienenstock, E. J., and Stoloff, J. A. (1995). 'An Empirical Test of the Cultural Capital Hypothesis', *Review of Black Political Economy*, 23(4): 7–27.

Kahneman, D., and Varey, C. (1991). 'Notes on the Psychology of Utility', in J. Elster and J. E. Roemer (eds), *Interpersonal Comparisons of Well-Being*. Cambridge: Cambridge University Press, 127–63.

Kant, I. (1964). *Groundwork of the Metaphysic of Morals*. New York: Harper and Row.

Keith, V. M., and Herring, C. (1991). 'Skin Tone and Stratification in the Black Community', *American Journal of Sociology*, 97(3): 760–78.

Kersten, F. (1956). *The Kersten Memoirs, 1940–1945*. Translated by C. Fitzgibbon and J. Oliver; introduced by H. R. Trevor-Roper. London: Hutchinson.

Kiesel, A. et al. (2006). 'Unconscious Manipulation of Free Choice in Humans', *Consciousness and Cognition*, 15: 397–408.

Kosfeld, M. et al. (2005). 'Oxytocin Increases Trust in Humans', *Nature*, 435(7042): 673–6.

Lang, K. L., and Vernon, P. A. (2001). 'Genetics', in W. J. Livesley (ed), *Handbook of Personality Disorders: Theory, Research, and Treatment*. New York: Guilford Press, 177–95.

Lees, J., Manning, N., and Rawlings, B. (1999). 'Therapeutic Community Effectiveness: A Systematic International Review of Therapeutic Community Treatment for

People with Personality Disorders and Mentally Disordered Offenders', York: NHS Centre for Reviews and Dissemination, University of York.

Liberzon, I., and Young, E.A. (1997). 'Effects of stress and glucocorticoids on CNS oxytocin receptor binding', *Psychoneuroendocrinology*, 22(6): 411–22.

Lieberman, M. D. et al. (2005). 'An fMRI Investigation of Race-Related Amygdala Activity in African-American and Caucasian-American Individuals', *Nature Neuroscience*, 8(6): 720–2.

Linehan, M., and Dimeff, L. (2001). 'Dialectical Behavioural Therapy in a Nutshell', *The California Psychologist*, 34:10–13.

Link, H., Dayanithi, G., and Gratzl, M. (1993). 'Glucocorticoids Rapidly Inhibit Oxytocin-Stimulated Adrenocorticotropin Release from Rat Anterior Pituitary Cells, without Modifying Intracellular Calcium Transients', *Endocrinology*, 132:873–7.

Locke, J. (1924). *An Essay concerning Human Understanding*. Edited by A. S. Pringle-Pattinson. Oxford: Clarendon Press.

Mill, J. S. (1979). *Utilitarianism*. Indianapolis, IN: Hackett.

Milton, J. ([1667] 2000). *Paradise Lost*, in J. Leonard (ed), *Paradise Lost*. London: Penguin Books.

National Institute of Clinical Excellence (NICE). (2009). 'Borderline Personality Disorder: Treatment and Management', London: NICE.

National Institute of Mental Health in England (NIMHE). (2003). 'Personality Disorder: No Longer a Diagnosis of Exclusion', London: NIMHE.

National Offender Management Strategy (NOMS). (2011). 'Working with Personality Disordered Offenders: A Practitioner's Guide', London: NOMS.

Neumark, D., Bank, R. J., and Van Nort, K. D. (1996). 'Sex Discrimination in Restaurant Hiring: An Audit Study', *Quarterly Journal of Economics*, 111(3): 915–41.

Paris, J. (2001). 'Psychosocial Adversity', in W. J. Livesley (ed), *Handbook of Personality Disorders: Theory, Research, and Treatment*. New York: Guilford Press, 231–41.

Pearce, S., and Pickard, H. (2009). 'The Moral Content of Psychiatric Treatment', *British Journal of Psychiatry*, 195:281–2.

Persson, I., and Savulescu, J. (2011). 'Unfit for the Future? Human Nature, Scientific Progress and the Need for Moral Enhancement', in J. Savulescu, Julian, R. Ter Meulen, and G. Kahane (eds), *Enhancing Human Capacities*. Oxford: Wiley-Blackwell, 486–500.

Persson, I., and Savulescu, J. (2012a). 'Moral Transhumanism: The Next Step', *Journal of Medicine and Philosophy*, 37(4): 405–16.

Persson, I., and Savulescu, J. (2012b). *Unfit for the Future: The Need for Moral Enhancement*. Oxford: Oxford University Press.

Persson. I. and Savulescu, J. (2013). 'Getting Moral Enhancement Right: The Desirability of Moral Enhancement', *Bioethics*, 27:124–31.

Phelps, E. A. et al. (2000). 'Performance on Indirect Measures of Race Evaluation Predicts Amygdala Activation', *Journal of Cognitive Neuroscience*, 12(5): 729–38.

Pickard, H. (2009). 'Mental Illness Is Indeed a Myth', in M. R. Broome and L. Bortolotti (eds), *Psychiatry as Cognitive Neuroscience*. Oxford: Oxford University Press, 83–101.

Pickard, H. (2011). 'Responsibility without Blame: Empathy and the Effective Treatment of Personality Disorder,' *Philosophy, Psychiatry, Psychology*, 18(3): 209–23.

Ramachandran, V. S., and Oberman, L. M. (2006). 'Broken Mirrors: A Theory of Autism', *Scientific American*, 295:62–9.

Ransford, H. E. (1970). 'Skin Color, Life Chances, and Anti-White Attitudes', *Social Problems*, 18(2): 164–79.

Rodgers, W. M., and Spriggs, W. E. (1996). 'What Does the AFQT Really Measure? Race, Wages, Schooling, and the AFQT Score', *Review of Black Political Economy*, 24(4): 13–46.

Santos, A., Meyer-Lindenberg, A., and Deruelle, C. (2010). 'Absence of Racial, but Not Gender, Stereotyping in Williams Syndrome Children', *Current Biology*, 20(7): R307–8.

Savulescu, J. (1994). 'Rational Desires and the Limitation of Life-Sustaining Treatment', *Bioethics*, 8:191–222.

Savulescu, J., and Persson, I. (2008). 'The Perils of Cognitive Enhancement and the Urgent Imperative to Enhance the Moral Character of Humanity', *Journal of Applied Philosophy*, 25(3): 162–7.

Savulescu, J., and Persson, I. (2011). 'The Turn for Ultimate Harm: A Reply to Fenton', *Journal of Medical Ethics*, 37(7): 441–4.

Silber, M. et al. (1987). 'The Effect of Oral Contraceptive Pills on Levels of Oxytocins in Plasma and on Cognitive Functions', *Contraception*, 36:641–50.

Smith, G. (2011). 'Steve Jobs Doomed Himself by Shunning Conventional Medicine until Too Late, Claims Harvard Expert', *Mail Online*, 14 October, http://www.dailymail.co.uk/news/article-2049019/Steve-Jobs-dead-Apple-CEO-shunned-conventional-cancer-medicine.html (accessed 7 December 2012).

Stock, S., Karlsson, R., and von Schoultz, B. (1994). 'Serum Profiles of Oxytocin during Oral Contraceptive Treatment', *Gynecological Endocrinology*, 8(2): 121–6.

Terbeck, S. et al. (2012). 'Beta-Adrenergic Blockade Reduces Implicit Negative Racial Bias', *Psychopharmacology*, 222(3): 419–24.

Terbeck, S. et al. (Under Review). 'Emotion in Moral Decision-Making: Beta Adrenergic Blockade Increases Deontological Moral Judgments'.

Thaler, R. H., and Sunstein, C. (2008). *Nudge: Improving Decisions about Health, Health, and Happiness.* New Haven, CT: Yale University Press.

Tse, W.S., and Bond, A. J. (2002). 'Serotonergic Intervention Affects Both Social Dominance and Affiliative Behaviour', *Psychopharmacology*, 161:324–30.

Watson, G. (1989). 'Free Agency', in J. Christman (ed), *The Inner Citadel: Essays on Individual Autonomy.* New York: Oxford University Press, 109–22.

Wood, R. M. et al. (2006). 'Effects of Tryptophan Depletion on the Performance of an Iterated Prisoner's Dilemma Game in Healthy Adults', *Neuropsychopharmacology*, 31(5): 1075–84.

Young, R. (1986). *Personal Autonomy: Beyond Negative and Positive Liberty.* London: Croom Helm.

3.2

Commentary

(Im)Moral Technology? Thought Experiments and the Future of 'Mind Control'

Robert Sparrow

Philosophers love thought experiments. A good thought experiment progresses intellectual enquiry by clearing away extraneous details and exposing the philosophical essence of a problem. By clarifying the issues at stake, thought experiments help distinguish different philosophical positions and reveal connections between different philosophical problems.

In some areas of philosophy, inventing a good thought experiment is its own reward: philosophers have made careers out of formulating problems that have kept other philosophers busy trying to solve them. However, in applied ethics, where the ultimate goal must be to contribute to solving real-world problems in all their messy complexity, arguments involving thought experiments are both especially tempting and especially problematic. They are especially tempting because it is hard to see how we can solve the messy complex issues we face in the real world if we cannot first develop our intuitions and principles in deliberately simplified test cases. They are especially problematic because of the difficulties involved in moving from real-world dilemmas to thought experiments and back again.

In order for an argument involving a thought experiment to progress debate in applied ethics three things must be true. First, the thought experiment must accurately represent and illuminate a pressing ethical dilemma. Second—and most obviously—the central claims of the argument regarding the thought experiment must be plausible. Third, it must be possible to apply or develop the arguments established with reference to the thought experiment to the real-world cases the experiment is intended to illuminate.

In their paper, 'Autonomy and the Ethics of Biological Behaviour Modification', Savulescu, Douglas, and Persson (in this collection) are discussing the ethics of a technology exist for improving moral motivation and behaviour, which does not yet exist and—as I will argue below—will most likely never exist. At the heart of their argument sits the imagined case of a 'moral technology' that magically prevents people from developing intentions to commit seriously immoral actions. It is not too much of a stretch, then, to characterize their paper as a thought experiment in service of a thought experiment. In this commentary, I will argue that there are serious reasons to question the extent to which their argument meets each of the challenges involved in the use of thought experiments in applied ethics, outlined above. While Savulescu et al. succeed in showing how behavioural modification might be compatible with freedom and autonomy—and perhaps justifiable even if it were not—in the fantastic case they consider, there is little we can conclude from this about any technology of 'moral bioenhancement' in the foreseeable future. Indeed, there is a real danger that their argument will license attempts to manipulate behaviour through drugs and brain implants, which raise profound moral issues that they barely mention.

Can we really make people 'more moral' through biomedical interventions?

Savulescu and his co-authors begin by pointing out that various drugs and other biological manipulations are capable of influencing human behaviour. In so far as human minds supervene on neurological systems with a significant chemical component, this is hardly surprising. What is more tendentious is whether or not any of the interventions they discuss are accurately characterized as affecting 'moral motivation and behaviour', let alone as 'moral bioenhancement'. Timely application of a sedative gas might prevent someone from getting up to mischief, but we would hardly want to characterize this as a 'moral enhancement'. At the very least, then, 'moral bioenhancement' would require modifying both behaviour *and* motivation. Moreover, because—as Savulescu et al. admit—both behaviour and motivations that may be virtuous in one person and/ or circumstance may be vicious in another, any biological manipulations touted as making people more 'moral' will need to be extraordinarily finely tuned. It is, I think, not incidental to the rhetorical—if not the logical—force of their argument that Savulescu, Douglas, and Persson rely heavily here on a small number of controversial studies involving 'sexy' but still determinedly 'medical' drugs, such as oxytocin, serotonin, and propranolol, where they might equally well have pointed to the potential for mundane—though regrettably, for enthusiasts for enhancement, illegal—drugs to be used to modify motivation and behaviour: cannabis for tolerance, ecstasy for beneficence, and alcohol for 'Dutch' courage. Of course, thinking about these more familiar cases very quickly reveals how unlikely it is that any chemical manipulation is going to reliably improve people's *moral* reasoning.

Indeed, as Savulescu, Douglas, and Persson themselves later note, 'one acts morally when one does the right thing, and for the right reason(s)' (Savulescu, Douglas, and Persson in this collection). I suspect that Savulescu et al. think of acting for the right reasons on an 'externalist' model, wherein it is only required that individuals act as would be required by correct moral reasoning in their particular situation whether they actually reason this way themselves or not. It is worth noting, however, that on some accounts of moral action—not least some Kantian accounts—in order to act morally, agents must themselves consciously embrace—if not rehearse—the reasons for their actions. It is hard to see how any drug could alter our *beliefs* in such a way as to track the reasons we have to act morally. More importantly, the idea that our motivations should track the reasons we have to act is internal to the idea that we are acting *for those reasons*. Such 'reason tracking' also requires appropriate sensitivity to counterfactuals. If we praise an individual for helping someone in distress, the judgement that this was morally admirable depends upon the thought that they should not have felt compelled to help them otherwise. It would be a good drug, indeed, that made us feel love only for what is worthy of love and brave only in the service of a just cause.

Ultimately, Savulescu, Douglas, and Persson concede that 'the technology to biologically influence moral motivation and behaviour is still in its infancy, or even pre-embryonic stages', yet they insist that 'it seems likely that science will afford ever more powerful interventions' and that 'it would be bold to rule…out' the development of this technology (Savulescu, Douglas, and Persson in this collection). The matter of how and why it has become the case that bioethicists feel compelled to discuss the ethics of every hypothetical technology that cannot be shown to be impossible is worthy of an essay in its own right. However, it is clear from this admission that their argument fails the first test that I suggested was necessary for arguments involving thought experiments in applied ethics—it does not illuminate a pressing moral dilemma.

Autonomy and the ethics of 'moral technology'

Savulescu, Douglas, and Persson then go on to consider the genuinely interesting philosophical question of whether moral bioenhancement would be wrong by virtue of restricting the 'freedom to do wrong' and thereby reducing personal autonomy—a criticism that has been put forward (somewhat bizarrely, given his enthusiastic advocacy for other forms of enhancement) by John Harris (2011).

The nature of 'freedom of the will' is one of the most ancient and difficult questions in philosophy. Savulescu and his co-authors attempt to bypass concerns about pharmaceutical interventions restricting freedom by highlighting two related cases where we tend not to think that people lack freedom: the 'naturally virtuous'; and moral education. There is an obvious tension between their description of the naturally virtuous person as someone for whom it is psychologically or motivationally out of the question to do wrong and their later claim that autonomy requires the vivid imagination of alternatives. Nor is it obvious that a pill that renders someone 'more open to the experiences and lives of others' achieves the same results as reading Tolstoy, as they suggest. Someone who reads Tolstoy arguably learns *reasons* to be less judgemental and in doing so develops greater understanding: someone who takes a pill has merely *caused* their sentiments to alter. In so far as moral action requires acting for the right reasons, the person who has learned tolerance from Tolstoy has more and better reasons for action.

In any case, the concern that biological interventions to shape motivation and behaviour threaten freedom and autonomy is not exhausted by arguments in metaphysics or philosophy of mind. The tension between God's omnipotence and man's freedom is a matter of politics as much as—or perhaps even more than—metaphysics. In asking whether someone is free we are also asking whether they may appropriately be held responsible for their actions.

Savulescu, Douglas, and Persson concede this when they admit that biomedical interventions to reshape the behaviour or motivations of other people constrain their freedom if they cause them to act or feel differently than they would otherwise have been inclined to do. Yet Savulescu et al. try to temper the opposition between freedom and moral enhancement by discussing the case of a hypothetical—and frankly fantastic—'moral technology' which would only intervene to prevent people forming the desire to carry out seriously immoral actions. By reducing the number of seriously immoral actions in societies in which it was introduced without significantly reducing people's freedom, such a device would, they suggest, constitute a powerful technology of moral enhancement. In most cases, they argue, when people chose to act morally they would also be doing so freely: in just a few cases would individuals' moral choices result from the coercive power of the magical moral technology.

However, Savulescu and his co-authors here underestimate the tension between the power of some and the freedom of others. This tension is highlighted by the notion of 'freedom as non-domination' that has been developed by Philip Pettit (1997) in the course of his explorations of the philosophical foundations of republicanism. Pettit argues convincingly that citizens of a society run by a benevolent dictator are, in an important sense, not free even if the dictator is genuinely benevolent and chooses never to exercise his dictatorial powers. To return to the case that so exercised Milton, if God could have intervened to prevent Man's fall, but didn't, then God seems as responsible for the fall as were Adam and Eve. God's power—and not just God's exercise of his powers—is incompatible with human freedom. Similarly, given that people who are subject to the magical 'moral technology' are *not* free to do anything other than act morally, this suggests that there is an important sense in which they do not act freely even when they choose to act in such a way that the technology does not intervene.

Savulescu, Douglas, and Persson's argument therefore fails the second test that arguments involving thought experiments must pass: it does not convincingly establish their central claim even in the context of the hypothetical technology they discuss.

Having said that, I do want to acknowledge that Savulescu and his co-authors succeed in establishing that biomedical manipulation of oneself is compatible with autonomy and may even promote it by making it easier for us to realize our higher-order goals. This is a not-uninteresting result and should indeed serve to undermine some of the reflexive hostility that the very idea of moral enhancement currently tends to evoke. Nevertheless, the 'Ulysses and the Sirens'-type cases that Savulescu, Douglas, and Persson discuss are a special case and leave the larger argument about the ethics of enhancing *other* people untouched.

The real world of 'mind control'

However, it is when we turn to the third test of arguments involving thought experiments in applied ethics—the extent to which their lessons can be applied to real-world cases—that Savulescu, Douglas, and Persson's argument is most deficient.

In the course of their discussion, Savulescu, Douglas, and Persson admit that previous efforts at 'mind control'—which include the drugging of children, military interest in 'brainwashing', and the history of attempts to 'cure' homosexuality—'were either used in the service of misguided goals or were performed without adequate protections for those subjected to them' (Savulescu, Douglas, and Persson in this collection). I can see no reasons—and certainly the authors offer us none—as to why either the motivations of governments or the protections they offer the vulnerable are likely to be better in the future.

In the context of a concern for the real-world prospects of any technology that could reliably alter behaviour or motivation, four things stand out in Savulescu, Douglas, and Persson's paper.

First, their discussion is introduced and justified by reference to a naive conservative account of social phenomena. It simply isn't true, for instance, to say that the public health problems they refer to in order to motivate the search for technologies of moral enhancement are the result of 'lifestyle' choices. They are the result of modern life-styles but these lifestyles aren't chosen by individuals so much as imposed upon them by their environments. Moreover, to the extent that it is possible to speak of some indi-viduals choosing these lifestyles, such claims play no role in the explanation of the public health phenomena which result from the aggregate impact of the behaviour of indi-viduals. There are a number of competing (though not, of course, entirely mutually exclusive) explanations for the increase in levels of obesity in wealthy nations since 1985—increases in the sugar and/or fat content of many foods due to developments in agriculture, food processing, and manufacturing; changes in the economics of food production and consumption; changes in patterns of daily activity as a result of lower prices of consumer electronics; changes in intestinal flora as a consequence of increased use of antibiotics; changes in the nature and distribution of paid employment; the devel-opment of an urban infrastructure that mitigates against physical activity, etc.—but the claim that this phenomenon can be explained by the idea that lots of people 'decided to eat more' is an obvious non-starter. The main role played by such claims about individu-als' responsibility for their health-care condition is in fact to justify the use of coercive measures to reshape behaviour.

Second, there is a pervasive aura of intellectually dubious and politically dangerous sociobiology surrounding their key claim that meaningful biological manipulation of moral behaviour will be possible. Their claim that women are naturally more inclined to self-sacrifice than men is based upon the research of one—controversial—researcher and elides both the possibility of alternative cultural explanations for such differences and the deeper methodological question of how we identify particular behaviours as selfish or selfless. Similarly, the idea that a large percentage of prisoners have a biologi-cal disorder that has a tendency to 'criminal behaviour' as one of its diagnostic criteria is both circular and brazenly denies a long history of sociological investigations of the social construction and medicalization of deviance. However, more important than the truth or falsity of these individual claims is the way in which construing social problems as rooted in biology both buttresses the existing social order—the foundations of which are clearly primarily ideological rather than biological—and positively invites govern-ments to undertake the project of drugging and electrocuting the poor, the desperate, and the marginalized. Indeed, there is a telling slippage in a sentence that appears early in the manuscript. The authors say that they aim to explore 'how ethics could justify the use of radical advances in the neurosciences for the purposes of modifying moral motivation and behaviour' (Savulescu, Douglas, and Persson in this collection). I presume they are interested in the intellectual possibility of an argument for moral enhancement. However, another, more cynical, reading would hear this as an invitation to those who feel that they know better than others what sorts of behaviours are desirable to cloak their interests in a facade of ethical argument. Moreover, the project of 'moral bioenhancement' invites this abuse: it assumes that we know what moral behaviour in various circumstances consists in, where in fact this is, within limits, controversial and should also remain so; it will almost certainly involve the powerful acting on the powerless.

Third, the role played by a rationalist account of autonomy in the final section of the paper also invites abuse. If only rational desires count as autonomous then interventions to thwart or reshape the desires of others that one holds to be irrational will not count as infringing their autonomy. It is all too likely then, that governments who wish to manipulate the behaviour of their citizens will mobilize this argument to insist that they do not violate any rights in doing so.

Fourth, by making crucial sections of their case using the imaginary example of their 'moral technology', the authors massively prejudice the argument in favour of their preferred conclusion that moral bioenhancement might be justified even where it does constrain freedom and autonomy. They may well be right about the ethics of their 'moral technology'. However, there is little, if anything, we can conclude about the ethics of plausibly real-world technologies to reshape motivation and behaviour from this idealized case.

Thus, not only does Savulescu, Douglas, and Persson's discussion do little to illuminate the many pressing moral and political concerns about the prospect of biomedical manipulation of motivation and behaviour (in particular, about who would control this technology and to what ends), it significantly misrepresents the relevant moral landscape. Rather than illuminate the ethics of a relevant real-world ethical dilemma, the thought experiment at the heart of their argument obscures it.

Conclusion

I have argued that the vision of moral bioenhancement that Savulescu, Douglas, and Persson put forward is a fantasy. Moreover, insofar as it neglects the many pressing moral issues that would arise the moment any putative technology of moral enhancement actually became available, it is a dangerous fantasy. However, in concluding I want to acknowledge that this interpretation of the import of Savulescu, Douglas, and Persson's argument relies on a substantive account of the proper role of thought experiments in applied ethics, which, I suspect, Savulescu and his co-authors reject. As a piece of philosophy their argument is indeed thought provoking and has significant merits. As a treatment of the bioethical issues we are likely to face in the next century as a result of progress in the neurosciences, however, it is much less compelling.

References

Harris, J. (2011). 'Moral Enhancement and Freedom', *Bioethics*, 25(2): 102–11.

Pettit, P. (1997). *Republicanism: A Theory of Freedom and Government*. Oxford: Clarendon Press.

Savulescu, J., Douglas, T., and Persson, I. (2014). 'Autonomy and the Ethics of Biological Behaviour Modification', in A. Akabayashi (ed.), *The Future of Bioethics: International Dialogues*. Oxford: Oxford University Press, 91–112.

3.3

Commentary
Some Remarks on Moral Bioenhancement

Masahiro Morioka

1 What is moral bioenhancement?

Julian Savulescu and his colleagues have recently advocated the necessity for developing moral bioenhancement technologies, and Peter Singer and Agata Sagan discussed a 'morality pill' in the *New York Times* (Singer and Sagan 2012). Moral bioenhancement is, according to Persson and Savulescu, 'moral enhancement not merely by traditional means, such as education, but by genetic or other biological means' (Persson and Savulescu 2013: 2). Savulescu, Douglas, and Persson argue that, in the future, in addition to pharmacological means, other non-pharmacological methods, such as transcranial magnetic stimulation, deep brain stimulation, genetic manipulation, and targeted optic stimulation could be used to influence one's moral motivation and behavior (Savulescu, Douglas, and Persson in this chapter).

Their argument on moral bioenhancement is eloquently presented in their paper, 'The Perils of Cognitive Enhancement and the Urgent Imperative to Enhance the Moral Character of Humanity' published in 2008. They argue that we are now living in an age of cognitive enhancement, and 'this expansion of scientific knowledge and cognitive ability will put in an increasing number of people's hands "weapons of mass destruction" or the ability to deploy them' (Persson and Savulescu 2008: 166). With these weapons, even a small terrorist group will be able to devastate the whole world. Hence, '[t]o eliminate this risk, cognitive enhancement would have to be accompanied by a *moral* enhancement which extends to *all* of us, since such moral enhancement could reduce malevolence' (Persson and Savulescu 2008: 166). They further argue that '[i]f safe moral enhancements are ever developed, there are strong reasons to believe that their use should be obligatory, like education or fluoride in the water, since those who should take them are least likely to be inclined to use them. That is, safe, effective moral enhancement would be compulsory' (Persson and Savulescu 2008: 174).

2 Social improvement and moral bioenhancement

Persson and Savulescu talk about two different kinds of moral bioenhancements: moral bioenhancement applied to individuals, such as criminals, and that applied to a group

Number of homicides

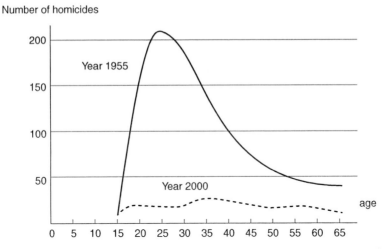

Figure 3.1 Number of homicides committed by men per one million people in Japan.

of people or to an entire population in an area. An example of the former is hormonal manipulation treatment prescribed to pedophiles, and an example of the latter is altruism-enhancing drugs blended in the tap water in an entire area for the purpose of preventing actual use of weapons of mass destruction by terrorists.

The former, a drug treatment for pedophiles and other criminals, has already been performed in some countries, and it may be effective in preventing future crimes. However, this kind of drug therapy targeting a single criminal individual is not the main theme Persson and Savulescu want to pursue under the name of moral bioenhancement. What they really have in mind is compulsory manipulation of the minds of a group of people by coercing them to take moral bioenhancement drugs. Their aim is moral bio*enforcement* of the whole population.

John Harris severely criticizes Persson and Savulescu in his paper titled 'Moral Enhancement and Freedom' (Harris 2011). He argues that human immorality, such as racism, has been 'reduced dramatically in the last hundred years by forms of moral enhancement including education, public disapproval, knowledge acquisition and legislation,' hence, 'racism can be defeated by such means without resorting to biological or genetic measures which might have unwanted effects' (Harris 2011: 105).

I agree with Harris's argument. Let me present an interesting example that might illustrate the relationship between moral enhancement and social improvement. Figure 3.1 shows the number of homicides committed by men per capita (per one million people) in Japanese society in 1955 and 2000.[1]

You can see a drastic reduction in the number of homicides during the 45 years, particularly by men in their twenties. This is attributable to Japan's economic prosperity and 45 years of peace in our society. (Japan has not directly waged war against any country in more than 55 years since the end of World War II.) Japan has succeeded

---

[1] This graph was created by the author, using the statistical data in Hiraiwa-Hasegawa (2005).

in reducing the number of homicides by improving social conditions and environments. This implies that social improvement is easier and more effective than moral bioenhancement.

Of course, in the future, by taking super cognitive-enhancement drugs people may have the capacity to run ten times faster, see in the dark, and instantly kill more than ten people by hand. They could easily steal dirty bombs and detonate them in cities. This appears to be one of the things that Persson and Savulescu fear. However, a coercive moral bioenhancement would not be able to prevent the occurrence of such events. The only way to prevent them would be to strictly control the access to those problematic pharmaceutical substances and establish laws to punish individuals for possession of those drugs. Japan has succeeded in prohibiting the possession of guns among ordinary citizens. (I have never seen a real gun in our country in my life.) Hence, prohibition should be possible in the case of cognitive-enhancement drugs or advanced technologies that could be detrimental to humans. (Nevertheless, it might not be possible in countries where people have the right to carry guns for self-protection. This suggests that gun control among citizens ought to be the first challenge for ethicists in favor of moral bioenhancement.)

3   Compulsory moral bioenhancement of all people is impossible

Persson and Savulescu insist that moral bioenhancement ought to be forced on all of us, but this is impossible because powerful, rich, and greedy people would use every conceivable method to avoid taking moral bioenhancement drugs. Even if drugs are blended into the tap water in an area, it is possible to get pure water from elsewhere. Furthermore, it is difficult to force moral bioenhancement on those who are in a position to force it on ordinary people. Hence, a moral bioenhancement policy will create two groups of people: those who are forced to take moral bioenhancement drugs, and those who can avoid taking such drugs. Then, what would happen among them?

Imagine lifeboat ethics. There are six people on a lifeboat with a capacity for five. One of the six individuals is a morally bioenhanced person. Savulescu, Douglas, and Persson argue that self-sacrifice and altruism are the two central characteristics of morality, and that these traits can be enhanced by biological determinants. If they are right, this morally bioenhanced person in the lifeboat would think that she has to sacrifice herself to save her fellow passengers by plunging into the sea. As a result, the other five greedy people would be saved. A lesson from this episode is that when there are both morally bioenhanced people and non-enhanced people, the latter could survive at the expense of the former. Is this what ethicists in favor of moral bioenhancement would aim at?

Savulescu, Douglas, and Persson suggest that oxytocin could be used to enhance morality, as, according to several studies, it enhances our pro-social attitudes, such as trust, sympathy, and generosity (Savulescu, Douglas, and Persson in this chapter). Is this really good news for moral bioenhancement? The answer is negative because after providing a group of people with oxytocin we could effectively dominate them, use them, and finally exploit them as slaves. This shows that moral bioenhancement can be used to control the minds of people who do not have social resources or social status to bypass the coercion to take moral bioenhancement drugs. Moral bioenhancement functions as a tool to divide our society into two layers.

Savulescu and colleagues might emphasize that moral bioenhancement should be mandatory for all without exception, but it is virtually impossible as mentioned above. Even if it becomes possible to force everyone to take moral bioenhancement drugs, there still remains a very difficult problem. Let us assume that everyone in a society becomes morally bioenhanced by drugs blended in the tap water. The morally bioenhanced people would become highly vulnerable to aggression, violence, and exploitation by other people. If a group of people immune to those drugs were to appear, who would never become morally bioenhanced by the drugs, they could easily dominate and exploit the morally bioenhanced people in the way that wild colonists enslaved empathetic and generous indigenous inhabitants in the past.

In the first place, can we imagine morally bioenhanced police or a morally bioenhanced army? If they are under the influence of moral bioenhancement drugs, they cannot accomplish their tasks properly. I am basically a pacifist who believes that the army should be reduced as much as possible; however, I do think that a society needs a well-organized police who perform their jobs in a law-abiding manner, and that they should even execute violence and aggression in order to save the lives and properties of ordinary citizens in emergencies. The police whose hearts are filled with empathy and generosity would never be able to complete their mission in emergency situations. Then, should the police be an exception? But if the police are considered an exception, it would open a route for them to become conquerors of society, thereby leading to police despotism.

In short, compulsory moral enhancement will lead to the exploitation of one group of people by another. Persson and Savulescu emphasize the danger of terrorist attacks carried out by a small terrorist group with weapons of mass destruction (Persson and Savulescu 2008: 166). However, I suspect that the most dangerous players in the contemporary world would still be the military forces, equipped with a variety of weapons, which take a multitude of lives every year. In this sense, it might be interesting to force moral bioenhancement only on top political and military leaders, CEOs of huge companies, and multimillionaires in order for them not to appropriate the world. However, even in this case, effective enforcement of moral bioenhancement drugs remains a problem.

4 Enhancement of moral sensitivity is not always good

Savulescu, Douglas, and Persson write that '[o]ur point is merely that, in many people, enhancing one or more of the traits we have discussed would, in many circumstances, result in that individual being more likely to act morally than would otherwise have been the case' (Savulescu, Douglas, and Persson in this chapter). This is a fairly naïve idea. Persson and Savulescu state that moral bioenhancement can be achieved by enhancing people's disposition of altruism and their sense of justice or fairness (Persson and

Savulescu 2008: 168–9). This means that moral bioenhancement requires the enhancement of one's moral sensitivity, but empirically speaking, the enhancement of moral sensitivity does not necessarily bring happiness. Consider the number of immoral and unfair acts we commit every day. Remember what you said to your partner last night when you were quarrelling. Remember the gorgeous dinner you had at a fabulous party, and think about how many starving people's lives in a developing country could have been saved if the cost of the dinner had been sent to them. Think about why you did not invite a stranger, who was standing outside your apartment shivering in the cold air, into your home. That person might have suffered hypothermia and frozen to death somewhere during the night. Without moral bioenhancement drugs, such ideas would only come to our mind for a very short period of time, quickly disappearing without any traces. However, morally bioenhanced people cannot easily escape these depressing ideas. They would be trapped in such moral dilemmas every day and become depressed day and night.

Morally sensitive people worry about every immoral and unfair deed they commit. They are not saints. They cannot save every suffering individual they encounter or call on every suffering individual residing in their neighborhood. They would think this is their own fault. Morally bioenhanced people might wish to escape from this kind of psychological stress and take other drugs to forget their painful memories and ideas. The reason why ordinary people can survive every day would be that they are not so morally sensitive as to worry about such 'small' things. Hence, at first, a society filled with morally sensitive people might be considered a good society, but in reality, against our expectations, people living in such a society might not necessarily be happy.

5   Conclusion

Several issues concerning moral bioenhancement remain to be discussed, but I will leave them for another paper.[2] My provisional conclusion is that moral bioenhancement might be effective in treating pedophiles and other criminals, but not in other cases. Compulsory moral bioenhancement is impossible, and if we want to improve our society, improvement of social conditions would be easier and more effective.

References

Harris, J. (2011). 'Moral Enhancement and Freedom,' *Bioethics*, 25(2): 102–11.

Hiraiwa-Hasegawa, M. (2005). 'Homicide by Men in Japan, and Its Relationship to Age, Resources, and Risk Taking,' *Evolution and Human Behavior*, 26:332–43.

Persson, I., and Savulescu, J. (2008). 'The Perils of Cognitive Enhancement and the Urgent Imperative to Enhance the Moral Character of Humanity,' *Journal of Applied Philosophy*, 25(3): 162–77.

---

[2] Undiscussed issues include arbitrariness of the idea of morality, the reason why moral enhancement by biological means appears problematic, the difference between moral bioenhancement and self-discipline, who needs moral bioenhancement drugs, and the meaning of immoral aspects of our dispositions.

Persson. I. and Savulescu, J. (2013). 'Getting Moral Enhancement Right: The Desirability of Moral Enhancement', *Bioethics*, 27: 124–31.

Savulescu, J., Douglas, T., and Persson, I. (2013). 'Autonomy and the Ethics of Biological Behaviour Modification', in A. Akabayashi (ed), *The Future of Bioethics: International Dialogues*. Oxford: Oxford University Press, XXX–XXX.

Singer, P., and Sagan, A. (2012). 'Are We Ready for a 'Morality Pill'?' *New York Times*, 28 January.

3.4

Commentary
Moral Technology and the Concept of 'the Self'

Tomohide Ibuki and Satoshi Kodama

Since the beginning of the twenty-first century, dramatic progress has been made in neuroscience, which has also enlivened the field of neuroethics. Neuroethics can be roughly divided into two major areas. The first is the neuroscience of ethics, which examines ethical and philosophical concepts in light of new findings in fields such as cognitive neuroscience. The second area is the ethics of neuroscience, which examines the ethical propriety of research and intervention in neuroscience (cf. Roskies 2002).

Savulescu, Douglas, and Persson discussed the ethics of neuroscience in the article 'Autonomy and the Ethics of Biological Behaviour Modification.' Specifically, they defended the ethical propriety of enhancing moral capacity and technologically manipulating human morality (i.e. moral technology; hereafter referred to as 'MT'[1]). In this commentary, we will critically analyze the discussion by Savulescu et al. on how MT affects freedom and autonomy and argue that advances in MT may endanger these basic human ideals.

1 Becoming 'virtuous' through MT

It is commonly believed that MT procedures violate human freedom and autonomy. John Harris argued that MT undermines the freedom to act in morally improper ways and restrains individual autonomy (Harris 2011). Savulescu et al. responded by arguing that a person who has undergone MT and, as a result, is incapable of immoral behavior, is no different to a virtuous person who is unable to act in morally improper ways. Virtuous people would not feel that their freedom was restricted, and therefore it cannot be concluded that morally enhanced individuals would have their autonomy restrained.

In general, we do not think of virtuous people as lacking the freedom to act immorally. According to Aristotle, virtue is 'not merely the state in accordance with right reason, but

---

[1] MT is used as a general term for all technologies that manipulate moral capacity, such as moral enhancement.

[rather] the state that implies the presence of right reason' (Aristotle 1980: VI, 13, 1144b). Although it may seem that virtuous people have limitations on their freedom, they do not because there is no desire for immoral behavior in the first place. Since no restrictions are placed on their desires, individual freedom is maintained and autonomy protected.

If virtue is viewed in an Aristotelian manner, those who received MT may not be similar to those who were virtuous without it. A virtuous person must have not only the desire to perform moral actions but also the tendency, and it is not clear whether MT operates in this manner. Consider the hypothetical case below.

CASE 1

Alex wants to hurt other people. Following a criminal incident, he is arrested and his moral capacity is enhanced by MT to reduce his desire to harm others.

Did Alex become a virtuous person? To answer this question, it is necessary to consider what individual capabilities and characteristics MT affects. If Alex is truly virtuous, then his freedom to act immorally has not been infringed upon. But for that argument to be valid, MT must function in a way where Alex achieves the desire to act morally in accordance with his new character. If MT truly operates in this fashion, however, individual autonomy may be threatened. We address this dilemma in the next section.

2 MT and the hierarchy of 'the self'

Savulescu et al. believed that although MT may modify individual desire and restrict the freedom to act immorally, it does not always violate autonomy. Specifically, MT does not threaten individual autonomy in situations where I) the improper behavior prevented by MT originated from inauthentic or irrational desires, or II) the individual voluntarily chose to receive MT.

The authors used the example of Ulysses and the Sirens to support these situations. According to Greek mythology, Sirens lured sailors with their beautiful singing voices toward rocks and caused them to shipwreck. Despite the danger, Ulysses wanted to listen to these creatures. By ordering his crew to plug their ears with wax and tie him to the ship's mast, Ulysses was able to hear the Sirens and avoid being shipwrecked. Savulescu et al. thus argued that when an individual's rational self gives prior consent to restrict the irrational self and limit personal freedom, autonomy has not been violated.

Acceptance of this argument requires a certain understanding of 'the self'; that is, the hierarchy of individual desires, where upper-level desires (or reason) control lower-level ones. The upper-level ones are considered to be the authentic self and associated with what Frankfurt calls second-order desires (higher desires) (Frankfurt 1971). Using MT to alter or control first-order desires (lower desires) based on these higher desires should not harm the authentic self.

Utilizing these distinctions, let us consider the conditions according to Savulescu et al. that do not harm autonomy. In Situation I, MT does not damage the authentic self because the individual was motivated by desires that were either irrational or did not originate from the authentic self. Therefore, MT does not threaten individual autonomy. In Situation II, consent to receive MT came from the authentic self, thus preserving individual autonomy.

3 What level of 'the self' is controlled by MT?

The previous section raised the question of whether MT controls not only lower desires but also higher desires as well. If higher desires and the authentic self are controlled, then individual autonomy could be harmed. Rather than attempt to determine which human desires MT will affect, let us instead contemplate two possible scenarios: A) MT controls only first-order desires, and B) MT controls both first- and second-order desires. The level of the self MT regulates will result in different problems for each scenario when implementing MT without an individual's consent. Consider the following example of Scenario A below.

CASE 2

Bob not only wants to hurt other people, but also wishes to maintain this desire. After a criminal incident, he is arrested and is subjected to MT to enhance his moral capacity. As a result, Bob no longer has the desire to harm others.

Because MT only altered his first-order desire (i.e. to harm others), Bob still retains his second-order desire (i.e. to maintain the desire to harm others). His second-order desire will continue to not be fulfilled for the duration of the effects of MT, but his authentic self will not have been compromised by other people. Savulescu et al. appeared to have this scenario in mind when they argued that autonomy is not harmed even if MT restrains an individual's freedom to act immorally.

If effective MT was implemented, the number of people who act immorally would decrease. Consequently, violence and crime would also be reduced and greatly benefit society as a whole. The tradeoff, however, is that people with tendencies to act immorally, like Bob, could become frustrated. The impact of this frustration on individuals should be carefully examined prior to considering the implementation of MT.

In consequence of implementation of moral enhancement, a defense mechanism could develop that modifies second-order desires and harmonizes them with the new first-order desires. Bob may eventually rationalize his feelings to appease his frustration and convince himself by saying, 'I never wanted the desire to harm others in the first place.' In this way, Bob's authentic self could be indirectly affected by MT. Therefore, if MT only alters first-order desires, the individual will either suffer the frustration of not being able to desire what s/he originally desired or try to avoid that frustration. The authentic self could thus be exposed to manipulation by others, and we should evaluate any possible modifications of it by MT. This challenge is particularly relevant to Scenario B, with an example below.

CASE 3

Cathy not only wants to hurt other people, but also wishes to maintain this desire. After a criminal incident, she is arrested and is subjected to MT to enhance her moral capacity. As a result, Cathy loses both the desire to harm others and her wish to maintain that desire.

The possibility of manipulating the authentic self by others exists in Scenario A, albeit indirectly. In Scenario B, however, first- and second-order desires of the individual are altered by MT and make the danger of manipulation more direct. The second-order desires, and thus the authentic self, of Cathy are explicitly altered by MT along with her first-order desires. However, modification of the authentic self in people with morally irrational or improper second-order desires, like Bob and Cathy, should not be completely dismissed. The potential value of manipulating an individual's authentic self should lead to discussions of whether it is always unethical.

While discussing the ethical propriety of modifying the authentic self, some may make a moral distinction between cases where modification is indirect (Scenario A) and cases where it is direct (Scenario B). If modification due to the rationalization of unfulfilled desires is permissible from the viewpoint of autonomy in Scenario A but not Scenario B, then the moral difference between the two scenarios should be clarified. Further analysis on the concepts of self and personal identity may be necessary.

To summarize this section, we believe that by controlling desires through MT as depicted in either Scenario A (i.e. only first-order desires are modified) or Scenario B (i.e. first- and second-order desires are modified), individual autonomy is threatened to a greater extent than Savulescu et al. hold. To address this point, we believe it is necessary to examine concepts related to the self and self-identity.

4 Conclusions

According to Aristotle, a virtuous person desires morally correct things and acts without conflict. In contrast, a person with strong self-control desires improper things but has the ability to suppress this desire. These two types of people may not need MT. MT may be necessary, however, for people with weak self-control who can be seduced to do improper things and fail to overcome lower desires, or people who unrepentantly desire improper things and act in immoral ways. Would such individuals even desire MT? In a series of previous articles, Savulescu and Persson argued for MT because appropriate use of current and future scientific technologies may require the enhancement of moral capacity in those who use such technology (Persson and Savulescu 2008; Persson and Savulescu 2010). This argument supports enhanced moral capacity in order to benefit society as a whole. Savulescu et al. also claim that MT may not alter individual autonomy or freedom, although their claim may need further limitations based on our analysis.

If we agree that MT violates freedom or autonomy to an extent, then it would be constructive to consider what justifies the use of MT. For example, should the liberty or autonomy of a few be sacrificed for the greater benefit of society? Arguments in favor of MT are sometimes criticized as they usually side with those who want to implement it rather than those who will receive it. Similar to public health practices, restraints on individual autonomy and freedom may be acceptable for social benefit. Thus, the ethical propriety of MT may need to be considered from the viewpoint of both the government and its citizens.

References

Aristotle. (1980). *Nicomachean Ethics*. Translated by W. D. Ross. Oxford: Oxford University Press.
Frankfurt, H. (1971). 'Freedom of the Will and the Concept of a Person,' *Journal of Philosophy*, 68(1): 5–20.

Harris, J. (2011). 'Moral Enhancement and Freedom,' *Bioethics*, 25: 102–11.

Persson, I. and Savulescu, J. (2008). 'The Perils of Cognitive Enhancement and the Urgent Imperative to Enhance the Moral Character of Humanity,' *Journal of Applied Philosophy*, 25(3): 162–77.

Persson, I. and Savulescu, J. (2010). 'Moral Transhumanism,' *Journal of Medicine and Philosophy*, 35(6): 656–69.

Roskies, A. (2002). 'Neuroethics for the New Millennium,' *Neuron*, 35: 21–3.

3.5

Response to Commentaries

Julian Savulescu, Thomas Douglas, and Ingmar Persson

In our chapter, we argued that moral bioenhancements could preserve autonomy even where they restrict the freedom to act wrongly. We suggested that this would most plausibly be the case where (I) the agent autonomously chooses to undergo the bioenhancement *and* (II) the bioenhancement operates by attenuating an autonomy-restricting desire. And we argued that even in those cases in which it does undermine autonomy, it could still be morally justified in certain circumstances.

Ibuki and Kodama invoke a Frankfurtian hierarchical account of autonomy to argue that MT could threaten autonomy even in the kinds of cases where we suggested it threatens only freedom. It could do this, they suggest, because it could alter the agent's 'authentic' or 'higher' self, which they associate with the agent's second-order desires—her desires regarding her other desires. Ibuki and Kodama suppose that we were imagining cases in which an agent has (i) a putatively contra-moral first-order desire, such as a desire to inflict harm, and (ii) a second-order desire to maintain this first-order desire. They then imagine two different ways in which MT might operate. First, it might directly attenuate only the contra-moral first-order desire. Second, it might directly attenuate the first-order desire *and* alter the second-order desire to align it with the agent's new first-order desire. Regarding the first case, Ibuki and Kodama worry that the agent might, as a 'defense mechanism', modify his second-order desire so as to bring it into line with his first-order desire. For example, if MT has weakened or eliminated an agent's desire to inflict harm, the agent might, over time, also eliminate his desire to possess this desire. In that case, MT would have indirectly influenced the agent's higher self. In the second case, the worry is more obvious: in this case, MT directly influences the agent's higher self. Ibuki and Kodama suggest that, because both of these kinds of MT would alter the agent's higher self, they might threaten autonomy. They would do so, for example, if imposed by one agent on another. The first agent would then, they suggest, be 'manipulating' the higher self of the other.

An initial problem with this argument is that it is not clear why altering another person's higher self entails restricting that person's autonomy. On minimalist Frankfurtian accounts of autonomy, all that is needed for autonomy is that one's first- and second-order desires are aligned—that is, that one's first-order desires are endorsed by one's second-order desires. Though both of the scenarios that Ibuki and Kodama imagine involve (directly or indirectly) altering second-order desires, neither ultimately leaves the agent with unaligned first- and second-order desires, thus neither would threaten autonomy, on the minimalist Frankfurtian view.

Admittedly, there are more sophisticated Frankfurtian accounts which posit more stringent conditions for autonomy. For example, on one view, autonomy requires not only alignment between one's first- and second-order desires but also that this alignment is not the result of inauthentic influences (Dworkin 1981). On this view, MT might restrict autonomy even if it leaves the agent's first- and second-order desires well aligned. However, it will do so only if MT itself qualifies as an inauthentic influence, and Ibuki and Kodama provide no argument to show that it must.

A second and more serious problem with Ibuki and Kodama's argument is that it does not bear on cases in which our suggested conditions—(I) and (II)—hold. In those cases, the agent autonomously chooses to use MT, so we would not have one agent manipulating the higher self of another. Rather, in these cases, the agent would be autonomously altering *her own* higher self, and this would not threaten her autonomy. On any plausible Frankfurtian account, an agent can autonomously adopt actions which alter her second-order desires without thereby compromising her autonomy. Consider a person whose second-order desires change because she chooses to read *Anna Karenina*. Surely there is no assault on autonomy in this case.

Perhaps Ibuki and Kodama's aim was merely to show that autonomy would be threatened in cases where (II) holds, but not (I)—cases, that is, where MT attenuates or blocks an autonomy-restricting desire, but is not undergone autonomously. This would be enough to establish that condition (II) is not sufficient for the preservation of autonomy, which would be an interesting result (though not one that we disputed).

Unfortunately, however, Ibuki and Kodama do not establish even this. This is because the scenarios they discuss are not ones in which MT is used to block or attenuate a non-autonomous desire. In their scenarios, the agent has a contra-moral first-order desire and a second-order desire *to maintain* that contra-moral desire. These cases are, if we accept a Frankfurtian account of autonomy, cases in which nothing is amiss at the outset, at least from the point of view of autonomy; the agent's first- and second-order desires are aligned.[1] In these cases, there is no autonomy-restricting desire for the agent to block or attenuate.

The cases that would most plausibly satisfy condition (II), on a Frankfurtian account, would be cases in which the agent has a contra-moral first-order desire and a second-order desire *to be without* that first-order desire. MT could then be used to block or attenuate the first-order desire. Ibuki and Kodama do not consider such cases, and it is not clear why they would be autonomy-restricting, on a Frankfurtian account.

A final difficulty with Ibuki and Kodama's argument is that it presupposes that a Frankfurtian account of autonomy is correct. In fact, such accounts are dogged with problems of how second-order desires are autonomously formed and regress problems (Thalberg 1978). There are other accounts of autonomy—such as the rationalist account we outlined—that are arguably more plausible and according to which it is irrelevant whether MT alters the agent's second-order desires.

---

[1] We assume here that the second-order desire to maintain the contra-moral first-order desire is not the result of inauthentic forces.

Ibuki and Kodama suggest that we are committed to accepting a Frankfurtian account; our 'argument requires a certain understanding of "the self"; that is, the hierarchy of individual desires, where upper-level desires (or reason) control lower-level ones' (Ibuki and Kodama in this chapter). We do not see why our argument requires this. It does require that some of an agent's desires can be autonomy-restricting, but this is something that can be accommodated by many accounts of autonomy, including the rationalist account that we outline.

Morioka argues we should pursue social rather than biological means to moral enhancement. He points to the dramatic drop in homicide over the last 60 years, which he attributes to increased prosperity and gun control laws. He then argues that future threats, such as the use of extremely powerful biotechnology to kill millions (Persson and Savulescu 2008), should also be addressed using social measures:

The only way to prevent them would be to strictly control the access to those problematic pharmaceutical substances and establish laws to punish individuals for possession of those drugs. Japan has succeeded in prohibiting the possession of guns among ordinary citizens. (Morioka in this chapter)

Sadly, gun control models are unlikely to be effective in tackling the existential threats we face. Modified smallpox virus could potentially obliterate the human population and, within a decade or two, hundreds of thousands of people may have the capacity to create such viruses, thanks to progress in genetic engineering and synthetic biology. It may take only one of these individuals to wreak catastrophic havoc.

The situation is urgent. Persson and Savulescu argued in a recent book (Persson and Savulescu 2012) that we must pursue all avenues open to us. We three have *never* argued against social means to moral improvement. Indeed, we have acknowledged that social means will typically be the most desirable means. However, it is doubtful whether social means will reduce the risk of catastrophic harm to negligible levels. Thus, once social means have been exhausted, there will remain a case for exploring the possibility of moral bioenhancement (Persson and Savulescu 2008). In fact, we tend towards the view that even once all acceptable social *and biological* means to moral improvement have been pursued, there will remain a significant risk of catastrophic harm due to the malevolent use of new technologies. Gun control is important, but it is a vanishingly small part of the existential challenges we face.

Morioka raises another common objection: exploitation of the morally enhanced.

Imagine lifeboat ethics. There are six people on a lifeboat with a capacity for five. One of the six individuals is a morally bioenhanced person. Savulescu, Douglas, and Persson argue that self-sacrifice and altruism are the two central characteristics of morality, and that these traits can be enhanced by biological determinants. If they are right, this morally bioenhanced person in the lifeboat would think that she has to sacrifice herself to save her fellow passengers by her plunging into the sea. As a result, the other five greedy people would be saved. (Morioka in this chapter)

Similarly, he sees people taking oxytocin as enabling others to 'effectively dominate them, use them, and finally exploit them as slaves' (Morioka in this chapter). The morally enhanced would be like indigenous people at the hands of 'wild colonists' (Morioka in this chapter).

And there would be no protection: 'The police whose hearts are filled with empathy and generosity would never be able to complete their mission in emergency situations' (Morioka in this chapter).

Morioka has a very narrow view of what moral enhancement would consist in. We gave altruism and empathy as examples of traits whose augmentation might produce, or be a component in, moral enhancement in some cases. But we explicitly acknowledged that *in some individuals and some circumstances* augmenting these traits would not produce a moral enhancement, and might even result in moral disenhancement. Morioka's examples illustrate this. It is not moral for an altruistic person to give up his life for a bad person. Arguably, it is wrong. It would be an altruistic act to give up his life for three innocent, normal children—and that would surely be laudable. Similarly, it is not moral to always follow the Christian ideal to 'turn the other cheek'. In some cases, aggression is warranted in the face of a grave injustice or wrong.

Moral enhancement is a complex and context-specific process to which many different factors might contribute: moral imagination, empathy, sympathy, altruism, general intelligence, strength of will, sense of justice, willingness to retaliate to moral wrongs, etc. Typical instances of moral enhancement will, we assume, involve altering a number of these traits. There may be some individuals, in some circumstances, who would be morally enhanced by augmenting only one of these traits. (Imagine a person whose only moral defect is a slight lack of empathy.) However, as we have been at pains to emphasize, there is no one of these traits whose augmentation would be sufficient for moral enhancement in all people and all circumstances.

A common strategy in the literature critical of moral bioenhancement has been to single out each of the traits suggested as possibly relevant to moral enhancement by its defenders and show that there are cases in which augmenting this trait would in fact produce moral deterioration (Harris forthcoming). However, this strategy misses the mark. To our knowledge, no one who has defended moral bioenhancement has simplistically posited the augmentation of altruism, sympathy, or any other single trait as a universal basis for moral enhancement.

Finally, Morioka worries that moral sensitivity would make us unhappy—instead of enjoying our expensive dinner we would think of starving people and it would spoil our enjoyment. 'The reason why ordinary people can survive every day would be that they are not so morally sensitive as to worry about such "small" things' (Morioka in this chapter).

People like Peter Singer would argue that morally we should worry more about our expensive selfish tastes and our obligations to others. The fact that our immorality makes us unhappy is, if not a good thing, perhaps a necessary thing for moral improvement. As Singer has argued (and shown), the moral life is in fact perfectly compatible with a truly happy and fulfilled life (Singer 1997).

Morality will inevitably require self-sacrifice. So it will at some deeper level cut into well-being. However, as Sidgwick argued (he called it the Dualism of Practical Reason (Sidgwick 1884)), how the reasons of self-interest are to be weighed against those of morality is one of the deepest questions for ethics. One minimal answer to this question is a duty of easy rescue: when the cost to you of performing some action is small, and the benefit to others is great, then all things considered, you should perform that action. Buying a £30 bottle of wine instead of a £300 bottle for the sake of helping someone else is surely not too much to ask.

There may be a point beyond which moral enhancement is no longer morally required, because it will result in more self-sacrifice than we are morally required to bring about. There may also be a point beyond which augmenting one's disposition to self-sacrifice for the sake of others would no longer qualify as a moral enhancement, say, because it would leave one permanently sick and thus reliant on others. But most of us have scope to morally enhance ourselves a great deal before reaching either of these points.

In any case, concerns about self-sacrifice involved in moral enhancement are not specific to moral *bio*enhancement. If there are limits to how far we must or may go in augmenting our disposition towards self-sacrifice, those limits will apply as much to moral enhancement via introspective reflection, engagement with literature, or moral discussion with others as the will to biological interventions.

Rob Sparrow is in eloquent form, moving gracefully back and forth between incompatible objections. He starts by laying out some criteria for thought experiments and complaining that our thought experiment fails to meet them. 'It is not too much of a stretch, then, to characterize their paper as a thought experiment in service of a thought experiment' (Sparrow in this chapter). But this *is* too much of a stretch. We constructed a thought experiment about being able to change people's intentions and behaviour without their knowledge. Clearly, it is not currently possible to alter people's intentions and behaviour in the fine-grained way that we imagined. However, it is possible to biologically alter intentions and behaviour—including morally relevant intentions and behaviour—in much messier ways. For example, propranolol, oxytocin, and SSRIs have all been shown to have influence on either morally significant behaviour, or moral judgements that are likely to have behavioural effects (Levy et al. forthcoming). Propranolol and SSRIs are widely used drugs, and oxytocin is an endogenously produced agent whose production and release are affected by widely used drugs including steroids. In addition, some drugs are already used in part for their effects on morally significant behaviour: in several European and North American jurisdictions, some sex offenders are offered testosterone-lowering agents ('chemical castration') to help prevent reoffending, and methylphenidate (Ritalin) is widely used in part in order to control what might be regarded as immoral behaviour in schools. Thus, our thought experiment is, like most thought experiments, simply a 'cleaned-up' version of something that is already possible, and indeed is already happening. It has relevance to the moral assessment of drugs that are used in part in order to control moral behaviour (as in the case of methylphenidate and testosterone-lowering agents) and of drugs that are used for other purposes but are likely to have effects on moral behaviour (such as propranolol and SSRIs).

Having criticized our argument for lacking practical relevance, Sparrow then takes the reverse tack, speculating that 'there is a real danger that their [our] argument will license attempts to manipulate behaviour through drugs and brain implants, which raise profound moral issues that they [we] barely mention' (Sparrow in this chapter). But if this is a thought experiment about a thought experiment, with no real-world application, how could it license attempts to use drugs or brain implants to manipulate behaviour? Either we are engaging in armchair philosophical speculation with no practical application or we are discussing something that could be real. Sparrow criticizes us for both at the same time.

Moreover, he does not substantiate either accusation. On the one hand, it is not clear why mere armchair speculation on the topic of moral enhancement would be a bad thing. After all, armchair speculation is the modus operandi of most philosophers outside practical ethics. Sparrow worries that our argument 'does not illuminate a pressing moral dilemma' and suggests that '[t]he matter of how and why it has become the case that bioethicists feel compelled to discuss the ethics of every hypothetical technology that cannot be shown to be impossible is worthy of an essay in its own right' (Sparrow in this chapter). But it is not clear what is positively wrong with such hypothetical speculation, and Sparrow seems to acknowledge that it does have some philosophical interest: 'As a piece of philosophy their argument is indeed thought provoking and has significant merits' (Sparrow in this chapter). Would Sparrow raise similar concerns regarding the work of most metaphysicians and logicians, which also illuminates no pressing moral dilemma but is hopefully of some philosophical interest?

On the other hand, Sparrow does not adduce convincing evidence that our argument is likely to be misused to devastating effect. As one of us (Julian Savulescu) argues in his response to Sparrow's chapter, any prediction that reasonable bioethical discussion will somehow lead to an atrocious outcome must be backed up by more than mere speculation.

We argued in our paper that some forms of moral enhancement would not undermine freedom because they could act, for example, by opening up someone to understanding the suffering of others, like reading Tolstoy. Sparrow objects: 'Someone who reads Tolstoy arguably learns *reasons* to be less judgemental and in doing so develops greater understanding: someone who takes a pill has merely *caused* their sentiments to alter. In so far as moral action requires acting for the right reasons, the person who has learned tolerance from Tolstoy has more and better reasons for action' (Sparrow in this chapter).

But learning is something that we can be more or less good at. Biological manipulations can enhance learning abilities. It is a common mistake to assume that all moral bioenhancements would directly alter sentiments and thereby directly alter behaviour, leaving our deliberative capacities entirely out of the picture. Actually, it may be the case for many that they act by augmenting the normal processes by which we form moral motivations and learn to be moral. Indeed, one of us has previously characterized the most plausible examples of moral enhancement as interventions that alleviate barriers to (among other things) sound moral reasoning (Douglas 2008). Just as steroids do not make a person stronger without physical training, just as cognitive enhancements do not produce enhanced knowledge or cognitive skill without learning, so too moral enhancements may not produce more moral behaviour without precisely the activities that Sparrow has in mind. They would just increase the magnitude or likelihood of the benefit from those experiences.

Sparrow suggests that 'There is an obvious tension between their description of the naturally virtuous person as someone for whom it is psychologically or motivationally out of the question to do wrong and their later claim that autonomy requires the vivid imagination of alternatives' (Sparrow in this chapter). But we do not see this tension. A person can vividly imagine an option while nevertheless being so strongly motivated not to pursue that alternative that it is rightly described as 'out of the question'. Indeed, the alternative might be 'out of the question' precisely because the agent imagines how horrible the consequences of that alternative would be. Moreover, it does not follow from the fact that it is motivationally out of the question for the agent to do an immoral act that he is unfree in any morally problematic way. It remains the case that the agent could have acted wrongly.

Of course, in our case of 'perfect mind control' the agent *is* unfree in a morally important way: he genuinely can't act wrongly. But we argued that even in these cases, the agent may still be fully autonomous. Regarding this case, Sparrow raises some interesting points. For example, he argues that 'given that people who are subject to the magical 'moral technology' are *not* free to do anything other than act morally, this suggests that there is an important sense in which they do not act freely even when they choose to act in such a way that the technology does not intervene' (Sparrow in this chapter). This assumes incompatibilism about free will. We do not wish to enter this complex debate, but according to compatibilism, freedom can exist even if determinism is true, that is, even if we could never have acted other than we did. If freedom is compatible with complete determinism, it is compatible with the moral technology we describe.

Sparrow closes with his political critique, similar in vein to his chapter in this volume. He argues that much choice is socially constructed, using the spread of obesity since 1985 as a case in point. The origin of behaviour—in individual free choice or through social construction—is indeed interesting. But it is not our target. We have not argued that 'social problems [are] rooted in biology' (Sparrow in this chapter). We are interested in how behaviour can be biologically modified, whether it is biological, psychological, or social in origin, or some combination of those. It is certainly true that social means can be effective at modifying behaviour. And it may even be true that all our problems are social in origin. We have sought to explore whether biological means can also be employed to deal with these problems and whether their employment would raise new or irresolvable ethical issues.

Sparrow worries that 'the project of "moral bioenhancement" invites…abuse: it assumes that we know what moral behaviour in various circumstances consists in, where in fact this is, within limits, controversial and should also remain so; it will almost certainly involve the powerful acting on the powerless' (Sparrow in this chapter).

There is certainly controversy about what is right and good. But there is also consensus (Smith 1994). Racism and sexism are wrong. Sexual abuse of young children is wrong. In our recent book, two of us (Ingmar Persson and Julian Savulescu) have focused on the collective action problem of climate change, gross global inequality, and threat of annihilation of the human race (Persson and Savulescu 2012). These are all uncontroversially bad states of affairs and we have sought to understand what role knowledge of human biology might play in the future in addressing these.

The powerful have many ways already ready at hand to oppress the powerless. It is hard to see how they need the project of moral bioenhancement to exercise their power. It is precisely the kind of oppression that Sparrow fears which is the target of our concerns: how could we use knowledge of the nature of the human animal to prevent the kind of oppression that already has occurred with relentless frequency and in atrocious magnitude? History has not been rosy (Glover 2001). With the exponentially increasing power of technology together with globalization, the tendency of humans to oppress and harm each other reaches critical mass. More than ever, we require a project of moral enhancement using our knowledge from medicine and science in general.

References

Douglas, T. (2008). 'Moral Enhancement', *Journal of Applied Philosophy*, 25(3): 228–45.

Dworkin, G. (1981). 'The Concept of Autonomy', in R. Haller (ed.), *Science and Ethics*. Amsterdam: Rodopi, 203–13.

Glover, J. (2001). *Humanity: A Moral History of the Twentieth Century*. New Haven, CT: Yale Nota Bene.

Harris, J. (Forthcoming). 'Moral Progress and Moral Enhancement', *Bioethics*, Advance online publication, 19 June 2012. DOI: 10.1111/j.1467-8519.2012.01965.x

Ibuki, T. and Kodama, S. (2014). 'Moral Technology and the Concept of "the Self"', in A. Akabayashi (ed.), *The Future of Bioethics: International Dialogues*. Oxford: Oxford University Press, 126–30.

Levy, N. et al. (Forthcoming). 'Are You Morally Modified? The Moral Effects of Widely Used Pharmaceuticals', *Philosophy, Psychiatry, and Psychology*.

Morioka, M. (2014). 'Some Remarks on Moral Bioenhancement', in A. Akabayashi (ed.), *The Future of Bioethics: International Dialogues*. Oxford: Oxford University Press, 120–5.

Persson, I. and Savulescu, J. (2008). 'The Perils of Cognitive Enhancement and the Urgent Imperative to Enhance the Moral Character of Humanity', *Journal of Applied Philosophy*, 25(3): 162–77.

Persson, I. and Savulescu, J. (2012). *Unfit for the Future: The Need for Moral Enhancement*. Oxford: Oxford University Press.

Sidgwick, H. (1884). *The Methods of Ethics*. London: Macmillan.

Singer, P. (1997). *How Are We to Live? Ethics in an Age of Self-Interest*. Oxford: Oxford University Press.

Smith, M. (1994). *The Moral Problem*. Malden, MA: Blackwell.

Sparrow, R. (2013). 'Im(Moral) Technology? Thought Experiments and the Future of "Mind Control"', in A. Akabayashi (ed.), *The Future of Bioethics: International Dialogues*. Oxford: Oxford University Press, 113–19.

Thalberg, I. (1978). 'Hierarchical Analyses of Unfree Action', *Canadian Journal of Philosophy*, 8(2): 211–26.

4.1

Primary Topic Article
Ethics, Eugenics, and Politics

Robert Sparrow

Introduction

Philosophers are often accused of having their heads in the clouds. The sight of bioethicists earnestly discussing the ethics of human enhancement is unlikely to disillusion anyone.[1] The ethics of human enhancement is perhaps the hottest topic in applied ethics and bioethics today. While this debate extends to include the ethics of enhancement using pharmaceuticals and biomedical implants, the core of the enhancement debate is discussion about the ethics of the 'new' eugenics—the project of enhancing future human beings using recombinant DNA technology, cloning, and preimplantation genetic diagnosis (PGD).

For most people outside the circles of professional philosophy and bioethics, talk about human enhancement—let alone about 'eugenics'—conjures up visions of Nazi scientists and other racists making nonsensical claims about Aryan supremacy. It therefore typically comes as a great surprise to people to learn that not only is there a serious discussion of human enhancement going on in these disciplines but that the majority of philosophers and bioethicists writing about human enhancement today support it.

Obviously, very few—if any—of the philosophers and bioethicists writing about human enhancement have any sympathy for National Socialism. The contemporary debate about enhancement is therefore premised on the idea that it is possible to describe and defend a 'new' morally defensible—or perhaps even praiseworthy—eugenics that is distinct from and will not lead to the 'old', bad, Nazi, and Fabian eugenics. While the precise details of what distinguishes this 'new eugenics' from the 'old' remain controversial (Kitcher 1996; Wikler 1999), two features may plausibly be taken to be characteristic of the new eugenics: first, the new eugenicists are concerned with the welfare of

---

[1] Major figures in the debate about human enhancement have discussed the ethics of the pursuit of 'radio-telepathy' (Silver 1999: 278–80), of introducing artificial chromosomes into the human genome in order to allow future individuals to choose whether and when to turn on and off particular genes (Stock 2003), and of genetically modifying human beings so that they are more 'moral' (Persson and Savulescu 2008). It is therefore hard to avoid the impression that this debate is at least somewhat fantastic.

Morton College Library Cicero, ILL

individuals rather than with the health or welfare of populations such as 'nations', 'races', or 'the species'; second, an insistence that the human rights of parents (and children) must not be infringed by the pursuit of eugenic goals (Buchanan 1996: 18–19; Wikler 1999; Agar 2004: 3–16).

In this chapter I want to suggest that the debate about human enhancement has, for the most part, taken place in a dangerously rarefied sphere and has neglected important political realities. While on paper it may be possible to sketch out visions of a world in which the pursuit of genetic enhancement of human beings does not lead to a renewed interest in racial hygiene and widespread violations of human rights, the political assumptions one must make in order to hold that this is possible in the real world are—I will argue—excessively optimistic. In reality, the pursuit of human enhancement is all too likely to lead us back to something that looks very much like the old eugenics wherein the state is, as a matter of routine, licensing who is allowed to have children and what sort of children they are allowed to have, and thus infringing the reproductive liberty of parents. Similarly, the notion that states will confine the use of technologies of genetic enhancement to the promotion of the welfare of those who are 'enhanced' and will resist the temptation to engineer some for the benefits of others also relies on a number of dubious assumptions about the political cultures of the societies in which genetic technologies are likely to be used.

This chapter will therefore sketch a political critique of recent arguments for human enhancement. I will argue that the intellectual distance between the old and the new eugenics is much smaller than contemporary advocates of human enhancement acknowledge. I will also suggest that in the absence of a naive faith in the resilience of liberal democratic political cultures there is a very real danger that genetic technologies will be used for social engineering and not just for the benefit of individuals. A more realistic politics should lead us to be much more cautious about defending the 'rights' of parents to enhance their children. This, in turn, has implications for the ethics of advocating human enhancement in the philosophical literature. At the very least, future discussions of the ethics of enhancement should pay much more attention to the political preconditions and presuppositions of claims about any putative moral obligation to enhance future human beings.

Technologies of genetic enhancement

The theoretical possibility of altering human genetics has existed since the first genetically modified bacteria were created in 1973 or perhaps even since Hermann Muller showed that it was possible to induce mutations in fruit flies in the late 1920s.[2] Certainly science fiction has featured 'enhanced', genetically modified, human beings from the late 1930s onwards.[3] However, recombinant DNA technology is still not reliable enough to use to modify human beings in any except the direst medical emergency. Moreover,

---

[2] See Carlson (1981). Muller himself wrote extensively about the implications of his work for the project of improving society through genetic manipulation. My thanks to Russell Blackford for suggesting the importance of Muller in this context.

[3] See, for instance, Wylie (1930). My thanks to Russell Blackford for directing me to this source.

demonstrating that any technology that involves manipulating human embryos *in vitro* is safe is extremely difficult given that ideally one would want to wait until a large number of people who had been modified *in vitro* had lived a full lifespan before venturing this assessment.[4] Thus it would be a brave parent indeed who set out to genetically modify their child.

Perhaps because of this, more recent discussions of enhancement have concentrated on the idea that it might become possible to enhance future human beings by using PGD. The Human Genome Project holds out the hope that we might come to learn which genes or combinations of genes are associated with desirable phenotypes. If we discover reliable associations then we might be able to improve the life prospects of future human beings by selecting embryos with genes for 'above species-typical' capacities. The power of PGD as an enhancement technology will itself be greatly magnified if—as recent results using human stem cells suggest—it becomes possible to derive ova from induced pluripotent stem cells. This would allow couples to overcome the limit on the number of embryos that they can create and choose amongst, which is currently imposed by the small number of ova that can be gathered in each cycle of IVF. Finally, were it to become possible, human cloning via somatic cell nuclear transfer would be a powerful technology of human enhancement in so far as it would allow us to bring people into the world with a known genotype.

A not-so-new eugenics?

Defenders of human enhancement may be arguing (1) that parents should be permitted to enhance their children or (2) that they are morally obligated to do so. Obviously, the second position includes and is significantly stronger than the first. However, a central question in thinking about the politics of human enhancement is whether the first position inevitably slides into the second. I will consider this matter below.

The second position also admits of at least two variations. Those arguing that there is an obligation to enhance may be arguing: a) that there is an obligation to provide particular enhancements or enhancements up to some threshold; or, b) that parents are obligated to provide all available enhancements so as to have 'the best children possible'.

The latter, stronger, claim plays a peculiar role in the contemporary debate about enhancement. One of the main figures in the enhancement debate, Julian Savulescu (2001a; 2005; 2008), has advanced this claim with particular enthusiasm and has been echoed in this by his various co-authors. John Harris (2007) also appears to be committed to this claim, as do some of *his* co-authors (Chan and Harris 2007). If the relevant metric by which to determine the 'best' child is the child's expected welfare—or

---

[4] In practice, medical researchers have proved surprisingly willing to trial reproductive technologies that must essentially remain experimental until a whole generation has passed. If one holds that individuals cannot be harmed by actions that bring them into existence, then such experiments will be justifiable as long as researchers have taken all reasonable precautions to prevent children being born with lives 'not worth living'. Alternatively, if one allows the willingness to risk the welfare of the first individuals created by, for instance, IVF to set the required standard of caution then further development of reproductive technologies may not appear unethical.

perhaps the child's parents' estimation of their expected welfare—then it may appear as though the desire to conceive the 'best child' follows inevitably from parents' concern for their child's welfare or perhaps even simply from the fact that rational agents are concerned to secure the best outcome in relation to their own desires (Savulescu 2001a; Savulescu 2008). Yet the authors of what is undoubtedly the most thorough attempt by professional philosophers to think through the ethics of human enhancement to date dismiss this idea as an obvious non-starter, pointing out that, when it comes to environmental interventions into the well-being of a child, very few, if any, parents do *everything* they can to provide their child with the best possible life, as doing so would deprive them of any time or resources to dedicate to their own interests (Buchanan et al. 2000: 161–2; Glover 2006: 54). The idea that we should *maximize* our children's welfare therefore appears to derive most of its currency in the enhancement debate from the desire of advocates of enhancement to court controversy by making the strongest possible claim and the fact that this claim then serves as a convenient stalking horse for critics of human enhancement.

I will begin by discussing the policy implications of the stronger case for human enhancement, that parents are morally obligated to enhance their children. As I have recently argued at length in the *Hastings Center Report*, there is a significant tension between the claim that parents are morally obligated to enhance their children and the claim that they should never be coerced to do so, especially where the first claim is founded in a maximizing, consequentialist, moral philosophy (Sparrow 2011a). Because my interest here is in the politics of the new eugenics, I will be mainly concerned with the question as to what sorts of *means* might be justified to ensure that parents live up to their obligations to 'enhance'. However, because our assessment of the ethics of means is inevitably and properly influenced by the ends to which they are directed, I will quickly note that the ends advocated by at least some leading proponents of the new eugenics are much less attractive than the literature generally acknowledges.

The claim that we are morally obligated to have the 'best child possible' more-or-less immediately has a number of startling implications.

First, as 'best' is a maximizing notion, in any given environment there will only be one 'best genome'. It would therefore appear that all the parents sharing an environment should aspire to bring into existence a child produced by cloning from the same, 'best', embryo. It also follows that parents do something wrong if they choose to reproduce naturally or even choose one of their own embryos after PGD rather than a clone of an embryo with a better genome. There are very few couples who could plausibly claim that even their best child was the 'best possible'.[5]

Second, in so far as our only concern is the expected welfare of the child and in the absence of the belief that the possession of normal human capacities marks out a morally significant point on the spectrum of possible genomes, parents will be morally obligated to shape their children to suit their expected social environment as much as their physical environment. Being born with the 'wrong' skin colour will severely reduce a child's

---

[5] In a recent discussion of procreative beneficence, Savulescu and Kahane (2009) limit the force of the putative obligation of procreative beneficence to choosing the best child from amongst the parents' possible biological children. However, they provide no justification for this qualification.

life prospects in a racist society; thus parents will have reason to ensure that their child is born with local marks of beauty and privilege (Sparrow 2007). Advocates of *enhancement* can hardly object that this would involve the use of medical technology to modify or select against a normal human trait. Arguing that parental obligations are properly responsive to concerns about what sort of society we wish to live in—for instance, by suggesting that parents should not reinforce injustice through their eugenic choices— undercuts the distinction between the old and the new eugenics by revealing the new eugenics also to be concerned with the character of the nation.

Third, as I have argued at length elsewhere, it appears that we should have a strong preference in relation to the sex of our children (Sparrow 2010a; Sparrow 2010c). The presence or absence of a Y-chromosome will have a much greater impact on the shape of a child's life than the vast majority of the genes that bioethicists have been concerned about in the enhancement debates. If we want our child to have the best prospects then we will need to decide whether they are more likely to have a better life if they are born male or female and then choose their sex accordingly (Sparrow 2011b).

Together, these observations imply that in societies wherein wealth and social power are associated with being white, male, and heterosexual, for example, parents who wish to have the 'best child possible' should choose to bring into existence only good-looking, heterosexual, white men (indeed, the first observation suggests that they should all procure a clone of the same 'perfect' child) (Sparrow 2007).

The more plausible claim that parents are obligated to enhance their children so that they achieve some threshold level of well-being need not have these problematic— some would say, repugnant—implications. The required threshold might be set at such a level as to allow that women (or men) or racial minorities may be judged to have sufficient expected well-being such that parents have no obligation to avoid bringing members of these groups into existence. Yet, equally well, any threshold account *may* have the consequence that members of minorities in unjust societies will not meet the threshold. Indeed, it seems likely that this will usually be the case for some minorities. Moreover, accounts that admit an obligation to enhance up to a threshold confront a serious difficulty in explaining why the obligation to improve our children's welfare should lapse once the particular threshold they advocate has been reached. It is for this reason that Harris and Savulescu argue that parents should maximize their children's welfare.

Already, then, we see how the real world of power and privilege impacts on arguments about enhancement so as to bring them to conclusions that are much more like those of the old eugenics than contemporary advocates of enhancement advertise. However, the small distance between the new eugenics and the old only really becomes apparent when we turn to consider the question of what sort of means would be appropriate for the state to adopt once we grant the existence of reasons for parents to have the best child possible.

By definition, 'enhancements' are good for those who receive them (Harris 2007). When we are considering alterations to the capacities of existing adults, it makes good sense to leave it up to individuals to decide whether particular changes to their capacities would be enhancements or not. However, as the technologies to modify the human genome require the manipulation of human life at the embryonic stage, the new eugenics involves shaping *future* persons. This has—at least—two important implications. First, it suggests that we must exercise significant caution in determining what sorts of change-es might count as enhancements to future persons. Only changes that could be expected to improve an individual's chances of success in pursuit of a wide variety of different life plans—or that could be argued to increase well-being according to some objective measure independent of individuals' desires—can unequivocally be classed as enhance-ments (Agar 1998; Dekker 2009). Second—and more importantly for the purposes of the current investigation—it establishes a prima facie case that the state should take an interest in parental decisions about enhancement. These decisions do not only—or even primarily—involve the interests of parents but also the interests of future citizens. And, in modern societies at least, the state is the organization that we have empowered to protect the interests of those who cannot currently protect their own interests, includ-ing future citizens. Thus, for instance, when it comes to the welfare of children, we do not typically grant that parents have unlimited authority in the matter. Where parents are wilfully and seriously neglectful of their child's well-being, the state may intervene in order to protect the interests of the child (Feinberg 1980). Were it to become possible, then, to significantly enhance future human beings the question would immediately arise as to whether these enhancements should be made mandatory.

John Harris (2007) and Julian Savulescu (2002) have independently argued that it would be wrong to establish *laws* requiring parents to enhance their children by draw-ing on an essentially libertarian account of when state coercion is justified. They hold that—as John Stuart Mill argued—the state is only justified in interfering with indi-vidual liberty when an individual's actions would otherwise generate harms to oth-ers. One might think that a parent's failure to enhance their child might constitute harm sufficient to justify legislation. However, a philosophical subtlety about the nature of the technologies involved in the new eugenics renders this unclear. As Harris and Savulescu point out, selection of embryos for above species-typical capacities using PGD and (possibly) genetic modification of embryos using recombinant DNA tech-nology both involve choosing *which* individuals will come into existence rather than altering the well-being of a determinate individual.[6] In Parfit's terminology, these are non-person-affecting decisions (Parfit 1984). What this means is that the people who are born as a result of these decisions are arguably unable to hold that they have been harmed (or benefited) by them. The counterfactual that normally underpins attribu-tions of harming or benefiting (what would their well-being be if the decision had been made differently?) fails in cases like this because had the decision been made differently they would not have existed at all (instead, another person would have existed in their place). Thus, while we may still have consequentialist reasons to enhance children based on a concern for the total amount of well-being in the world, if this analysis is correct then the failure to enhance children will not harm them and so legislation requiring enhancement will not be justified—as long as we adopt a Millian account of the limits of the appropriate use of state power.

---

[6] The later claim, about genetic modification, is controversial and depends upon the thesis that genetic modification of the early-stage human embryo would alter the identity and not just the traits of the person who is born as a result (Zohar 1991).

In a moment, I will query whether we can rely upon the assumption that legislators will abide by the strict restrictions that Mill placed on the exercise of their power.[7] However, first, I want to note that even if parents' decisions about enhancement cannot harm their children, they may harm other existing citizens and that these harms might justify state intervention. In any society that maintains a system of redistributive taxation, bringing children into the world who will have a lower standard of well-being by virtue of not being enhanced will impose avoidable costs on other citizens, whose tax dollars will flow towards these new poor. Even in the absence of such redistributive flows, to the extent that social inequality impacts negatively on the quality of life of all members of the society, parents who allow their children to be born with lower life prospects than other citizens will harm their compatriots.

Of course, whether these harms would be sufficient to justify state intervention is unclear: it would depend upon a myriad of details about particular cases. However, a more important question is why we should expect the state to refrain from regulating parents' choices around enhancement even granted that these do not harm existing persons.

Let me begin by noting that there is at least one important set of cases where we already allow that it is appropriate for the state to legislate in order to prevent non-person-affecting consequences: pollution of the environment. As Parfit observed, some forms of pollution may generate negative impacts mainly for future generations. If the emission of the pollution also alters (by subtly affecting who has children with whom and at what time) which people are born, then these impacts will not be person-affecting. Yet it seems entirely fair to point to the impact of the pollution on the welfare of the future population as justification as to why the state should legislate to prevent such pollution.

It is also worth observing that the consequentialist arguments that Harris and Savulescu provide for embracing enhancement provide little support for the idea that we should always accept a Millian restriction on the limits of the proper exercise of the power of the state in the context of non-person-affecting harms. If non-person-affecting enhancements do not harm anyone, neither do they benefit anyone. Thus if we are going to have reason to pursue them this must derive from their contribution to the total welfare existing (in the world? in our society?) in the future. And once we adopt a consequentialist perspective then we should respect rights and liberty only in so far as such respect leads to better consequences than the alternative. If enhancing future individuals would make a sufficiently large difference to total welfare then the state *would*— on consequentialist grounds, at least—be justified in legislating to ensure that parents enhance their children (Sparrow 2011a).

Regardless of whether the exercise of state power is justified, though, the new eugenics presumes that it will not be used. This relies on a number of assumptions about the

[7] Elsewhere, I have argued that there are various measures short of coercion that the state or, indeed, groups of concerned citizens might adopt to try to encourage parents to have 'better' babies (Sparrow 2011a). While these measures would not threaten the reproductive liberty of parents, the existence of public campaigns, whether organized by the state or by private individuals, to encourage parents to have certain sorts of children should be a cause of extreme discomfort to those aware of the history of eugenics.

political cultures of the societies in which human enhancement may become possible, several of which seem to be extremely dubious. These assumptions also play a critical role in the arguments surrounding less ambitious endorsements of the new eugenics. I will therefore return to them after first discussing the philosophical logic of 'liberal eugenics'.

The logic of liberal eugenics

Not every writer discussing the ethics of human enhancement embraces the idea that we are morally obligated to enhance our children once it becomes possible to do so. A number of authors have argued for the weaker—and more plausible—position that it would be morally permissible for parents to use genetic technology to enhance their children (Robertson 1994; Buchanan et al. 2000; Agar 2004). These authors emphasize the freedom of parents to make decisions about whether or not to enhance their children and what sorts of enhancements to pursue; for this reason their position has come to be known as 'liberal eugenics'.[8] However, because parental genetic interventions might severely constrain the life options available to their children, advocates of liberal eugenics must also be concerned with the liberty of children.

In another context, I have argued that both a concern for the liberty of parents and a concern for the liberty of future citizens ground powerful arguments for a strong role for the state in any future wherein enhancement is possible (Sparrow 2010b). In order to avoid collective action problems arising out of the free choices of parents and, in particular, to avoid the prospect of a 'genetic rat race' wherein parents must enhance their children in order to avoid them being disadvantaged by other parents' pursuit of positional goods for *their* children, it may be necessary for the state to regulate access to enhancements. And in order to prevent parents from locking their children into the pursuit of the parents' chosen way of life through genetic manipulation, the state must regulate to defend the future liberty of children (Feinberg 1980; Davis 2001; Agar 2004; Fox 2007).

For these reasons, a plausible liberal eugenics must include a very strong role for the state in regulating genetic interventions—a result that further problematizes the distinction between the new and the old eugenics. Nothing I have said so far suggests that a liberal eugenics need lead to egregious human rights violations of the sorts associated with the old eugenics. However, even in the absence of such violations, the pervasive and routine involvement of the state in deciding what sort of people will be born is profoundly problematic for at least three reasons.

First, it would involve widespread violation of 'reproductive liberty'. As a number of authors have argued, the intimate nature of human reproduction, and the centrality

---

[8] Because, as I discussed above, advocates of an obligation to enhance typically resile from the conclusion that the state should legislate to ensure that parents meet this obligation, they may also be described as defending a version of 'liberal eugenics' although, as I have argued, in this case the connection with liberalism is merely contingent. To the extent that advocates of an obligation to enhance wish to insist upon retaining a liberal institutional framework for regulating genetic interventions, the criticisms developed in this section will also apply to the arguments discussed above.

of decisions about reproduction to individuals' life plans establishes a strong presumption that people should be allowed to make these decisions themselves (Dworkin 1993; Brock 1994; Robertson 1994). It may appear odd to invoke a concern for reproductive liberty in the course of a critique of human enhancement given that advocates of enhancement themselves typically highlight the importance of reproductive liberty in order to motivate the idea that parents have a right to determine the genetics of their children (Savulescu 1999; Savulescu 2001a; Harris 2004). Yet if a liberal eugenics is to promote both the liberty of parents and the liberty of future citizens, it must both claim the right to interfere with parental choices *and* routinely interfere with them in order to prevent worse outcomes for the liberty of both children and parents.

Second, if the state is going to take on this role, it must draw upon a substantive and therefore controversial account of the range of plausible conceptions of the good life in order to do so. There is no way to determine whether a particular genetic intervention reduces or increases the modified individual's prospects of achieving a good life for themselves that does not—whether explicitly or implicitly—make reference to evaluations about what sorts of lives might reasonably be held to be good. Similarly, if less obviously, deciding whether or not to restrict individual choice in order to prevent a destructive genetic rat race requires a judgement as to whether the benefit that parents might pursue for their children is a positional or an absolute good, which cannot be determined except by reference to an account of what sorts of things contribute to an individual's well-being. Thus not only will the state be interfering in parents' reproductive liberty but it will be doing so in the service of a controversial account of what will improve the lives of its citizens.

Third, regulation to avoid collective action problems—typically to preserve public goods—requires paying attention to the aggregate consequences of uncoordinated individual decisions (Brock 2005). That is to say, the state will need to be concerned with the character of the society or nation that might be produced if parents make various eugenic choices. This significantly undercuts the idea that the new eugenics can be distinguished from the old by virtue of its focus on the welfare of individuals rather than collectivities. Even if the motivation for this concern remains the welfare of the individuals within the society, this is not sufficient to distinguish a liberal eugenic policy from more obviously problematic eugenic projects such as, for instance, that described in Huxley's *Brave New World*.

The argument of this section has been concerned with the philosophical logic of a liberal eugenics. Again, we have seen how the fact that people live in societies and the ways in which their decisions may affect each other—in other words, politics—transforms the new eugenics into something much closer to the old. Yet, as I intimated above, the real worry about the new eugenics is not its philosophical logic but rather its cultural or political logic.

Politics and eugenics

The writers I have been discussing believe that the pursuit of human enhancement would be justified if it respected the human rights of individuals and if it were dedicated to improving the welfare of enhanced individuals. Yet a crucial question, which is largely neglected in the literature on the new eugenics, is how likely it is that these two conditions would be realized in practice. The last time nations tried to use their knowledge of genetics to improve human beings was a disaster. What reasons do we have for thinking it would be any different if we took up this project now?

There are strong prima facie grounds for concern about the interaction between politics and technologies of genetic selection, especially in the light of the historical experience of eugenics. The project of genetic human enhancement risks encouraging elitism, discrimination, and social engineering.

Genetic selection risks encouraging elitism and discrimination because of the cultural and political slippage between claims about genes and claims about those who possess them. A number of authors, writing in the debate about the 'expressivist' critique of prenatal testing, have argued that there is no *necessary* connection between the belief that it would be better to be born with (or without) particular genes and the belief that those people born with particular genes are inferior persons (Buchanan et al. 2000: 276–81; Steinbock 2000). However, while the distinction between an evaluation of the impact of genes on individuals' welfare and an evaluation of their implications for their worth may be plausible at the level of individual belief, there are powerful social forces in most, if not all, contemporary societies that make it difficult to sustain this distinction at the level of social beliefs. In divided and inegalitarian societies, those at the top of the social heap have a strong interest in promoting the idea that the current social hierarchy is natural. The same research that has sparked the contemporary philosophical interest in genetics has also contributed to an increasing geneticization of human life, which in turn encourages the idea that genetics is destiny. If people with better genes have 'better lives', then it is a small step indeed to the thought that they are better people. The fact that leading philosophers (Harris 1998; Savulescu 2005) have described enhanced human beings as a 'new breed', as though there would be a qualitative difference between enhanced and unenhanced human beings, is a telling indication of just how tempting is this slippage.

There are a number of ways in which the development of the power to shape the genetics of future human beings is likely to encourage the use of this power to achieve social goals and not just to advance the welfare of enhanced individuals. As I observed above, once technologies of genetic human enhancement become available, states will not be able to avoid paying attention to their aggregate impacts if they wish to avoid various negative outcomes. Yet as soon as states begin to regulate parental choices with an eye to their social consequences it will be extremely tempting to focus directly on what sort of society they wish to govern and to engineer people to achieve this goal. It is already the case that an important reason why some governments subsidize access to prenatal testing in order to allow parents to terminate the pregnancy if they receive a diagnosis of a condition associated with disability is to reduce the social costs associated with caring for people with disabilities. There is also, I think, more 'folk' support for such social engineering than the debate about human enhancement typically acknowledges: I am repeatedly surprised by how many of my students studying genetics or bioethics advance arguments about the evolution or the progress of the species in support of human enhancement. The role played by consequentialist reasoning in the arguments for human enhancement is significant here both because of the focus of consequentialism on total social welfare rather than respect for individual rights and also because of the historical association between utilitarianism and utopian programmes of social engineering.

On the other hand, there are two reasons that I can see why one might hold that the future of eugenic selection will be brighter than its past. First, one might hold that the new eugenics is based upon superior science to the old. Second, one might hold that contemporary societies have deeper and more resilient cultures of respect for human rights than those that violated human rights in the service of eugenic goals in the past.

There is an obvious sense in which the first of these claims is clearly correct. Human genetics has advanced in leaps and bounds since the turn of the twentieth century. More importantly, in some circles at least, the vital lesson that genotype only produces phenotype in a given environment has been well and truly learnt.

However, again, there is a large gap between the claim about scientific progress and a claim about the extent to which this progress is likely to be reflected in politics. Many popular discussions of genetics continue to be bedevilled by a failure to distinguish between biological phenomena that might plausibly be explained with reference to genes and social phenomena that may not. Thus, the media flock to report claims about a 'gay gene', despite the fact that while there might be a gene for being attracted to people of the same sex, being gay is a social identity that can shift with context and circumstance and is thus incapable of being explained by biology (not every individual who has sex with people of the same sex either identifies themselves as gay or is identified by others as gay). Similarly, the claim that there is a genetics of aggression is increasingly popular even though whether behaviour is classified as aggressive or not will depend upon the social context (on the rugby field or in the philosophy seminar) in which it takes place. Indeed, this confusion between social and biological categories seems even to infect some of Savulescu's work, where he has argued for eugenic selection against genes 'for criminality' (Savulescu 2001b; Savulescu et al. 2006). Yet criminals share nothing in common other than that their activities have been ruled by the state to be illegal (legislators can create or abolish criminals with the stroke of a pen!). Thus, while there may well be genes that make various behaviours (assuming that these can be suitably described without reference to social classifications) more or less likely, there cannot possibly be a gene that determines whether or not someone is 'a criminal'. If science journalists and bioethicists can make these sorts of errors, there is little cause to hope that the broader population will not seize upon genetic explanations for social phenomena and then demand that politicians adopt genetic solution to social problems. In this context, it is also worth noting that in many supposedly advanced industrial societies the level of scientific literacy in the broader community is woefully low.

It is the second of the two claims introduced above—that contemporary societies are more deeply committed to respecting individual freedom than those that embraced the old eugenics—that, I believe, mostly explains philosophers' willingness to reconsider the possibility of genetic selection. Ideas of moral and intellectual progress are deeply entrenched in the political cultures of 'Western' nations as well as in the self-understanding of the discipline of moral philosophy. It is therefore extremely tempting for intellectuals in these traditions to believe that the extensive violations of human rights that occurred when eugenic ideas were taken up in the early 1900s could not happen again. Unfortunately, this belief reflects both a selective understanding of historical politics and a rose-tinted view of contemporary political circumstances. The nations that embraced eugenics in the 1920s and 1930s included societies with strong democratic traditions and social forces—in the form of organized labour movements—that were better placed to resist the systematic infringement of human rights than the equivalent organizations today. Meanwhile, in the same period as the debate about human enhancement has been taking place, supposedly liberal societies have embraced extended detention without trial, the organized kidnap, secret imprisonment and torture of enemies of the state, and routine and extensive surveillance of the conversations and correspondence of their citizens, in response to a 'terrorist' threat that has been exaggerated out of all reasonable proportion. It has also seen a reinvigoration of racist and xenophobic politics around the globe and the emergence of neofascist and extremist political parties as significant political forces in a number of European nations.

The idea that an authoritarian government could not come to power in the countries in which the debate about the new eugenics is taking place is a comfortable fantasy but a fantasy all the same.[9] And if such a government should come to power when technologies of human enhancement have been developed and come to be socially accepted, it is naive to believe that it would not put them to use to entrench its power at the expense of the human rights of those deemed to be 'unfit' or a threat to the unity of the social body.

The political responsibilities of bioethicists

I have been arguing that the new eugenics is all too likely to collapse into a morally repugnant 'old eugenics'. There is an obvious response available to the defenders of the new eugenics at this point: they may simply insist that should this collapse occur then they would not support the pursuit of human enhancement. Is it not wrong for me to criticize them for the nature of a position they do not support?

It would indeed be if there was little or no connection between the new eugenics and the old. However, my argument above is that the attempt to realize the new eugenics is likely to lead to repugnant consequences. As a vision of how actual societies might respond to the development of genetic technologies of human enhancement, the new eugenics is extremely implausible. Moreover, the same social circumstances and forces that seem likely to transform the new eugenics into the old in the future also problematize the ethics of advocating human enhancement today. Whether they intend to be or not—and I presume they do not—advocates of the new eugenics are contributing to intellectual currents that make an old-style eugenics more likely. When Harris and Savulescu write about the coming 'new breed' of enhanced human beings they unwittingly reinforce racist and elitist strands of thought that are already all too present

---

[9] It is also worth pointing out that it is naive to think that when/if technologies of genetic human enhancement become available they will only be adopted in societies that might currently be described as liberal or democratic. Both China and Singapore, for instance, are technologically advanced societies wherein the state has a history of concerted interest in eugenics.

in our contemporary social milieu. Consider another illuminating example, the cover illustrations of three of the most influential recent books in the debate about human enhancement. The 2007 hardcover version of John Harris's *Enhancing Evolution* features an image that twice references fascist iconography: a human arm in a blue uniform flexing its biceps in front of the expanding rays from a rising sun (Harris 2007). The cover of Nick Agar's *Liberal Eugenics* consists in an image of the muscled torsos of three men marching in unison, presumably into the future (Agar 2004). Meanwhile, Savulescu and Bostrom's edited collection, *Human Enhancement*, displays the silhouettes of three groups of six hyper-muscled men in various bodybuilding poses that are also iconic poses of martial victory (Savulescu and Bostrom 2009). Thus despite these philosophers' advocating various versions of an essentially liberal eugenics, the presentation of their work in the public sphere also functions to advance ideas about the nature of enhancement and genetic superiority that are closely associated with the old eugenics.[10] Importantly, the political resonances of contemporary claims about eugenics are entirely predictable. It is therefore not unjust to expect that philosophers thinking about the new eugenics should consider how their work is likely to be received and how it will contribute to the future development and application of technologies of human enhancement.

Conclusion

The ethics of human enhancement has now been much discussed by many different philosophers and bioethicists. However, the politics of human enhancement, both in terms of the political assumptions that underpin the ethical debate and the political consequences of this ethical debate itself have been relatively neglected. I hope I have shown here that paying attention to these issues reveals the 'new eugenics' to be much more problematic than the bioethical literature currently acknowledges and calls into question the wisdom of the enthusiasm with which some philosophers have advocated human enhancement in the public sphere. If we wish to avoid the nightmare of genetic technologies being used for social engineering in the twenty-first century in violation of important human rights, it will be vital for future investigations of the ethics of human enhancement to address its politics with equal rigour.[11]

References

Agar, N. (1998). 'Liberal Eugenics', *Public Affairs Quarterly*, 12(2): 137–55.

Agar, N. (2004). *Liberal Eugenics: In Defence of Human Enhancement*. Oxford: Blackwell.

Brock, D. (1994). 'Reproductive Freedom: Its Nature Bases and Limits', in D. Thomasma and J. Monagle (eds), *Health Care Ethics: Critical Issues for Health Professionals*. Gaithersburg, MD: Aspen Publishers, 43–61.

[10] Given how the publishing industry works, these images may well have been chosen *against* the wishes of the authors by publishers intent upon generating sales for the works by highlighting the controversy they court. This does not, however, alter the fact of their semiotics.

[11] My thanks to Catherine Mills for reading early drafts of this manuscript.

Brock, D. (2005). 'Shaping Future Children: Parental Rights and Societal Interests', *Journal of Political Philosophy*, 13(4): 377–98.

Buchanan, A. (1996). 'Choosing Who Will Be Disabled: Genetic Intervention and the Morality of Inclusion', *Social Philosophy and Policy*, 13(1): 18–46.

Buchanan, A. et al. (2000). *From Chance to Choice.* Cambridge: Cambridge University Press.

Carlson, E. A. (1981). *Genes, Radiation, and Society: The Life and Work of H.J. Muller.* Ithaca, NY: Cornell University Press.

Chan, S., and Harris, J. (2007). 'In Support of Human Enhancement', *Studies in Ethics, Law, and Technology*, 1(1): Article No. 10. DOI: 10.2202/1941-6008.1007.

Davis, D. S. (2001). *Genetic Dilemmas: Reproductive Technology, Parental Choices, and Children's Futures.* New York: Routledge.

Dekker, T. J. (2009). 'The Illiberality of Perfectionist Enhancement', *Medicine, Health Care, and Philosophy* 12:91–8.

Dworkin, R. (1993). *Life's Dominion: An Argument about Abortion, Euthanasia, and Individual Freedom.* New York: Knopf.

Feinberg, J. (1980). 'The Child's Right to an Open Future', in W. Aiken and H. LaFollette (eds), *Whose Child? Children's Rights, Parental Authority, and State Power.* Totowa, NJ: Littlefield, Adams, and Co: 124–53.

Fox, D. (2007). 'The Illiberality of Liberal Eugenics', *Ratio*, 20:1–26.

Glover, J. (2006). *Choosing Children: Genes, Disability, and Design.* Oxford: Oxford University Press.

Harris, J. (1998). *Clones, Genes, and Immortality: Ethics and the Genetic Revolution.* Oxford: Oxford University Press.

Harris, J. (2004). *On Cloning.* London: Routledge.

Harris, J. (2007). *Enhancing Evolution: The Ethical Case for Making Better People.* Princeton, NJ: Princeton University Press.

Kitcher, P. (1996). *The Lives to Come: The Genetic Revolution and Human Possibilities.* New York: Simon and Schuster.

Parfit, D. (1984). *Reasons and Persons.* Oxford: Clarendon Press.

Persson, I., and Savulescu, J. (2008). 'The Perils of Cognitive Enhancement and the Urgent Imperative to Enhance the Moral Character of Humanity', *Journal of Applied Philosophy*, 25(3): 162–77.

Robertson, J. A. (1994). *Children of Choice: Freedom and the New Reproductive Technologies.* Princeton, NJ: Princeton University Press.

Savulescu, J. (1999). 'Sex Selection: The Case For', *Medical Journal of Australia*, 71:373–5.

Savulescu, J. (2001a). 'Procreative Beneficence: Why We Should Select the Best Children', *Bioethics*, 15(5): 413–26.

Savulescu, J. (2001b). 'Why Genetic Testing for Genes for Criminality Is Morally Required', *Princeton Journal of Bioethics*, 4(Spring): 79–97.

Savulescu, J. (2002). 'Deaf Lesbians, "Designer Disability", and the Future of Medicine', *British Medical Journal*, 325:771–3.

Savulescu, J. (2005). 'New Breeds of Humans: The Moral Obligation to Enhance', *Ethics, Law, and Moral Philosophy of Reproductive Biomedicine*, 1(1): 36–9.

Savulescu, J. (2008). 'Procreative Beneficence: Reasons Not to Have Disabled Children', in L. Skene and J. Thomson (eds), *The Sorting Society: The Ethics of Genetic Screening and Therapy.* Cambridge: Cambridge University Press, 51–68.

Savulescu, J., and Bostrom, N. (eds). (2009). *Human Enhancement*. Oxford: Oxford University Press.

Savulescu, J., and Kahane, G. (2009). 'The Moral Obligation to Create Children with the Best Chance of the Best Life', *Bioethics*, 23(5): 274–90.

Savulescu, J. et al. (2006). 'Behavioural Genetics: Why Eugenic Selection Is Preferable to Enhancement', *Journal of Applied Philosophy*, 23(2): 157–71.

Silver, L. M. (1999). *Remaking Eden: Cloning, Genetic Engineering, and the Future of Human Kind*. London: Pheonix.

Sparrow, R. (2007). 'Procreative Beneficence, Obligation, and Eugenics', *Genomics, Society, and Policy*, 3(3): 43–59.

Sparrow, R. (2010a). 'Better than Men? Sex and the Therapy/Enhancement Distinction', *Kennedy Institute of Ethics Journal*, 20(2): 115–44.

Sparrow, R. (2010b). 'Liberalism and Eugenics', *Australasian Journal of Philosophy*, 89(3): 499–517.

Sparrow, R. (2010c). 'Should Human Beings Have Sex? Sexual Dimorphism and Human Enhancement', *American Journal of Bioethics*, 10(7): 3–12.

Sparrow, R. (2011a). 'A Not-So-New Eugenics: Harris and Savulescu on Human Enhancement', *Hastings Center Report*, 41(1): 32–42.

Sparrow, R. (2011b). 'Human Enhancement and Sexual Dimorphism', *Bioethics*, 26(9): 464–75.

Steinbock, B. (2000). 'Disability, Prenatal Testing, and Selective Abortion', in E. Parens and A. Asch (eds), *Prenatal Testing and Disability Rights*. Washington, DC: Georgetown University Press, 108–23.

Stock, G. (2003). *Redesigning Humans: Choosing Our Children's Genes*. London: Profile Books.

Wikler, D. (1999). 'Can We Learn from Eugenics?' *Journal of Medical Ethics*, 25(2): 183–94.

Wylie, P. (1930). *Gladiator*. New York: Knopf.

Zohar, N. J. (1991). 'Prospects for "Genetic Therapy": Can a Person Benefit from Being Altered?' *Bioethics*, 5(4): 275–88.

4.2

Commentary

Eugenics in Society: A Sociological and Historical Consideration

Yasutaka Ichinokawa

In this commentary, I will address three issues about eugenics from a sociological perspective.

1 Disability studies: social model of disability

I have been engaged in disability studies in Japan for nearly ten years. The Japan Society for Disability Studies was established in 2003, and since then I have been on the board. In addition to academic activities, I have been involved in the independent living movement of people with disabilities as a personal assistant for more than 20 years.

Professor Jun Ishikawa (University of Shizuoka), the first president of our society, is a sociologist and is blind. Professor Yoichiro Asahi (Nagano University), the second president, is a professor of social work and has some impairment due to cerebral palsy. Professor Satoshi Fukushima (University of Tokyo), one of my colleagues, is a professor of pedagogy and disability studies. He is blind, and also became deaf at the age of 18. We communicate with him using finger Braille.

In the various activities of our society, we continuously put the concepts of disability studies into practice, based on the social model of disability (Oliver 1990). In contrast to the individual (or medical) model, the social model finds the cause of disability not in an individual's physical or mental impairments, but in the lack of accommodations that people surrounding the individual should have arranged. The social model defines 'dis-ability' as the social deprivation of an individual's abilities. For example, to the question 'Why can't they read my paper?' the individual model says, 'Because they are blind.' The social model says instead, 'Because I don't provide it in Braille, etc.' Likewise, to the question 'Why can't they understand my speech?' the individual model says, 'Because they are deaf,' while the social model says, 'Because I don't use sign language.'

In this way, the social model urges the reform of social environments. It urges more appropriate accommodations rather than enhancement of an individual's physical or mental qualities, which is the primary goal of eugenics.

Neither I nor the Society claims that every disability could be removed using the social model. There is a limit, but there is room within this limit for social reform that is not yet sufficiently fulfilled. It seems to me that people supporting so-called 'liberal eugenics' overemphasize the limit and do not pay sufficient attention to the potential for social reform.

2 'Old' and 'new' eugenics

Concerning the aim or final goal, I think there is no difference between 'old' and 'new' eugenics. Alfred Ploetz (1860–1940), one of the leaders of German eugenics (or racial hygiene), said in his book:

Reproductive hygiene (*Fortpflanzungshygiene*) is a science about the influence of the variation of the germ cells and their artificial selection. The conflict between the opinion against selection and that for it could disappear, if we could displace the moment of human selection and exclusion from the level of the grown-up to that of the cells from which they come into existence, or if we could artificially select the germ cells. (Ploetz 1895: 231)

In short, the prenatal selection and elimination of human beings from the medical point of view was the final goal of Ploetz's 'reproductive hygiene.' Therefore, Fritz Lenz (1887–1976), one of Ploetz's students, insisted that 'euthanasia [suggested by K. Binding and A. Hoche] is by no means the essential method for racial hygiene (eugenics)' (Lenz 1932: 306–7). Why? Because eugenics should aim at the prenatal selection of human beings while euthanasia applies to the postnatal.

However, in the age of Ploetz and other eugenics supporters, there was no medical technology for precise prenatal selection. The only possibility was the sterilization of adults supposed to have 'hereditary' diseases or disabilities. In other words, they had to make a postnatal detour for prenatal selection. The emergence of prenatal diagnostic technology since the late 1960s enabled what Ploetz had been eager for at the end of the nineteenth century. From the beginning, eugenics aimed at prenatal selection (or elimination) of human beings.

On the other hand, we should recognize the difference between old and new eugenics according to the dichotomy 'coercive' or 'voluntary'; in other words, whether the method is practiced against one's will or based on individual choices. However, we should be careful on this point. Today we think that most of the old eugenic practices were coercive, as in Nazi Germany, but at that time it was not considered coercive when people who were sterilized were those considered to lack legal competence for decision-making, consent, etc., due to mental or intellectual disorders. They were not supposed to have sufficient will from a legal perspective, and therefore it was assumed that there could be no coercive practices violating their autonomy.

In current discussions of bioethics, there are some arguments that exclude a certain group of human beings from the category of 'person.' According to H. T. Engelhardt (1986), not every human being is a person whose autonomy should be respected and protected, and people with severe mental handicaps, for example, cannot be recognized as persons. Naturally, Engelhardt would condemn the coercive eugenic practices in

Nazi Germany, but the basic structure of his argument seems to me not so different from that of K. Binding and A. Hoche (1920), who approved the extermination of those who were considered lacking legal competence for consent. The bioethical principle of autonomy is nearly always accompanied by a limitation of those who have autonomy. Once someone is excluded from this circle of autonomy (or being a person), there can be no coercive measures, though those who disagree with this exclusion might think the measures coercive.

3   Eugenic legislation in Japan

The National Eugenic Act was passed in Japan in 1940. The level to which the Japanese law was influenced by the 1933 Nazi German sterilization act is controversial, but it would have been impossible if it had not been preceded by the German law.

Article 6 of the National Eugenic Act legalized coercive sterilization 'for the public interest.' However, this article was not implemented and no sterilizations were recognized as coercive from 1941 to 1948 in Japan. One reason for this was the objection from conservative people who claimed that the individual family (*Ie*), which passed from father to eldest son, formed the basis of Japanese society. Like the Japanese imperial system (*Tennou-Sei*), the continuity of each family should be preserved. Forced (eugenic) sterilization endangered this Japanese ideology.

Eugenic sterilization was practiced on a small scale (538 cases) from 1941 to 1947, and all cases were classified as voluntary. In contrast, more than 400,000 people were sterilized in Nazi Germany. The Nazis also had an ideology of family, but the nation (*Volk*) or the race (*Rasse*) always took priority, and the reproduction of families that could interfere with the biological enhancement of the German race was easily and coercively prohibited. This was not the case in Japan until at least 1945. The name of the 1940 Japanese sterilization act, 'National Eugenic Act,' seems ironic because the national logic collapsed in the face of the social importance of family continuity.

In Japan, it was only after 1945 that this conservative idea of family became less important and eugenics had its time. The Eugenic Protection Act was passed in 1948, which legalized (1) voluntary and non-voluntary sterilization (newly including Hansen's disease), and (2) eugenic and non-eugenic abortion.

In Japan, non-voluntary, or coercive, eugenic sterilization was practiced after 1945 in the age of and in a society of democracy and further modernization. I do not hesitate to use the word 'coercive,' because the official directives concerning the 1948 act clearly permitted coercive methods, such as physical constraint, use of anesthesia, and fraud. From 1949 to 1996 there were more than 16,000 non-voluntary eugenic sterilizations in Japan (Figure 4.1).

Eugenic abortion in the 1948 act referred to abortion when it was supposed that the mother, not the baby in her body, had a hereditary disease or disability.

Generally speaking, there are two models for legalization of abortion. One is the periodic model that establishes until what stage of pregnancy abortion can be legalized. The other is the indication model that establishes in which case (or why) abortion can be legalized, and there are at least four indications: (1) medical indication (for the

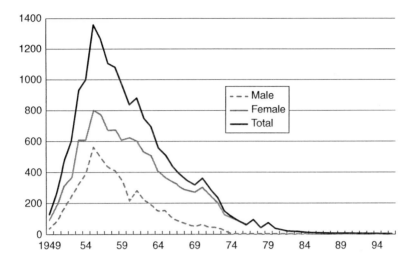

Figure 4.1 Non-voluntary eugenic sterilization in Japan

protection of the health and life of the pregnant woman); (2) criminal indication (rape); (3) social or economic indication (poverty); and (4) eugenic indication (in cases where the fetus is suspected to have an incurable disease or disability).

The Japanese 1948 Eugenic Protection Act and 1996 Act for Protection of Mothers' Bodies are based on the indication model. However, there has been no eugenic indication in Japan, although in the UK the Abortion Act 1967, in France the Abortion Act 1975, and in Germany the Reformed Criminal Law 1976 introduced it. I think lack of the eugenic indication is one reason why prenatal diagnosis has been practiced on a smaller scale in Japan than in Europe and the US.

Why is there no eugenic indication in Japan? The radical social movement and criticism from people with disabilities in Japan are often mentioned as factors. Indeed, as the introduction of the eugenic indication (coupled with the elimination of the economic indication) was discussed in the 1970s, there was strong opposition from people with disabilities. However, opposition was primarily raised not by people with hereditary diseases (spina bifida, hemophilia, etc.), but by those with non-hereditary disabilities (especially cerebral palsy) that can hardly become the target of prenatal diagnosis. The latter criticized eugenics radically, and in this process the meaning of the word 'eugenics' in Japanese changed and acquired a unique connotation. It came to mean discrimination against all people with disabilities. Whether the disability was hereditary (genetic) or not was put aside. This expansion of meaning is one of the sociological characteristics of the word 'eugenics' in Japan.

There are also some people in Japan who advocate liberal eugenics, claiming that there is no problem with abortion after prenatal diagnosis and for other reasons, if the parents want it. I myself cannot find strong reasons to prohibit this kind of abortion. However, if we really respect the individual right of autonomy, we should at the same time recognize the violation of it in the form of eugenic coercive sterilization after 1945, and make appropriate compensation to the victims publicly.

References

Binding, K., and Hoche, A. (1920). *Die Freigabe der Vernichtung lebensunwerten Lebens*. Leipzig: F. Meiner.

Engelhardt, H.T. (1986). *The Foundations of Bioethics*. Oxford: Oxford University Press.

Lenz, F. (1932). *Menschliche Auslese und Rassenhygiene (Eugenik)*. 4. Aufl. München: J. F. Lehmanns.

Oliver, M. (1990). *The Politics of Disablement*. Bakingstoke: Macmillan.

Ploetz, A. (1895). *Die Tüchtigkeit unsrer Rasse und der Schutz der Schwachen*. Berlin: Fischer.

4.3

Commentary

Are 'Brave' Parents Practicing Eugenics, Enhancement, or Something Else?

Michelle L. McGowan

In 'Ethics, Eugenics, and Politics' Robert Sparrow problematizes the ethics of promoting human enhancement (Sparrow 2013). The expert bioethics debate on human enhancement has focused on the moral permissibility of and obligations associated with enabling parents to decide whether and how to enhance their offspring. It has also addressed the potential for enhancement technologies to facilitate genetic selection, designer babies, a genetic class divide, and state investment in the make-up of its population. Sparrow is particularly concerned with the ways in which philosophers and bioethicists have engaged in thought experiments in which they promote human enhancement using a liberal individualist rationale. Sparrow's cautionary critique of a liberal eugenics approach to human enhancement is logically sound, and effectively demonstrates how the fantastical preoccupations of academics with human enhancement may be out of touch with social and political realities.

However, in focusing on the expert discourse of liberal eugenics, Sparrow himself seems to fall prey to the same criticism that he wages against the promoters of liberal eugenics, as he too has an entirely futuristic orientation to his argument. Ruminating about how to reform the ways in which philosophers and bioethicists promote liberal eugenics has its place in the bioethics literature; however, it is entirely speculative when it need not be. If bioethics is meant to be an applied field, the expert discourse on human enhancement may be informed and grounded by the perspectives of users of so-called enhancement technologies. Sparrow argues that only 'brave' parents would seek to genetically modify their children via gene therapy. Thus, he speculates that in practice PGD may be the more likely technological intervention involved in human enhancement. Given this, the perspectives of PGD users may be pertinent here as their viewpoints may help to address the question of whether human enhancement has already begun and what weight Sparrow's argument of the slippery slope of liberal eugenics might carry.

Assisted reproductive technologies now comprise 1 percent of all births in the United States (Centers for Disease Control and Prevention 2007). Of these births, an increasing number utilize PGD, which has been available clinically for more than 20 years now (Handyside et al. 1990). Yet the perspectives of users of this technique seem to be missing from Sparrow's argument on the social and political implications of liberal eugenics. This raises the question as to how the perspectives of users of PGD might contribute to Sparrow's argument on the moral permissibility and appeal of human enhancement. To address this question I will rely upon empirical research conducted in the United States that I have published elsewhere (McGowan 2008; Sharp et al. 2010; McGowan 2011; McGowan and Sharp submitted) to explore PGD users' motivations and experiences as they may relate to human enhancement. Participants in these qualitative research studies were interested in or had already made use of PGD for genetic selection to select against heritable disease traits or chromosomal anomalies or to select embryos for a specific sex.

In the first study, women who were interested in selecting against disease traits in their offspring came to genetic selection only after suffering a range of reproductive frustrations and losses ranging from prolonged infertility and multiple miscarriages to medically indicated terminations of wanted pregnancies (McGowan 2008; McGowan 2011). These women understood PGD as a responsible choice and an obligation to their families to manage known genetic and chromosomal risk factors (McGowan 2011). The participants in this study were all women and prospective mothers, and they actively feminized the responsibility for reproductive outcomes; for these women using PGD was seen as an expression of 'good' motherhood (McGowan 2008; McGowan 2011). These users of PGD were primarily concerned with:

the potential to find 'strong embryos'—embryos that are genetically and chromosomally 'normal' and hearty enough to withstand life in a petri dish, embryo biopsy, manual transfer to the uterus, and the two-week wait for the pregnancy to 'stick.' (McGowan 2008: 101)

These 'strong' embryos were presumed to be the most likely to allow the women to achieve their goals of becoming mothers to healthy babies. However, in pursuit of strong embryos, participants in this study made clear that they were aware of the controversial nature of their actions. The couples raised concerns about how their families, friends, and children resulting from PGD might feel about their choice to choose their offspring by screening embryos to select against disease traits, and they expressed conflicted selfishness, guilt, and familial obligation related to using a controversial technology that would judge or place 'value' on their prospective children based on their genetic traits (McGowan 2011).

A comparable set of tensions existed in the second study, which evaluated the moral attitudes and beliefs of prospective users of PGD for non-medical sex selection who had enrolled in a family balancing program (Sharp et al. 2010). While the couples who participated in this study were enthusiastic about the possibility of enrolling in a family balancing program and using PGD to create a balanced gender ratio in their families, they understood sex selection as an individual and familial choice rather than as a decision with broad social implications. Couples echoed liberal eugenicists' rhetoric promoting procreative liberty peppered with appeals to the private nature of reproductive decision-making, and some justified sex selection as a way to enhance their family dynamics and relationships (Sharp et al. 2010). The moral concerns that prospective users raised about using PGD for non-medical sex selection were also focused on how their families, friends, and existing children would feel about the decision to deliberately select the sex of the next child. Despite these concerns, participants had widespread support for a liberal approach to reproductive autonomy. However, they generally questioned an unlimited approach to procreative liberty, particularly when it came to the idea of extending to using genetic engineering to create the desired family (McGowan and Sharp submitted). It was seen by some couples as morally problematic to select traits that are not naturally occurring, and would constitute crossing a boundary of acceptability that may call into question an unlimited presumption of reproductive liberty because it might extend too much control to parents to 'play God.'

With these perspectives in mind, one might ask whether 1) selecting against genetic traits to reduce disease burden on an individual and family or 2) selecting for a normal human trait to ensure gender balance in the family should be considered forms of enhancement. Perhaps neither of these applications fits Sparrow's definition of enhancement as selecting embryos for 'above species-typical capacities.' Though with the rhetoric of strong embryos and idealized families mirroring the imagery that Sparrow uses to describe the cover art of liberal eugenics theorists' books, it may be hard to argue that users of PGD are not somehow engaged in personal eugenics, if not human enhancement. However, it is doubtful that users themselves would consider their use of PGD enhancement of their offspring and some would disavow any association between their actions and morally questionable genetic engineering. The rhetoric of personal autonomy that dominates the liberal eugenics literature resonates with the perspectives of seekers of non-medical sex selection but seems muted in users' qualitative perspectives on PGD in relation to concepts of moral obligation for disease avoidance. Hence, the slippage toward moral obligation to enhance one's offspring that Sparrow's addresses may be more mundane than he predicts. Rather than enhancement technologies creating a technological imperative to enhance one's offspring, perhaps the perspectives of PGD users suggest that attitudes toward moral obligation may inhabit a smaller scale in the confines of familial decision-making rather than on the social and political stage. This is not to argue that the use of PGD is without social consequences. Actually, I agree wholeheartedly with Sparrow's argument that the use of PGD has the potential to reinforce existing social hierarchies and generate new forms of social inequality. However, my previous research suggests that these concerns are not shared by the actual and prospective users of PGD. Thus, the expert bioethics discourse on PGD and other enhancement technologies may be out of step with the matters of importance to the users of the technologies.

In order for bioethical debate on liberal eugenics to be grounded in the social and political realities of technologically mediated reproductive decision-making, philosophers and bioethicists should take into consideration culturally situated values, understandings, and enthusiasm for the uptake of enhancement technologies by those most likely to be in a position to utilize them. Engaging prospective users on their values regarding the morality of human enhancement and the attitudes and worldviews that would contribute to their willingness to enhance their children would contribute tremendously to our collective understandings of how human enhancement may proceed. Users' perspectives also have the potential to contribute to or diminish the fears that Sparrow has presented on the potential for liberal eugenics to slide toward social engineering, and would provide a valuable grounding of the liberal eugenics debate as it relates to contemporary applications of human enhancement technologies.

References

Centers for Disease Control and Prevention. (2007). '2005 Assisted Reproductive Technology Success Rates: National Summary and Fertility Clinic Reports,' http://www.cdc.gov/art/artreports.htm (accessed 11 December 2012).

Handyside, A. H. et al. (1990). 'Pregnancies from Biopsied Human Preimplantation Embryos Sexed by Y-specific DNA Amplification,' *Nature*, 344:768–70.

McGowan, M. L. (2008). 'Producing Users of Preimplantation Genetic Diagnosis: Dominant and Marginalized Discourses in the US Context,' in A. Bammé, G. Getzinger, and B. Wieser (eds), *Yearbook 2007 of the Institute for Advanced Studies on Science, Technology, and Society*. Munich: Profil, 95–110.

McGowan, M. L. (2011). 'Constructions of Good Motherhood in an Online Forum for Users of Preimplantation Genetic Diagnosis,' in M. Moravec (ed), *Motherhood Online*. Newcastle upon Tyne: Cambridge Scholars, 180–99.

McGowan, M. L., and Sharp, R. R. (Submitted). '"We're Just Trying to Equal It Out": Reproductive Justice in the Context of a Family Balancing Program.'

Sharp, R. R. et al. (2010). 'Moral Attitudes and Beliefs among Couples Pursuing PGD for Sex Selection,' *Reproductive Biomedicine Online*, 21:838–47.

Sparrow, R. (2014). 'Ethics, Eugenics, and Politics,' in A. Akabayashi (ed.), *The Future of Bioethics: International Dialogues*. Oxford: Oxford University Press, 139–53.

4.4

Commentary
Therapy, Enhancement, and Eugenics

D. Gareth Jones

In commenting on Sparrow's paper (Sparrow 2013), I shall take to heart a remark that came at the conclusion of the preceding paper by Lysaght and Campbell (Lysaght and Campbell 2013). If I am allowed to paraphrase it for the purposes of this paper, it might read something like this: 'Bioethics needs to move beyond the contested philosophical issues surrounding human enhancement, and move towards more practical clinical issues. While bioethics should not be merely pragmatic, our critical analysis has to start and end with dilemmas that medicine encounters in the clinics and in everyday practice.'

As I read Sparrow's paper the issues that dominate his discussion and indeed any discussion of the prospects opened up by the enhancement debate revolve around what he terms the 'dangerously rarefied sphere' of the discussion, allied to which is a neglect of political realities. As a scientist with clinical interests I am constantly bemused by the first of these. Is this the real world of the clinic and consulting room, or is it far closer to the realm of intriguing—and even idle—philosophical speculation? As I ponder on this, I cannot help but think of the world of therapy, and its relationship to enhancement. True, the two are usually seen in opposition; therapy is merely attempting to rectify that which has gone wrong, returning an individual to normal health, while enhancement goes beyond the normal, extending the individual into new territory. Therapy is mundane, the world of the present; enhancement is exciting, the world of the future. From my perspective this contrast is unhelpful, since cutting-edge therapy can throw light onto our assessment of enhancement.

Linked to this is the ease with which so many analyses of enhancement skirt around definitions of what any specific enhancement might encompass. The enhancement debate is mired in an unwillingness to commit to any clear definitions of what enhancement will entail, leaving commentators unclear as to what sorts of changes might count as enhancements. In precisely the same way we often do not know what counts as normality—whether normal health, normal behavior, or normal expectations—and hence are unable to determine when we are moving from therapy into enhancement. Additionally, enhancement is frequently viewed as a homogeneous phenomenon, lacking the nuances of the diverse ways in which individuals will probably respond to any particular procedure. Neither do we hear about probable unpleasant and even unwanted side effects, which in turn may vitiate the thrust of the enhancement. If only we paid more attention to therapy, we would not be so cavalier about the beneficial effects of enhancements. While these are not areas that Sparrow has tackled, they complement his many concerns about implementing procedures to produce 'the best children possible' with 'above species-typical' capacities, the obligation to enhance, violation of reproductive liberty, and the liberty in future of enhanced children. Consideration of therapy is also relevant to the sliding of the new liberal eugenics, which I take as being inherently pro-enhancement, into the old immoral eugenics.

Between therapy and enhancement

In order to set the scene I shall make reference to cystic fibrosis (CF), a very clear genetic condition that is reasonably common, and is the subject of intense research that has produced revolutionary therapies. Nevertheless, it continues to be associated with demanding ethical quandaries that span the alleged dividing line between therapy and enhancement.

Some time ago a boy was born to a young couple, and within two days of his birth he underwent a major operation. This immediately suggested the diagnosis of CF, a diagnosis confirmed by genetic analysis a couple of weeks later. The treatment he received at the time and has subsequently received has been state of the art, and his progress has been as good as could possibly be expected.

The ongoing trajectory of growth and development has been therapy dependent, since the little boy has been intimately dependent for his daily needs upon a very high level of technological expertise. Not only this, if the facilities had not been available, he would have died as a neonate. The resources necessary to save the life of a child like this, and hopefully provide him with an ongoing good quality of life, are a *sine qua non*. This is science and technology at its most impressive. It is also science and technology in the service of humanity.

As one considers CF one soon encounters the central place of research in its treatment. The life expectancy of those with this genetic condition that affects all the exocrine glands has been transformed over the past 15–20 years, so that many of those who receive sophisticated treatment from birth (involving enzymatic, antibiotic, and gene-based therapies) can live well into their 40s (Elborn, Shale, and Britton 1991; Davis 2006; Dodge et al. 2007). Inevitably, this has profound implications for patients and family alike, and may also be of relevance when negotiating the treacherous waters of therapy and enhancement.

What then of the parents as they look ahead, and begin to contemplate the birth of a *second child*? They would prefer not to have another child with this condition because the demands on them, let alone on the affected child, are immense. Many of the considerations raised in the enhancement debate surface here as well. Are the parents, both CF carriers, able to provide any future child with the 'best possible life'; what might that mean in a situation such as this one? Indeed, what criteria do we have for determining what is the best possible life? It may be easy to categorize a life with CF as substandard, but this has overtones of evaluating an individual with CF as substandard and therefore of less value. This is an illustration of the social and political slippage between claims about genes and about those who possess them, as highlighted by Sparrow.

Should these parents have the liberty of bringing into existence a child with the 'wrong' genetic make-up, knowing that he or she will suffer from ill health and will impose financial burdens on the state as well as on themselves? What are we to think of parents who might 'allow their children to be born with lower life prospects than other citizens' with consequences beyond themselves? Are they to be prevented from acting in what some would consider an irresponsible manner? The tension between liberal and mandatory eugenics emerges with striking clarity in these very real clinical situations. After all, this child will not meet a 'threshold level of well-being' unless that is placed very low on a genetic scale.

The parents currently have *four options*, to which I shall add *a fifth* with enhancement in mind.

Option 1. They could decide against having another child; the one-in-four prospects of another child with CF are more than they can bear. Neither do they want to bring into the world another individual with a debilitating condition like CF. Is this their choice alone, or should the state take an interest in it and make it mandatory?

Option 2. They could take a one-in-four chance, and hope their next child will be unaffected. Whatever eventuates, they will continue with the pregnancy even if it means having a second child with CF. In accepting whatever comes, are they acting in the child's best interests?

Option 3. They could take a chance, knowing that they can have an abortion if the fetus when tested at nine to ten weeks' gestation using chorionic villus biopsy turns out to be affected. They would only go down this path as a very last resort, especially since in their eyes it may demean the inherent value of their little boy who has CF and whom they love very deeply.

Option 4. They could go in the direction of IVF and PGD. If this dual procedure is carried out and shows that an embryo at the four- or eight-cell stage does not have the CF gene it will be transferred to the woman's uterus in the normal way. On the other hand, if the CF gene is present in an embryo, that embryo will be discarded and the same procedure will be carried out on a second embryo, and so on until an embryo lacking this gene is found. They are prepared to consider this as a possible way forward but feel they are treading a very delicate and uncertain path. It is also an expensive option and an impersonally clinical procedure for a couple with no fertility problems.

Option 5. What might enhancement mean for a CF individual? Imagine gene therapy for an affected embryo or fetus that, rather than rectifying the dysfunctional ion transport system, enhances mucosal enzyme secretion in the lung and gut, allowing the individual to break down the excess mucous. Should this or some variant of it work, the condition is in effect being treated by enhancing other capacities and not by correcting the dysfunction. An alternative one could envisage would be the use of gene therapy to improve the dysfunctional ion transport system causing CF, and hence augmenting function beyond what is 'species typical'. The intended result would be a decrease in mucosal viscosity, thereby providing enhanced resistance to mucosal diseases. Any of these speculative possibilities involves a slide from highly sophisticated therapy into enhancement-tinged therapy.

Against this backdrop there are five issues that warrant additional discussion. The *first* is that the distinction between options 2, 4, and 5 is less clear than frequently imagined. But can the notion of enhancement apply to an individual with a genetic condition like CF? After all, these individuals are functioning below the species norm, no matter what currently available treatment is provided. On the other hand, their life prospects are already being dramatically improved by state-of-the-art treatment. While this can easily be dismissed as mere therapy, there can be little question that it is life changing for these individuals and the communities to which they belong. Their lives are enhanced even if they continue to function below the species norm after treatment. Options 2, 4, and 5 slide into one another, so that some of the well-worn distinctions between therapy and enhancement are unhelpful. In practice, therapeutic regimes may display strong 'enhancing' qualities.

The *second* issue is that, since all three options are expensive, the state may decide against funding any of them. This would immediately make them the preserve of the rich; and any inkling of equality of treatment would disappear. Alternatively, the state may mandate against couples like this, and determine that option 1 is the only acceptable avenue open to them, since this represents the least financial drain on the state. It would also, of course, be an illustration of non-liberal eugenics in action. The point I am making is that the possibility of state-mandated eugenics is not confined to enhancement vistas, but is also raised by therapeutic ventures such as the ones encountered in this CF scenario. Sparrow is correct in asserting that eugenics of the strong sort is alive and well, and should not be seen as merely a tragic historical aberration.

Third, closely related to this question is the liberty of the parents against the liberty of the children, as brought out by Sparrow in the enhancement debate. Even if we accept that parents are free to bring into existence a child with CF (Bosslet 2011), what of the future individual who will suffer even with the best therapy available and will have a limited lifespan? Would these future CF individuals have chosen this life for themselves or would they have opted for non-existence? We do not know, but by the same token neither do we know how enhanced individuals will respond to choices made on their behalf by their parents. We need to beware of indulging in elitist notions of eugenics.

The *fourth* issue comes back to what is regarded as 'normal'. In the case of CF it is obvious that those with CF are not genetically normal. But again there are problems. How do CF individuals regard themselves? What counts as normality? It appears that many children and young adults with CF regard themselves as normal (Williams et al. 2009). While this is a multifaceted issue ranging from 'normal to self' and 'normal for self', to 'normal to others' and 'normal for others', it points to the complexity of the 'normality' concept and of the way in which individuals with chronic illness have multiple meanings for these terms and engage in behaviors that play to different audiences. It behoves us, therefore, to take great care that we do not assume too readily that we know how individuals and communities regard themselves.

The well-known story of Alexander Stobbs in the UK attests to the importance of this response. Although having a severe form of CF, this musically gifted young man pushes himself to and beyond the limits, even to the point of conducting a performance of Bach's *St Matthew Passion*, a daunting project for any young person, let alone someone with severely limited lung function. The titles of two chapters in his book, *A Passion for Living*, sum up his attitude: 'I'd rather not be seen as someone with CF' and 'I strive to be the same as everyone else' (Stobbs 2009). One can speculate that enhancement in his case would include therapy that increased his lifespan far beyond that typical even today for CF sufferers in order to give him far more scope for displaying his prodigious musical abilities, and in turn developing these abilities well beyond those normally encountered.

Even this would not be enhancement in the sense of moving beyond species norms or generally accepted species boundaries, and yet it would be enhancement for an individual who commences from a markedly subnormal baseline according to species norms. This is a perennial problem in this area, since so much of the enhancement debate errs towards population norms and expectations, and ignores the fact that ultimately it comes down to issues raised by the enhancement of individuals. A high-profile illustration of this tension is that of Oscar Pistorius, the South African athlete, the double-amputee world record holder in the 100, 200, and 400 metres for that class of athlete. Born without a fibula in each of his legs, at the age of 11 months his legs were amputated halfway between the knees and ankles. He runs with the aid of Cheetah Flex-Foot carbon-fibre transtibial artificial limbs.

Are his prostheses an enhancement or are they a therapeutic device that enables him to live a relatively normal existence? Outside the sporting arena they give every appearance of being therapeutic, in that they enable him to walk relatively normally. However, once sporting prowess enters the picture the enhancement conundrum raises its head, since the prostheses enable him to run just as fast as world-class athletes with normal limbs. Were someone with normal legs to have them amputated in order to use these particular prostheses, with the intention of improving their running ability, this would be classic enhancement. But Pistorius is not in that category. While this may be regarded as nothing more than an unusual problem for sporting authorities, it brings to the fore the uneasy boundary between therapy and enhancement.

Fifth, Sparrow alludes to the manner in which technologies, once available, have social and political consequences barely envisioned when originally developed. One does not have to look far in biomedicine to see countless examples of this. The multitude of uses to which IVF and its offshoots have been put have transformed a procedure developed within the narrow therapeutic context of the alleviation of infertility into one with profound social consequences for the notion of family relationships. Interestingly, these have not been driven by states but by commercial enterprises and individual choice. It would be surprising if the same did not take place once enhancements became available. It is this aspect of them that will be difficult to envisage, let alone control. In other words, the social engineering may be driven by two forces—the population at large as well as the state.

What if I had been enhanced?

So much of the enhancement literature assumes that all concerned will know and agree on what will class as enhancement, and that there will be general agreement that it is good and will be welcomed by those who will discover as they grow up that they have been enhanced. What would I think if I discovered that I had been enhanced in some way? I would know that I had been predestined to walk in steps preordained for me by someone else, in all probability my parents. In reality, of course, their plans and prospects would probably not work out as they anticipated, and I would be more of a free agent than they had contemplated. Perhaps this is where enhancement and therapy diverge. Enhanced individuals are not meant to be free or to experience the world for themselves; the notion of enhancement has within it a built-in lack of freedom of expression. This is not generally the case with therapy that has as its goal the well-being of the individual undergoing treatment. Liberal eugenics morphs all too readily into old-fashioned compulsory eugenics, particularly when aiming at enhancement.

At a more personal level, what if I had been enhanced in the expectation that I would enter the world of international banking? But I rejected this and turned instead to academia, and became a professor neither of banking nor of finance. Some elements of the enhancement would be detectable in my abilities in finance. And yet one imagines I would have been a disappointment to my parents in the academic role. That was not what they envisaged as the way ahead for me. Alternatively, I may have become an unsuccessful and dispirited international banker, enhanced, and rebellious at the all-too-obvious infringement of my freedom. Or I may simply have tossed aside what I knew were my parents' fantasies and become a poet!

These possibilities point to a reality so often ignored in discussions about enhancement; it may prove profoundly disappointing, as disappointing as so many of our other ventures. As with therapy, we may be disillusioned. When the enhancement debate is brought down to the level of the individual, the messiness of ordinary life rudely intervenes, and so it is pertinent to ask ourselves how we would respond to walking in the footsteps of others, a life foreordained by others, determined by the whims and aspirations of others. The notion of liberal eugenics seems frivolous when confronted by a life of coercion.

References

Bosslet, G.T. (2011). 'Parental Procreative Obligation and the Categorisation of Disease: The Case of Cystic Fibrosis', *Journal of Medical Ethics*, 37(5): 280–4.

Davis, P. B. (2006). 'Cystic Fibrosis since 1938', *American Journal of Respiratory and Critical Care Medicine*, 173(5): 475–82.

Dodge, J. A. et al. (2007). 'Cystic Fibrosis Mortality and Survival in the UK: 1947–2003', *The European Respiratory Journal: Official Journal of the European Society for Clinical Respiratory Physiology*, 29(3): 522–6.

Elborn, J. S., Shale, D. J., and Britton, J. R. (1991). 'Cystic Fibrosis: Current Survival and Population Estimates to the Year 2000', *Thorax*, 46(12): 881–5.

Lysaght, T., and Campbell, A. V. (2014). 'The Ethics of Regenerative Medicine: Broadening the Scope beyond the Moral Status of Embryos', in A. Akabayashi (ed.), *The Future of Bioethics: International Dialogues*. Oxford: Oxford University Press, 5–26.

Sparrow, R. (2014). 'Ethics, Eugenics, and Politics', in A. Akabayashi (ed.), *The Future of Bioethics: International Dialogues*. Oxford: Oxford University Press, 139–53.

Stobbs, A. (2009). *A Passion for Living*. London: Hodder and Stoughton.

Williams, B. et al. (2009). 'I've Never Not Had It So I Don't Really Know What It's Like Not to: Nondifference and Biographical Disruption among Children and Young People with Cystic Fibrosis', *Qualitative Health Research*, 19(10): 1443–55.

4.5

Commentary

The Nature of the Moral Obligation to Select the Best Children

Julian Savulescu

I have argued for a principle of procreative beneficence (PB): that couples have a moral obligation to use genetic selection to have the best child, of the possible children they could have (Savulescu 2001b; Savulescu 2008). This is different to liberal eugenics, which claims that couples should be free to use genetic selection technologies, but it is silent on whether there is a moral obligation to use such technology. Sparrow speculates that 'the new eugenics is all too likely to collapse into a morally repugnant "old eugenics"' (Sparrow in this chapter). He calls this speculation a 'political critique'. I will argue that both ethics and politics speak against his speculation. He claims that this is in part because the enhancement debate has been conducted in the 'dangerously rarefied sphere and has neglected important political realities' (Sparrow in this chapter).

I, and more recently with Guy Kahane, have responded to many of the criticisms made by Sparrow (for example, we addressed his objections to maximization and how strong or exclusive our reasons to have the best child are in Savulescu and Kahane 2009). He raises the problem of children being born with the 'wrong' skin colour and the social determinants of best. Again we have addressed these arguments in Savulescu 2001b, Savulescu 2008, and Kahane and Savulescu 2009. I have also responded directly to his arguments about the moral relevance of sex (Savulescu 2001a) and his concerns about increasing inequality and justice (Savulescu 2006; Savulescu 2009). I will here focus on his claim that making PB a moral obligation increases the chance of a slide to the old eugenics and that 'there is a significant tension between the claim that parents are morally obligated to enhance their children and the claim that they should never be coerced to do so' (Sparrow in this chapter).

PB as a moral obligation

When I say moral obligation, I mean pro tanto moral reason, which must be weighed against other moral reasons to determine what we have most reason to do (Savulescu and Kahane 2009). The obligation is a defeasible obligation or prima facie moral obligation. It would be absurd to suggest, as some writers have tried to argue I have suggested, that our overriding moral obligation or ultimate moral reason is to have the best children. It is a moral obligation, which must be weighed against our other moral obligations to decide what we have as moral obligation. Of course, there are other reasons—e.g. parental interests and societal interests (including commitments to equality and non-discrimination).

Rob Sparrow, along with many other people, objects to the claim there is a moral obligation to select better children. He thinks calling these reasons 'moral obligations' will increase the likelihood of the slide from new to old eugenics. Let me defend the claim that there is a moral obligation to select the best children.

Since the actions of parents in procreation are not purely self-regarding but affect others (that is, the children born of their actions), they fall in the moral, not prudential, realm. Many people, including me, claim that reproduction should be a private affair—but this does not remove it from the moral. Procreation and childrearing are moral affairs. Thus abortion and child abuse are appropriately seen as moral issues. The fact that many actions in procreation and childrearing are not subject to moral evaluation and parents enjoy great liberty does not show that these are always removed from the non-moral realm. Parents do have obligations towards their children when what are at stake are fundamental interests, significant liberties, or opportunities.

There are many things which parents do which fail to maximize their children's well-being that we do not think are moral failings. Thus buying a car without airbags when you could afford one which is safer is not seen as a moral failing, even if there are no countervailing good reasons. It is the parents' prerogative or freedom to make such decisions. Selection of a child's genes is like that, opponents of PB claim.

I am inclined to disagree that these decisions which impose small foreseeable, avoidable risks for no good reason are not moral decisions. I believe they are but that the fact that they involve small risks means that moral censure, punishment, blame, etc. are not appropriate. Still, if someone asked, 'Should I (or ought I) buy a safer car for my children?' the answer is yes, unless you have something better to do with the money.

But let us grant for argument's sake that decisions which involve small risk of or no decrement in well-being of children are not moral decisions. So, on this view, there is no moral obligation to select darker skin which is more resistant to melanoma in sunny climates, even though it would advantage the child.

This would imply that parents do not have a moral obligation to select the best child. Nonetheless, they would still have reason to use many genetic selection technologies to select children who are expected to have substantially higher levels of well-being. They will have moral obligations to select better children. For it is clear that parents do act morally wrongly when they significantly harm their children, say by emotional or physical abuse. Parents who failed to install baby seats correctly, contributing to the serious disablement of their child in a car accident, would be acting morally wrongly.

If there are genetic dispositions which affect well-being to a similar level as dispositions to disease, then there exist moral obligations to select the more advantageous disposition. I have argued that self-control or ability to delay gratification is a trait which is highly correlated with well-being. There would be a moral obligation to select in favour of its genetic basis, if there were a significant genetic contribution.

So even on a narrow reading of moral obligation, there will still be moral obligations to select certain genes which are highly important to well-being and opportunity.

But this is in significant part a terminological matter. It may not be essential to determine what parents have moral reason or obligation to do. It may be enough to decide what they should do or ought to do. Genetic selection is an important reason for action and grounds what we should do, absent other important countervailing reasons. Even if parents are not under a moral obligation to select a darker-skinned child in a sunny climate, they should/ought/have reason to do so.

Other moral obligations

PB is not a special moral obligation. It is similar to other moral obligations and this comparison is useful in evaluating some of Sparrow's claims. Compare the following moral obligations of the form 'You should do A in order that X has a good life.'

Helping. You have a moral obligation to help John who is starving in Africa. You should do A in order that John lives a good life (A = give money, time, expertise, etc.).

Selecting. You have a moral obligation to select the best embryo of the embryos available. You should do A in order that James exists and lives a good life (A = IVF plus PGD, or some other selection procedure).

One might object that *Helping* makes John better off and involves a person-affecting benefit. *Selecting* in contrast does not make anyone better and involves impersonal benefits. We do not have a moral obligation to provide impersonal benefits.

As Sparrow correctly notes, we do commonly accept impersonal reasons for action when we argue that people should care for and conserve the climate and environment. Such actions are frequently identity affecting in the same way as selection decisions, yet we still claim that people have a moral obligation to, say, reduce carbon emissions for the sake of future generations.

Conservation. You have a moral obligation to reduce carbon emissions. You should do A so that people exist in the future with good lives (A = reducing air travel, using clean energy, etc.).

Importantly, in *Conservation*, one's individual actions to reduce climate change will have very little effect on the lives of future generations. The tiny absolute contribution each of us makes by reducing carbon emissions has in itself negligible effect on future generations. Yet a personal moral obligation is still said to exist. Even though the impersonal value we contribute and the difference each of us makes is negligible, a moral obligation is still said to exist. The difference we make in *Selection* is much greater. So if a moral obligation exists in *Conservation*, then a moral obligation exists in *Selection*.

Even though a moral obligation exists in each of these three cases, the obligation is prima facie or defeasible. What we have most reason to do depends on what all our reasons for action are at the time. We might have an all-things-considered obligation to fly in a plane to help our sick mother.

Is there evidence that a slide from the new to the old eugenics is likely?

The targets of old eugenics were the intellectually disabled, people with psychiatric diseases, and criminals. The current testing of fetuses and embryos for genetic disorders, especially intellectual disability (including Down syndrome), fits within the classic target of the old eugenics.

The weakness of Sparrow's speculations can be seen by the fact that the new eugenics is already widely practiced and accepted. It shows no signs of sliding into the old eugenics. Eugenics has occurred ever since prenatal and preimplantation diagnosis were offered to couples over 20 years ago to give them the freedom to have a child without a serious genetic disorder. It was precisely such people who were the objects of Nazi extermination and involuntary sterilization programmes in the United States and Europe earlier last century. The political reality is that any pressure to move to old eugenics can be and has been blocked by a strong commitment to procreative liberty within Western liberal societies.

One other common objection to PB is that people will be held responsible if they do not avail themselves of selection technologies. Again, the 'natural experiment' of genetic testing for Down syndrome and other genetic disorders in the last few decades is informative. One complaint labeled at such testing is that couples who do not employ testing are blamed by others in society for not using it, and for thus giving birth to a child with Down syndrome. However, this situation is clearly not so grave that it warrants withdrawing testing for genetic disorders.

Moreover, testing for genetic dispositions through the use of behavioural genetics would be expected to lead to less of this kind of problem for the reason that such tests are only probabilistic, whereas genetic testing for genetic disorders is fully predictive. It is obvious that someone has not used genetic testing to select against genetic disorder because genetic disorders like Down syndrome and cystic fibrosis are both obvious and purely genetically determined. In the case of, say, testing for genes for intelligence, self-control, or aggression, since the trait has both genetic and environmental determinants, it would not be obvious whether testing had been employed or not. Responsibility would be lessened and attribution would be difficult if the decision to test or not test remained private.

Sparrow touches on the issue of responsibility when he worries that 'parents who allow their children to be born with lower life prospects than other citizens will harm their compatriots' (Sparrow in this chapter). Clearly this is already occurring when people do not use very effective genetic screening technologies for expensive-to-treat diseases. Yet there is no significant coercion or reprobation of people who impose these costs on others. We believe and show that liberty is an important value to uphold. Moreover, everything we do, including eating a hamburger, drinking alcohol, smoking, engaging in risky sports, etc. has these indirect effects on others through consumption of resources. Such indirect effects, tout court, should not be the basis for invoking the liberal harm principle to employ coercion.

Sparrow worries that these technologies could be abused by authoritarian regimes. In the 1990s, China did pass its 'Eugenics Law' or the Infant and Maternal Health Care Law. This required mandatory genetic testing, abortion, and childlessness for those at risk of a genetic disorder. This was old-style eugenics. But China also had a one-child policy. Should we then ban contraception, or not argue in its favour, to prevent abuse of contraception? Sterilization was used in old-style eugenics—should we then fear a slippery slope from voluntary to involuntary sterilization? Indeed, medicine and surgery, including psychosurgery, were abused by the Soviets (and Americans) to pursue ideological ends. Is this an argument against their value or appropriate use? No.

Any authoritarian (or other illiberal) government can abuse any technology. Genetic selection technologies are no different from any other powerful technology. Indeed, they are less prone to abuse because for the vast majority of cases, genes only contribute but do not determine traits. There are many more effective ways of determining what kind of people there are, as the Nazis realized when they used the very simple method of killing to realize their fascist, social Darwinist, racist ideals. The risk of authoritarian abuse is no reason for us not to advocate and use technology, though it might be a reason to limit access to it.

Any moral obligation can be twisted by governments to coerce people in the name of the same goal. Consider *Helping*. Governments could unreasonably increase taxation, or still worse move to slavery, to increase foreign aid to developing countries. There are abundant historical precedents of the state subjugating people and their labor to realize its moral ideals. One recent, familiar case was socialism. The fact that authoritarian states might abuse the use of the labour of their citizens should not stop talk of helping or contributing to some global collective ideal of equality.

Sparrow claims my ideas are contributing to a slide to the old eugenics. As evidence, he is worried that my book with Nick Bostrom (Savulescu and Bostrom 2009) and Nick Agar's book, *Liberal Eugenics* (Agar 2004), both have musclemen on the front. In our case, the image was chosen by the publisher, presumably to provoke people to buy the book. I always thought our cover looked slightly ridiculous, but I am no aesthetic expert. But I hardly think it is about to bring about a new Nazi eugenics.

An example

Let's consider an example in this debate. Imagine a couple is having IVF for infertility. They produce ten embryos and utilize PGD to test for chromosomal disorders and genetic dispositions to major diseases. In the near future, they will be able to test not merely for major genetic disorders, but to use whole-genome analysis to test for minor conditions and the genetic dispositions to personality type, cognitive abilities, physical abilities, and behaviour in general. In a case in which IVF and PGD are already being undertaken, testing for non-disease genes imposes no extra costs or risks to the couple or the embryo.

Currently, the UK, the Australian state of Victoria, and many other jurisdictions, if they allow PGD at all (Germany does not), only allow it to be used to detect serious diseases. Couples are denied available information for their reproductive choices. I have argued that not only should they be allowed to access this full range of information but that they should access it and choose that embryo, or range of embryos, which have the best chance of the best life.

An example might be a genetic disposition to poor impulse control. Impulse control (or ability to delay gratification) has been strongly correlated with academic and social success, higher socio-economic status, and lower risk of imprisonment. If some set of genes were associated with poor (but within the normal range) impulse control, couples should select other embryos with a better impulse control profile, if that were possible and other things were equal. The reason is that embryos with genetic dispositions to better impulse control are likely to become future people who are more likely to have better lives, whatever they choose to do.

Sparrow believes that selection would require different kinds of decisions: 'parents who wish to have the "best child possible" should choose to bring into existence only good-looking, heterosexual, white men (indeed, the first observation suggests that they should all procure a clone of the same "perfect" child)' (Sparrow in this chapter).

This of course conflicts with his claims elsewhere that PB is committed to selecting only women because they live longer. Does Sparrow really believe that people would enjoy and flourish more in a world of only women, or only white heterosexual men, or single clones? Such a world would be boring and sterile.

Virtually all goods have a mixture of positional and non-positional value. Sparrow treats good as purely non-positional. This is the opposite of the common tendency to treat goods as purely positional, e.g. claiming intelligence or height are only of value if one has them and others do not. Yet there can be advantage, as well as disadvantage, in difference. In Scandinavian countries, dark skin and dark eyes may be valued because they are different; in Latin countries, blond hair and blue eyes.

As Sparrow notes, individual actions have collective effects and those effects need to be taken into account when making selection decisions about what will be best for the child. It may be advantageous to make different decisions.

Moreover, collective effects can be bad, as Sparrow notes. He rightly claims that any plausible non-libertarian system of reproductive decision-making will include some state-imposed constraints. That is exactly right. I have always maintained that there are other reasons for action besides PB. The public interest is one example.

We already have state-imposed constraints on reproduction. In many jurisdictions, no more than two embryos can be transferred, and in some, only one. Indeed, parents cannot access any genetic tests for non-disease genes in Europe and Australia. These are severe limitations—too severe. So the claim that there might be state limitations of procreative autonomy if PB were adopted misses the point that there are already very severe limitations.

It would be legitimate for liberal democracies to place some constraints on selection decisions to prevent adverse collective effects and to limit parents to choosing genes which are plausibly related to increased chances of a good life, or at least not clearly associated with a decreased chance of a good life. So, for example, it might be legitimate to prevent doctors assisting with the deliberate transfer of an embryo known to become anencephalic, or to have Trisomy 18.

If one were very nervous, as Sparrow appears to be, about the risk of abuse, one could limit selection decisions to genes for which there is good evidence of significant effect on future well-being, such as genes for adequate impulse control. And if one were concerned that selection decisions might be made in the interests of the state, but associated with lower personal well-being, one might exclude selections of this kind.

The interesting debates to be had are not about PB, but about what constitutes well-being and which genes are significantly associated with increased chances of well-being. As a first step towards PB, one could limit access to selection for non-disease genes to those for which a consensus exists on their value.

This would be an advance on all current regimes. At present, no testing is allowed, even when IVF and PGD are otherwise being undertaken, such as in Europe or Australia; or there is a free market with no constraints, with people buying supposedly superior eggs and sperm, employing any genetic test, for any purpose, on an ability-to-pay basis, as occurs in the US. The first is a kind of involuntary, naturalistic eugenics; the second rampant libertarianism.

Sparrow claims the idea that parents should aim to maximize their child's well-being is 'an obvious non-starter', citing Buchanan et al.'s observation 'that when it comes to environmental interventions into the well-being of a child very few, if any, parents do *everything* they can to provide their child with the best possible life, as doing so would deprive them of any time or resources to dedicate to their own interests' (Sparrow in this chapter). I made it clear (Savulescu and Kahane 2009) that it is irrational to aim at submaximization. Yet this claim is different from recognizing that there are other reasons besides PB and costs to gaining more information.

Sparrow also criticizes the idea that parents, if they could, should aim at the best. '[A]s "best" is a maximizing notion, in any given environment there will only be one "best genome". It would therefore appear that all the parents sharing an environment should aspire to bring into existence a child produced by cloning from the same, "best", embryo' (Sparrow in this chapter).

The very formulation of PB anticipates this objection when it reads 'or at least as good as others'—best denotes a range, perhaps a very broad range, of possible lives. It would be absurd to think that a single genome would be uniquely best. Is it better to be introverted or extroverted? Presumably each can be advantageous—and disadvantageous—in certain environments. Is it better to be a manic depressive genius, or a euthymic ordinary Joe? It is hard to say. There will be many cases in which there either is no clearly superior genome, or we cannot know which is superior. But that should not stop us saying that some genomes are clearly worse, say for example one having a tendency to very poor impulse control or self-control.

Weighing person-affecting and impersonal reasons

To see why a slide from the new eugenics to the old eugenics should not occur, it is important to distinguish two kinds of reasons. The reason, as Sparrow recognizes, that is captured by PB is an 'impersonal' reason. Derek Parfit first described this reason with this example.

The Medical Programmes. There are two rare conditions, J and K, which cannot be detected without special tests. If a pregnant woman has condition J, this will cause the child she is carrying to have a certain handicap. A simple treatment would prevent this effect. If a woman has condition K when she conceives a child, this will cause the child to have the same particular handicap. Condition K cannot be treated, but always disappears within two months. Suppose next that we have planned two medical programmes, but there are funds for only one; so one must be cancelled.

Parfit supports the No Difference View: he believes that each programme is right and there are equally strong reasons to pursue each. This I believe is wrong. I will call the programme to treat condition J, *Treatment*, and the programme to detect condition K, *Prevention*. The reasons involved in these cases are of different kinds, of different moral significance and weight.

In the case of *Treatment*, there is person-affecting harm. If you fail to treat, a future person is made worse off than he or she would otherwise have been. In *Prevention*, the harm is impersonal—the world is worse for having more suffering than it could have contained, but no person is worse off than he or she would otherwise have been.

In my view, there are both person-affecting reasons and impersonal reasons. However, person-affecting reasons are stronger than impersonal reasons, even though the latter are reasons for action.

Some people are sceptical that impersonal reasons are reasons at all. However, the justification of environmental policies such as carbon reduction strategies are based partly on impersonal reasons. Environmental policies subtly change the timing of reproduction by changing the course of events, and so change the identity of future generations. Parfit realized this in Part IV of his *Reasons and Persons* (Parfit 1984). For this reason, a policy of depletion rather than conservation of natural resources, or of emission of large amounts of carbon rather than reduction, will not harm any person in the future (assuming their lives are still worth living), because those people would not have otherwise existed. Environmental policies are identity affecting.

Many people speak of 'future generations' as if they were now identifiable individuals who will exist in the future. This is a mistake. The choices we now make will determine which possible future generation will come into existence. If we believe their lives should be better rather than worse, then we believe in the existence of impersonal reasons. Sparrow accepts the existence of such impersonal reasons.

As I said, Parfit believes that there is as much reason to pursue *Prevention* as there is to pursue *Treatment*. This is a mistake. Imagine a deaf couple who wish to have a child who will be deaf like them and a part of the Deaf Community. In the case of *Poison*, they give their newborn baby a poison which selectively destroys the nerve cells in the ear. In *Selection*, they use IVF and genetic testing to select an embryo they know will be deaf. In both cases, a deaf child results. But the wrong which the parents do in *Poison* seems significantly worse. If this is true, this could at least in part be because personal harms are much worse than impersonal ones.

Compare selecting a child with mild intellectual disability with failing to treat mild intellectual disability. The latter seems worse. It would not only be wrong for a parent to fail to treat their child's intellectual disability or pain or disability, a court would order treatment on behalf of the child. There is both a moral and a legal obligation.

Such a legal obligation does not exist in the case of genetic selection. According to Mill's harm principle, the sole ground for interference in the liberty of another is because that person's actions harm or risk harming another person. Although wrong, procreative decisions to deliberately select a disabled or disadvantaged embryo do not harm anyone, provided the child's life is worth living. They are impersonally wrong but there is no person-affecting harm.

For this reason, I have argued that deaf people and dwarfs should be free to deliberately select offspring with genetic forms of deafness or dwarfism. Even though such choices are wrong, they should be permitted (Savulescu 2002).

In general, proscriptions against person-affecting harm should be much stronger than those against impersonal harms. We should not significantly harm individuals now to bring about a better world, where the betterness is impersonal.

Impersonal reasons then could be rather weak when pitted against personal reasons. Requirements of PB and to preserve and protect the environment are reasons, but should not require major person-affecting harms. Nor should they require major sacrifices from prospective parents or others existing now in society.

Invasion of personal liberty is a serious harm. According to Mill, it is only justified when that person threatens to directly and seriously harm another. I would add, when that harm is personal in nature.

If our reasons to have the best children (and best future environment) are relatively weak, they are easily overridden by person-affecting reasons. Not only does interfering in procreative liberty constitute a harm, there are other harms involved in forcing or compelling people to have certain kinds of children. These are psychological and involve loss of dreams, plans, aspirations, etc.

There are strong philosophical grounds to hold that procreative liberty should extend to people selecting less than the best child. Sparrow's failure to distinguish between person-affecting and impersonal harm leads him, I believe, to make claims like: 'If enhancing future individuals would make sufficiently large difference to total welfare then the state *would* on consequentialist grounds, at least, be justified in legislating to ensure that parents enhance their children' (Sparrow in this chapter).

Sparrow seems to derive this from the correct observation that states have already legislated certain environmental policies and this is on the ground of impersonal reasons. However, such legislation is misplaced—we should encourage individuals to behave better, develop better energy sources and solutions but not require them by law to curtail their behaviour in ways which significantly harm them. And of course such legislation could be justified on the grounds other than the impersonal value to future generations, for example by encouraging solidarity, protecting the environment itself, etc.

In some ways, our obligation as parents to have the best child is like our obligations as citizens to preserve the environment and resources for future generations. I have argued that these obligations are weak compared to obligations to presently existing persons. Nonetheless, they are obligations. Sparrow's worries about authoritarian abuse seem particularly misplaced when we realize our obligations generated by procreative beneficence are like obligations to future generations. Of course authoritarian governments *might* subjugate the present generation to promote welfare of future generations (or some other impersonal ideal). But that is both unethical and unlikely to succeed in the long term. As is well known in the politics of the environment, future generations have no presence or vote or power today. Presently existing individuals have the voice of power.

Genes for criminality

Sparrow claims that I am in 'error' talking about genes for criminality. 'There cannot possibly be a gene that determines whether or not someone is "a criminal"' (Sparrow in this chapter).

There cannot be a gene that determines whether any human behaves in a certain way. He grants that genes can make certain behaviours more or less likely. But that is all 'genes for criminality' could mean. And it is indeed how I have discussed it. There is a large amount of evidence that the nonsense mutation of the gene for the enzyme MAOA (responsible for the metabolism of neurotransmitters in the brain) is highly correlated with criminal behaviour (Brunner et al. 1993a; Brunner et al. 1993b).

More surprisingly, there are two common variants of MAOA: the low-activity polymorphism (MAO-L) is possessed by 30 per cent of people, the high-activity variant (MAO-H) by 70 per cent (Baum and Savulescu forthcoming). Caspi and colleagues (Caspi et al. 2002) followed 1,037 New Zealand male children at regular intervals as they grew to 26 years of age. Antisocial behaviour was measured by convictions for violent crime, diagnosis of adolescent conduct disorder, psychological assessment of violence acceptance, and third-party-reported antisocial personality disorder (ASPD) symptoms. Neither MAO-L nor MAO-H correlated significantly with later antisocial behaviour alone. Maltreatment, however, did (8 per cent of boys experienced severe maltreatment, and 23 per cent probable maltreatment between the ages of three and 11).

However, a deeply surprising result emerged when the maltreated boys were further grouped according to MAOA variant. Childhood maltreatment had its expected increase in risk of later antisocial behaviour in boys who possessed the MAO-L variant, but maltreated boys with MAO-H were not statistically more likely to exhibit future antisocial behaviour than boys who were not maltreated. Maltreatment significantly predisposed the boys to later antisocial behaviour *if and only if* they possessed MAO-L. If the boys were not maltreated, genotype had no effect.

Only 12 per cent of boys were maltreated *and* possessed the MAO-L genotype, but this group was responsible for 44 per cent of convictions for violent crime. The authors point out that the effect was similar in magnitude to 'major risk factors associated with cardiovascular disease' (Caspi et al. 2002: 854). This was the first example of a gene–environment interaction correlating with a violent behaviour.

As we have argued (Baum and Savulescu forthcoming), MAO-L is a gene that plausibly correlates disadvantage in conditions of abuse. Of course, we should try to ensure children are not abused or maltreated. But social protection is never perfect. The MAO-H confers resilience to abuse. And MAO-L is apparently not correlated strongly with any advantage in any situation (though there is some weak evidence it might reduce chances of depression).

In my view, the evidence of the effects of MAO-L and MAO-H is strong enough to warrant the claim that MAO-H is better than MAO-L, though of course this should be the subject of further debate. However, if these results are further confirmed (and meta-analysis has supported them—Baum and Savulescu forthcoming), this would be a candidate gene for selection, not mainly because of the risk of harm to others (though that is a relevant consideration—Savulescu 2001c), but because imprisonment plausibly reduces well-being. Importantly, this genetic science has been used in mitigation in recent criminal cases (see Baum and Savulescu forthcoming), acknowledging its role in causation of crime.

Couples accessing IVF and PGD for reasons of infertility or genetic disorder should also be able to test for MAOA and they should select the MAO-H variant. Far from being a far-fetched example, perhaps one of the best examples of the use of current genetic knowledge is related to 'genes for criminality'.

Responding to moral obligations

I would like to make one concession to Sparrow. Thanks to discussions with him, I have realized that ordinary talk of moral obligation often is conflated with ideas of what people *must* (rather than should) do, and invites blame and punishment for failure to meet obligation.

That is not how I see moral obligation but I grant that by saying we have a moral obligation to select, many people will misunderstand that I mean that they must select, they should be blamed and possibly even punished if they don't select. On the view I have proposed, people who choose not to have genetic screening are doing the wrong thing when they have a child with a disability. It is offensive to say to someone you should have had a different child.

I agree with this criticism. But I have two responses. Firstly, if someone has a child with a disability, that child now exists and deserves equal respect and concern. It is wrong at that point to say, 'You should have had a different child.' It would be offensive to the child. In this way, the moral obligation to select should only operate prospectively, not retrospectively.

Secondly, the nature of our response to normative reasons and obligations depends on the strength or weight of those reasons and obligations. Response can vary in the gravity with which it restricts liberty on a sliding scale:

provision of choice—provision of information—persuasive argument—harnessing biases and heuristics—inducements—taxes/levies—punishment—imprisonment—coerced medical treatment—invasive surgery

As I have argued elsewhere, we should always choose the least liberty-infringing intervention necessary to protect third parties or the public interest. In the case of selection decision, perhaps because a child will exist who should be loved and accorded equal concern and respect, we should only provide choice and information to select, without encouragement or attempted persuasion.

This would require making tests for important non-disease genes like MAO-H available and providing information about them, but not attempting to strongly direct people to the right choice. The nature of our response to normative reasons is a large issue which I have not addressed in detail.

In this response, I have argued that our reason to select the best child is an impersonal reason and as such grounds a weak moral obligation. It is easily defeated by person-affecting moral obligations. Since our obligations to select better children are weak, there is little risk of a slide back to the old eugenics. Because of the need to protect the interests of present people with disability and genomes which disadvantage those people, the nature and strength of our obligation to select may only ground the provision of the possibility of selection together with information on the consequences of that choice.

It remains true that people should select the best child. Though that claim should not be silent, it should not be especially loud. People should remain free to select less than the best child and they should not be especially pressured to select. Nonetheless, if a gene or genes are correlated with a better chance of a better life, you should choose those genes.

References

Agar, N. (2004). *Liberal Eugenics: In Defence of Human Enhancement*. Oxford: Blackwell.

Baum, M., and Savulescu, J. (Forthcoming). 'Behavioural BioMarkers: What Are They Good for?' in I. A. Singh and W. Sinnott-Armstrong (eds), *Bio-Prediction of Bad Behaviour*. Oxford: Oxford University Press.

Brunner, H. G. et al. (1993a). 'Abnormal Behavior Associated with a Point Mutation in the Structural Gene for Monoamine Oxidase A', *Science*, 262(5133): 578–80.

Brunner, H. G. et al. (1993b). 'X-Linked Borderline Mental Retardation with Prominent Behavioral Disturbance: Phenotype, Genetic Localization, and Evidence for Disturbed Monoamine Metabolism', *American Journal of Human Genetics*, 52(6): 1032–9.

Caspi, A. et al. (2002). 'Role of Genotype in the Cycle of Violence in Maltreated Children', *Science*, 297:851–4.

Kahane, G., and Savulescu, J. (2009). 'The Welfarist Account of Disability', in A. Cureton and K. Brownlee (eds), *Disability and Disadvantage*. Oxford: Oxford University Press, 14–53.

Parfit, D. (1984). *Reasons and Persons*. Oxford: Clarendon Press.

Savulescu, J. (2001a). 'Justice and Health Care: A Right to a Decent Minimum Not Equality of Opportunity', *American Journal of Bioethics*, 1(2): 1a–3a.

Savulescu, J. (2001b). 'Procreative Beneficence: Why We Should Select the Best Children', *Bioethics*, 15(5): 413–26.

Savulescu, J. (2001c). 'Why Genetic Testing for Genes for Criminality Is Morally Required', *Princeton Journal of Bioethics*, 4: 79–97.

Savulescu, J. (2002). 'Deaf Lesbians, "Designer Disability", and the Future of Medicine', *British Medical Journal*, 325:771–3.

Savulescu, J. (2006). 'Justice, Fairness, and Enhancement', *Annals of the New York Academy of Sciences*, 1093:321–38.

Savulescu, J. (2008). 'Procreative Beneficence: Reasons Not to Have Disabled Children', in J. Thompson and L. Skene (eds), *The Sorting Society: The Ethics of Genetic Screening and Therapy*. Cambridge: Cambridge University Press, 51–68.

Savulescu, J. (2009). 'Enhancement and Fairness', in P. Healeyand and S. Rayner (eds), *Unnatural Selection: The Challenges of Engineering Tomorrow's People*. London: Earthscan, 177–87.

Savulescu, J., and Bostrom, N. (eds). (2009). Human Enhancement. Oxford: Oxford University Press.

Savulescu, J., and Kahane, G. (2009). 'The Moral Obligation to Create Children with the Best Chance of the Best Life', *Bioethics*, 23(5): 274–90.

Sparrow, R. (2014). 'Ethics, Eugenics, and Politics', in A. Akabayashi (ed.), *The Future of Bioethics: International Dialogues*. Oxford: Oxford University Press, 139–53.

4.6

Response to Commentaries
The Real Force of 'Procreative Beneficence'

Robert Sparrow

My primary topic article is critical of the contemporary philosophical enthusiasm for human enhancement and argues both that, were this technology to be realized in reality, its consequences are likely to be much more disturbing than this debate acknowledges, and—perhaps more importantly—that the politics of this debate are more problematic than many of those participating in it perhaps realize. Since writing it, and in the course of subsequent debate about these claims, I have become more and more convinced that when philosophers debate the ethics of genetic human enhancement—a prospect that remains largely imaginary—what the public hears is that 'genes matter' and by implication that those who are wealthy and successful must have better genes than those who are not. That is to say, the most likely consequence of the current debate about human enhancement is to reinvigorate Social Darwinism. I am pleased that three of my correspondents also share my concerns about the ethics of human enhancement and the manner in which the current philosophical debate is being conducted. Unsurprisingly, Professor Savulescu, who is arguably the single philosopher most responsible for the current vogue for writing about enhancement, disagrees. Inevitably then, most of this response will focus on the arguments Professor Savulescu has made in his criticisms of my chapter.

However, before I move to consider Professor Savulescu's objections let me first note a number of valid criticisms and useful additions from the other correspondents as well as a few places where I am inclined to dispute particular claims.

Professor Ichinokawa (2014) offers a valuable account of the history of eugenic sterilization in Japan, which dramatically illustrates the dangers associated with eugenic ideas and the power they have to motivate infringements of individual liberty even in the relatively recent past. His observation that many of the historical instances of sterilization that we today think of as being coercive were actually justified with reference to a lack of capacity in those being sterilized to consent to the decision and are therefore susceptible to being brought within a 'liberal' framework is particularly insightful. He also reminds us that a concern for the welfare of future individuals should motivate us first and foremost to be concerned with the *social* environment into which future citizens are born.

Dr McGowan (2014) agrees that the enhancement debate has the structure that I suggest but questions the extent to which my own argument suffers by virtue of having 'an entirely futuristic orientation' (in this chapter). She draws upon her own empirical research into the motivations and experiences of those undertaking PGD to suggest that some of the dangers I identify regarding the ways in which social expectations might shape decisions about genetic selection are already being realized in the context of PGD for selection against disease traits and for gender selection. She also notes that users themselves have complex and conflicted understandings of their own practices, which simultaneously emphasize reproductive liberty, acknowledge social and medical pressures to avoid known genetic and chromosomal risk factors, and disavow the pursuit of an ideal family. While I agree that such empirical investigations of user perspectives have a role to play in informing our understanding of the likely future of human enhancement, I remain confident that what we already know about the relationship between social context and individual decision-making is sufficient to suggest that, were meaningful genetic human enhancement to become available, individuals are less likely to remain 'free' to resist enhancement for their children than advocates of enhancement typically allow.

Professor Jones (2014) also insists on the primacy of 'dilemmas that medicine encounters in the clinics and in everyday practice' (in this chapter). I have much sympathy for this thought but would also defend the legitimacy of engaging in debates about more speculative possibilities, as I have done here, especially when the purpose of doing so is to reveal how these debates have real-world political consequences. Jones also calls attention to the likelihood of significant negative side effects of enhancement as well as a number of other arguments against enhancement I did not have space to discuss in my primary topic article. Two issues in this generally sympathetic discussion, in particular, deserve comment. First, Jones is obviously right that many of the issues about the obligations of parents and the dangers of social coercion already arise in the context of therapeutic interventions. Second, while the line between therapy and enhancement is indeed hard to draw, as his series of scenarios demonstrates nicely, I would nevertheless insist that we need to, as far as we can, affirm the moral significance of the therapy/enhancement distinction as being the only plausible place to draw a line that might help resist the social pressures towards enhancement I identified in my original paper (see also Sparrow 2010a; Sparrow 2010c; Sparrow 2011b). I am especially cynical about any definition of enhancement as anything that increases an individual's well-being even if such an increase leaves the individual's functioning below that which is species typical.

Let me turn now to Professor Savulescu's more critical discussion (Savulescu 2014). Much of his commentary rehashes arguments he has made elsewhere in defence of the putative obligation of procreative beneficence (Savulescu 2001a; Savulescu 2001b; Savulescu 2002; Savulescu 2005; Savulescu et al. 2006; Savulescu 2008; Savulescu and Kahane 2009) and to which I have previously responded (Sparrow 2007; Sparrow 2010d; Sparrow 2011a). Like him, I am happy to leave it up to the interested reader to refer to that larger literature (see also: de Melo-Martin 2004; Häyry 2004; Herissone-Kelly 2006; Parker 2007; Stoller 2008; Bennett 2009; Elster 2011) and decide for her- or himself where the burden of the argument lies. However, in this latest contribution by Savulescu, there are: a number of points of substantive disagreement that have not been as evident elsewhere; several places where he has missed the point of my original criticism and thereby failed to respond to it; a couple of outright contradictions; and an extremely useful clarification of both the content and force of the 'obligation' of procreative beneficence and the idiosyncratic nature of the terminology Savulescu has used in the course of asserting it. Each of these is worthy of some further, brief, comment in this context.

Disagreements

To begin with the straightforward, substantive, disagreements.

Professor Savulescu notes, as does Professor Jones, that any danger of the new eugenics sliding into the old eugenics should arise just as much in relation to therapeutic uses of genetic technologies as in relation to enhancement. Savulescu sees no evidence that this has occurred and insists that 'a strong commitment to procreative liberty within Western liberal societies' will continue to prevent this from happening (Savulescu in this collection). Like Jones, I believe there is ample evidence that couples confronting reproductive decisions around disability are subject to a range of subtle and not-so-subtle social and institutional pressures to make particular sorts of decisions, sufficient to call into question the extent to which their decisions may be said to be truly 'free'. However, Savulescu is correct that, with rare exceptions such as the UK Human Fertilization and Embryology Act 2008, Western 'liberal' governments have as yet mostly shied away from directly legislating parental responsibilities in this regard. However, this may well be due to the relatively small number of parents who confront these decisions and the even smaller number who proceed to knowingly bring into existence children with severe impairments.[12] Should it become possible to achieve significant improvements in human welfare via genetic human enhancement, the pressure to coerce those individuals who wish to refuse such enhancements for their children may well, as I have argued, prove irresistible. In this context, Savulescu's insistence that testing for genetic dispositions is unlikely to generate such pressures either because it would sometimes not work or because it would often be unclear whether it had worked is surprising given the large claims made for genetic human enhancement elsewhere in the literature (Harris 1992; Silver 1999; Stock 2003; Green 2007). Moreover, Savulescu himself goes on to endorse state regulation justified on the basis of concern for the welfare of children later in his own argument! Similarly, his suggestion that parental freedom should be limited where unrestricted choice would threaten diversity betrays a surprising willingness even in this supposedly staunch defender of reproductive freedom to sacrifice liberty for social benefits.

I am also inclined to continue to insist that the fact that many of the societies in which contemporary arguments for human enhancement are being heard and read are not 'Western liberal societies' is significant for our ultimate assessment of the plausibility of arguments within this debate. The example Savulescu chooses serves him ill here: the

---

[12] It is also worth observing that the supposed commitment to 'procreative liberty' has not been sufficient to secure women a right to abortion on demand as yet in many jurisdictions in 'Western liberal societies'.

abuses of egalitarian arguments by authoritarian regimes should indeed give us cause to think carefully about how or whether we should advance them. Think here, too, of the role played by concerns that 'rogue states'—and not just peace-loving nations like the United States (!)—will develop nuclear weapons in discussions concerning technologies related to nuclear proliferation. One need not agree with the detail of these arguments or endorse their conclusions to acknowledge that the actual nature of the world in which technologies are being developed is relevant to discussions about the ethics of their development and application.

Missing the point

Savulescu completely misses the point of my argument that 'there cannot possibly be a gene' for criminality. The issue here is not whether the penetrance for genes associated with antisocial behaviour is high or low or whether the genes only code for certain behaviours in certain environments, as his discussion implies.[13] Rather, my point was simply that 'criminal' is a social category, the limits of which are specific to historical and social context. In some jurisdictions if you smoke marijuana you are a criminal, in others you are an ordinary law-abiding citizen. There may well be genes that predispose individuals to enjoy getting high, but there cannot be a gene that predisposes them to being a criminal 'dope fiend'—as membership in the latter category is not a function of behaviour per se but rather of social context. Indeed, this point goes for behaviour more generally: same gene, same bodily actions, in a different context will be a different behaviour. Thus, if the child with the gene for MAO-L who is a victim of abuse grows up to join the police force or an irregular militia, where their predisposition to violence on a short fuse may even be a virtue, they may never be identified as involved in 'antisocial' behaviour. The point here is not that their antisocial behaviour is not singled out—it is that violence and intimidation in defence of law and order are not 'antisocial'. A gene for 'criminality' would have to somehow track these sociopolitical differences, which is impossible.

Savulescu also misses the point of my argument that his account implies that parents should all choose clones of the one 'best' embryo and that—at the very least—they should all choose embryos of the same sex.

Savulescu's protestations that many different genomes may be 'equally good' (of which, more below) notwithstanding, there seems to be no reason to rule out the possibility that one particular genome might be clearly superior to all others available—in which case all parents would indeed be obligated to choose clones of an embryo with this genome. In any case, the key point here is that any obligation on parents to maximize their child's welfare will radically constrain the range of morally permissible options available to them.

---

[13] Although, in passing, in the context of Savulescu's reliance on claims about the implications of a genetic predisposition to poor impulse control for the future welfare of children, it is interesting to note the recent publication of a paper (Kidd, Palmeri, and Aslin 2013) suggesting alternative, non-genetic, mechanisms whereby what at least at first appears to be 'poor impulse control' in young children might correlate with poor socio-economic outcomes in later life.

Preimplantation (or preconception) sex selection for 'enhancement' is an important test case for arguments about 'procreative beneficence' because it is the one case where parents can wield significant influence over their child's life prospects through non-therapeutic selection on the basis of our existing (parlous) knowledge of human genetics. Whether procreative beneficence implies that parents have reason to select male or female children will depend on whether we believe they should take the impact of systemic social injustice into account in their deliberations about the implications of their reproductive decision for the welfare of their future child. There is therefore nothing inconsistent in my having pointed out that, strictly speaking, if parents wish to maximize the welfare of their child in racist, homophobic, and sexist societies they should choose to have 'good-looking, heterosexual, white men' and that, if they are obligated to neglect the implications of injustice for welfare in making this calculation, then they should all choose female children (because of their longer life expectancy). Whether injustice should figure into these calculations or not is a problem for advocates of enhancement. Again, what is important here is that whatever obligations parents have in relation to the sex of their children will bear on all couples. That is to say, parents should all make *the same* choice.

The fact that parents acting on their obligation to choose the 'best child' would be disastrous for diversity, as Savulescu rightly observes, is precisely why this is an interesting and problematic consequence of the argument for 'procreative beneficence'. A concern to preserve diversity is relevant at the level of law or public policy but does not alter the content of parental obligations, given that social homogenization would occur as the aggregate consequence of hundreds of thousands of uncoordinated reproductive choices and not as the result of any particular couple's decision. The fact remains, then, that each and every couple would be obligated to choose a child of whatever sort (and sex!) is judged to have superior life prospects. Moreover, to insist as Savulescu does here, that a concern for diversity would justify regulating to prevent these sorts of collective action problems is to argue that parents should be required to sacrifice the welfare of their children for the sake of social benefits. However, once this principle was admitted, what principled grounds do we have to object to more radical programmes for improving social welfare by engineering individuals to fit predetermined social roles? This disjunct between the implications of his account for the obligations of parents and the public policy implications of the threat to diversity remains to be addressed by Savulescu.

Finally, Savulescu has failed to appreciate the significance of my observation about the fascist iconography on the front covers of various key texts in the enhancement debates. Granted that the publication of these books will not in itself bring about a coercive eugenics, the fact that the editors and/or publishers of these books would choose such images independently of the desires of the authors is a vivid illustration of my argument that the politics of the debate about human enhancement transcends the intentions of those participating in it.

Contradictions

The nature (and force) of the obligation of procreative beneficence, given the non-person-affecting nature of the decisions to which it applies, is one of the most contested questions in the debate surrounding human enhancement. Two contradictions in Savulescu's response to me suggest that even he remains confused about it. First, Savulescu insists that 'PB is not a special moral obligation' whilst simultaneously arguing, in his discussion of Parfit, that non-person-affecting reasons are 'of different moral significance and weight' to person-affecting reasons (Savulescu in this collection). This tension is reflected in his equivocation regarding the force of the obligation of procreative beneficence more generally. Second, and relatedly, Savulescu agrees that 'It would be legitimate for liberal democracies to place some constraints on selection decisions to prevent adverse collective effects and to limit parents to choosing genes which are plausibly related to increased chances of a good life, or at least not clearly associated with a decreased chance of a good life' but also argues that 'a legal obligation does not exist in the case of genetic selection' for 'a disabled or disadvantaged embryo [sic]'; elsewhere he suggests that coercion is only justified when harm 'is personal in nature' (Savulescu in this collection).[14]

Revealing clarifications

Despite these various disagreements with Professor Savulescu, I am extremely pleased that this exchange has prompted him to clarify several key points in the increasingly muddy debate around 'procreative beneficence'.

Perhaps Savulescu's most striking admission is that there is no such thing as 'the best child', at least as this phrase would ordinarily be understood. In many cases, he now acknowledges, there is no answer to the question as to which of various genomes is superior. Although he doesn't use the term, his discussion makes it clear that many different bundles of genetically influenced capacities are incommensurable when it comes to evaluating well-being. This admission is striking because: A) Savulescu's published work has repeatedly referred to an obligation to choose *the* best child, which invites the interpretation (the *single* best child) that he now claims is a misinterpretation; and, B) it risks effectively voiding the force of the obligation by allowing that any genome that would allow a child a life 'worth living' is as 'good' as any other, as scholars associated with the disability critique of prenatal testing have long argued.

In fairness, as Savulescu points out, the original formulation of the principle of procreative beneficence did allow for the possibility that there would be no single clear winner of the title of 'best embryo'—in which case parents would be obligated only to choose from amongst the set of embryos that were not worse than any others. However, I have always interpreted this as a concession to the problem that there might be no highest-ranked choice in rare cases of ties (such as when embryos are genetically identical), which besets any account of a maximizing principle, rather than—as it now turns out—a recognition that there will be no answer as to which embryo is best *in many cases*. Moreover, I believe my mistake was a reasonable one, shared by many others, given the emphasis on maximization in the key papers on procreative beneficence

---

[14] Note that the collective effects of reproductive decisions are not person-affecting in so far as they will, harm, individuals who do not yet exist.

and the references to 'the best' in the text of these papers and occasionally in their titles (Savulescu 2001a; Savulescu and Kahane 2009). Indeed, even in this most recent treatment Savulescu's opening sentence affirms 'that couples have a moral obligation to use genetic selection to have *the best child*, of the possible children they could have' (Savulescu in this collection; italics added). Given that he has now conceded that in many cases there will be no such thing as *the* best child, a less misleading statement of parents' obligations would be 'not to have any child worse than another child they could have had'.

However, the real significance of allowing that, in many cases, there is no answer to the question of which genome is 'best' is that it concedes the possibility that procreative beneficence may seldom, if ever, be relevant to parents' reproductive decisions. Theorists from the disability community have argued forcefully on the basis of their own experience that the lives of those with even quite severe genetic conditions can be just as good as the lives of individuals with putatively 'better' genes (Kaplan 1993; Asch 1999; Hurst 2009; Oliver 2009). Even if we wish to insist that it is always 'better' to be born without impairments, we might still hold that any 'normal' genome is as good as any other.[15] This would be the case, for instance, if the presence of an allegedly 'superior' trait in an individual, which conveys advantages in relation to the pursuit of some range of projects, always comes at the cost of their capacity to succeed in other projects (Sparrow 2010b). Conceding the possibility of the incommensurability of the life prospects of embryos therefore calls into question the entire project of genetic human enhancement.

It is also extremely useful to have it openly acknowledged that procreative beneficence is compatible with regulation 'in the public interest', including regulation that requires parents to have children with significantly worse welfare than others that they could have had (as would be the case where parents are expected to have a male child with a five-year shorter life expectancy for the sake of 'diversity' or a 'less boring world'). This is precisely why I worry about the development of a more coercive regime of regulation of reproductive decisions as a result of contemporary philosophical enthusiasm for human enhancement. The more we emphasize the importance of the public interest in deliberations about reproductive technology, the more likely it is that states will intervene in more reproductive decisions.

Although, as I noted above, there remains significant lack of clarity therein, Savulescu's discussion of the force of the 'obligation' of procreative beneficence is also timely. It is now abundantly clear that procreative beneficence provides us with only 'some reason' to choose the better embryo and that this reason is easily defeated by a wide range of other considerations. A key question now is whether *any* countervailing reason, such as the parents' desire to have another sort of child, is sufficient to vitiate the obligation of procreative beneficence—in which case it is extremely unlikely ever to determine parents' all-things-considered obligations (Sparrow 2007)—or whether countervailing person-affecting reasons must reach some particular threshold before they can outweigh reasons arising out of procreative beneficence—in which case we are owed a further

---

[15] Interestingly, this is what people appear to think when the question of whether it is better to be born male or female is posed.

account of what this threshold might be and why procreative beneficence should have this force precisely.

Finally, I am grateful for Savulescu's acknowledgement that his use of the language of obligation in the debate surrounding procreative beneficence has, to date, been somewhat idiosyncratic. As Savulescu admits, 'a moral obligation' would ordinarily imply that those who fail to act upon it 'do the wrong thing' and consequently should be blamed and criticized for doing so. Moreover, *obligations* are usually thought to have an especial weight relative to the other reasons that might bear upon us (for instance, prudential reasons or mere preferences) such that to insist that we are obligated to do something is to say more than just that we have a reason to do it. Finally, while not all obligations should be enforced by law, the question of the appropriateness of regulation at least arises with regards to individuals' failure to meet their obligations, where it typically does not if they merely fail to act on the basis of their interests or desires. Savulescu's admirable sensitivity to the feelings of the parents of children with disabilities and his suggestion that the moral obligation to select might only operate prospectively, not retrospectively, do indeed go some way to mitigate the implications of these consequences for those who fail to meet their reproductive obligations.

While these clarifications should be of significant interest to those who have followed the debate about human genetic enhancement, unfortunately they do not directly address my larger argument that the real significance of this debate is the encouragement (and the veneer of respectability) it provides for advocates of cruder—and more politically troubling—eugenic arguments. Of course, if the original publication advocating 'procreative beneficence' had argued that there is no such thing as a 'best child' but that parents have 'some' reason to choose genes that would be likely to increase the welfare of their children—a point that seems to me to be trivially true—one wonders whether we would be having this exchange at all today.[16]

References

Asch, A. (1999). 'Prenatal Diagnosis and Selective Abortion: A Challenge to Practice and Policy', *American Journal of Public Health*, 89(11): 1649–57.

Bennett, R. (2009). 'The Fallacy of the Principle of Procreative Beneficence', *Bioethics*, 23(5): 265–73.

de Melo-Martin, I. (2004). 'On Our Obligation to Select the Best Children: A Reply to Savulescu', *Bioethics*, 8(1): 72–83.

Elster, J. (2011). 'Procreative Beneficence: Cui Bono?' *Bioethics*, 25(9): 482–8.

Green, R. M. (2007). *Babies by Design: The Ethics of Genetic Choice*. New Haven, CT: Yale University Press.

[16] I am extremely grateful to Professor Savulescu, Professor Ichinokawa, Dr McGowan, and Professor Jones, for their commentaries on my original paper, as well as to Professor Akira Akabayashi, Associate Professor Satoshi Kodama, Dr Hitoshi Arima, and Dr Keiichiro Yamamoto for their assistance with the production of this (and my other) contribution(s) to this volume.

Harris, J. (1992). *Wonderwoman and Superman: The Ethics of Human Biotechnology*. Oxford: Oxford University Press.

Häyry, M. (2004). 'If You Must Make Babies, then at Least Make the Best Babies You Can?' *Human Fertility*, 7(2): 105–12.

Herissone-Kelly, P. (2006). 'Procreative Beneficence and the Prospective Parent', *Journal of Medical Ethics*, 32(3): 166–9.

Hurst, R. (2009). 'Are Disabled People Human?' in P. Healey and S. Rayner (eds), *Unnatural Selection: The Challenges of Engineering Tomorrow's People*. London: Sterling, VA: Earthscan, 60–6.

Ichinokawa, Y. (2014). 'Eugenics in Society: A Sociological and Historical Consideration', in A. Akabayashi (ed.), *The Future of Bioethics: International Dialogues*. Oxford: Oxford University Press, 154–8.

Jones, D. G. (2014). 'Therapy, Enhancement, and Eugenics', in A. Akabayashi (ed.), *The Future of Bioethics: International Dialogues*. Oxford: Oxford University Press, 163–9.

Kaplan, D. (1993). 'Prenatal Screening and Its Impact on Persons with Disabilities', *Clinical Obstetrics and Gynecology*, 36(3): 605–12.

Kidd, C., Palmeri, H., and Aslin, R. N. (2013). 'Rational Snacking: Young Children's Decision-Making on the Marshmallow Task Is Moderated by Beliefs about Environmental Reliability', *Cognition*, 126(1): 109–14.

McGowan, M. L. (2014). 'Are "Brave" Parents Practicing Eugenics, Enhancement, or Something Else?' in A. Akabayashi (ed.), *The Future of Bioethics: International Dialogues*. Oxford: Oxford University Press, 159–62.

Oliver, M. (2009). *Understanding Disability: From Theory to Practice*. 2nd ed. Basingstoke: Palgrave Macmillan.

Parker, M. (2007). 'The Best Possible Child', *Journal of Medical Ethics*, 33(5): 279–83.

Savulescu, J. (2001a). 'Procreative Beneficence: Why We Should Select the Best Children', *Bioethics*, 15(5): 413–26.

Savulescu, J. (2001b). 'Why Genetic Testing for Genes for Criminality Is Morally Required', *Princeton Journal of Bioethics*, 4(Spring): 79–97.

Savulescu, J. (2002). 'Deaf Lesbians, "Designer Disability", and the Future of Medicine', *British Medical Journal*, 325:771–3.

Savulescu, J. (2005). 'New Breeds of Humans: The Moral Obligation to Enhance', *Ethics, Law, and Moral Philosophy of Reproductive Biomedicine*, 1(1): 36–9.

Savulescu, J. (2008). 'Procreative Beneficence: Reasons Not to Have Disabled Children', in L. Skene and J. Thomson (eds), *The Sorting Society: The Ethics of Genetic Screening and Therapy*. Cambridge: Cambridge University Press, 51–68.

Savulescu, J. (2014). 'The Nature of the Moral Obligation to Select the Best Children', in A. Akabayashi (ed.), *The Future of Bioethics: International Dialogues*. Oxford: Oxford University Press, 170–82.

Savulescu, J., and Kahane, G. (2009). 'The Moral Obligation to Create Children with the Best Chance of the Best Life', *Bioethics*, 23(5): 274–90.

Savulescu, J. et al. (2006). 'Behavioural Genetics: Why Eugenic Selection Is Preferable to Enhancement', *Journal of Applied Philosophy*, 23(2): 157–71.

Silver, L. M. (1999). *Remaking Eden: Cloning, Genetic Engineering, and the Future of Human Kind*. London: Phoenix.

Sparrow, R. (2007). 'Procreative Beneficence, Obligation, and Eugenics', *Genomics, Society, and Policy*, 3(3): 43–59.

Sparrow, R. (2010a). 'Better than Men? Sex and the Therapy/Enhancement Distinction', *Kennedy Institute of Ethics Journal*, 20(2): 115–44.

Sparrow, R. (2010b). 'Liberalism and Eugenics', *Australasian Journal of Philosophy*, 89(3): 499–517.

Sparrow, R. (2010c). 'Should Human Beings Have Sex? Sexual Dimorphism and Human Enhancement', *American Journal of Bioethics*, 10(7): 3–12.

Sparrow, R. (2010d). 'Why Bioethicists *Still* Need to Think More about Sex ...', *American Journal of Bioethics*, 10(7): W1–3.

Sparrow, R. (2011a). 'A Not-So-New Eugenics: Harris and Savulescu on Human Enhancement', *Hastings Center Report*, 41(1): 32–42.

Sparrow, R. (2011b). 'Human Enhancement and Sexual Dimorphism', *Bioethics*, 26(9): 464–75.

Stock, G. (2003). *Redesigning Humans: Choosing Our Children's Genes*. London: Profile Books.

Stoller, S. E. (2008). 'Why We Are Not Morally Required to Select the Best Children: A Response to Savulescu', *Bioethics*, 22(7): 364–9.

5.1

Primary Topic Article
The Misguided Quest for *the* Ethics of Enhancement

Thomas Murray

The title of this essay refers to the "misguided quest for the ethics of enhancement." The problem is not with the quest, which is important, or with ethics, which are urgently needed in discussions of enhancement. No, the problem is with the definite article "the," denoting a singular all-purpose ethics for every form of human enhancement. We will argue that the ethics of each particular enhancement is not determined by the technology or method used, or by whom it is employed. Rather, understanding the ethics of enhancement is deeply dependent on context. We will argue further that a fruitful way to describe what is important about a particular context is by elucidating the values that are sought in or served by that sphere of human endeavor, and by the meaning ascribed to that sphere by people who participate in it.

Unpacking "enhancement"

We can begin with a brief account of ambiguities in the concept of enhancement. The Oxford Online Dictionary offers this definition: "an increase or improvement in quality, value, or extent." What possible objection could a reasonable person have to some intervention that increases quality or value? Take an example often given by commentators. Vaccinations have helped hundreds of millions of people escape the ravages of infectious diseases. Vaccines typically work by enhancing the responsiveness of an individual's immune system to antigens presented by an infectious microbe. This is surely an enhancement to be celebrated and provided to all who can benefit from it.

Imagine a strategy that reasoned the following way. With ever more vaccines coming available, the trouble and expense entailed in vaccinating large populations becomes an increasing challenge. What if, rather than going disease by disease, we fashioned a vaccine that resulted in a general amplification of the immune system, increasing its ability to fight off all disease-causing organisms? Would that be an enhancement we should welcome?

As knowledgeable physicians understand, a person's immune system can turn on its own body, resulting in nasty syndromes known collectively as autoimmune diseases. A generalized amplification of a person's immune system caused by the hypothetical all-purpose vaccine could have disastrous consequences if it triggered attacks against one's own tissues and organs. So, even if it successfully enhanced the body's ability to resist infection, it may jeopardize the person's overall prospects for a long and healthy life. The pan-vaccine example shows that context and consequences matter in evaluating proposed enhancements. An enhancement can aim at something nearly universally regarded as good, and we can applaud the intentions of those promoting the enhancement; but a wise and comprehensive evaluation of any such proposed enhancement must take into account its overall impact, including unintended consequences.

We also have an example of a supposed "enhancement" that has become notorious. Some time after the destruction of the World Trade Center towers on September 11, 2001, the Bush administration approved the use of "enhanced interrogation" techniques on certain prisoners that included waterboarding, "stress positions," and other tactics that many international agreements and bodies classify as torture (Shane, Johnston, and Risen 2007). Officials such as former Vice President Dick Cheney continue to defend so-called "enhanced interrogations" and claim that they were distinguishable from torture and, furthermore, effective (Diamond 2011). Both claims have been widely disputed by experts in the US and elsewhere (Schneiderman 2011).

The point here is not whether "enhanced interrogation" is or is not torture. Assume for the moment that the "enhanced interrogation" techniques served their intended purpose: that they resulted in truthful and important information that could not otherwise be obtained. What does this use of the "enhancement" honorific tell us about the concept?

To begin with, not everyone may agree with the enhancement's goal or with the means employed to reach it. Indeed, the example of "enhanced interrogation" shows that any claim that something "enhances" assumes satisfactory answers to several prior questions, such as: What end is this particular enhancement meant to reach? What values does it serve, and what values may it violate? In the individual case, and if the practice were to be generalized, what would be the implications for our integrity and our values?

A case study: why do we play? Drugs, values, and sport

The use of performance-enhancing drugs in sport is an intriguing problem in both practical ethics and public policy. In a project begun more than 30 years ago at The Hastings Center, I learned one vital lesson very quickly: that good ethics begins with good facts. The second lesson, at least as important, took much longer to fully take in: that evaluating the ethics of enhancement in any given sphere of human endeavor requires understanding the values sought in and through that sphere, and its meaning in the lives of the people who participate in it.

Gathering the relevant facts meant employing simultaneously two very different strategies. On the one hand, we analyzed the scientific literature about patterns of drug use in sport, along with the effectiveness of the drugs for the purposes athletes appeared to be using them and their side effects. On the other hand we spoke with athletes, coaches, and others in sport to understand why athletes were using—or refusing—performance-enhancing drugs, and their beliefs about the drugs' impact on them.

The sport scientists and physicians looked to as "experts" at the time tended to endorse two claims: first, that the drugs did not enhance athletic performance; and, second, that they were very, very dangerous to athletes' health. The athletes with whom I spoke scoffed at the first claim and were skeptical of the second. They had seen their competitors suspected of using anabolic steroids suddenly put on masses of muscle and their performances improve sharply, even as the stigmata of steroid use appeared: acne, mood swings, and in women, deeper voices and hair growing in places more commonly seen on men. Athletes and coaches were convinced that some drugs, especially anabolic steroids and stimulants, were highly effective. Nor did they believe that the drugs were as harmful as the experts were claiming. Their competitors were not dropping dead. The short-term side effects, though unpleasant, did not seem to be catastrophic, and no one had convincing evidence of long-term health risks. In any case, the experts had lost their credibility with the athletes, so their warnings were far less persuasive than they might have been otherwise (Murray 1983: 24–30).

Another critical insight emerged when I asked athletes and coaches why their competitors used performance-enhancing drugs. In hindsight, the point seems obvious, but at the time it helped to make sense of the honest athlete's predicament. Sport is an inherently, relentlessly, competitive activity. Particularly among elite athletes, the difference between winning and losing often is measured in fractions of seconds or meters. The highest-performing athlete may have a 1 percent advantage over his or her closest competitors. The math is straightforward: a drug that gives a 2 percent performance boost can turn a less talented athlete into a winner, eclipsing the efforts and talent of the best athlete. Two percent beats 1 percent.

When athletes believe that some of their competitors are using drugs that give a notable performance edge, they face mostly unhappy options. Some athletes choose not to use drugs and compete at a disadvantage, hoping their talent and dedication will prevail. Connie Carpenter Phinney won the first Women's Olympic bicycle road race against riders who were blood-doping—and who happened to be her teammates on the US squad (Rostaing and Sullivan 1985). Edwin Moses dominated the hurdles for many years with his astonishing talent and self-discipline. But other athletes, such as Doug Glanville, who played center field for several Major League baseball teams, have wondered if their careers were shortened because they declined to use the drugs that enabled other ballplayers to hit more home runs (Glanville 2010).

The second option an athlete has is to cease competing at the level at which their talents and dedication would have permitted them to be successful if they did not have to face off against competitors using drugs. We hear very little about such cases, but occasionally we learn of an athlete who made that choice, such as an American bicycle racer I met recently. He had been identified as exceptionally talented and sent to Europe for seasoning. He learned quickly that he was expected to use without questioning the assorted nostrums thrust upon him by trainers and soigneurs. Soon after, he decided to pursue a career in science instead (Kelly undated).

The third option has been, in certain epochs in particular sports, the most common: do as the others do: use whatever drugs are needed to be competitive. This has been the general response in sports from weightlifting to cycling at various times, and likely accounts in part for the eruption of home runs in baseball during its steroid era.

Smart "doping control" employs a combination of measures from education and testing to policies meant to discourage the manufacture, importation, and selling of performance-enhancing drugs. Its goal is to allow athletes to compete without resorting to drugs in the reasonable expectation that the other athletes in the competition are likewise drug free. That is, the point of doping control is to provide athletes a fair contest.

Is doping control unjustified paternalism?

If you want to see athletes roll their eyes in disbelief, tell them that they should careen down snow-covered mountain slopes at 70 miles per hour or collide at full speed with a 350-pound lineman blocking for the kick returner in a National Football League game—but don't use drugs because you might hurt yourself! Athletes are quick to sniff out hypocrisy. Paternalism is a sound justification for preventing children and youth from using drugs; but it fails miserably with mature adult athletes.

Public health ethics provides a far more robust and cogent argument against doping in sport. The Institute of Medicine in 1988 defined public health as "what we, as a society, do collectively to assure the conditions in which people can be healthy" (Institute of Medicine 1988: 1) This is not garden-variety paternalism, which defends infringing on an individual's liberty with the intention of promoting the best interest of that individual regardless of his or her preferences. The goal of public health is not to advance any particular individual's best interest, but rather to promote the well-being of a population (Beauchamp and Steinbock 1999: 25). The assumptions and principles underlying public health ethics are better suited than paternalism's individualistic focus to address circumstances in which the individual actions have significant adverse consequences for others—very much the case in drug use in athletic competition. Three often used justifications of public health principles support anti-doping in sports.

The first is John Stuart Mill's harm principle, which articulates an important distinction between justified and unjustified infringements on individual liberty. According to Mill, "the only purpose for which power can be rightfully exercised over any member of a civili[z]ed community, against his will, is to prevent harm to others" (Mill 1975: 11). The ban on cigarette smoking in public venues became much more defensible and acceptable once evidence emerged that second-hand smoke was a danger to others.

Mill's harm principle is not always a neat fit: consider mandatory helmet laws for motorcyclists. Second-hand smoke harms bystanders, but it is not as clear how noncompliance with helmet laws puts others at risk. The effort to explain the connection leads at times to rather awkward arguments; for instance, a Florida court insisted cyclists who fail to wear protective head and eye gear could potentially get hit by a bug or flying object, lose control, and become a hazard for other vehicles (Jones and Bayer 2007: 211). Does prohibiting doping in sports satisfy the harm principle?

At first glance, it may seem that an athlete's choice to use performance-enhancing drugs does not cause any harm to others. But this ignores the inescapable reality of competitive athletics, where athletes are pitted directly against one another. To see how Mill's harm principle applies to the use of drugs in competitive athletics, consider it within the context of a further public health consideration, the fact of human interdependence. The reality of human interdependence, manifest in sport by the ever-present pressure to match or exceed the efforts of your competitors, makes it clear that doping threatens the health and well-being of the population of athletes.

According to the "Principles of the Ethical Practice of Public Health," human interdependence is a central tenet in the practice of public health, which entails that "rightful concern for the physical individuality of humans...must be balanced against the fact that each person's actions affects other people" (Public Health Leadership Society 2002). The competitive nature of sports is inherently coercive to individual athletes; when one person attains a significant competitive advantage, other participants are pressured to seek out similar advantages (Murray 1983: 27). Mill's harm principle, coupled with the interdependence of competition, provides a strong public health justification for banning doping in sports.

An additional insight from public health ethics is the principle of collective action and efficiency (Faden and Shebaya 2010). This principle takes into account that certain ends require near-universal compliance to be achieved. There are circumstances in which modest degrees of non-compliance could seriously threaten the committed efforts of the aggregate community. The drive to eradicate tuberculosis (TB) is an example (Bayer and Fairchild 2004: 489). Complete eradication of TB requires that nearly everyone follow proper protocol when exposed to TB. If enough infected persons choose not to seek treatment, their unwillingness to cooperate would jeopardize the collective goal of eliminating TB. Such collective action and efficiency may also be required if the goal is to ensure fairness and eliminate the distortion of sports competitions. Because collective action is the only way to preserve such balance, restricting the individual liberty to use performance-enhancing drugs may be justified as a necessary means to achieving a communally valued end.

The decision to ban doping in sports on the basis of public health ethics does restrict freedom of choice for those individuals who would otherwise choose to use drugs. But the more we know about what motivates athletes to use such drugs, the more clearly we see a parallel with arms races between nations where competition among nations forces each county into actions that threaten its own well-being and increase the risks of harm to all.

The ethics of public health does not rest on paternalism. Instead, it invokes the harm principle, the fact of human interdependence, and the need for collective action and efficiency. These principles are relevant and weighty in the case against performance-enhancing drugs in athletic competition.

On meanings and values in sport: data from a US survey

If we take seriously the adage that good ethics begins with good facts, and we advance an argument that makes claims about what people value in sport, it would be useful to know what meanings and values people, in fact, find or aspire to in sport. Fortunately, a recent US survey provides some insights (US Anti-Doping Agency 2011). The survey was sponsored by the US Anti-Doping Agency (USADA) and conducted by Discovery Education. The survey focused on youth sport. The survey divided youth into three subgroups: children, tweens, and teens, and reached out to three categories of influential adults: parents, teachers, and coaches. It further divided respondents into those with a link to an Olympic sport association as compared with the general population with no such link.

When adults from the general population were asked what values sport should reinforce, six values were endorsed by more than 80 percent of respondents: honesty, fair play, respect for others, doing your best, teamwork, and fun. Of the list of 16 values, the two at the bottom were competitiveness and winning—the latter endorsed by fewer than a quarter of all respondents.

Ask what values sport actually reinforces, though, and the results are in stark contrast. Competitiveness is now at the top followed by winning. Fair play, respect for others, and honesty are near the bottom.

Every group—young and old, with and without involvement in Olympic sports—overwhelmingly identified "fun" as the most important motivation for becoming involved with sport.

Finally, respondents were asked to rate the seriousness of problems facing sport today. The biggest problem, according to the 4,443 general-population adults answering the question, is the use of performance-enhancing substances, followed by the focus on money and the criminal behavior of well-known athletes.

A few points stand out. First, sport is capable of supporting and reinforcing important values, and there is remarkable agreement on what those values should be. But as currently practiced, youth sport in the US fails to reinforce those values deemed most important. We do not reward what we value. Second, the way to draw young people into becoming involved with sport, and the way to keep people active as they grow older, is to keep it fun. Third, the American public believes that drugs in sport are a very serious problem.

Adults say that we play sport in order to learn values like honesty, hard work, fair play, respect for others, and doing your best. Children say we play for fun, friendship, and exercise. These are all good reasons to play sport. We can add to that list the drive to do a thing well, to master a skill. A consequence of learning to play well is that we develop our character. That may not be the reason young people take up sport, but if they devote themselves to improving their skills and perfecting their talents, it will happen in due course. And it would be a serious oversight to leave out the beautiful things that come occasionally with playing sport: glimpses of excellence when you do a thing just right—for a golfer, hitting a perfect drive; for a basketball player, launching a jump shot with backspin and hearing it zip though the netting suspended beneath the rim. In such moments, we experience a harmony of body and mind that is precious and rare in modern life.

Technologies of enhancement, meanings, and the importance of context

A brief detour will help establish the significance of context. Many years ago I created an absurd hypothetical, which, like most of my absurd hypotheticals over the years, turns out to be not so fanciful (Murray 1983). Imagine a drug that quiets the small, natural tremor in a surgeon's hand. Imagine further that an inquisitive surgeon tries this drug that, in our hypothetical at least, has no known significant risks at the dose sufficient to still the tremor. Our surgeon is pleased with the results but, being a well-trained scientist, organizes a double-blind, placebo-controlled, crossover design randomized clinical trial. The results? Patients operated on by surgeons taking the drug had fewer complications and more rapid recoveries.

Sugden and colleagues' research on modafinil's ability to improve the performance of sleep-deprived surgeons has clear parallels to my hypothetical. Their recent study concludes that "fatigued doctors might benefit from pharmacological enhancement in situations that require efficient information processing, flexible thinking, and decision making under time pressure." Not all outcomes were positive: they found no improvement in "basic procedural tasks" (Sugden et al. 2012: 222).

There are surely ethical questions to be raised about surgeons' use of modafinil or other drugs. Some of the questions will resemble those raised by athletes' drug use, such as the coercive pressure that may be exerted on surgeons to use enhancing agents. But context makes an enormous difference. The crucial values sought in the practice of surgery are centered in the patient's health and well-being. The meaning or point of surgery is to heal patients. Technologies that promote that end are presumptively welcomed, whether they be practices like sterilization, tools like precision scalpels or imaging devices—or, perhaps, a drug that helps a fatigued surgeon make good decisions.

This is not an argument for giving modafinil to sleepy surgeons; we can just as well eliminate the practices that produce sleep deprivation. And we would need far more evidence that using the drug improves outcomes reliably without harming the surgeons who take them. In any event, this not-so-hypothetical is sufficient to show that assessing the ethics of enhancement technologies in any particular sphere of human endeavor must be grounded in an understanding of the meaning and values in that sphere. The question is never whether taking a performance-enhancing drug is justified or not; rather, the question is whether it supports or undermines what we value in that particular sphere. In surgery, we want patients to get well; what do we want in sport?

We gain insights about meaning and values in sport through examining how it deals with equipment and rules, including drugs intended to enhance performance. Sport's attitude toward a wide range of technologies provides abundant clues to the meaning of sport. Sport has banned many technologies from being used in competitions including golf balls designed to fly straight rather than hook or slice and clubs with deep rectangular grooves that afford more control when hitting out of tall grass. Swimming has banned many buoyant and slippery full-body suits that diminish the water resistance swimmers would otherwise encounter (FINA 2009). Ultralight bikes can be hugely expensive even as their durability and dependability decrease.

In case after case, sport has resisted technologies and rules that make it easier to perform. Is this simple perversity? Anyone who insisted that surgeons use nineteenth-century instruments—or forgo sterile procedures—would be instantly dismissed as ignorant, crazy, or evil. What makes sport different when it refuses to indulge in "deskilling?" Many innovations are eventually accepted such as plant boxes and flexible poles in the pole vault (VerSteeg 2005: 103). But many, many others, including performance-enhancing drugs, are rejected. What is it about the meaning of sport that guides it through the shoals of innovation, however lurching and uncertain the journey seems at times?

Our claim here is that arguments over whether to accept innovations in sport are about something rather than nothing—specifically about deep, shared convictions about what matters in that sport. The "nothing" school emphasizes the arbitrariness of rules in sport. Why must the goals on a football (known as soccer in America) pitch be eight feet tall and 24 feet wide? Some people complain about the lack of scoring. Widening the net to 40 feet would lead to many more goals scored. I asked a group of European bioethicists if they would welcome such a change. They reacted with horror. The tension, the balance between goalie and striker would be thrown completely off. Goalies would be nearly helpless to prevent a score no matter how skilled they were. I also asked about shrinking the goal to the size of an ice hockey net, four by six feet. The response was similar. Scoring would be effectively impossible, no matter how brilliantly the kicking team played.

The rules of any sport worthy of the name are "arbitrary" only in the harmless sense that they could be a bit different without changing what matters in that sport. But for people who play, love, and understand a sport, its rules are essential for calling forth whatever talents that particular sport values and celebrates. Consider what happened to baseball in 1968.

Don Drysdale, of the Los Angeles Dodgers, had one of the greatest seasons ever for a pitcher in Major League baseball including 58 2/3 consecutive scoreless innings. Bob Gibson, pitching for the St. Louis Cardinals, had an even more impressive year, giving up just over one earned run per game in his 34 starts, 13 of which were complete game shutouts. The distance between the pitcher's rubber and home plate was, at 60'6," unchanged for 75 years, but pitchers had increased their dominance. To restore competitive balance between hitters and pitchers, baseball lowered the height of the mound by one-third—from 15 to 10 inches, reducing the pitcher's advantage.

In a 1981 letter to his friend Owen Fiss, John Rawls (2008), the preeminent political philosopher of his era, explained why baseball is the best of all sports:

First: the rules of the game are in equilibrium: that is, from the start, the diamond was made just the right size, the pitcher's mound just the right distance from home plate, etc., and this makes possible the marvelous plays, such as the double play. The physical layout of the game is perfectly adjusted to the human skills it is meant to display and to call into graceful exercise.

One does not have to agree with Rawls on the superiority of baseball to see that he understands what makes it worthwhile: it displays and calls into graceful exercise certain human skills. We could give a similar account for any sport. The particular skills and talents will vary enormously from sport to sport and even within many team sports such as football, basketball, and baseball where different positions call upon different skills. But a common theme runs through them: the rules of sport, including its attitude toward technologies of enhancement, must stand the test of calling forth the skills and talents valued in that sport.

Why resist doping in sport?

When sports have to decide on rules and technologies, three categories of moral appraisal stand out: to promote fairness; to prevent harm; and to preserve meaning. For each of the three, we will look briefly at what the critics say and at how that category of appraisal can be rescued from its critics.

Fairness. Critics say that doping is unfair only because it is banned, with the result that some athletes gain surreptitious advantages from drugs while others compete without such advantages. If the ban was lifted and every athlete had access to the same drugs, they argue, doping would not be cheating and using drugs would cease to be unfair. (Kious 2008: 224–5).

Can fairness be rescued from this attack? First, as a point of logic, as long as doping is prohibited, doing it constitutes cheating and this is unfair to other athletes. But, a more thoughtful response to the critics must go deeper than this to the prior question whether doping *should* be banned in sport. And that, as we've argued, is a question of meaning, to be taken up again in a moment.

Harm. The critics have several arguments to offer here. They claim that trying to prevent adult athletes from using drugs on the grounds that they may harm themselves is unjustified paternalism (Fost 1986: 9). Some critics defend certain drugs as safe (though they disagree with one another as to which drugs are safe and which are not) (Kayser and Smith 2008: 87). And some have argued that athletes' health would be better protected by a policy of medically supervised drug use (Kayser, Mauron, and Miah 2007: 8–9).

Can we rescue harm as a reason to continue to prohibit performance-enhancing drugs? Here it is crucial to recall the relentlessly competitive nature of sport. An individual athlete's actions are not merely self-regarding; they affect all who compete against that athlete. A sound ethical foundation for preventing harm to athletes will be found in public health ethics, not in paternalism.

What of the claim that some drugs are not harmful and therefore should be permitted? It's worth noting that EPO, not long ago touted as "safe" for enhancing endurance, now carries a "black box" warning in the US, placed there by the FDA because of mounting evidence that EPO and similar drugs impose life-threatening risks to patients (Pollack 2007). Whether healthy young athletes are also at risk is an unanswered question, but we know that athletes strive for much higher concentrations of red cells than patients typically reach. What may seem safe today may not be, especially when athletes are taking multiple drugs, some of them at dosages far higher than their clinical usages. Lifting the prohibition against doping in sport is likely to increase sharply the scope and intensity of the uncontrolled massive pharmaceutical "experiment" we are now witnessing in sport.

Meaning. Critics have had less to say about meaning. A notable exception was a 2004 paper by Savulescu, Foddy, and Clayton (2004: 667) where maximum performance is proposed. They assert that "the athletic ideal of modern athletes is inspired by the myth of the marathon. Their ideal is superhuman performance, at any cost" (Savulescu, Foddy, and Clayton 2004: 666). There is much to think about here. For one thing, it appears they are referring only to elite athletes rather than the hundreds of millions of people who play sport at other levels. But even if we limited this proposition to elite athletes it seems to be as much an empirical claim about athletes' beliefs as a moral one. I've met many elite athletes. Though I've not taken a formal survey of their views, I've yet to meet one who embraces the principle Savulescu advocates. They want to do their best, and they want a fair chance to succeed, but not to emulate the marathoner of the myth who, it should be remembered, dropped dead.

A more promising approach to understanding meaning in sport is to recall what John Rawls admired about baseball: "the game is perfectly adjusted to the human skills it is meant to display and to call into graceful exercise." Every sport has its own inventory of talents and skills that make for success. Different sports call forth quite different inventories. The largest weightlifter is no more likely to excel in the marathon as the lithe marathoner is to be a superb weightlifter. Sport is a commodious tent welcoming many different forms of human embodiment under its folds. Young and old, large and small, many, many people can find a sport and a level to play it that will be fun and that will allow them to experience moments of excellence and grace. When we live up to our values, sport can be a celebration of ways of being human, and of human excellence in body and spirit.

If we are persuaded that drug-free sport is the path to follow, we must accept the responsibilities that go with that choice. We will need to provide level playing fields for athletes. This will require vigilance to unearth cheating, a fair and transparent system for adjudicating cases where cheating is suspected, and a sound scientific basis for understanding the effects of drugs and for detecting their use. We must pay careful attention to the concerns of athletes, and enlist them effectively in the effort to assure fair, drug-free competitions. In my experience, athletes are very intolerant of drug use among their competitors. It's not a surprise. They are the people most directly hurt when other athletes gain an illicit advantage.

We should continue to focus on values and meaning in sport, on what we value in each particular sport, and on the values we promote through participating in sport. In the end we must take seriously why we play. Bill Bradley was a star basketball player at Princeton, a Rhodes Scholar, a key member of the NBA champion New York Knicks team, then a US Senator. In a memoir, *Values of the Game*, Bradley (1998: 6) had this to say about why he played:

The only thing I had to do was allow the kid in me to feel the pure pleasure in just playing. In plenty of games, I played simply for the joy of it, shooting and passing without thinking about points. I forgot the score, and sometimes I would go through a whole quarter without looking at the scoreboard.

From my decades of basketball—with at best a tiny fraction of Bradley's talents and dedication to the game—I understand exactly what he means. And I suspect that just about everyone who has ever played a sport important to him to her does as well.

References

Bayer, R., and Fairchild, A. L. (2004). "The Genesis of Public Health Ethics," *Bioethics*, 18:473–92.

Beauchamp, D. E., and Steinbock, B. (eds). (1999). *New Ethics for the Public's Health.* New York: Oxford University Press.

Bradley, B. (1998). *Values of the Game.* New York: Artisan.

Diamond, M. (2011). "Cheney Defends Torture, Says Administration 'Not Up to the Task' in Libya," *Think Progress*, May 8, http://thinkprogress.org/security/2011/05/08/164419/cheney-defends-torture-says-administration-not-up-to-the-task-in-libya/?mobile=nc (accessed January 24, 2012).

Faden, R., and Shebaya, S. (2010). "Public Health Ethics," *Stanford Encyclopedia of Philosophy*, http://plato.stanford.edu/entries/publichealth-ethics/#ColAct (accessed January 25, 2012).

FINA (Federation Internationale de Natation). (2009). "Dubai Charter on FINA Requirement for Swimwear Approval," http://www.fina.org/H2O/docs/PR/the dubai charter (accessed February 1, 2012).

Fost, N. (1986). "Banning Drugs in Sports: A Skeptical View," *Hastings Center Report*, 16:5–10.

Glanville, D. (2010). *The Game from Where I Stand: A Ballplayer's Inside View.* New York: Henry Holt.

Institute of Medicine, Committee for the Study of the Future of Public Health. (1988). *The Future of Public Health.* Washington, DC: National Academy Press.

Jones, M. M., and R. Bayer. (2007). "Paternalism and Its Discontents: Motorcycle Helmet Laws, Libertarian Values, and Public Health," *American Journal of Public Health*, 97:208–17.

Kayser, B., and Smith, A. (2008). "Globalisation of Anti-Doping: The Reverse Side of the Medal," *BMJ*, 337:85–7.

Kayser, B., Mauron, A., and Miah, A. (2007). "Current Anti-Doping Policy: A Critical Appraisal," *BMC Medical Ethics*, 8:1–10.

Kelly, B. (Undated). "One Cyclist's Experience," *Anti-Doping Research,* http://www.antidopingresearch.org/LockerRoom_athletes_stories.php (accessed January 25, 2012).

Kious, B. M. (2008). "Philosophy on Steroids: Why the Anti-Doping Position Could Use a Little Enhancement," *Theoretical Medicine and Bioethics*, 29:213–34.

Mill, J. S. (1975). *On Liberty.* Edited by D. Spitz. New York: W.W. Norton.

Murray, T. H. (1983). "The Coercive Power of Drugs in Sports," *Hastings Center Report*, 13:24–30.

Pollack, A. (2007). "F.D.A. Warning Is Issued on Anemia Drug's Overuse," *New York Times*, March 10, http://www.nytimes.com/2007/03/10/washington/10fda.html (accessed January 26, 2012).

Public Health Leadership Society. (2002). "Principles of the Ethical Practice of Public Health. Version 2.2," http://www.phls.org/home/section/3-26/ (accessed January 25, 2012).

Rawls, J. (2008). "The Best of All Games," *Boston Review*, March–April, http://bostonreview.net/BR33.2/rawls.php (accessed January 24, 2012).

Rostaing, B., and Sullivan, R. (1985). "Triumphs Tainted with Blood," *Sports Illustrated*, January 21, http://sportsillustrated.cnn.com/vault/article/magazine/MAG1119061/index.htm (accessed January 25, 2012).

Savulescu, J., Foddy, B. and Clayton, M. (2004). "Why We Should Allow Performance Enhancing Drugs in Sport," *British Journal of Sports Medicine*, 38:666–70.

Schneiderman, R. M. (2011). "Human Rights Watch: Prosecute Bush, Cheney over Torture Crimes," *The Daily Beast*, July 12, http://www.thedailybeast.com/articles/2011/07/12/human-rights-watch-prosecute-bush-cheney-over-torture.html (accessed January 25, 2012).

Shane, S., Johnston, D., and Risen, J. (2007). "Secret U.S. Endorsement of Severe Interrogations," *New York Times*, October 4, http://www.nytimes.com/2007/10/04/washington/04interrogate.html?fta=y (accessed January 24, 2012).

Sugden, C. et al. (2012). "Effect of Pharmacological Enhancement on the Cognitive and Clinical Psychomotor Performance of Sleep-Deprived Doctors: A Randomized Controlled Trial," *Annals of Surgery*, 255: 222–7.

US Anti-Doping Agency. (2011). "What Sport Means in America: A Study of Sport's Role in Society," http://www.usada.org/outreach-research (accessed December 11, 2012).

VerSteeg, R. (2005). "Arresting Vaulting Pole Technology," *Vanderbilt Journal of Entertainment and Technology Law*, 8:93–117.

5.2

Commentary
Thomas Murray's Enhancement of a Bioethics of Enhancement

Carl Becker

Overview

Dr. Thomas Murray has spearheaded research on enhancement issues for 30 years now, so his views are not to be taken lightly. His surveys that highlight the gaps between the socially held goals of amateur sports and the commercially promoted goals of professional sports deserve particular attention and concern. His essay is as much a literary paean to the joys of sport as a rigorous critique of enhancement. He begins by "unpacking 'enhancement'" as "improvement," illustrating the potential dangers of "improved" biological immunity and the immorality of "improved" interrogation techniques. Yet the very flexibility of his arguments on enhancement reveals potential ambiguities, or at least requires clarification.

Murray suggests that *some* enhancements may be acceptable, if they follow the principles of:

(M1) promoting fairness;
(M2) preventing harm;
(M3) proffering meaning.

This Murray mantra resembles the Beauchamp/Belmont/Bioethics mantra:

(B1) first do no harm;
(B2) autonomy;
(B3) fairness.

M's major obvious variation from B is the move from autonomy to meaning-making—a noteworthy advance!

I have argued elsewhere that the bioethics mantra presupposing "self-made" individualism downplays three vectors central to human society and civilization (Becker 2011):

(C1)   Long-term sustainability (cf. Murray's "unintended consequences");
(C2)   Social/other-awareness (cf. Murray's "principle of collective action");
(C3)   Psycho-spiritual satisfaction (cf. Murray's "meaning-making").

Murray significantly improves the B mantra in the following respects:

(M1)   fairness extends (B3) by including (C2) social awareness/values;
(M2)   harmlessness extends (B1) by including (C1) long-term effects;
(M3)   revises (B2) autonomy to include (C3) meaning-making.

So it is no surprise that I deeply agree with Murray's analysis. Murray's position is more socially, temporally, and ethically robust than the individualistic "maximize today for tomorrow we die" tendencies latent in the B mantra. Let us clarify the above outline in more detail, while asking further clarification of Dr. Murray.

1   Fairness

Opponents of the "fair playing field" ideal have argued that society already is swamped with a plethora of unfairnesses, ranging from genetic differences at birth to social, economic, and educational differences throughout one's life. Since the world already allows those who can ride or yacht from childhood to outperform those who lack horses or yachts, so the argument goes, there is nothing inconsistent in allowing those who can drug themselves to outperform those who lack the access to drugs.

We might use the "two wrongs don't make a right" idea here; the fact that society (or fate) is already imbalanced is not a reason to artificially make it more so. Yet a gradually growing literature is showing that both simian and human societies are happier when there is greater equality than when there is greater disparity in wealth and opportunity or ability. A wide range of religious values advocate *noblesse oblige*: that the privileged distribute their benefits to the poor rather than acquiring more for themselves. Yet many people waver, wondering where to stand between "free competition" and "social justice." I wonder if Dr. Murray might advance guidelines to distinguish between fairness and artificial intervention. In spheres other than sport, for example, is it morally acceptable to allow some elite group indefinitely to enhance their abilities unchecked, if the rest of the society has no opportunity to pursue the same enhancement, and feels significantly disadvantaged by this unfairness?

2   Dangers

Dr. Murray appropriately cites Sugden's London research suggesting that fatigued doctors might benefit from modafinil. In fact, six years ago, Gill and colleagues at Loma Linda already pointed out the danger of modafinil causing doctors' insomnia (Gill et al. 2006). More recently, Indiana's Drabiak-Syed has warned about addiction to and abuse of modafinil, especially among doctors (Drabiak-Syed 2011). So each new drug needs to be carefully evaluated and followed.

I intuit that Dr. Murray's guidelines might accept drugs to slow the progress of diseases, as opposed to those that enhance certain abilities above the drugless norm. It may be that society chooses to allow some recreational drugs, such as alcohol, to be used with appropriate age and behavioral limitations (e.g. not while driving or operating machinery), but I concur with his wariness toward jumping on to each new drug bandwagon. Clearly, criteria for "harm" must include not only the number of rats that die shortly after imbibing drugs under clinical testing, but longitudinal studies looking at the longer-term effects of relying on particular drugs or enhancements.

Murray is quite right to suggest that good ethics begins with "good facts." However, most medical prescriptions must be made in the face of more uncertainties than facts. What levels of certainty must be sought in order to decide whether a drug is harmful or beneficial? This becomes a question not only of fact but of value judgment.

Bioethicists must participate in clarifying the guidelines to be used in considering the safety of legalization and prescription of behavior-enhancing substances, both for athletes and ultimately for the general population. The clarity of this discussion becomes increasingly important as public demand for such substances grows. I wish he might speak or write more fully about any other kinds of guidelines that should be cleanly drawn.

3 Values

While we bioethicists continue to debate enhancement in the literature, major pharmaceutical corporations are devoting funds that trivialize our paltry salaries toward developing and marketing mind- and body-enhancing drugs, ranging from tranquilizers in classrooms and modafinil in operating rooms to steroids in sports. Murray's analysis of enhancement also leads in this direction. He points out the dangers of unintended consequences, and the impotence of paternalist arguments to stop competitive athletes from seeking to self-enhance.

All of our language is fruitless if it has no impact on the real world. While I recognize the need for further debates on the bioethical playing field, I am even more concerned about what average citizens (like mere bioethicists) can begin to do to counterweigh the overwhelming economic incentives to sell drugs.

Among his valuable exhortations, Dr. Murray appropriately advocates everything from first-rate science and vigilant adjudication to enlisting athletes to remember and remind us what we value in sport. If we do nothing, society will most surely bend to the pressure of the media and markets, toward the animalistic least common denominators of sex and consumption, rather than to the higher values of self-cultivation and cooperation. Here I should like to pick Dr. Murray's brain further, about what citizens, educators, and bioethicists can practically *do* in order to influence the future of our societies' policies toward drugging and enhancement.

4 Further questions on sports and values

Murray argues that positions on enhancement should not be monolithic, but rather ask whether enhancement "supports or undermines what we value in that particular sphere" (Murray in this chapter). Then he argues that, since pharmaceutical enhancement does not support but rather undermines what society (ought to) value in sport, we ought to reject pharmaceutical enhancement. Our dialogue opens further questions:

4.1 The unity or difference of values in the sphere(s) of sport

Is "sport" indeed a single sphere with a single set of values, or is commercial competition actually a superficially similar but fundamentally different sphere of activity from amateur sport, with a different set of values? For example, the same superficially similar act of homicide is condemned within society for the sake of personal advantage but (however unwittingly or unethically) lauded in wars against foreigners or gangsters for the sake of social or national advantage. Might it be the case that sport, while consisting of superficially similar activities, in fact consists of two distinct spheres: amateur recreation, which prioritizes fun, grace, and social values; and professional competition, which (however unwittingly or unethically) prioritizes overcoming opponents at all costs? Might this account for the differences between Murray's and Savulescu's accounts of athletes' value preferences? If so, how are we to distinguish legitimately different spheres of social value? If not, how are we to persuade the more belligerent spheres that they are in fact socially unacceptable?

4.2 The grounds for social values

I concur with Dr. Murray's grounding his discussion of enhancement in the values that society wants to promote. But in a sense, his stance begs the question: *how* should we argue for *what* society *ought* to value (in sport or any other arena)? Murray's impassioned personal examples laud model athletes who focus on the joy of basketball swishes and teamwork, or those who resign from sports under pressure to take drugs. Yet his cameos are more appeals to a leap of faith than criteria for public policy. Here I should beg to insert my own cameo, and then connect it to reasons why it justifies certain values over others.

I had been raised in university communities in Chicago and Honolulu to believe subconsciously that a "Big Gulp" (liter of liquid) was more satisfying than a sip of tea, that typing rapidly was superior to handwriting slowly, and that teenage Miss Universes were more beautiful than octogenarians.

My first month living in a temple in Japan 38 years ago transformed that worldview. I sat on my heels for hours in a tea room to receive a sip of tea more deeply memorable and satisfying than any liter of cola. I witnessed an 88-year-old calligrapher brush a scroll which combined art and wisdom in a way no typing could. I watched the withered hands and face of an octogenarian classical dancer perform with more grace and beauty than any Miss Universe.

As media's blinders fell from my eyes, I gained hope for humanity. If size, speed, and youth were all that mattered, then all adult humanity must forever remain wretchedly longing to be bigger or swifter or younger than they can ever be—and people who are slower or smaller or older are forever doomed to inferiority. But it is precisely these animalistic values that Japan has transcended, in the classical arts and lifestyle that it has cultivated.

Once our basic needs for hydration, food, and shelter are achieved, it is more sustainable—and more human—to appreciate the grace of making a single cup of tea, rather than to consume far more calories or resources than our bodies need. With locally made paper and brush, an elderly Japanese calligrapher communicates elegance and self-cultivation that all can admire and seek to cultivate in themselves. To be sure, the teen-age is the most biologically desirable time for human bodies to reproduce—but this is no reason that our entire value system need be debased to a worship of youth and biological reproduction. For our species, that lives longer after than before reproduction, to cultivate grace and elegance in movement can proffer a more fulfilling goal for the remainder of our days.

Max Weber devastatingly critiqued the devaluation of the Protestant work ethic from an ethic that valued good work in itself to an ethic that reduced value to the by-product of work (capital). Now it may be time for us to critique the devaluation of the sports ethic from an ethic that valued sportsmanship and self-cultivation in itself to an ethic that reduces it to the by-product of sports (viz. winning, and ultimately capital). If all human values become reducible to competition for capital, then the environment and the majority of the human race are in grave danger.

When our greed for capital wealth destroys our environment; when our self-aggrandizement destroys human (or international) relationships; when our search for eternal youth destroys our understanding of what it means to mature as a human— then bioethicists must challenge these social values and seek to balance them with wisdom, compassion, and understanding of the human condition.

This is not to say that humans should not try to improve ourselves, but rather that our search for personal or national cultivation should constantly seek to be aware of the long-term and social consequences, and also to avoid depriving others of avenues for similar self-cultivation.

Education has been peculiarly incapable of elevating cooperation and fairness in the face of mass-media marketing which continually touts being the first, the fastest, the richest, or the strongest. In our hospitals today, we are faced with constant claims from families who expect the same impossible miracles of us that they saw on *ER* (TV) last week, while psychological side effects of bereavement are taking a toll unthinkable in former ages when every family cared for its own dying parents and children.

Sport remains one arena which, at least in the popular mind, continues to value fairness and cooperation, applauding exemplary performance over ill-won points, money, and self-aggrandizement. With Rawls and Murray, I do hope that it will remain so. To that end, I hope this dialogue can continue to demarcate spheres of activity, clarify their ethical values, and advance methods by which they may be sought and maintained.

References

Becker, C. B. (2011). "Neuroethics, Bioethics, and Health," *Journal of Philosophy and Ethics in Health Care and Medicine*, 5: 5–38.

Drabiak-Syed, K. (2011). "Reining in the Pharmacological Enhancement Train: We Should Remain Vigilant about Regulatory Standards for Prescribing Controlled Substances," *Journal of Law, Medicine, and Ethics*, 39(2): 272–9.

Gill, M. et al. (2006). "Cognitive Performance Following Modafinil versus Placebo in Sleep-Deprived Emergency Physicians: A Double-Blind Randomized Crossover Study," *Academic Emergency Medicine*, 13(2): 158–65.

Murray, T. (2014). "The Misguided Quest for *the* Ethics of Enhancement," in A. Akabayashi (ed.), *The Future of Bioethics: International Dialogues*. Oxford: Oxford University Press, 193–204.

5.3

Commentary
Arguments for and against Enhancement in Sports

Renzong Qiu

The concept of enhancement

Enhancement involves the use of technological or artificial means to overcome limits in performance or capacities imposed by the normal human body. For example, the traditional concept of health means that the functions of the human body are within the statistical norms of the human species. However, according to the concept of enhancement, health in its original sense is limited and defective; like a computer, the human body needs to be updated from time to time. So unlike improvement only up to the point we would classify as "perfect health," enhancement goes beyond the natural limits of human capacities, functions, and even structure. Enhancement uses technological means to enable the human body to acquire new capacities that have never before been possessed by members of the human species. Cognition, mood, physical strength, physical beauty, lifespan, and intelligence are among the features often considered targets for enhancement.

Buchanan et al. (2000, chapter 4) tell us that in bioethics, a line is drawn between treatment and enhancement. The line is useful for distinguishing between interventions which aim to prevent or cure disease or impairment, and interventions which aim to enhance a condition viewed as a normal function of members of our species (*homo sapiens*). Buchanan et al. go on to argue that the distinction between what is treatment and what is enhancement does not necessarily help us decide what services are obligatory and what are supernumerary. I agree. The grounds for identifying services as obligatory should be moral considerations such as preventing harms, promoting justice and equality of opportunity, and promoting the fundamental values in sports or health care. For example, the human species has no inherent immunity to HIV. If we were able, without taking serious risks, to enhance the human immune system so that we could resist HIV infection, then it might well be considered obligatory to provide such increase in immune responsiveness, even though this could be classified as enhancement rather than treatment. Conversely, in some specified condition the treatment could be withheld or withdrawn if it is futile and imposes more suffering on the patient.

Enhancement in sports: history and status quo

Thomas Murray has written: "Drug use for performance enhancement among athletes has become a recognized problem in sports. In USA the 2007 Mitchell Report found that several Major League baseball players had used performance-enhancing drugs; other reports have found doping prevalent in cycling, track and field, and other sports" (Murray 2008: 153). In the period between 1994 and 2009, there were ten major cases of doping in sports in China, including swimming, track and field, weightlifting, cycling, triathlon, and others. The enormous financial and commercial pressures on athletes provide motivation for such illegal drug use.

Quinn Norton has argued that sport is the area that is pioneering the moral debate about human enhancement, because so much is now spent on helping elite performers to perform. "The modern elite player," she writes, "is an isolated cyborgian construct with barely room for a life and identity away from their sport" (Norton 2010).

There are divergent opinions on enhancement in sports. In what follows, the arguments for and against enhancement in sports will be examined respectively.

Arguments for enhancement in sports

One argument says that athletes are just giving people what they want. If enhancement can produce performance that makes fans more joyful, why not do it? Murray rebutted this argument very well as follows: "The fans in the Roman Coliseum may have loved to see lions tearing the arms off Christians or gladiators hacking each other to death. So 'what the fans desire' is not an ethically robust defense" (Murray 2008: 153).

Two further arguments have been put forward in favor of allowing enhancement. The first, identified by Murray, that it is up to each individual athlete to decide what happens to his or her body and how to balance the risks and benefits. The second, advanced by Andy Miah (2006), claims that enhancement enriches sport by improving performance. Murray (2008: 153) has forcefully countered the first argument: what one athlete does affects all in the competition, and a few athletes using enhancers while others abstain would undermine the "level playing field" that is so important to at least many athletes. The second argument ignores or misunderstands the core values in sports. Enrichment of the practice is not the core value, nor does it make the protection of the natural human less relevant.

Arguments against enhancement in sports

There are several arguments against enhancement in sports; we will examine them one by one and see which one among them is ethically tenable.

Rule argument

Murray (2008: 154) argued that every sport has rules, and the rules determine which features can legitimately be changed or developed and which cannot. Murray considers the Tour de France, the rules for which stipulate a minimum weight for all bikes. This rule, he suggests, prevents the use of expensive bikes that would be beyond the reach of all but the richest cyclists, thus ensuring a wider range of potential competitors. It also protects cyclists from the pressure to use cycles so light that they would not be safe in the mountainous terrain (Murray 2008: 155).

However, rules are made by humans, and may be defective. Indeed they are changed from time to time. Norton provides a counterargument to Murray's argument. She asks: "What makes a hypobaric chamber OK, but an injection [of erythropoietin] a firing offense?" She answers: "Because we said so" and "After all, the rules of sports are arbitrary" (Norton 2010). She goes on to argue in the following way: erythropoietin (EPO) is a naturally occurring substance that regulates the number of red blood cells. Injecting synthetic EPO to increase the number of red blood cells and hence boost performance is considered doping. However, athletes can produce EPO in other ways: by sleeping in a hypobaric chamber, or pitching a tent halfway up Everest. The body responds to these stimuli by producing its own EPO. Despite the end result being the same as that of injecting synthetic EPO, neither of these activities would be considered cheating (Norton 2010). Another example Norton gives where what is legal seems arbitrary is Tommy John surgery, "an operation that replaces the ligament in the elbow that tends to suffer most in baseball pitchers" (Norton 2010). This surgery, which increases pitching ability, is perfectly legal. "On the other hand," she continues, "strengthening the arms by supplementing with a combination of testosterone and weight training is prohibited" (Norton 2010).

Norton's examples do not prove that the rules of sport are arbitrary, since there might be good reasons for the differences that she identifies. She has offered a "legal" argument against enhancement in sports by showing that the fact that certain enhancements are outlawed by the rules of sport can be considered sufficient justification for why competitors should avoid those enhancements. However, she has not provided an ethical argument. A robust ethical argument would engage with the justification for the rules in sports. As Murray pointed out, "rules are changed at times to preserve a sport." Even when rules are changed there is something deeper that is preserved: that is, the essential features of the sport (Murray 2008: 155). An ethical argument against enhancement in sport would show why enhancement threatens to undermine these essential features.

"Arms race" argument

Murray also considers an "Arms Race" argument. He wrote, "the dynamics of drugs in sport bear more than a superficial resemblance to an arms race: each party drives the other further, lest either be left behind," and "athletes, caught in the sport arms race, would be pressed to take more and more drugs, in ever wilder combinations and at increasingly higher doses" (Murray 2008: 156). This argument is essentially a consequentialist argument. As such it is a robust ethical argument against enhancement only if the consequences of enhancement are shown to be sufficiently negative, for example if the drug race in sport could potentially result in a public health catastrophe or lead to the loss of the most graceful, beautiful, and admirable things about sport.

Giftedness argument

Michael Sandel (2002; 2007) argued that life is a gift that is not subject without limit to our mastery or dominion. Enhancement in general, and genetic enhancement in particular, will deprive us of what the theologian William F. May calls an "an openness to the unbidden" (Sandel 2002; Sandel 2007). William Saletan (2007) objected that this "is a particularly awkward posture for a philosopher like Sandel, who infers norms and virtues from the way people live." "Once gene therapy becomes routine," he suggests, "the case against genetic engineering will sound as quaint as the case against [athletics] coaches" (Saletan 2007). Sam Crane (2007) has argued that Saletan's argument "relies too heavily on a biological definition of human nature," and that biology is only part of the story: human nature must be enacted socially as well. Indeed, both Sandel and Saletan are genetic determinists to some degree.

In what follows I will argue that the robust arguments against pharmaceutical, machinery, and genetic enhancements in sports are the harm (or safety) argument, the fairness argument, the core value argument, and the humanity-diminishing argument.

Harm argument

The harm (or safety) argument against enhancement in sports observes that it is reasonable to believe that doping would harm the physical and mental health of athletes, and that these harms may be lifelong and irreversible. The problem is that hard evidence for this claim needs to be obtained through scientific testing. It may not be ethical to conduct clinical trials with humans using performance-enhancing drugs, but we can legally conduct *in vitro* or animal experiments. As Murray has pointed out, "While the scientific evidence that the drugs athletes use are harmful is often less conclusive than opponents of drugs in sport portray, that is little reason for comfort" (Murray 2008: 156). In view of the fact that athletes often take drugs in much greater doses than have been properly studied, or in bizarre combinations, we should be concerned about risks to athletes, and we should perform whatever epidemiological and observational studies are possible under the circumstances (Murray 2008: 156).

Sandel claimed that "[t]he safety argument is the least controversial and least interesting objection," and that "it leaves open the question whether these practices are troubling in themselves" (Sandel 2002). The harm or safety argument is, then, inadequate as an argument against enhancement in sport because it tells us nothing about whether such enhancement would be objectionable if it were risk free.

Fairness argument

If the harm argument focuses on the athlete her/himself, the fairness argument, or level playing field argument, addresses the sporting community as a whole. In sports the play should be fair. The concept of the level playing field applies not only in sports but also in other fields, such as education, health care, business, and research.

One way of overcoming the fairness argument against drug enhancement would be to allow all athletes to take whatever drugs they want, and to make performance-enhancing drugs available to all players who wish to use them. Thus "[w]e could do away with the cat and mouse game between drug users and testers, saving money and aggravation"

(Murray 2008: 156; see also Sandel 2002). However, as Murray has pointed out, these purported advantages would come at some cost: sports would lose their core values (Murray 2008: 156). Thus the fairness argument is interrelated with the next argument: the core value argument. According to the principle of fair play, or level playing field, the winners in sports must be the smarter, harder working, more devoted, more diligent, more ingenious competitors. The fans will enjoy the performances that demonstrate the athletes' talents, excellence, and perfection.

Core value argument

Alice Dreger asks the question: "Sex, drugs and prosthetic legs. Who would have thought they could have so much in common? Yet all three are posing ever more challenges to sports officials, and all have at their root the same conundrum: *what is sport really about?*" (Dreger 2009; italics added).

Murray makes a similar point: "When performance-enhancing drugs have the power to overcome differences in natural talents and the willingness to sacrifice and persevere in the quest to perfect those talents, we cannot avoid confronting the question, What do we value in sport?" (Murray 2008: 155)

The core values of sport have always been, and will continue to be, socially constructed. In China, what we call the "spirit of sport" or the "spirit of the Olympic games" is intensive training, hard work, smart tactics, conscientious dedication, and strong will. All these can improve one's performance and all of them are regarded as admirable ways of perfecting one's natural talents. The rules may be revised, the diversity of sport may be proliferated, but the core values or the spirit of sport will remain constant; they will only be reinterpreted as times and technology change.

Without the core values, without the spirit of sport, sport will lose its essence or degenerate into something inferior.

Humanity-diminishing argument

The final argument against enhancement in sports in what Sandel has called the humanity-diminishing argument. Sandel (2002) argues as follows:

One aspect of our humanity that might be threatened by enhancement is our capacity to act freely, for ourselves, by our own efforts, and to consider ourselves responsible—worthy of praise or blame—for the things we do and for the way we are ...The more the athlete relies on drugs, the less his performance represents *his* achievement. At the extreme, we might imagine a robotic, bionic athlete who, thanks to implanted computer chips that perfect the angle and timing of his swing, hits every pitch in the strike zone for a home run. The bionic athlete would not be an agent at all; "his" achievements would be those of his inventor. According to this account, enhancement threatens our humanity by eroding human agency. Its ultimate expression is a wholly mechanistic understanding of human action at odds with human freedom and moral responsibility. (Sandel 2002)

Sandel's humanity-diminishing argument indicates that enhancement in sports is relevant not only to sport itself, but has much wider implications for what it means to be human.

Future of enhancement in sports

I believe that there are two areas that are particularly important in future research. The first arises from the prospect of gene doping, i.e. the prospect that athletes will be genetically enhanced. Murray has explained as follows:

The same techniques being perfected for gene therapy may be used to give athletes a genetically programmed boost. Progress in gene therapy is in a relatively early stage of development, but the doping control agencies have realized that they need to engage the interest and creativity of top scientists, who are now working on a variety of promising strategies to detect gene doping. (Murray 2008: 157)

The second area for future research arises from the need to address the culture of doping. It could be very helpful to learn more about the culture of sports doping—why athletes dope, who influences their decisions, and the like. Chinese experiences suggest that the commercialization of sports and related incentive systems are strong factors that cannot be ignored or neglected, and that are underestimated.

In conclusion I wish to endorse Murray's three Ps as a basis for an ethical approach to sports:

Promote fairness;
Prevent harms;
Preserve meaning—the meaning of sport and the meaning of humanity.

References

Buchanan, A. et al. (2000). *From Chance to Choice: Genetics and Justice*. Cambridge: Cambridge University Press.

Crane, S. (July 2007). "Against Perfectionism," *The Useless Tree*, http://uselesstree.typepad.com/useless_tree/2007/07/against-perfect.html (accessed December 3, 2012).

Dreger, A. (2009). "Science is Forcing Sports to Re-Examine Their Core Principles," *New York Times*, September 12, http://www.nytimes.com/2009/09/13/sports/13dreger.html?ref=sports (accessed December 3, 2012).

Miah, A. (2006). "Rethinking Enhancement in Sport," *Annals of the New York Academy of Sciences*, 1093:301–20.

Murray, T. H. (2008). "Sports Enhancement," in M. Crowley (ed), *From Birth to Death and Bench to Clinic: The Hastings Center Bioethics Briefing Book for Journalists, Policymakers, and Campaigns*, Garrison, NY: Hastings Center, 153–8. http://www.thehastingscenter.org/Publications/BriefingBook/Detail.aspx?id=2206 (accessed December 3, 2012).

Norton, Q. (February 2010). "Sports Enhancement and Life Enhancement: Different Rules Apply," *H+ Magazine* [online magazine] http://hplusmagazine.com/2010/02/22/sports-enhancement-and-life-enhancement-different-rules-apply/ (accessed December 3, 2012).

Saletan, W. (2007). "Tinkering with Humans," *New York Times*, July 8, http://www.nytimes. com/2007/07/08/books/review/Saletan.html?pagewanted=all&_r=0(accessed   December 3, 2012).

Sandel, M. (2002). "What's Wrong with Enhancement," http://bioethics.georgetown.edu/pcbe/ background/sandelpaper.html (accessed December 3, 2012).

Sandel, M. (2007). *The Case against Perfectionism: Ethics in the Age of Genetic Engineering*. Cambridge, MA: Harvard University Press.

5.4

Commentary

What We Can—and Cannot—Learn about the Ethics of Enhancement by Thinking about Sport

Robert Sparrow

In 'The Misguided Quest for *the* Ethics of Enhancement,' Tom Murray (2013) makes two related claims. First, he argues that 'understanding the ethics of enhancement is deeply dependent on context' (in this chapter). Second, he suggests that, as a consequence, we should not look for 'a singular all-purpose ethics for every form of human enhancement' (in this chapter). In this brief response, I will argue that while Murray is correct in the first of these claims, there is an important sense in which he is wrong in the second. His focus on the ethics of enhancement in sport serves him well in illustrating how our reasons to embrace or resist technological change as it impacts on athletes and players depends crucially on 'why we play' and in particular on nature of the excellences made possible by the current rules of the game. However, the thing about life is that the 'rules' are unknown and the meaning of participation and the excellences it makes possible are widely disputed. For this reason, a focus on the ethics of sport serves us less well when it comes to the larger question of the attitude we should take towards 'human enhancement.' In the context of the profound disputes about the nature of the good in modern liberal societies, we may indeed need a single, robust, theoretical framework through which to resolve questions about enhancement—although whether this is best thought of as an 'ethics' or a 'politics' of enhancement is a further (and difficult) question. Regardless of how such a framework is conceived, Murray's observations about the importance of context, the significance of competition, and the attractions of a 'public health ethics' approach all serve to alert us to just how difficult the task of developing an ethics for human enhancement more generally is likely to be.

Murray begins his essay with some timely reminders of just how difficult it is likely to be to resolve even the question of whether a particular technological intervention to improve upon human capacities is an 'enhancement' or not. The ultimate impact of such changes must be evaluated in the context of a realistic appreciation of the complexity of human biology, in the long term, and in an awareness that the social consequences of technology are often unpredictable and hard to evaluate. All of these qualifications and hard tasks are routinely skipped over in the contemporary literature on human enhancement, which all too often blithely proceeds from an optimistic interpretation of a few early studies involving rats or nematodes to a confident claim about the benefits that these technologies will provide in humans. However, at a deeper level, these cautionary notes leave the larger philosophical debate about enhancement untouched. Sensible advocates of enhancement will simply concede that it is important to be appropriately confident that particular technologies do constitute enhancements before we proceed to embrace them.[1]

The bulk of Murray's chapter consists in a nuanced discussion of enhancement in sport, with which I find myself entirely in agreement. His treatment of the topic shows clear traces of—and benefits from—an extended history of engagement with actual sports people and sporting organizations, which, again, has been sadly lacking in the larger debate about enhancement in sport. He argues convincingly that whether the introduction of particular technologies into particular sports should be embraced or resisted depends upon the extent to which they enhance or detract from the values that participants seek to realize in these sports—and also on their implications for the health and safety of athletes understood through a public health framework. As an interested observer of the emergence of the debate about enhancement in sport in the last decade, I must admit that I have struggled to understand how anyone could believe otherwise. Even the pursuit of 'maximum performance,' which Savulescu, Foddy, and Clayton (2004) have advocated—and which Murray rightly dismisses as a plausible account of what athletes are seeking—requires a non-trivial account of what "performance" consists in and therefore both of the goals of participants and of our intuitions about why participation in a particular sport is something to be admired. If the goal in, for instance, the 100-metre dash was simply for a person to cover a distance of 100 metres in the shortest time possible, there would be nothing incongruous about the suggestion that we should fire the athletes out of cannons, or allow them to take their place at the track behind the wheel of Formula One racing cars. There is nothing wrong with Formula One racing, of course, but it is a different sport to sprinting and makes possible different excellences. Similarly, competition between genetically enhanced athletes—or athletes taking performance-enhancing pharmaceuticals—is a different sport than competition between athletes allowed only a more modest range of performance-enhancing techniques. Would the former be a better sport than the latter? Well, that depends, as Murray points out, on how much we value the skills and excellences athletes could demonstrate in each (the skill of the genetic engineers who

---

[1] There is, of course, an important and difficult debate to be had about just how confident we need to be in order to be 'appropriately confident' that an intervention counts as an enhancement and about who should make this decision. Given the many uncertainties that beset technological interventions in the cause of therapy and, indeed, our adoption of technology more generally, the level of confidence necessary that enhancements will be beneficial may in fact be quite low. Moreover, in liberal societies there is at least a prima facie ground to believe that it should be up to individuals to decide how much risk they are willing to take on in pursuit of some desired benefit. Advocates of enhancement tend to be those individuals who—on paper at least—are willing to accept larger risks in the hope that some particular technology will ultimately prove beneficial. On the other hand, the fact that many enhancements will produce significant negative externalities argues in favor of a democratic process of determining which (purported) enhancements individuals should be allowed to trial.

'enhanced' them versus strength of will in training?) and also—importantly—on the impact that participating in one sport rather than the other would have on the health and safety of athletes. As, in many cases, there will be little to choose between two closely related sets of excellences, or there may only be historical reasons for prefer-ring one to another, judgments as to which technological enhancements to permit in sporting contests will often rightly turn on the implications for the health and safety of athletes of allowing participants to use some new technology.

Yet the clarity of Murray's discussion and the strength of his conclusions are made possible in a large part precisely by the fact that sports do have rules and traditions that make possible some excellences rather than others and that also may serve as a resource and a basis to ground arguments about which excellences they promote—and their value. If there is room for argument as to whether it is good bowling or good batting that constitutes the highest form of excellence in cricket, there is no question that it is not skill at sword fighting or the ability to lift heavy weights. That is to say, if arguments about the ethics of enhancement must make reference to context, we are fortunate enough in the debate about enhancement in sport to have access to a rich and determi-nate context.

When we turn from the ethics of enhancement in sport to the ethics of human enhancement more generally, the attempt to resolve ethical questions with reference to claims about context is immediately much more controversial. In modern multi-ethnic, multicultural, and multi-faith societies, there is little consensus on the point of life, on which are the highest human excellences, or on anything approaching the 'rules of the game.' Arguments based on context may well therefore founder on a lack of agreement about the relevant context and its content.

Of course, there may be specific areas of human life where the range of disagree-ment is narrower and reference to context can therefore do slightly more work. It is doubtful that a drug that promoted hysterical laughter would find much of a market as a 'sexual enhancement' or that a carcinogen would be lauded as a 'health enhancement.' But most of the enhancements with which the 'enhancement debate' is concerned will have impacts across a range of different spheres of human life, such that the appropriate 'context' to use to assess them will be a whole human life. Moreover, even in the special cases where technological interventions affect only a specific arena of human life there is likely to be deep disagreement about the nature, meaning, and value of goods within the arena. Is sex 'about' reproduction, love, or fun? Is it 'healthier' to live a longer life with a moderate quality of life each day or a shorter life with a higher daily quotient of well-being? Different answers to these questions will generate different conclusions as to what counts as an enhancement in the relevant sphere and about the value of differ-ent enhancements.

The traditional liberal solution to problems which involve questions about the mean-ing of human life is to leave it up to individuals to resolve these for themselves as long as their chosen solutions do not prevent others from doing the same or harm others in some other way. It is tempting to conclude that to adopt this approach to enhance-ment is already to propose 'a singular all-purpose ethics for every form of human enhancement' of the sort that Murray denies we need. At the very least it is to con-verge upon a single all-purpose theoretical and policy framework for general-purpose enhancements in a liberal society.[2] Strictly speaking, though, at least in its most plausible and well-known variant, this liberal approach motivates a political rather than an ethical framework for enhancement. That is to say, it tells us that people should be *permitted* to adopt enhancements unless their doing so harms others or restricts their freedom—it does not settle the question of the ethics of their doing so. Still, if context cannot play the role that Murray attributes to it, this may be all that is available to us.

However, Murray's discussion of the ethics of enhancement in sport also touches upon two related phenomena which together suggest that this liberal solution is much more problematic than is generally acknowledged.

First, Murray draws attention in passing to the role played by competition in sport in driving the uptake of performance-enhancing technologies. Those who wish to be able to win against others who have the option of adopting performance-enhancing technology must embrace enhancement even where the enhancement concerned is known to be dangerous to those who use it. Second, Murray recognizes that the fact of 'human interdependence' means that this dynamic needs to be taken seriously as a way in which the actions of those embracing enhancement impact upon the well-being of others and suggests that a 'public health ethics' will sometimes justify restricting individual access to enhancement for the sake of 'the well-being of a population' (Murray in this chapter).

The first of these observations is also relevant to enhancement outside the context of sport. There are significant aspects of life in contemporary capitalist societies, such as the pursuit of wealth or social status, that are also 'inherently, relentlessly competitive' (Frank 1985). Indeed, the ideology of such societies encourages the idea that this is true even of parts of life that are not. Thus, the moment citizens begin to feel that particular enhancements can provide a competitive advantage in the struggle for these goods, they will feel compelled to adopt them (Kavka 1994). Moreover, establishing a rat race or arms race is not the only way in which individuals' adoption of enhancements may affect others. The relationship between enhancements and the context of the human activity that they enhance works both ways. If it becomes possible to love someone by taking a drug that produces love, then the meaning of love, and how we respond to it, would change dramatically. As Erik Parens (1995) and Bill McKibben (2003) have each argued convincingly, the meaning of many of our most rewarding experiences is intimately related to our limits: by what we can't do, as much as what we can. Importantly, such changes in context and meaning are not confined to the individuals who choose to adopt or not adopt enhancements. Because meanings are social, once a significant percentage of the population has altered their capacities by adopting an enhancement, the meaning of related activities and experiences will be changed for everyone.

In life, even more than in sport, then, the fact of human interdependence means that we cannot afford to look at the ethics of enhancement solely at the level of individual choices. This, in turn, means that the "liberal" approach to the ethics of enhancement

---

[2] For an attempt to defend a framework of this sort in the context of debates about genetic human enhancement, see Agar (2004). For a critique, see Sparrow (2010).

described above is manifestly inadequate. Many, perhaps even most, enhancements are likely to both harm and restrict the liberty of others, by generating destructive rat races and through their consequences for social meanings that play a vital role in constructing a good human life.

Yet the 'public health model' that Murray advocates as a way of negotiating the tension between individual liberty and public good in the context of enhancement in sport is also extremely problematic when we turn to the larger question of the ethics of human enhancement. When sporting organizations and officials are regulating sport, it is uncontroversial that the health and safety of athletes and players should be a pre-eminent concern. However, the values that government should promote in society as a whole are highly contested. Indeed, once we move away from the promotion of 'health'—itself a more plural concept than is often acknowledged—the very idea that we are justified in sacrificing individual liberty for the sake of public benefit is controversial. It should be especially controversial in the context of debates about human enhancement given the shameful record of human rights violations for the sake of the 'nation' or 'population' in the history of eugenics (Sparrow 2011).

Should significant human enhancement become possible, therefore, the fact of human interdependence means that decisions about enhancement should not be left up to individuals. We will, indeed, need a more-or-less-general 'ethics of enhancement' of the sort that Murray disavows. Yet we cannot rely straightforwardly upon a 'public health' model to provide one. We are left, then, with Murray's original insight about the importance of context in determining what counts as an enhancement and how we should respond to the prospect of changes in the sorts of excellences that participation in important social practices makes possible. The relevant 'context,' however, will be the whole of human life. Debate about the ethics of enhancement will therefore require discussions about the projects and values we, as a society, think that it is valuable to pursue. Similarly, settling upon the nature of the 'public good' that should constrain the individual liberty to adopt enhancements will require engaging in arguments about deeply contested matters of value. These are both projects that modern multicultural societies have tended to shy away from.

The main lesson that thinking about enhancement in sport can teach us, then, is just how difficult it will be to come up with the necessary 'ethics of enhancement' once we move from the relatively narrow and uncontroversial context of sport to the larger context of human existence. Yet there is a further lesson here for politics more generally. Human interdependence is not confined to enhancement. Other technologies impact upon the context in which we make our choices and the sorts of values it is possible to pursue. Indeed, many forms of social, cultural, and political action, carried out by individuals and groups, either are intended to reshape the stock of meanings and values that constitute the context of our cultural and political lives or inevitably do so regardless of their initiators' intentions. Perhaps surprisingly, the lessons—both positive and negative—that we can draw from Murray's thoughtful discussion of the ethics of enhancement in sport generalize. Context matters, both for how we evaluate our lives, and for what it is possible to do in them. Any politics that does not recognize this will fail to adequately safeguard both individual liberty and the public good. Taking context seriously, as Murray insists we should, on the other hand, requires a broader and more vigorous political debate that confronts questions about meaning and value that a traditional liberal politics abjures.

References

Agar, N. (2004). *Liberal Eugenics: In Defence of Human Enhancement*. Oxford: Blackwell.

Frank, R. H. (1985). *Choosing the Right Pond: Human Behavior and the Quest for Status*. Oxford: Oxford University Press.

Kavka, G. S. (1994). 'Upside Risks: Social Consequences of Beneficial Biotechnology,' in C. Cranor (ed.), *Are Genes Us? The Social Consequences of the New Genetics*. New Brunswick, NJ: Rutgers University Press, 155–79.

McKibben, B. (2003). *Enough: Staying Human in an Engineered Age*. New York: Times Books.

Murray, T. (2014). 'The Misguided Quest for *the* Ethics of Enhancement,' in A. Akabayashi (ed.), *The Future of Bioethics: International Dialogues*. Oxford: Oxford University Press, 193–204.

Parens, E. (1995). 'The Goodness of Fragility: On the Prospect of Genetic Technologies Aimed at the Enhancement of Human Capabilities,' *Kennedy Institute of Ethics Journal*, 5(2): 141–53.

Savulescu, J., Foddy, B., and Clayton, M. (2004). 'Why We Should Allow Performance Enhancing Drugs in Sport,' *British Journal of Sports Medicine*, 38: 666–70.

Sparrow, R. (2010). 'Liberalism and Eugenics,' *Australasian Journal of Philosophy*, 89(3): 499–517.

Sparrow, R. (2011). 'A Not-So-New Eugenics: Harris and Savulescu on Human Enhancement,' *Hastings Center Report*, 41(1): 32–42.

5.5

Response to Commentaries
Laments, Limits, and Liberalism

Thomas Murray and Cameron R. Waldman

It is nothing less than a considerable honor to read and reflect on the commentaries by Professors Becker, Qiu, and Sparrow. Each of the commentaries demonstrates a close and careful reading of the arguments in "The Misguided Quest for *the* Ethics of Enhancement" and each offers an opportunity to clarify and expand the arguments offered there.

Carl Becker draws on his experience of nearly 40 years as an American living in Japan to explain his concerns about how the quest for enhancement can go wrong. Yet, in that same experience, he finds inspiration, beauty, grace, and meaning. Renzong Qiu shows a remarkable command of the literature on ethics, drugs, and sport from the most recent scandals to the principal philosophical arguments used to defend, and to condemn, athletes' use of drugs to enhance performance. He worries that certain "enhancements" may, in the end, diminish our humanity. Robert Sparrow praises the topic article's emphasis on context, but challenges the claim that we should not expect to find "a singular all-purpose ethics for every form of human enhancement." He believes that (classical) liberalism is insufficient as a guide for navigating through the thickets of enhancement technologies. He argues that we need to talk "about the projects and values we, as a society, think that it is valuable to pursue" (Sparrow in this chapter).

Laments: Carl Becker calls our attention to a variety of ways in which we debase that which has value. The consumerism epitomized in the "Big Gulp" soft drink, where mere quantity is treated as a good in itself, misunderstands the nature of what should be valued, even in the simple act of consuming a beverage. His evocative description of the meaning of a sip of tea in the course of an elaborate ritual shows the utter lack of correlation between quantity and value. The ancient calligrapher he observed creating, slowly, a work of great beauty and lasting significance demonstrated the value of creative work itself, apart from the utility or market value of the object created. And the classical Japanese dancer he describes showed that grace and beauty are not the exclusive province of the young, despite contemporary society's celebration of youth's vigor and the relative absence of the marks a lifetime of work and struggle inscribe upon a person's body and spirit.

In an otherwise very sympathetic paper, Becker describes the stories and hypotheticals in "The Misguided Quest for *the* Ethics of Enhancement" as "cameos...more appeals to a leap of faith than criteria for public policy" (Becker in this chapter). He expresses a desire for guidelines for "behavior-enhancing" drugs, which, he correctly notes, the paper does not provide. His observations invite clarification on the role such stories play in the broader argument the paper attempts to develop. His request also requires an expanded discussion of the relationship between ethical analysis and public policy—including the sort of guidelines Becker asks for.

We have avoided trying to specify or explicitly defend the method used in "The Misguided Quest for *the* Ethics of Enhancement." But it can plausibly be described as a hybrid between the "thick description" Geertz employed in his analysis of Balinese cockfighting (Geertz 1972) and the "reflective equilibrium" Rawls used so skillfully in his *A Theory of Justice* and in *Political Liberalism* (Rawls 1971; Rawls 1993). The analysis begins with an exploration of what values people seek through sport. The relevant inputs range from public opinion polling data to detailed narratives by athletes, coaches, and others who love and understand their sport. Those tentative conclusions are then tested against whatever challenges we can identify. People are born with vastly different talents for sports: Is that unfair? People play for many different reasons, including popularity and money: Does the multiplicity of motives undermine any effort to find consistent values or meaning in sport?

The account of values is honed and refined in response to such challenges; the list is much longer than the handful just mentioned. The goal is to provide an account that represents robustly why we play: what values we pursue in and through sport, and what meanings we find there.

At the same time, we must examine these values critically: Are they worthy of being valued in a comprehensive account of a fully human life? In many different comprehensive accounts, even if not all possible ones? What legitimate human desires and needs does sport, rightly understood, help us satisfy? What does sport do for our developing character and our relationships, not merely for our body? Here we move from description to normative analysis and critique.

All along the way we try to extract whatever general principles best account for the values and meanings that emerge from the interaction between description and moral assessment. Those principles are meant to help distinguish between acceptable and unacceptable forms of enhancement. Thus far, the inquiry has led us to propose three such principles: promote fairness; prevent harm; preserve meaning. We make no claim that these are the comprehensive set of ethical principles for analyzing every possible candidate enhancement technology in sport; but they have proven useful so far. And, although they have not been exhaustively tested in other spheres of human endeavor, they may prove a helpful starting point for ethical evaluation of putative enhancement technologies outside sport.

That, in short, is as close as "The Misguided Quest for *the* Ethics of Enhancement" comes to having a formal "method." Becker wants us to go beyond the realm of sport and offer policy guidance for substances intended to enhance behavior in other spheres of life.

In a book whose working title is *Why We Play*, one of us, Murray, examines in much more detail the implications for public policy on drugs and sport of the principles described here. But ethics and public policy are not the same thing. One can have a thoroughly defensible—even essential—public policy without any judgment that a particular action is morally wrong per se. Driving on the left-hand side of the road is public policy in Japan, the UK, and many other nations. In North America, we drive on the right. No intrinsic wrongness or rightness attaches to driving on one side or the other: but once enough vehicles take to the roads, it's absolutely necessary to choose one or the other lest cars and trucks career head first into one another.

On the other hand, a well-founded, even universally shared judgment that some particular action is wrong does not, in itself, provide sufficient reason to create a formal public policy such as a law to prohibit or regulate it. It's generally believed that telling a lie or making a promise one has no intention of keeping is wrong. And so it is. When two people meet in a bar, and one promises to call by the end of the week—knowing all along that no such call would be made—this is an instance of a false promise. But no serious student of human relationships and the law would advocate passing a statute that routinely punished such false promises with fines or prison. Other promises—of the kind we call contracts—are meant to be kept, and the law provides a variety of forms of redress if they are broken.

Using ethical principles or judgments to shape public policies requires discerning how such principles are to be interpreted and applied. Principles are not self-interpreting. Everyone can agree that preventing harm is a good thing to do. But what counts as a harm? Do small nicks and scratches count or should we limit our policy concerns to significant, long-term harms? What if the risks are a known and widely accepted part of the sport? American football players collide violently with one another on every play. Boxers pummel their opponent's body and head. Alpine skiers are always at risk of falls, twisted joints, and broken bones. These examples should not lead to hopelessness. Sports can and do alter rules and equipment in order to reduce the likelihood of injuries. A principle such as "prevent harm" guides us toward some practices and away from others. But the principle needs to be interpreted in the light of complex empirical assessments and the overall context in which it is to be applied.

In addition to the demands of interpretation, important procedural considerations arise. Whose voices should be heard in deciding what policy to institute, and what weight should we give these voices individually and collectively? When the World Anti-Doping Agency (WADA) considered the use of hypoxic environments to increase endurance, it determined that this technology was not simply equivalent to taking EPO, but was nevertheless inconsistent with what the WADA code calls the "spirit of sport." But the community of athletes, sport scientists, coaches, and trainers was consulted and firmly opposed a ban. They have a legitimate voice in such decisions, and their views were heeded.

Finally, in the voyage from ethical principles to public policy, a variety of practical matters must be taken into account. If a ban were enacted, would it be enforceable? What of collateral damage to other values such as privacy? And what are the opportunity costs of the policy? What could be achieved if the resources required to monitor and enforce a policy were used in other ways toward the same goal? For example, would investments in education on values, drugs, and sport be more cost effective than relying on drug tests and sanctions?

Each of these factors—interpretation, procedural considerations, and practical challenges—needs to be taken into account when ethical principles are being translated into public policy.

One last observation on Becker: His three "cameos"—the tea service, calligraphy, and traditional dance—bear important similarities to sport. Each one constitutes a performance within a structure of rules that foster the development and expression of particular forms of human excellence. Those excellences are perfected through a harmonious combination of physical and mental discipline. All of this is likewise true of sport.

Limits: Renzong Qiu devotes most of his commentary to describing recent developments in the use of performance-enhancing drugs by athletes and the arguments in defense of and against enhancement in sport. In point after point, Qiu appears to endorse the arguments and analyses I have offered, so, not surprisingly, I have no significant disagreements with him. My main response is to thank him for his scholarly analysis and support.

Near the end of his article, Qiu describes Sandel's concern that as we rely ever more on technologies that substitute interventions designed and controlled by others for our natural human capacities, we risk becoming more like a "robotic, bionic athlete" whose performance approaches or achieves perfection, but at the price of loss of agency. The bionic athlete's conquests are more properly credited to his inventor than to himself, Sandel asserts. Qiu worries that such scenarios lead to "a wholly mechanistic understanding of human action at odds with human freedom and moral responsibility" (Qiu 2013 in this chapter).

We are then forced to confront the libertarian enhancement paradox. Libertarian commentators defend the athlete's freedom to use any and all technologies of enhancement she or he wishes to use. Various experts (often self-described) and gurus are likely to control access to and administration of many of these technologies. Athletes often have little understanding or knowledge of the details. Consider the East German coaches and scientists who gave powerful hormones to adolescent swimmers and other young athletes, telling them they were receiving "vitamins." Or the head of the BALCO laboratory who supplied novel drugs to US athletes along with detailed schedules instructing them when to take each one.

When athletes exercised their liberty in this way, they became increasingly the manipulated product of others. The more they freely give away control over their bodies and lives, the less agency they can claim for their performances. As agency erodes, responsibility and freedom go with it.

Every sport imposes limits on how individuals may improve their performance. If the sport is wise and well governed, those limits help to prevent harm, promote fairness, and preserve meaning. That meaning provides a structure within which persons are free to develop the particular human excellences the sport celebrates, and the virtues that come from the disciplined effort to perfect our individual talents. Those limits can and should protect against the loss of agency that worries Sandel and Qiu.

Liberalism: Robert Sparrow offers the most direct challenge to "The Misguided Quest for *the* Ethics of Enhancement" in two ways. He shows why generalizing a public health ethics model beyond sport to other realms of human enhancement would be problematic. And he argues that the claim that we should not expect to find "a singular all-purpose ethics for every form of human enhancement" is, in an important sense, wrong. We agree that a public health ethics framework is not appropriate for thinking about every possible form of enhancement, and did not propose it as a universal, generalizable way of assessing the ethics of enhancement. Sparrow's elaboration of his reasons for thinking that the "all-purpose" assertion is wrong suggests that, in fact, we agree firmly on the central thrust of his argument—that understanding the ethics of enhancement requires that we take seriously substantive questions about what deserves to be valued and what forms of public good justify limits on individual liberty.

First, the appropriate use and limitations of public health ethics in thinking through the ethics of enhancement: When the conditions that justify a public health ethics approach are met, then we should look to it for insights. But that will not be true in a great many instances. I introduced it into the sports context as a rebuttal to the liberal/libertarian claim that athletes' decisions to use performance-enhancing drugs are self-regarding decisions and therefore solely the legitimate expression of each individual's liberty. The relentless competition in sport and the often minute differences that distinguish winners from losers power the drug race in sport much as the arms race drives nations to waste resources as well as risk their own futures and those of their neighbors and putative enemies. Public health ethics will provide insights into the ethics of enhancement when the conditions that motivate it, such as those specified in the topic article, are met. When they are not, we will need to look elsewhere.

Sparrow sets a particularly difficult challenge. He reminds us that sport is a rule-governed activity and that in the debate over enhancement in sport we "have access to a rich and determinate context" (Sparrow 2013 in this chapter). He contrasts the relative clarity and agreement on values he believes sport exhibits with other vital spheres of human life such as sex, reproduction, and ideas about health and the quality of life, where we are likely to find sharp disagreements over values, and, therefore, much greater difficulty coming to grips with the ethics of enhancements in those spheres. In these ways he stresses the differences between sport and other spheres, suggesting that it was relatively easy to deal with the ethics of enhancement in sport, but far more difficult to do so elsewhere.

I believe that Sparrow overestimates the gap between sport and all other spheres of human life. One problem is the conflation of rules and values. Yes, sports are rule governed, but that is in an important sense epiphenomenal. Rules themselves are morally trivial (although breaking them intentionally is cheating and that is a moral offense). The topic article argues that rules in sport are fundamentally dependent on shared understandings about values and meaning in each sport. That persistent, endlessly contestable conversation about values and meanings goes on every time there is a change in strategies, equipment, players, or proposed rules. And, for what it's worth, one can easily find sharp disagreements about the ethics of enhancement technologies in sport. A similar conversation over values and meanings must go on each time some enhancement technology is used or proposed for any sphere of human endeavor, including but in no way limited to sport.

Take an easy case: EPO enhances endurance and is banned in sport; but endurance is a vital attribute in other spheres, e.g. ski patrols. Suppose we could be confident that ski rescue workers' health was not endangered by taking modest doses of EPO and that the enhanced endurance it provided protected them on long treks to rescue persons and also increased the likelihood of a successful rescue. Would it be ethical to take EPO in such a context? Of course! If we had moral reservations they would be about the ski patrol members' health, not about the meaning of the sphere—which includes, after all, saving lives without needlessly risking your own.

Other spheres may be more difficult to reason through; Sparrow is certainly correct about that. But we must do our best to understand values and meanings in whatever context the supposed enhancement emerges. In each sphere, for each enhancement or category of enhancements, we can look at the ends of that particular sphere of human activity and the relationship of the proposed "enhancements" in light of those ends and the values relevant to that sphere. We do not need to agree on the ultimate meaning of life to agree that rescue workers ought to rescue. When it comes to enhancements in other spheres, we are advocating an approach—careful attention to context and particulars, values and meanings. This is something other than the "singular all-purpose ethics for every form of human enhancement" Sparrow calls for, but it is far from nothing.

It may also be the case that the three broad principles I identified in sport will turn out to be applicable in many, perhaps all, analyses of putative enhancements. If true, this would take us even further in the direction of a generalized ethics of enhancement. But our argument here does not depend upon that being the case. Reflective equilibrium will be a valuable strategy for understanding the reach and adequacy of these or other principles that may appear helpful.

Now, to the politics of enhancement: Sparrow offers a helpful analysis of what he calls the "traditional liberal solution" for questions about values and meanings: "leave it up to individuals to resolve these for themselves as long as their chosen solutions do not prevent others from doing the same or harm others in some other way" (Sparrow in this chapter). He observes that this is more a political than a moral solution. Allowing individuals to choose without interference may "solve" a policy problem, but it fails to address whether those choices are ethically defensible or wise. Asking such ethical questions requires engaging with fundamental questions about values, meanings, human good, and human flourishing. It also requires plunging deeply into context and particulars so that we may know what this particular "enhancement" means for people seeking whatever is valuable in that sphere.

We agree completely with Sparrow that any cogent discussion of the "ethics of enhancement" has to grapple simultaneously with fundamental matters of moral substance as well as with the welter of particulars in which the "enhancement" is being considered—the context. Where we may disagree—or not in the end—is over the resources available for substantive ethical engagement over ends and values in particular spheres of human life. We agree with Sparrow that in certain spheres, especially those with less defined rules and traditions than in the sphere of sport, such agreement may be more difficult to find. But there are rich and abundant resources for serious dialogue on values and meanings just about everywhere we look. We should expect that some would-be enhancements will be difficult to assess either because we don't agree on how they mesh with the ends and values of the particular practice, or because we don't agree on what those ends and values are. Those are conversations worth having—necessary conversations, we would argue, about ethics.

But we also need to attend to politics—a sphere much broader and arguably more complicated than that of sports. Even at the level of political discourse, we believe there is still room to derive meaning from context that is helpful in guiding the debate. Sparrow rightly points out that liberal political solutions that remain neutral on matters of human flourishing and ends will likely fail at addressing the underlying moral concerns of the enhancement debate. Fortunately, however, the liberal tradition does not stop at libertarianism. John Rawls provides a helpful framework anchored in political liberalism for thinking about the interplay between ethics and public policy. Rawls shows us that liberal political discourse and rich moral debate need not exclude one another. For Rawls, moral appeals, including appeals to valued ends and the good life, are encouraged so long as they *overlap* with "public reasons," that is, the reasons that would be universally agreeable for citizens participating within the political sphere. The lessons that we take from Rawls are twofold: first, our approach to enhancement need not necessarily be at odds with more nuanced theories of liberalism, and second, Rawls demonstrates that even within a sphere as broad as the political domain, there is opportunity to infer implicit moral values. Such values can be used to help shape our collective moral understandings on matters of politics, enhancement, as well as for other complex spheres of human endeavor.

The line Sparrow takes the paper to task on—about not looking for "a singular all-purpose ethics for every form of human enhancement"—could have been framed less provocatively, perhaps. It may be more clearly expressed in the following two statements:

1. Understanding whether any particular biomedical enhancement is or is not morally justified cannot be determined without an inquiry into the values and meanings of that particular sphere of human activity; the same performance-enhancing technology, e.g., may justly be morally condemned in one context and tolerated or praised in another.

2. Because context is so central to the full moral analysis of any putative enhancement, we should not expect broad generalizations of the form "enhancement technology X is always good/bad, justifiable/unjustifiable" to be valid. In the end, we must engage with fundamental questions about values, meanings, and flourishing.

I, Murray, and my co-author of this response, Waldman, are very pleased to join our esteemed commentators, Carl Becker, Renzong Qiu, and Robert Sparrow, on a quest to illuminate the ethics of enhancement technologies grounded firmly in each relevant context, and which engages eagerly and forthrightly with those fundamental questions.

References

Becker, C. (2014). "Thomas Murray's Enhancement of a Bioethics of Enhancement," in A. Akabayashi (ed.), *The Future of Bioethics: International Dialogues*. Oxford: Oxford University Press, 205–10.

Geertz, C. (1972). "Deep Play: Notes on the Balinese Cockfight," *Daedalus*, 101:1–37.

Qiu, R. (2014). "Arguments for and against Enhancement in Sports," in A. Akabayashi (ed.), *The Future of Bioethics: International Dialogues*. Oxford: Oxford University Press, 211–17.

Rawls, J. (1971). *A Theory of Justice*. Cambridge, MA: Harvard University Press.

Rawls, J. (1993). *Political Liberalism*. New York: Columbia University Press.

Sparrow, R. (2014). "What We Can—and Can't—Learn about the Ethics of Enhancement by Thinking about Sport," in A. Akabayashi (ed.), *The Future of Bioethics: International Dialogues*. Oxford: Oxford University Press, 218–23.

SECTION C

Emerging Problems in Research Ethics

6.1

Primary Topic Article

Redefining Property in Human Body Parts: An Ethical Enquiry

Benjamin Capps

1 Introduction

1.1 Ethical debate about property in human tissues and cells often refers to the seminal legal US case of John Moore.[1] Between 1976 and 1983, Moore was a patient undergoing treatment for hairy-cell leukaemia. However, unbeknownst to him, during this time his doctor and others were working in cahoots to isolate and patent what would subsequently be known as the 'Mo' cell line.[2] On finding out about the existence of the cell line, Moore sought a share of the profits: the cell line, after all, was derived from *his* body; it was, he claimed, his property. Ultimately, however, the Supreme Court of California rejected any property claim he might have; finding instead that only after human cells have been modified in some significant way could they be considered as property. Property, therefore, rested with the scientist able to apply skill, regardless of how the original cells came to be in their possession.

1.2 *Moore* has permeated the case law of many jurisdictions, and has thereby propagated the curious circumstances in which no one can *own* the cells removed from their own body, yet anyone else who is capable of modifying them can. (One could only own their own cells if they themselves had the ingenuity to modify them, and a licence allowing one to do so.) It is easy to see why *Moore* continues to be conceptually troubling, and this disconcert was revived in the recent UK case of *Yearworth*.[3] This case challenges the remarkably enduring precedent of *Moore*, because it suggests that a person *can*

---

[1] *Moore* v. *Regents of the University of California* (1998) 249 Cal Rptr 494; 215 Cal.App. 3d 709; (1990); 271 Cal Rptr 146; 793 P2d 479; cert denied (1991) 111 SCt 1388 (hereafter *Moore;* citations will refer to 51 Cal.3d 120 unless otherwise indicated).

[2] In this paper, I focus on property in respect to human parts: cells and tissues. For the remainder of this paper, I will refer to cells and tissues interchangeably. Tissue refers to a cellular complex which can be grouped to form respective organs.

[3] *Yearworth and others* v. *North Bristol NHS Trust*, EWCA Civ 37 (2009); QB 1. (2010) (hereafter *Yearworth*). Lord Judge CJ described the bifurcation of property rights in *Moore* as 'not entirely logical'; para. 45(d).

be the owner of his or her own cells, despite the cells, at the time, being cryopreserved and held within a medical trust facility.

1.3 The reason for rooting this discussion in these two legal cases is because the pressures to commodify body parts are inevitably going to increase over the next decades, yet so far there is neither ethical nor legal consensus on how to resolve the issue of property. In many jurisdictions, the idea of property remains a 'contradictory jumble of legal principles' (George 2004: 17).[4] And *Yearworth*, in this respect, is another legal approach that is grounded in uncertain ethical terms; while *Moore* is broadly utilitarian, *Yearworth* appears at first blush to be about rights. My paper, therefore, is about the future of property in light of a growing bio-business.

1.4 Locke wrote: 'There cannot be any one moral rule be propos'd, whereof a Man may not justly demand a reason' (Locke 1975: I, III, 4). My intention in this chapter is modest: I intend to enquire about the reasons given to justify the approach taken in each of the cases, and in particular, my intention is to review the *ethical* notion of property so as to understand what we expect a *theory* of property to do in moral interactions involving human body parts (and in this respect, this is a separate debate from that concerning trade in organs).[5] This is not intended to be a study of law: such an analysis would require tracing the legal steps, taking into account the idiosyncrasies in different jurisdictions, to surmise where we are now with respect to property and the human body.

1.5 My analysis assumes that linking together these seemingly disparate legal scenarios is possible, and in this respect it is of note that in both cases a property solution was pursued despite presumably there being legal misgivings from the outset (the traditional view is that the common law does not recognize any rights of property in a body). To make this possible, I use the European Convention on Human Rights and Biomedicine 1997 as a conflationary device to analyse the conceptual inference of property across jurisdictions. I conclude that the 'property right' model emanating from *Yearworth*, although needing further theoretical work, is a welcome challenge to the archaic reasoning in *Moore*.

2   The future of body parts

2.1 Many writers have resisted the property paradigm when talking about the human body and its parts because it relies on antiquated principles of Cartesian Dualism; simply stated, the body and the mind cannot be consistently separated so that the former can become someone's property (cf. Campbell 2009). But, as I will later argue, property remains a valid concept when one is talking about removed body parts. This is because the reasons that we might expect to protect the integrity of the human person are no

---

[4] I note that a number of cases from common law jurisdictions and the USA have returned to *Moore* to guide their considered judgments.

[5] I steer clear of the issues that arise from organ transplantation: this debate is about demands which outstrip supply and health risks and benefits to donors and recipients. Accordingly, legal principles are grounded in the ethical validity of comprehensive commodification, moderated rules of reimbursement or compensation, and contractual costs payable to those who make the transplantation possible. When organs are grown *ex vivo*, many of these objections will dissolve.

longer persuasive when talking about the interests we still have in such artefacts. While it is reasonable to find that a physical injury to the body is an actionable harm, one cannot register the same kind of response when damage is inflicted on human parts already removed. Therefore, if any interest remains in removed parts, it becomes necessary to consider them as protected on grounds conceptually different from those that protect the person. It is therefore proper to talk of these parts as 'things' or property. By property, I mean a legally enforceable or morally authoritative prescription that evinces control of an object. This control might include rights to use, the right to any benefit, a right to transfer or sell, and a right to exclude others. If an object can be properly considered as property, then the kinds of rights attached to it will be determined by an underlying moral principle.

2.2 The law of property in human body parts has become unwieldy: there are too many exceptions allowed under *sui generis* laws, and each one is grounded by bewildering and inconsistent reasoning. For instance, contemporary English and American law does not recognize property rights in living persons (Scott 1981). The moral object of such provisions is to preclude, among other things, forced or willing subjection into slavery, marital ownership, or the transfer of debt to the body of the debtor. This is based on the idea that 'What is possessed must under the definition be a thing',[6] and the living person as such cannot be possibly conceptualized as something which can be owned in the way that property is. Sometimes our bodies are *used* by others. For the most part this is according to prior agreement, for example when one willingly enters a profession that entails the waiver of certain rights (e.g. military service). But although the law does not allow the absolute conditions that would allow ownership of oneself, sometimes individuals are for all intents and purposes owned by the state, for example in national service, or are temporarily possessed to reconcile conflicts of interests arising from the 'need' to use another person (see Calabresi 1991[7]).

Likewise, cadavers are precluded from straightforward property interests. The law is anchored in the notion that society should be reverent in the proper treatment of 'embodied persons' subsequent to death (see Porter 2003: 223). This normally meant a quick and respectful burial or cremation of a worthy soul; but coincidently the dead body also held little tangible value and could be hastily and properly disposed of to avoid spreading disease. But the idea that the body had no worth would be dispelled with the advent of a sound medical basis for cadaveric dissection, and as a response to the unwelcome digging up of corpses to be procured by anatomists, the law has limited rights of possession of dead bodies to those involved with burial, licensed dissections, and forensics.

2.3 However, when it comes to body parts, the conceptual ideas shift to controversially endorsing property under specific conditions.[8] We can 'gift' parts of our bodies, such as organs, but we cannot normally sell them. This rule might be justified in terms of

---

[6] *Regina* v. *Bentham* (Appellant) UKHL 18, (2005), para. 8.

[7] On the problems of using another person's body, see Thomson 1971.

[8] Cf. 'An object need not be "property" before society can regulate it, and premature questions about the existence of property rights provide an unhelpful distraction from the substantive issue of whether or not individuals should be permitted to buy, sell or otherwise trade their body parts' (George 2004: 17).

repugnance or the risks of exploitation that result if we commodify such things, but also promulgates the impossibly vague idea of altruism. But, barring some exceptions (hair, for example, can be sold by the person it is cut from), cells and tissues are *res nullius*, no one's thing, or as matter abandoned *until claimed by someone else with an interest in owner-ship*. What this amounts to is that once cells are removed from the body, the person they came from cannot claim to be the owner; yet those same cells can be the property of an industrious, and as we shall see, a possibly mischievous researcher. In this respect, five steering features are important to my ethical analysis:

(a) That the removal of cells does not normally harm the patient, or at least does not result in permanent injury or alteration beyond that which is expected as part of the condition being treated.

(b) Removal does not need to be subject to consent for the object removed to be considered as property. One way to dismiss any similarity between *Moore* and *Yearworth* would be that consent was or was not given for the parts to be removed. Yet we are not normally so divisive in terms of the conditions for asking (or not) when talking about the appropriation of other things that are normally consid-ered as property.

(c) After their removal from the patient, one might expect that cells normally will be either discarded as waste or kept by the hospital for the purpose of future treat-ment, diagnosis, or medical education. Yet cells may also be taken as a biopsy as part of, or in addition to, an indicated medical procedure, or collected from surgi-cal waste, and this allows the opportunity for researchers to access and use them without direct consent from the patient. If they are kept for any reason, they will be modified from their originating state, either to preserve them or to capture some biological characteristic.

(d) The stored cells may be so ubiquitous that they have little use beyond the con-venience of a laboratory slide for diagnosis or education purposes. However, they are likely to be valuable if they display some atypical characteristics spotted by a physician or scientists, have some special function (thus have therapeutic or diagnostic value), or become finite (i.e. the cells are the last of their kind). This sets up two competing claims: the person who asserts ownership of the valu-able cells because they came from their body—this is likely to be a patient with neither the means nor licensed permission to keep the cells themselves—and the researcher already in possession of the cells and who demands ownership as a reward for their creative or industrious efforts. The cells also contain a unique genetic fingerprint of the source, thus a conflict also arises when the source wants to preclude access to or use of the information that they hold.

(e) Thus, patients might expect to retain some kind of interests in the removed cells, which may be expressed by controlling their use, or demanding knowledge about what purpose they are used for, and by whom.

I have two final caveats. One, some cells, such as oocytes, will require harvesting that entails a direct material risk to the source. However, while the act of removal might dif-fer, property remains a feature of *any* part previously part of a human body. Two, I intend to focus on removed cells and tissue from living adult patients. This is because post mortem appropriation dissipates consent as a procedural signal from the source, and such tissue also tends to have an additional emotional significance (The Wellcome Trust and Medical Research Council 2001).

2.4 In *Yearworth*, Lord Judge, C. J. states:

The law…has to some extent begun to be refined in relation both to a human corpse and to *parts of the human* corpse; but it has remained silent about *parts or products of a living human* body, probably because until recently medical science did not endow them with any value or other significance. (*Yearworth*, para. 29; italics in the original)

This shift makes property a pressing ethical issue. Up to now, there have been a handful of cases which presupposed that human parts and products thereof could be property in certain circumstances.[9] But if an *a fortiori* justification can be made to treat human material as property (rather than considering it as something else conceptually different), then one might expect that increasing complexities in the transfer of human cells and tissues will result in ever more exceptions to the 'no property' rule.

2.5 For example, commodification, referring to the contested status of human material within the context of a bio-economy, has changed the way in which we make financial deals with respect to body parts and allowing persons to engage in trade with them. For instance, the demand for human oocytes to meet research needs has intensified the debate about payment or provision of subsidized treatments as 'benefits in kind' as potentially ethical means to encourage women to provide them. This is despite the risks of harvesting and the implications for coerced and exploitative monetary transfer.[10]

2.6 It is also evident that individuals are often unaware that human tissue is used in a profit-driven industry, and moreover, that patients are oblivious to the fact that it is routinely retained by researchers for research purposes (Andrews and Nelkin 1998; Katches et al. 2000; Retained Organs Commission 2004). For this reason, one might expect that the business of bioscience will encourage the kinds of clandestine appropriation justified by *Moore* in a future of increased transfer of body parts.

Yet a further concern is that one may well also suppose that the increasing pervasiveness of technologies into medicine will create ever more reasons and opportunities to 'own' human body parts. For example, the practice of storing cells for future therapy is already big business; and where there is a perceptible value in an object, a desire to keep control can materialize: witness, for example, the growing incentive to store cord blood in commercial banks (see Rei 2010). Research biobanks have also been set up on the

---

[9] For example, and this is by no means an exhaustive list: In the UK, courts have treated body parts separated without permission, such as hair and urine, as property in the criminal law of theft or battery; see: *Regina* v. *Herbert* (1961) 25 J.C.L. 163; *Regina* v. *Welsh* [1974] R.T.R. 478. US courts have found that a decedent's preserved sperm has a property interest because the donor has the authority to use it for reproduction; see: *Hecht* v. *Superior Court*, 16 Cal. App.4th 836, 20 Cal. Rptr. 2d 275 (2d Dist. 1993). In *York* v. *Jones* (717 F. Supp 421, 1989), the court treated frozen embryos possessed by an IVF clinic as property owned by the parents and held under a bailment contract by the clinic.

[10] The demand for oocytes has led to a change in many jurisdictions to the conditions for procuring eggs as marketable artefacts; see Capps and Campbell 2007.

understanding that the contents are owned.[11] But this drive to capture the value in cells and tissues has also meant that the interest in bio-repositories has expanded to include many potential users. These repositories may initially be set up as research resources with the consent of the donors, but they have later been cosseted by their owners to limit their interests.[12] Furthermore, they are easily accessed by third parties wishing to draw on the inclusive data. In this sense, these collections create certain privileges for their owners, and subsequently, these freedoms can be passed on to users and third parties despite the possible objections of the providers of the samples. This is a particular concern when commercial or crime prevention interests are isolated from those of the donor.[13]

2.7 Moreover, in an era in which stem cell progress is reported almost daily, one might imagine that we are on the precipice of a vast regenerative industry, creating ever more property relationships (Tubo 2007). For example, it is clear that property claims are likely to be extended to *ex vivo* organs, because one might expect that some time in the future these body parts will become an insurance policy, pre-ordered and grown in vast repositories of human biological artefacts, each in its own bioreactor (Chang et al. 2009). How such organs are grown will likely influence the ethical debate—for instance, whether they are formed in 'brainless' vesicles modelled on the experiments that created headless frogs. Importantly, this raises questions about what we understand by 'person', and whether these kinds of human complexes can be owned.[14] However, when the 'body' is taken out of the property debate, it is likely that such a venture will be considered in the terms established for cells and tissues. It is therefore probable that notions of ownership of *ex vivo* organs will evolve in dissimilar ways from the 'no property' rule currently employed in respect to those derived from the human body.

One might surmise, therefore, that in an imagined regulatory future not all ownership interests will be surrendered, willingly or not; and neither will interests be so easily

---

[11] 'Consent will be based on an explanation and understanding of, amongst other things: the fact that UK Biobank will be the legal owner of the database and the sample collection, and that participants will have no property rights in the samples [section I.B.1] ...Such ownership conveys certain rights, such as the right to take legal action against unauthorised use or abuse of the database or samples, and the right to sell or destroy the samples. Participants will not have property rights in the samples' (UK Biobank Ethics and Governance Framework.Version 3.0 (October 2007) sec. II.A).

[12] Cf. *Washington University* v. *Catalona*, 490 F.3d 667 (2007), 676–7. (Rights of ownership of the contents of a tissue repository are with the institution in which the research was carried out, and not with the researcher who alleges that the samples were donated to him personally.) In *Catalona*, the Supreme Court's opinion was that patients did not have continuing property rights in the research samples they had donated: 'Thus, the district court properly concluded the research participants made informed and voluntary decisions to participate in genetic cancer research, and thereby donated their biological materials to Washington University as valid *inter vivos* ('between the living') gifts. This voluntary transfer of tissue and blood samples to [Washington University]—without any consideration or compensation as an incentive for doing so—demonstrates WU owns the biological samples currently housed in the Biorepository.'

[13] Cf. Those 'who should feel like a citizen ...—responsible and in control—feel instead like a suspect or recidivist' (Anderson et al. 2009: 9).

[14] Such bioreactors would have to avoid the possibility of being 'persons', otherwise engaging quite proper opposition to human ownership and slavery. The way around this is allegedly already in sight: scientists have created headless frogs by using gene-modification techniques to damage the gene that codes for the development of a head, and then inserted this modified DNA into the nucleus of a frog egg (Morton 1997).

dispelled by perfunctory and disjointed reasoning. It is likely that patients, who normally suppose excised tissues and cells to be disposed of by the hospital as a matter of course, and if kept, only used for future diagnostic purposes (or possibly medical teaching and training) will increasingly want an explanation for the asymmetrical rights awarded by *Moore*. And rather than passive approbation, one might expect to find dismay that they are included in profitable research, or banked indefinitely, or that the cells form the basis of a multimillion-dollar product. Modern biotechnology now imbues cells with value, and this raises these entities from triviality to significance.

3 *Moore*, then *Yearworth*: whither property?

3.1 The US case of *Moore* is a defining moment in the legal understanding of property. John Moore's complaint was that although he consented to the removal of his spleen and subjection to other post-operative procedures, he was under the impression that they were entirely for medically indicated reasons. He did not agree to his doctor and others using the cells from his spleen to create a profitable cell line. Of course, the conspiracy necessary to mislead Moore failed the test of *informed* that is normally necessary to make consent valid; and it was on this ground that the Supreme Court of California[15] found a breach of fiduciary duty against his doctor, David Golde. Moore, the patient, had the right to exercise control over his own body and therefore to determine whether or not to submit to medical treatment.[16]

But while it is easy to argue that taking a biopsy without consent would be an insult to the body (and inexcusable as such), the *Moore* case also concerned the concealment of commercial motives behind consented medical treatment.

3.2 The fiduciary duty does not exist between researchers and patients, so Moore's claim was also an alleged transgression of his property rights. The problem for Moore was that the Majority had *reason to doubt* that he had property rights in the cells taken from his body because there was no precedent that a person retains a sufficient interest in them.[17] In the circumstances, it was easy for the court to presuppose that once cells were removed from his body, Moore did not have the slightest concern in their fate; but more importantly, nor should one expect any of his interests to be preserved as a matter

[15] Four judges constituted the Majority opinion, written by Panelli, J. (Lucas, C. J., Eagleson, J., and Kennard, J. concurred); Arabian, J. wrote a separate concurring opinion; Broussard, J. concurred in part and dissented in part from the Majority; Mosk, J. dissented.

[16] David W. Golde, the attending doctor, failed in his fiduciary duty to disclose all information material to the patient's informed consent. It did not matter that the research was unrelated to the patient's health or that potential commercial value was unknown at the time. See *Moore*: 128–33, sections 2a and 2b. Golde denied misleading Moore about his intentions, because although he was interested in what might be found in his spleen as part of his ongoing research, he had no idea about the potential value of the T-lymphocytes, and therefore was unable to disclose any commercial interests (according to Golde, at the time he was more interested in the B-line cells as the cause of hairy-cell leukaemia) (Golde 1991). The court begged to differ, finding that 'the existence of a motivation for a medical procedure unrelated to the patient's health is a potential conflict of interest and a fact material to the patient's decision' (*Moore*: 133).

[17] 'No court, however, has ever in a reported decision imposed conversion liability for the use of human cells in medical *research*' (*Moore*: 135). The tort of conversion is an unauthorized act which deprives another of his property permanently or for an indefinite time.

of law.[18] Thus, the fact that the researchers acted without his consent was immaterial. The case is remarkable because in finding no grounds for conversion, it was concluded that there could be no actual interference with Moore's ownership or right of possession of cells removed from his body. This created a perplexing situation: someone (a scientist) could have property rights in cells, but yet these same cells could not be owned by the source. The court was able to make sense of this by manoeuvring the fiduciary duties of the doctor to one side and thereby offer a remedy to Moore,[19] and separately consider the *removed* parts within an ex post property right only after the application of skill.

3.3 The recent case of *Yearworth* reached a quite different solution to property in human body parts. Six men who were about to undergo chemotherapy were offered the possibility to store sperm within a National Health Service (NHS) hospital facility. However, prior to any attempt to use the sperm, the storage facility failed because of a procedural oversight, and the sperm thawed and subsequently perished irretrievably. The case was decided in an unexpected way: the men were to be compensated because the NHS Trust failed to look after the sperm that was transferred to it under the law of gratuitous bailment. Briefly,[20] the obligation of bailment arises because, the court stated, 'the taking of possession in the circumstances involves an assumption of responsibility for the safe keeping of the goods' (*Yearworth*: 48(c)); and 'If a gratuitous bailee holds himself out to the bailor as able to deploy some special skill in relation to the chattel, his duty is to take such care of it as is reasonably to be expected of a person with such skill' (*Yearworth*: 48(g)). There was no indication that the sperm would be used for any other purposes (nor could there be without further consent), and it would be returned to the men under the conditions of the Human Fertilisation and Embryology Act 1990 (amended in 2008) to assist their future fertility decisions. Therefore, although storage and use were subject to licence under the Act, it did not derogate from the men's rights to direct the fate of their stored sperm or to establish rights in relation to any other person. To make this stick, the court was required to find that the men had 'sufficient rights in relation to it as to render them capable of having been bailors of it' (*Yearworth*: 47). However, it would be a fiction to argue that the loss of sperm constituted a bodily or personal injury, therefore they successfully claimed for loss to property because they had legal ownership when the damage occurred, and the Trust was thereby liable to compensate them for any psychiatric injury foreseeably consequent on the breach of bailment.

3.4 Of course, the particularities of *Yearworth* led to the peculiar judgment: in wanting to find a way to compensate the men's distress, the court found it desirable to consider the sperm as property.[21] This was remarkable because, arguably, there were other avenues

[18] 'Moore clearly did not *expect* to retain possession of his cells following their removal, [and] to sue for their conversion he must have retained an ownership interest in them' (*Moore*: 136–7).

[19] The court intentionally set up the dichotomy between property in the body and property in removed tissue. Perhaps it was confident that the law of persons would protect Moore and other patients from surreptitious actions of this sort in the future. This remains a curious predicament: consent is central to the doctor–patient relationship such that its presumption or waiver can allow what would normally be considered as trespass or assault, but we are led to believe that researchers are not subject to the same conditions as long as they don't touch or otherwise interfere with the patient (see Fletcher 1996: 109).

[20] For further discussion, see Hawes 2010.

[21] This was not the first time that property interests in sperm were recognized. In the Californian case of *Hecht* v. *Superior Court* it was held that sperm is 'a unique type of 'property'; 20 Cal.Rptr.2d 275 (Cal.App. 2 Dist. 1993) (stored sperm bequeathed to girlfriend).

for legal redress (cf. Northern 1998; Priaulx 2010). But the judgment, although strictly adhering to the facts of the case, hinted at its intention:

In this jurisdiction developments in medical science now require a re-analysis of the common law's treatment and approach to the issue of ownership of parts or products of a living human body, whether for present purposes (viz. an action of negligence) or otherwise. (*Yearworth* para. 45(a))

On the one hand, one might envisage that other jurisdictions, themselves not immune to the novel applications of technology to the human body, are also vulnerable to such tensions. Yet one might also contend that the case lacks international interest, because judges are likely to be fastidious in the kind of precedent admissible to their jurisdiction. It is indeed important to note that the two cases emerged from different jurisdictions and contained very different factual circumstances. And in this regard, any resemblance between *Moore* and *Yearworth* dissolves on its own special facts: that consent was not given to take the cancer cells, but was fully informed to take the gametes; and the expected fate of the cells, which would be either to be discarded post operatively or to be given back to the men at a point yet to be determined. Indeed, commentaries on *Yearworth* have been critical about its legal importance because it allegedly encapsulates a very narrow conception of the property debate, offers limited ethical guidance, and therefore its import into a general dialogue is potentially restricted (Harmon 2010). Yet such a view is perhaps disingenuous to the leeway given to judges to interpret statutes and manoeuvre through case law, and which allows them to resolve hard cases, especially when the background jurisprudence to the material facts is itself questionable. Perhaps most importantly, in this respect *Yearworth* concerned reproductive cells, and this plausibly opens up the debate to the regenerative characteristic of *all* cells given their propensity to be induced into a reprogrammable state (a stem cell-like state), and then used to clone the source or to create *de novo* gametes (see Hübner et al. 2003; Wilmut and Paterson 2003; Nayernia et al. 2006). Moreover, to date *Yearworth* has not been tested further within the UK legal system, and has drawn even less attention outside this jurisdiction. Thus, the case might yet become the catalyst for moving away from *Moore*, a US case that has transcended borders, as a basis for such ethico-legal justifications. Lastly, although one must be careful to not take this judgment further than legal bounds would permit, there is a great deal more one can say about the ethical insight it provides.[22] In this respect, it is an important case that challenges the remarkably persistent grounds for current practice that is unmistakably utilitarian in offsetting patient rights for the sake of perceived commercial benefits. And in this respect, some have argued that the courts' handling of property in biological materials must depart from its tendency to see such matters in purely monetary terms otherwise they will continue to obscure the human concerns at stake (Gold 1996). *Yearworth* is therefore a continuation in the debate about property rights, and for this reason it cannot reasonably be considered (or remain) as an isolated anomaly.

To take the ethical debate forward, I now only focus on the two principal and coincidental circumstances of the cases: a) that cells were in a state separate from the person; and b) that in both cases a claim of property was employed to find a resolution.

---

[22] Nicolas Stallworthy (representing the respondent in the case, and paraphrased by Lord Judge, C. J.): 'warns us against any piecemeal and ill-considered attempt to develop [common law] in order to cater for modern conditions' (*Yearworth*: para. 29).

4 The ethical grounding of property in *Moore*: avoiding the 'big' decisions

One can surmise that the Majority disposition in *Moore* considered the following as telling ethical deductions.

4.1 *To avoid conflating property in cells with the status of organs*

The court appeared unwilling to endorse wholesale commodification of the human body; perhaps such an idea incurred an association to exploitation and the understandable objections to how far this can go once it is no longer immoral to sell human body parts for profit.[23] Therefore, the Majority expressly set out to make sure that it did not damage established policy goals that to date had dealt with human biological materials as objects *sui generis* (*Moore*: 137). Where the law says anything substantive about human parts it has normally done so through statutes, and finding the law of conversion applicable in this case would have risked abandoning any human material not covered elsewhere to the general law of personal property. An alternative outcome could have been to merge laws which concern human organs with those of human cells and tissues, thus risking the conflation of politically welcome goals (commerce in cells) with ethically contentious norms.

Separation was achieved in two steps.

Firstly, the court endorsed a presumption of *abandonment*, which is well-known in UK and US law.[24] This presumption is prospective, and grants, for example, hospitals the powers to dispose of any tissue remaining after a consented medical procedure for public health and safety reasons. But this also opens up the possibility of someone, other than the source, acquiring the cells without informing the patient. The conditions under which this would occur would normally limit claims to those trained and authorized to handle such material.

Secondly, the court used the precedent of *process or other application of skill* to limit the scope of property to those who they believed warranted ownership rights: in this case, the scientists who had used 'human ingenuity' and 'inventive effort'.[25] This also got around the existing 'no property' rule by metaphorically severing any association between the body and organs, on the one hand, and cells and tissues on the other. In this respect, skill had transformed the diseased spleen into patentable blood cell line, and this line was 'factually and legally distinct' from any cells to be found in Moore (*Moore*: 141). Moreover, Moore's claim did not sit easily with the fact that the Mo cell line had already been granted patent status. This appeared to be an 'authoritative determination' that it was the product of human ingenuity and not a naturally occurring entity (*Moore*: 142).

---

[23] As alluded to in the concurring opinion of Arabian, J. (*Moore*: 149), and criticized by the dissenting view of Broussard, J. (*Moore*: 160).

[24] See also: 'By the force of social custom, we hold that when a person does nothing and says nothing to indicate an intent to assert his right of ownership, possession, or control over such material, the only rational inference is that he intends to abandon the material.' USA: *Venner v. State of Maryland* 354 A. 2d 483, (Md. Ct. of Spec. Apps.), (1976), 498–9. Also see UK's Human Tissues Act 2004, s. 44.

[25] This condition is also found in the UK's Human Tissue Act 2004, 32(9)(c).

4.2 To avoid overstepping the courts' remit into matters rightly reserved for policy

The Majority expressly set out to make sure that it did not damage established policy goals, particularly those which prohibited the trade in organs (*Moore*: 137). Despite the troubling conceptual incoherence in the judgment (expressed in trenchant terms in the dissenting opinions) it was a stopgap pending proper direction from the legislature.[26] Thus it successfully restricted the worst kinds of economic-driven commerce in human bodies, but did so without stifling ongoing research.

4.3 To preserve the public good of research

The Majority was convinced that to allow property in the intermediate stages, that is when the cells are said to be abandoned, would 'destroy the economic incentive to conduct important medical research' (*Moore*: 146). Others at the time concurred, defending the judgment because it would otherwise result in the 'chaotic disruption of the industry built on research in cell lines' (Curran 1991). The researcher would have to seek a waiver every time they used another person's cells, and this might encourage an environment of bargaining between the vendor and the researcher, and a welter of impeding contractual arrangements.[27]

Finding in favour of the defendants was possible by employing a distinctly utilitarian argument that resulted in protecting the commercial interests of an up-and-coming biotech industry. Such an approach is appealing to a culture biased to biotech commerce because it can adapt to the needs of the industry despite the opposition of individuals affected. In *Moore* it was implied that 'too many proprietary stakeholders interfere with the progression of the research and delay the delivery of its benefits' (Brownsword 2009: 99), allowing the judges to shut the door on the source having any property rights at all.[28]

4.4 Dissatisfaction in the judgment

The dissatisfaction in the judgment was clearly stated in the dissenting opinion of Broussard, J. He pointed out the absurdity of the Majority's opinion:

> Far from elevating these biological materials above the marketplace, the majority's holding simply bars *plaintiff*, the source of the cells, from obtaining the benefit of the cells' value, but permits *defendants*, who allegedly obtained the cells from plaintiff by improper means, to retain and exploit the full economic value of their ill-gotten gains free of their ordinary common law liability for conversion. (Broussard, *Moore*: 160; italics in the original)

---

[26] Cf. In *Yearworth*, the representative of the respondent (Stallworthy) 'invites us to rely on Parliament either to update the concept of ownership in this connection or to make further provision which, without updating it, would remedy any perceived injustices in other ways' (para. 29).

[27] Cf. 'with every cell sample a researcher purchases a ticket in a litigation lottery' (*Moore*: 146).

[28] In support of this approach, one of the responses to the Retained Organs Commission Consultation Document stated: 'If procedures designed to satisfy the emotional requirements of handling post mortem tissue were to be applied to all human tissue the result would be disastrous for teaching and research. This would work against the common good and hence damage the very individuals the regulations are attempting to protect' (Academy of Medical Sciences 2002).

Mosk, J., also expressing his despondency, stated:

> The most abhorrent form of such exploitation, of course, was the institution of slavery...Yet their specter haunts the laboratories and boardrooms of today's biotechnological research–industrial complex. It arises wherever scientists...claim...the right to appropriate and exploit a patient's tissue for their sole economic benefit—the right, in other words, to freely mine or harvest valuable physical properties of the patient's body. (Mosk, *Moore*: 173–4)

This idea that the law can protect commercial interests for the 'common good' has also been criticized as 'embarrassingly' pro-business (Annas 1990), and has contributed to the disempowerment of other would-be (and unwitting) cell sources (cf. Jasanoff 2005). The judgment is clearly not intended to appease any rights-orientated thinkers: although the idea of consent was fundamental to the illegitimate actions of Golde, the judgment left the scientists untouched. We might therefore expect that the law will continue (and to date, has done so unabated) to protect specific interests by rolling out familiar arguments found in *Moore*: ones which we are led to believe are justified by the 'good of science'. Yet the bifurcation of industry interests from the sources of cells establishes a model of supply and demand, perhaps adapted to a paradigm borrowed from neoclassical economics. In such a framework, one need not be too concerned with the rights of individuals, as any harm caused (which itself is in doubt because such cells and products hold little interest for the originator and therefore can be procured without much intrusion) is appreciably less than the potential harm to the biotech industry (or the benefits are significantly less than those that a vibrant research industry can generate).

Yet this condones an ethos in which it is considered quite normal for the source to be unaware of the interest in his or her cells, and because of the proximity to a consented medical procedure this can quite easily be kept secret: why disclose an 'extra' biopsy, sharing samples after diagnostic interest has waned, or scavenging tissue from the floors of operating theatre? It is perhaps trite to argue that too much is expected of utilitarian reasoning: in this respect, the Majority's judgment is 'fraught with irony' (*Moore*: 166). But despite the Majority's own moral recoil from encouraging commercial organ trading (something that other utilitarians have not shied away from), they appear comfortable in resolving the 'property question' under the same ethical banner. This is perhaps because within such a framework, rights are only as good as they contribute to what counts, and therefore, with no particular commitment to consent (or any other side constraint), one's authorization is only required depending on the exiguities of the particular situation. If a rule requiring consent contributes to utility then it is likely to be upheld, but adequacy of this rule can change as circumstances and consequences dictate.

5 The ethical grounding of property in *Yearworth*: finding a remedy in rights

5.1 Despite the habit of legal scholars to point out the limits of presenting unlike cases alike, *Moore* has become a defining feature in cell transactions, and, moreover, has permeated widely through many jurisdictions and disparate cases. Significantly, the Human Tissue Act 2004 cleared the way for cell and tissue commercialization in the UK, and on the face of it this appeared to impose formally (although it was already the case through precedent) certain features of the Majority's disposition in *Moore*.[29] However, the recent legal provocation of *Yearworth* must be seen as a first step in challenging this legal orthodoxy. Notwithstanding that consent alone may have properly served to protect the interests of the men in *Yearworth*, the court took an uncertain path of finding a solution in property rights: this suggests an acknowledgement that people do have certain expectations about what is going to happen to cells removed from their body because of their ordinary ownership of them. Although the case says nothing explicitly about the expectations of appropriated research material, it hints at the conditions under which others can be in possession thereof: there can be no ethical justification for taking cells without consent, and it is presumably therefore unlawful to take or use them contrary to this norm (and subject to the conditions of statutory law).

In *Yearworth*, these expectations are easily distinguishable from supposed disinterest in abandoned tissue. But do other patients have any similar expectations? It is my contention that if *Moore* is stripped of the shamelessly pro-industry ideology, a different picture emerges: the possibility that if a patient reasonably expected to maintain control over his cells upon removal, a property interest would have to be recognized as a matter of right.[30]

5.2 Patients' expectations and property rights. *Moore*'s bifurcation of consent and property has persisted at the cost of fundamental equality in the scientific endeavour, the prevention of unjust enrichment, and a failure to protect patients' rights (cf. Nelkin and Andrews 1995; Boulier 2005). *Yearworth*, however, shows that when a patient specifies the parameters of storage and use of cells prior to removal from their body, he or she should not be precluded from claiming a property interest in them, thus potentially redressing such disparity. *But it should not matter* that John Moore was not able to specify the conditions of removal, because in terms of property, the fact that he did not know the cells were taken does not preclude his ownership of them. *Nor does it matter* that the men in *Yearworth* were given such an opportunity because it was only them (and not a scientist, or anyone else) that had an interest in the fate of the cells. I will argue that an interest in property may be broadly construed (as has been the case in interpreting, for example, the significance of privacy in the European Convention on Human Rights 1950), so as to encompass rights to autonomy and dignity. Thus, not only is *Moore* a compelling case of misappropriation and deceit, it is also a befuddling legal artifice.[31]

---

[29] The Act prohibits commercial dealings in the human body and body parts as 'controlled material' (sec 53 (1)). However, 'relevant material' may be the subject of property because of an application of human skill. This excludes gametes, embryos outside the human body (both covered by the HFE Act 2008), and hair and nail from the body of a living person (which are unconditionally fungible). Importantly, the Act makes consent a central requirement prior to its alteration. Under section 44, 'Surplus tissue': '(1) It shall be lawful for material to which subsection (2) or (3) applies to be dealt with as waste. (2) This subsection applies to any material which consists of or includes human cells and which has come from a person's body in the course of his—(a) receiving medical treatment, (b) undergoing diagnostic testing, or (c) participating in research. (3) This subsection applies to any relevant material which—(a) has come from a human body, and (b) ceases to be used, or stored for use, for a purpose specified in Schedule 1.' Part 1 of Schedule 1 states the: 'Purposes requiring consent: general', and lists '6. Research in connection with disorders, or the functioning, of the human body.'

[30] Cf. Dissenting opinion of Mosk in *Moore*.

[31] And responsible for a legal framework described as 'ambiguous' at the time by the National Bioethics Advisory Committee in the US (National Bioethics Advisory Commission 1999).

5.3 *Yearworth* suggests a different property paradigm from *Moore*: one in which a patient does not give up *all* claims on his or her cells. In *Moore*, it was presumed that the source could have no objection to someone else appropriating or using his cells so that his consent applies. But in fact, for various reasons to be explained below, patients often do expect to control parts of their bodies after removal as a matter of right. However, this right cannot be effectively or logically subsumed under a right of bodily integrity (what *Yearworth* referred to as a 'fiction') (*Yearworth*, para. 23), and without this solution available, patients must look elsewhere to protect their interests from misappropriation. Therefore, property can be put to work to protect rights as a function of the patient's relationship to a thing, and this relationship, I argue, is one of rights protection.

5.4 In this respect, The Convention on Human Rights and Biomedicine (CHRB) 1997 is unambiguous in conveying that consent is central to transactions involving human body parts. In fact, a surprising ethical commonalty can be found between it and *Yearworth*.

5.5 To begin with, the CHRB establishes the conditions for financial gain:

Article 21: The human body and its parts shall not, as such, give rise to financial gain.

The Explanatory Report includes two conditions under which financial gain may occur: one, the test of the application of skill is used to justify 'reasonable remuneration' (para. 123); and two, the Convention excludes 'such products as hair and nails, which are discarded tissues, and the sale of which is not an affront to human dignity' (para. 133).[32] The idea of reasonable remuneration is described in paragraph 132 of the Explanatory Report, where it says that the 'human body and its parts' are precluded from financial gain 'as such'.[33] This serves to allow: a) 'technical acts (sampling, testing, pasteurisation, fractionation, purification, storage, culture, transport, etc.) which are performed on the basis of these items may legitimately give rise to reasonable remuneration'; and b) 'does not prevent a person from whom an organ or tissue has been taken from receiving compensation which, while not constituting remuneration, compensates that person equitably for expenses incurred or loss of income'.

5.6 Skill. Explanations of this legal precedent have often turned to John Locke (1632–1704). The idea of Lockean property stems from his oft cited assertion: 'by his labour [an agent] does, as it were, enclose it from the common' (Locke 1988: Second Treatise, Chapter V, s. 32). Locke's argument theorizes a 'state of nature' (Locke 1988: Second Treatise, Chapter V, s. 27) to convey the idea that bounty ('The Earth, and all that is therein' (Locke 1988: Second Treatise, Chapter V, s. 26)) is suspended and initially

---

[32] The exclusion of dead cellular material may have been justified during the drafting of the Convention because techniques at that time were limited to recovering mitochondrial DNA from such material. The kind of information that is obtainable from all human genetic sources has improved with effective techniques of isolating endogenous DNA (see Cline et al. 2003; Graham 2007).

[33] There are three possible meanings to 'as such': relating to something's inherent nature; being exactly or similar—i.e. the same nature—to what is mentioned or suggested; or considered alone or by itself: its natural state. In this case, all three are plausible as an explanation of a cell's unmodified state subsequent to removal from the body. Although 'as such' is used incorrectly in a transitional phrase, it appears to be used here to describe something with respect to its innate nature (type, sort, or description of quality), with the result that if one changes the subject matter, the same rule does not apply.

without a claim upon it ('no body has originally a private Dominion'); thus portraying the contemporary notion of something like *public goods*.[34] From this idea, a modern analogy to allow the 'Industrious and Rational' (Locke 1988: Second Treatise, Chapter V, s. 34) exclusive rights to appropriate and cultivate biological material, to 'improve it for the benefit of Life'[35] is straightforward:

> The *Labour* of [a person's] Body and the *Work* of his Hands, we may say, are properly his. Whatsoever then he removes out of the State that Nature hath provided, and left it in he hath mixed his *Labour* with, and joyned to it something that is his own, and thereby makes it his *Property*. (Locke 1988: Second Treatise, Chapter V, s. 27)

It does not justify violating the integrity of the person (that is, attacking the person to gain property), since 'every Man has a Property in his own Person' (Locke 1988: Second Treatise, Chapter V, s. 27)—thereby justifying a set of rights which are fundamentally distinguishable from those that we have in common things—but it does mean that anyone can acquire property by mixing one's labour with objects: that is, defining property in terms of the application of skill. The purpose of Locke's theory of property was to show that 'labour makes the far greatest value of things' (Locke 1988: Second Treatise, Chapter V, s. 42); that 'Land [*qua* that which is left suspended and unclaimed] that is left wholly to Nature ... is wast[e]; and we shall find the benefits of it amount to little more than nothing' (Locke 1988: Second Treatise, Chapter V, s. 42).

In contemporary imaginations, this appeals to the supposed mutual benefits that accrue from allowing certain people dominion over that which is unclaimed, abandoned, or fallow, or that which is 'perishable' unless captured by industrious effort (Locke 1988: Second Treatise, Chapter V, s. 47), and the expected utility that flows back into society as a result of securing its value (e.g. jobs, investment, economic growth, and plausibly 'medical research of importance to all society' (*Moore*: 135)). It allegedly follows that if society privileges scientists access to human material, we can expect that their career achievements will benefit the community with better medicines and enhanced economies (but I would not for one minute expect that the financial rewards for good science are not also an incentive to pursue research).

5.7 This can be objected to on the grounds that the privilege this affords scientists unjustly excludes them from consent transactions involving patients.[36] By creating these advantaged positions (which cannot signify the same privilege as that of the doctor–patient relationship), it merely advocates the industry-sanctioned mongering of expected public goods. Yet these 'goods' are intimately bound up with the interests of patients, who are forced into serving a public market. These patients, therefore, become resource utilities against their will. This possibility suggests that the labour thesis (or at least the 'commons' version, discussed above) is inapplicable to the legitimate appropriation of cells, because for it to work, it must be that human material is chanced upon chattels, cast adrift from the body to which it has no further link, and can be brought in from the

---

[34] 'that which God gave Mankind in common' (Locke 1988: Second Treatise, Chapter V, s. 25).

[35] 'Benefit' here is meant in terms of libertarian self-interest (Locke 1988: Second Treatise, Chapter V, s. 32).

[36] Indeed, Locke argued against the dishonesty of taking too much from the common, and 'For in Governments the Laws regulate the right of property' (Locke 1988: Second Treaties, Chapter V, s. 50). Yet this also could have implied, or overtly justified, capitalist accumulation (see Macpherson 1962: 209–10).

commons by industrious scientists working for or sponsored by industry. However, one can expect that such ring-fencing can erode principles of equity[37] —the 'tragedy of the commons'[38] —and moreover, it justifies the exploitation of the source ex ante because the labour thesis typically ignores the interests of the 'unskilled' source.[39] This sanctioned pro-research agenda, however, is now an antithesis to rights: consistency requires subjugating every policy to supporting this kind of privileged public-market interest, but with perhaps rather more unwelcome consequences for some.[40] One might also contend that ordinary and unusual human artefacts—those which are the cause or result of the patient's illness—are the focus of scientific interest because they are the products of circumstance, and genetic and environmental causes, not innovation, thus diluting any claims of investigative credit to be the 'inventor'.[41]

5.8 Remuneration. Remuneration is familiar to the organ donation debates, and I need not rehearse them in any detail here. For example, Neil Duxbury raises some familiar concerns of creating a market in human organs, such as the potential for abuse, exploitation, displacing need in favour of ability to pay, and discouraging gift donations (Duxbury 1996). On the other hand, Peter Sýkoria finds little wrong with payment, but admits the consequential dangers of an unregulated organ market (Sýkoria 2009). Whether these harms materialize will require some guesswork and careful scrutiny of existing systems. If, however, there can be property in cells and tissues, then it would be necessary to consider the kind of monetary arrangements that are possible and ethically justifiable.

5.9 The CHRB states that remuneration is only possible in instances of skill, ruling out in most cases the monetary transfer of unaltered biological material. Thus, the only recourse for the source is to 'gift' or unconditionally surrender the cells to those trained and authorized to handle them. If we put aside for one moment the asymmetrical rights issues, is it possible to say whether John Moore *was* owed anything for the use of his cells, and if yes, how is this to be calibrated in contemporary society? Firstly, commercial

---

[37] Cf. 'The business of business is to make money ...and the mode is secrecy, a proprietary control of information and the fruits of research. The motive force of the university is the pursuit of knowledge and the mode is open exchange of ideas and unrestricted publication of the results of research' (*Moore*: 215 Cal. App. 3d 709, 40).

[38] The idea here is that acquisition of common property becomes exploitive because the conditions of acquisition also mean that the costs are borne by the individual tissue sources and not the scientists. To use another example, it is personally efficient for an industrialist to pollute a river because the benefits accrue to him or her personally while everyone shares the costs; cf. 'The individual benefits as an individual from his ability to deny the truth even though society as a whole, of which he is a part, suffers' (Hardin 1968).

[39] Cf. 'Far from elevating these biological materials above the marketplace, the majority's holding simply bars ...the source of the cells, from obtaining the benefit of the cells' value, but permits defendants who allegedly obtained the cells from the plaintiff by improper means, to retain and exploit the full economic value of their ill-gotten gains free of their ordinary common law liability for conversion' (*Moore*: 160).

[40] In their commentary to an article promoting the socially responsible use of neurotechnologies, Capps and Carter argue that if utilitarian thinking is tied into aggregate notions of ethics, then it risks superseding all rights to vague calculations of the greater good (Capps and Carter 2010).

[41] This is in contrast to the argument offered by George, J. in the Appeal Court: 'it [the spleen] evolved into something of great value only through the unusual scientific expertise of the defendants, like unformed clay or stone transformed by the hands of a master sculptor into a valuable work of art' (*Moore*: 215 Cal. App. 3d 709).

interests are likely to argue that privileged access to markets in human material are possible because the majority of cells and tissues are going to be unexceptional, and therefore limits any economic value in raw material.[42] The source, therefore, deserves nothing. But, even if the cells have little value, can there be reason to compensate the donor?

Many have commented on the conceptual difficulties of conceptualizing 'costs' with commensurability when it comes to human bodies (Radin 1996: Chapter 13). Compensation, for instance, can be for both harmless loss and damages. Remuneration, on the other hand, indicates the affirmative character of payment. The CHRB rules out financial gain for the donor; but does allow compensation for certain losses. On the facts, Moore was not himself in a position to recognize the value in his cells or to use his skill to exploit them for commercial gain, and in granting conditional access to the cells, he was also unlikely to lose out significantly (but of course, could gain considerably). It does seem likely that he was subjected to and endured further prodding and poking, and this might amount to something worth compensating in terms of time, discomfort, and inconvenience.[43] Notwithstanding that compensation need not be monetary in value, some writers have sought alternatives to financial exchanges. Perhaps they are motivated by redefining market rhetoric to benefit those providing material, or because of deeply entrenched intuitions concerning the incommensurability of human parts.[44] Would recognizing Moore's role lead to the kinds of commodification that the Convention warns against (and at which the Majority baulked)?

5.10 Firstly, if compensation in some form is just (for instance, because the idea of altruism appears so conceptually flawed it cannot be relied upon to provide the raw material for valuable research), then one might find the idea of 'benefit sharing' appealing as a proposal for remodelling science in society. This is what Radin calls 'corrective justice' to indicate required changes in an unjustified state of affairs (Radin 1996: 187). The idea has become prevalent in other asymmetrical relationships, such as those which result from bio-prospecting and gene piracy. The United Nations recognized that communities, targeted by biotech companies for their biodiversity and genetic resources, were due compensation and recompense in the form of funds for economic development and technology transfer.[45] The threat of genetic exploitation is also a concern for families with genetic peculiarities, and legal cases have shown the

[42] However, one might also think that speculation has some merit, since the Majority in *Moore* also argued that the plaintiff's case was based on a 'highly theoretical windfall'; yet it turned out to be much more than that (*Moore*: 147).

[43] One might also want to include reimbursement for direct costs (expenses incurred), such as travel to attend the examinations.

[44] Some biobanks, for example, have offered health screens as a way to encourage participation. UK Biobank, on the other hand, perseveres with an idea of public good to secure the legacy of better health for future generations, by engaging with participants so that their involvement is seen as a benefit for them and for society as a whole. What distinguishes a 'public goods' approach from those which are more market driven is an insistence that resources are equally accessible to public and commercial researchers, and that commercial interests are balanced by direct benefits to the community (for example, requiring cell lines to be publicly available, or perhaps even by limiting the scope of patents using these cell lines); see Capps et al. 2008.

[45] See: *UN Convention on Biological Diversity* 1992. The subsequent *Bonn Guidelines* (2002) stated that benefit sharing should include both monetary (fees, joint ownership of patents) and non-monetary (sharing of research results); Secretariat of the Convention on Biological Diversity, *Bonn Guidelines on Access to Genetic Resources and Fair and Equitable Sharing of the Benefits Arising out of their Utilization* (Montreal: Canada 2002).

kind of questionable processes that are possible in this respect.[46] Therefore, we might find that all such benefits should be excluded from the sources of research material. The next step is to offer compensation to encourage participation in research wholeheartedly.[47] By this I mean that patients—at least those who have interesting or unique conditions—may willingly give up everything (or nearly everything) for the benefit of science: cells, tissues, medical records, personal history, time, and effort, and therefore ought to be compensated accordingly. Lastly, there is the concern that encouragement—especially reimbursement—secures materials and participation by implicating the kinds of coercion that follow from misconceptions about reward and personal benefits.

5.11 Secondly, one must be clear why commodification is sometimes resisted. The Nuffield Council on Bioethics (NCB) warned of the dangers of commerce in human tissue which 'are strongest where difficult medical decisions are being made at vulnerable times in patients', and lists securing 'genuine consent', the distortion of supply (for more valuable, and perhaps rare, tissue), and the discouragement of 'criminal or morally reprehensible methods of procuring human tissue, and would certainly have to be hedged with many restrictions to prevent unacceptable use being made of the tissue collected' (Nuffield Council on Bioethics 1995). But this did not stop the NCB from regarding cells and tissue as abandoned, and therefore intentionally conflating consent to treatment to 'refer to the possibility that removed tissue may be discarded or stored; and, if stored, that it may at some time be used for diagnosis, further treatment, research, teaching or study' (Nuffield Council on Bioethics 1995: 126, para. 13.13). The NCB suggested that this second condition may only need to be *implied*, thus relinquishing the researcher from asking at all.[48] But this will not do if consent is taken seriously. If consent to treatment is conflated with tacit research considerations, it means that the only way that a person can object to further uses of tissue is to refuse treatment. This introduces a considerable element of coercion. And if, as is suggested by the NCB, consent is indeed implicit to the agreement to undergo treatment, this still creates the kind of lopsided market favouritism which exploits and deceives patients. Moreover, an incoherent perception of instrumentalization, separating non-commodifiable organs from commodifiable cells and tissue, risks becoming so persuasive that all body parts (as long as they remain separable from the kinds of harms noted for organ donation) can be sold with little or no moral indignation. What, then, is to stop a market in *ex vivo*-grown

---

[46] Cf. *Greenberg* v. *Miami Children's Hospital Research Institute*, 264 F. Supp. 2d 1064, 2003, section E (hereafter *Greenberg*) (patenting of a test for the Canavan disease). A researcher enjoyed considerable cooperation from the families affected by Canavan disease who voluntarily donated tissues and funds to the research. Subsequently, the researcher filed a patent to license a test for the disease. The plaintiffs reportedly felt betrayed by the fraudulent concealment of the researchers' real intentions. The court relied heavily on the reasoning in *Moore* to find for the defendants (including dismissing ownership of the cells by the source) in all but the motion of unjust enrichment (the defendants obtained a benefit from the provision of cells and should therefore pay for the time and resources provided).

[47] Indeed, *Greenberg* introduced this remedy in terms of 'unjust enrichment' because the numerous actions in support of the research might deserve compensation. However, because the parties reached a settlement outside court, the merits of this approach as a legal solution remain untested.

[48] For example, if he had access to the operating theatre subsequent to an operation (Nuffield Council on Bioethics 1995: 126, para. 13.12).

organs? Dickenson considers this as a telling problem: 'the untrammelled commodification of practically everything' (Dickenson 2007), and she argues that control ought to be passed back to the donor to ward off unauthorized taking and reaffirm rights of control. However, reasserting control may implicate the right to sell, and it will be necessary, if commodification is at least partly unobjectionable, to build in exceptions so that, at a minimum, trade would be specific to the kinds of objects involved in any two-way transaction. Although this might lead to a mechanism of equitable transfer between people, the implications of *real control* in terms of coercion and exploitation would need consideration in light of a growing, and likely to remain inequitable, business model of cell and tissue commerce.

5.12 Article 22: 'Disposal of a removed part of the human body'. The idea that, upon removal, cells are considered as *res* (a thing) that is abandoned to research interests is likely to be opposed by rights talk.[49] Thus, Article 22 of the CHRB continues:

When in the course of an intervention any part of a human body is removed, it may be stored and used for a purpose other than that for which it was removed, only if this is done in conformity with appropriate information and consent procedures.

The approach may be described as employing a *consent strategy*, because it reflects the relationships that develop as a result of property transactions.[50] Importantly, the stipulation for consent is open: there are no conditions attached or requirement for specific interests, thus suggesting a 'rule-preclusionary' basis for empowering whoever is legitimately *in control* of the property.[51] Since it is impossible for persons to be the property of another, the only owner in the case of human body parts is the person to whom they are attached. In section 6, below, I will go further, and argue that if ex ante the conditions of property still prevail (that human parts *can* be owned at all), this control must remain with the source until such rights are waived. Therefore, while it appears entirely appropriate for skill to bestow upon an object property rights (as stated in Article 21) as long as significantly different attributes are endowed to the body part (see Sulston December 2002), it cannot bypass the act of appropriation. This is because the application of skill can also reflect *art* (Day 1966). It is not just a claim of toil (or even chancing upon the cells), but recognition of the feats of skill and diligence. This allows personal proficiency and dedication to flourish and for one to receive reward for creativity. But it does not justify taking raw materials for one's own surreptitious gain. More importantly, while the 'skill' proviso does its work after the event, Article 22 suggests that property also applies prior to any kind of alteration (again, skill now reflects a more meaningful interaction with an object; and in fact may signify the terms of bailment that allowed the men in *Yearworth* to remain in possession of minimally altered artefacts). Consent also operates with respect to the *purpose* of removal, and therefore is not absent in relationships

---

[49] Indeed, one might consider the conditions under which the tissues are removed become manifestly important to the rights of those affected (see Kennedy 2000: Annex B para. 66).

[50] From the Explanatory Report: '136. This provision thus establishes a rule consistent with the general principle in Article 5 on consent.'

[51] '"Because it is mine!" functionally means "It is so related to me that I do not have to say why I should be able to use it or why I may exclude others from using it!"' (Beyleveld and Brownsword 2001: 178)

which are established by happenstance or chancing upon presumptively abandoned cells. The Explanatory Report makes the reasons for this clear: 'Parts of the human body are often removed in the course of interventions, for example surgery. The aim of this article is to ensure the protection of individuals with regard to parts of their body which are thus removed and then stored or used for a purpose different from that for which they have been removed.' Why, then, is there a concern that implied abandonment is unethical in terms of rights?

6 Rights and property

6.1 Firstly, research using cell biopsies, routinely retained as a result of medical indications or amassed from that which is discarded, is not primarily a *material* risk to the original tissue provider's health (Van Diest 2002). However, research does represent a different set of adverse downstream consequences, characterized as *personal* harms (Ashburn et al. 2000). At the moment, the vacuity in property rights is acutely felt by those exploited for research material (cf. *Greenberg*: note 46). The undisclosed fate of excised tissue entails a loss of control of the tangible *and* intangible objects which are connected to one's interests. It is telling that a significant minority of patients want their authority to make choices about body parts to be respected (Goodson and Vernon 2004[52]); moreover, the plaintiffs' complaints in *Catalona* (note 12) and *Greenberg* (note 46) arose out of a perceived powerlessness to stop researchers and institutions from doing what they wanted with their cells and tissues. Therefore, there appears to be a proclivity to want to control access and use to the material removed from one's body. This might transpire as a desire to control what happens to the material (to direct its use or to at least be asked what it is used for), to ensure that its use remains within the original conditions of consent (or to be recontacted if deviation is planned), or to protect secondary interests that arise out of unauthorized access. This has particular ramifications for patients with unusual illnesses or scientifically intriguing genomes; they might well be anxious about the unchecked freedom of science to pry, own, and profit from their uniqueness.[53] The seeming inability to stop access rights opening up entire pathology archives or other donated resources highlights the powerlessness that some feel (see *Catalona*: note 12). For these groups, it is not enough for them to be obliged to remain 'silent partners': for some, recognizing their 'contribution to the venture is absolutely crucial' (*Moore*: 175).

Yet the significance of DNA has already mushroomed as a result of next-generation genomic technologies, providing faster, cheaper, and better resolved analysis, widening the risk of such exploitation to everyone. Concurrently, the courts have shown willingness to vest property interests with ever more benefactors outside a fiduciary duty.[54] With

---

[52] This paper failed to specify the kind of 'tissue or organs' that those asked would object to. It is likely that specifying the kinds of cells, tissue, or organs (hair, as distinct from a heart) will elicit different responses (see Clayton 2005). I stress that although some people want to be asked to donate, there is a higher level of disinterest in what happens to the samples once they are donated (Hoeyer et al. 2005).

[53] Cf. Dissenting opinion of Mosk, J.: the 'rush to patent for exclusive use has been rampant' (*Moore*: 171).

[54] A process of property incrementalization in which 'body parts are capable of being property for the purposes of s.4 [of the UK Theft Act 1968], even without the acquisition of different attributes, if they have a use or significance beyond their mere existence.' *Regina v. Kelly* [1998] 3 All E.R. 741, at 749.

the escalating use of reliable and more precise technologies within a growing surveillance culture, it is ever more difficult to maintain firewalls opposing 'bio-informational creep' and the expansion of the ways in which industrious agents can use data extracted from cells (see Lyon 2001: 111–13).[55] The Explanatory Report confirms: 'Such a provision [Article 22] is necessary in particular, because much information on the individual may be derived from any part of the body, however small (for example blood, hair, bone, skin, organ). Even when the sample is anonymous the analysis may yield information about identity' (para. 135).[56] One might expect, therefore, that if asymmetric property rights are maintained, the micro-event of transfer will remain outside the conditions of consent. The result is likely to be an unwillingness to legislate for the possibilities of using data on the grounds that we can ignore how it was come by.

6.2 Secondly, by becoming stealthily engrained in scientific culture, it glosses over questions about the need for covertness or collusion that allows researchers access to parts of the body in the first place. Access to the body under terms which lack consent are met by the fiduciary duty, but there remains no recourse for the patient who objects to their tissues being used once they are already removed.[57] However, one might expect consent to do more than preclude direct access to the body: it may also function to safeguard a person's ability to control proximate decision-making as a component of their rights. When choices are made in circumstances of selective nondisclosure or compulsoriness, they are not normally held to be irrevocable because the agent lacks the freedom to make voluntary decisions (Gewirth 1978: 32). But, if misappropriation (taking and using the cells without the knowledge or consent of the patient) is characterized as *no choice*, one might equally argue that the indicative elements of autonomy that are lost in circumstances of nondisclosure or compulsoriness might be the same as those of fraud or conspiracy: the researchers, in collusion with the physician, *intentionally* deprive the patients of their autonomy for their own gain. Not asking, therefore, is ethically unacceptable, because *access to the cells* is proximate to the *taking of them*, and if the cells are taken without consent, one might expect that *using* them without authorization falls into the same genus.

6.3 But what does *Yearworth* say about rights? In the case, the Lord Judge, C. J. argued that ownership signifies 'no more than a convenient global description of different collections of rights held by persons over physical and other things' (*Yearworth*: para. 28). He then alludes to what a description of ownership might include (relying in part on the ideas of Honoré) (Honoré 1986: 161–92). The judgment, however, has been argued to give short shrift to the extant academic literature, and fails to articulate clearly the scope of the rights involved; indeed, with so little articulation in the disposition, Harmon considers that it carries little moral weight or direction for future cases (Harmon 2010). Indeed, Harmon appears to suppose that the mere mention of the spectre of instrumentalization (quoting the work of Alastair V. Campbell) is enough to extinguish the ethical content of the judgment, and instead we should look elsewhere for an 'alternative

---

[55] My use of 'bio-informational' creep is derived from an idea of 'functional creep', discussed by Lyon.

[56] In respect to the potential to identify individuals DNA masked within a mixture (see Homer et al. 2008).

[57] Cf. Broussard, J.: 'in other factual settings an unlawful interference with a patient's right to control the use of his body part may occur in the absence of a breach of fiduciary duty' (*Moore*: 158).

metaphor'. Yet, it is exactly because Lord Judge, C. J., in part, harkens back to *Moore*, noting in particular the 'Two dissenting judgments [that] were expressed in trenchant terms' (*Yearworth*: para. 39), and the inference that the Majority's disposition therein was not 'entirely logical' (*Yearworth*: para. 45(d)), that it requires us to unpack the idea of property 'on a broader basis' (*Yearworth*: para. 45(e)). But we have to do this work ourselves!

6.4 So, a certain amount of legwork is required to fill in the gaps left by Lord Judge, C. J. The discussion of rights in the judgment is indeed patchy. Yet for my purposes it is sufficient to remind the reader that the normative grounding of rights has become the bedrock in many jurisdictions, and therefore there is a great deal of scholarly work which can aid us (Beyleveld and Brownsword 2001: 79–86). Moreover, a number of works have addressed the conceptual gap of ownership of 'other things' by expanding it to ideas of the intangible; and, indeed, have argued that it makes sense to talk of the 'bundle of property rights' by appeals to the morally weighty concept of dignity.[58] If these appeals are persuasive, then it signals a profane indication of the gravity of property. Indeed, the overturned judgment of the California Court of Appeal in *Moore* rather sounded like an appeal to the CHRB, by anchoring their judgment in favour of John Moore on the bases that (a) the recognized rights and interests that persons have in their bodies is so akin to property that to call them anything else would be 'subterfuge'; and (b) not to grant persons the right to control what happens to their tissue would lead to violation of rights to privacy and human dignity. Likewise, Mosk, J., dissenting from the subsequent Supreme Court of California disposition, disparagingly opined:

the majority cite no case holding that an individual's right to develop and exploit the commercial potential of his own tissue is *not* a right of sufficient worth or dignity to be deemed a protectable property interest. (*Moore*: 166)

Thus, the rights to property—if construed widely to include privacy and dignity—become appealing if one wants to bring the plight of John Moore and others deprived of control to the fore, because it encompasses the psychological as well as physical aspects that might signal the ownership of intimately personal things.

6.5 This is also a somewhat different approach from that characterized by Honoré's eleven relational factors, because, unlike his attempts to identify the necessary and sufficient conditions for something *to be* property (a list of liquorice allsorts that one can apparently pick and choose from), rights create questions about what property is expected to do as a feature of relationships. Thus, *Moore* was decided by stating what property *is* (in this case, cells were property after being subjected to scientific skill), but in terms of an ethical relationship it failed to denounce the lopsided one created between the scientist and the patient; and moreover, it condoned the failure of the scientists to get consent for what they planned to do. In contrast, a rights framework would be unlikely to let the scientists off so lightly,

---

[58] Dignity remains a notoriously troubling concept. Many would unashamedly recoil at my suggestion of deploying it here because it often serves to limit free choice; that it opposes utilitarian, as well as rights, thinking. They would be correct to point out that dignity has been used as a social or collective constraint—what has been pinned to the flag of 'Dignitarian Alliance'—and which elsewhere has been used to close down the freedom to take advantage of technology (see Ashcroft 2005). On the Dignitarian Alliance, see Brownsword 2003.

regardless of the claim that this will disincentivize potentially socially beneficial research. Moreover, in cases like *Moore*, far from being innocent to the misappropriation, scientists become conspicuous and complicit, and therefore accountable for the deception necessary to preserve the surreptitious relationship that they have with the patient. To ground rights, however, it is necessary to work out what we expect property to do in moral interactions. Thus, property rights are often considered as separate incidents within a 'bundle' and thereby conceptualized according to Hohfeld's correlatives (what he calls 'claim rights', 'privilege', 'power', and 'immunity') (Hohfeld 1964). The most important of these—claim rights—are not self-evident, yet a detailed synthesis of what might ground these rights is beyond this chapter. But one might expect that the non-consensual appropriation of cells would be excluded by the strongest of these correlatives: a claim right that entails correlative necessary duties to forebear with interfering with a person's freedom and well-being. Therefore, one might consider that a justified claim can be asserted in instances of coercion or nondisclosure. Working down a hierarchy of rights (Gewirth 1978: 63), one might find that a *power* to control access to removed cells is persuasive in discouraging inappropriate acts, or a *privilege* to transfer one's property empowers the donors in the ethical transfer of human material.

6.6 One might thereby find property doing the work of a 'right to autonomy' in terms of a right to choose: a 'gate-keeping mechanism to legitimate certain dealings associated with the human body'.[59] Accordingly, Beyleveld and Brownsword make a convincing argument that dignity in biolaw appeals to an idea of empowerment (Beyleveld and Brownsword 2001). They argue that dignity as empowerment is the basis of legal barriers to pursuing (or inflicting on others) certain goals that are contrary to dignity—it is a theory of rights. This rights inclination is also hinted in the judgment in *Yearworth* (without itself using the conceptually troublesome concept of 'dignity') by formulating property in terms of control. The case might also operate alongside a set of privacy rights.[60] In this sense, with ever more ways that technology can pry, we might feel even more strongly that privacy is about protecting one's quintessential capacities as a rights-holding agent.

This rights approach finds that rather than forcing the 'round pegs of 'privacy' and 'dignity' into the square hole of 'property' (*Moore*: 140), a framework of rights finds them as worthy allies (cf. Ackerman 1992[61]). A rights framework takes consent seriously; but that is not to say that we should become fixated on the consent proviso above all else. Under certain circumstances, the requirement for consent may be legitimately waived, such as in well designed, non-interventional epidemiological research (see Beyleveld and Pattinson 2008). Yet this same justification cannot ride roughshod over consent for purely commercial interests. Thus *Moore* appears wholly inadequate as an explanation

---

[59] This idea is discussed in Harmon and Laurie (2010: 492).

[60] There are two conceptions that are useful in this respect: spatial privacy and informational privacy. *Spatial privacy* is a state of non-access to the individual's physical or psychological self. This is prospectively violated by the non-consensual taking of biological samples and fingerprints, and, to a lesser extent, by unwanted surveillance of the individual. Informational privacy would protect the contents—the data gleaned from DNA analysis and turned into accessible profiles.

[61] 'The only real difference between the two concepts is the kind of relationship that is protected from interference—"property" principally protects market relationships while 'privacy' protects more spiritual ones. Yet surely this fact should not prevent recognition of "privacy" as a dimension of constitutional "property in its widest sense"' (Ackerman 1992: 347).

for property, because it fails to protect the rights of potential donors as easily undermined by utilitarian goals.[62]

7 Concluding remarks

7.1 I have argued that the archaic reasoning of *Moore* never did provide an ethical solution to the conditions of property in human cells and tissues. This is salient because it is now necessary to recognize the implications of routine cell and tissue appropriation *for the source*; and indeed, many biobank initiatives have begun to do so by providing the terms on which participation occurs, including whether or not there is a transfer of property. *Moore* was justified in terms of the expected utility of commercial interests, and as a justification to subsume individual interests into the 'good of science'. However, those taking note of the negative implications of the circumvention of consent requirements argue that we should be more suspicious of commercial interests, and, indeed, should think about implementing a 'more direct, traceable (re)distribution of the fruits of research' (Heyden 2007). In this paper, my intention has been to empower the unwitting source of cells and tissues. Under the rights framework, I have advocated that scientists, far from being innocent to the misappropriation, are complicit in the deception necessary to exploit the patient. It is because people want to extend control to what they have an interest in, rather than allow an undeclared privilege to dictate the fate of body parts, that autonomy and privacy might be conceptualized, among other rights, as one of property.

7.2 Where might this lead us? Will we see more cases decided in terms of *Yearworth*? On the one hand, one might see *Yearworth* as a model to find remedies in cases of unjust use and access to biological materials. In doing do, one might find that participation becomes the grounds on which research is built (section 5.9, above). A rights framework empowers patients because they have control of their property *in the first place*; and this allows them to waive any rights to ownership as they see fit. This does not mean that broad consent absolves the researcher from any further wrongdoing; or, for that matter, that it is always necessary if a defined public interest is applicable beyond lazy justification on the part of the owner. More importantly, taking consent seriously will perpetuate the kinds of control that I have argued for in terms of rights, inevitably leading to the strong claim that individuals will have property rights in respect to body parts, including *ex vivo* organs (section 2.7). On the other hand, the commodification that inevitably follows property interests may signal the progressive erosion of principles that have traditionally kept the human body out of economical transactions. My hope is that the first of these possibilities is more likely; and in this respect, dignity-grounded rules are more likely to resist policies that exempt researchers from requiring a patient's voluntary approbation to use cells. Yet the risk is that consent becomes an impediment to worthwhile research. However, the fact that over 500,000

---

[62] The targets of intentional circumstances that deprive human rights are most persuasively absent in a state of slavery or *owning* another human agent (see Bloustein 1964).

people are participating 'on terms' in UK Biobank suggests that there is little to be concerned about.[63]

7.3 There are a number of policy options that take this idea of property forward, and which have been variously tested by precedent. One, transfer is an *inter vivos* gift to the proprietors of a biobank or future bio-factory, who in return confirm limited rights to withdraw from a study or agreed access rights to the growing specimens and organs, but retain property in the cells themselves (*Catalona*: note 12, 676–7). Two, patients can sell their cells to interested buyers, thus giving up any further interest.[64] This model is limited by the arguments offered in respect to non-commodification or infungibility, and sets up difficult questions in respect to exactly how much human cells are worth. However, many jurisdictions already recognize the legitimate transfer of blood or semen by way of sale (and many other cells, such as oocytes, are open to transfer by means of payment or 'benefits in kind'). Both models also fall foul of the current Office for Human Research Protections (OHRP) guidelines, in which it is prohibited for researchers to use language that suggests that prospective participants relinquish legal rights (presumably including property rights) in terms of its exculpatory nature.[65] However, under the framework I have put forward, an agent may waive these rights if the projects or deals are explained to them properly.

A third option is to use the research process to strengthen bonds between the scientists and participants, or, in the future, between the customer and service provider at the bio-factory, by characterizing the relationship within a stewardship or bailment model, the terms of which will be fixed by ongoing consent. If consent becomes a focal point for transfer, then it requires those involved to be acutely aware of the fine details of that agreement: any litigation position must be consistent with the underlying documents and their actions, which are the best indications of what the parties intended at the time of the donations. This may be presented in terms of narrow opportunities (e.g. to withdraw samples not already in the legitimate possession of researchers);[66] and limitations may be built in such as statutory licensing requirements (for example, as found in the Human Fertilisation and Embryology Act in the UK). In this third option, the source maintains a property interest until a legitimate transfer of rights.

7.4 Advances in biotechnology since *Moore* require us to rethink our ethical notions of legal property simply because a new set of interests are at stake (such as disputed ownership of factory-manufactured organs or the implications of a participatory role in biobanking initiatives). In this respect, we can expect *Moore* to provide little legal consolation to the encumbered source. Yet the consequences of empowering the source would have far-reaching implications for the 'business' of science. But as things stand,

---

[63] As of 11 a.m. Monday 1 November 2010.

[64] Ted Slavin sold samples of blood containing unusually high levels of hepatitis B antibodies for research purposes (see Skloot 2006).

[65] '[T]he OHRP affirmed that participants could not be asked or required to relinquish putative property rights in tissue due to the "lack of clarity in the law"' (Hakimian and Kron 2004). Also see: Office for Protection from Research Risks; Cooperative Oncology Group Chairpersons Meeting, 15 November 1996. 'Exculpatory Language' in Informed Consent. US Department of Health and Human Services; Office for Human Research Protections. Exculpatory Language in Informed Consent Documents.

[66] See UK Biobank Ethics and Governance Council (June 2007).

abandonment appears to be an inappropriate way to treat an object, because both the source and the scientists can be aware of its potential value as a scientific opportunity, source of wealth, or window to information. And in the face of misuse, it is difficult, as a result of *Moore*, to evince rights to integrity to stave off unwelcome intrusions. In this respect, *Yearworth* suggests that property is about control, and this is a welcome addition to future ethical and legal discourse that engages with the idea of 'property in the human body'.

References

Academy of Medical Sciences. (2002). 'Responses to the Retained Organs Commission Consultation Document on "Unclaimed and Unidentifiable Organs and Tissue and a Possible Regulatory Framework"', http://www.acmedsci.ac.uk/p100puid39.html (accessed 21 January 2013).

Ackerman, B. (1992). 'Liberating Abstraction', *University of Chicago Law Review*, 59:317–48.

Anderson, R. et al. (2009). *Database State: A Report Commissioned by the Joseph Rowntree Reform Trust Ltd.* York: Rowntree Reform Trust Ltd.

Andrews, L., and Nelkin, D. (1998). 'Whose Body Is It Anyway? Disputes over Body Tissue in a Biotechnological Age', *Lancet*, 351:53–57.

Annas, G. (1990). 'Outrageous Fortune: Selling Other People's Cell', *Hastings Center Report*, 20:36–9.

Ashburn, T., Wilson, S., and Eisenstein, B. (2000). 'Human Tissue Research in the Genomic Era of Medicine: Balancing Individual and Societal Interests', *Archives of Internal Medicine*, 160:3377–84.

Ashcroft, R. (2005). 'Making Sense of Dignity', *Journal of Medical Ethics*, 31:679–82.

Beyleveld, D., and Brownsword, R. (2001). *Human Dignity in Bioethics and Biolaw*. Oxford: Oxford University Press.

Beyleveld, D., and Pattinson, S. (2008). 'Moral Interests, Privacy, and Medical Research,' in M. Boylan (ed). *International Public Health Policy and Ethics*. Dordrecht: Springer, 45–57.

Bloustein, E. (1964). 'Privacy as an Aspect of Human Dignity: An Answer to Dean Prosser', *New York University Law Review*, 39:962–1007.

Boulier, W. (2005). 'Sperm, Spleens, and Other Valuables: The Need to Recognize Property Rights in Human Body Part', *Hofstra Law Review*, 23:693.

Brownsword, R. (2003). 'Bioethics Today, Bioethics Tomorrow: Stem Cell Research and the "Dignitarian Alliance"'. *Notre Dame Journal of Law, Ethics, and Public Policy*, 17:15–51.

Brownsword, R. (2009). 'Property in Human Tissue: Triangulating the Issue', in M. Steinmann, P. Sýkoria, and U. Wiesing (eds), *Altruism Reconsidered: Exploring New Approaches to Property in Human Tissue*. Farnham: Ashgate, 93–104.

Calabresi, G. (1991). 'Do We Own Our Bodies?', *Health Matrix*, 1(1):5–18.

Campbell, A. (2009). *The Body in Bioethics*. London: Routledge.

Capps, B., and Campbell, A.V. (2007). 'Why (Only Some) Compensation for Oocyte Donation for Research Makes Ethical Sense', *Journal of International Biotechnology Law*, 4:89–102.

Capps, B., Campbell, A.V., and ter Meulen, R. (2008). 'Access to the UK Biobank Resource: Concepts of the Public Interest and the Public Good', Commissioned Report for the Ethics and Governance Council of UK Biobank/Wellcome Trust.

Capps, B., and Carter, A. (2010). 'Standing on the Precipice: A Cautionary Note About Incremental Goods', *American Journal of Bioethics*, 1:46–8.

Chang, E. et al. (2009). 'Tissue Engineering Using Autologous Microcirculatory Beds as Vascularized Bioscaffolds'. *FASEB Journal*, 23:906–15.

Clayton, E. (2005). 'Informed Consent and Biobanks', *Journal of Law, Medicine, and Ethics*, 33:15–21.

Cline, R. E., Laurent, N. M., and Foran, D. R. (2003). 'The Fingernails of Mary Sullivan: Developing Reliable Methods for Selectively Isolating Endogenous and Exogenous DNA from Evidence', *Journal of Forensic Sciences*, 48:328–33.

Curran, W. (1991). 'Scientific and Commercial Development of Human Cell Lines: Issues of Property, Ethics, and Conflict of Interest', *New England Journal of Medicine*, 324:998–1000.

Day, J. P. (1966). 'Locke on Property', *Philosophical Quarterly*, 16:207–20.

Dickenson, D. (2007). 'Consent, Commodification and Benefit–Sharing in Genetic Research', *Developing World Bioethics*, 4:109–24.

Duxbury, N. (1996). 'Do Markets Degrade?' *Modern Law Review*, 59:331–48.

Fletcher, G. (1996). *Basic Concepts of Legal Thought*. Oxford: Oxford University Press.

George, A. (2004). 'Is 'Property' Necessary? On Owning the Human Body and Its Parts', *Res Publica*, 10:15–42.

Gewirth, A. (1978). *Reason and Morality*. Chicago: Chicago University Press.

Gold, R. (1996). *Body Parts: Property Rights and the Ownership of Human Biological Material*. Washington, DC: Georgetown University Press.

Golde, D. (1991). 'Commercial Development of Human Cell Lines: Property, Ethics, and Conflicts of Interest', *New England Journal of Medicine*, 324:1745–6.

Goodson, M., and Vernon, B. (2004). 'A Study of Public Opinion on the Use of Tissue Samples from Living Subjects for Clinical Research', *Journal of Clinical Pathology*, 57:135–8.

Graham, E. (2007). 'DNA Reviews: Hair', *Forensic Science, Medicine, and Pathology*, 3:133–7.

Hakimian, R., and Kron, D. (2004). 'Ownership and Use of Tissue Specimens for Research', *Journal of the American Medical Association*, 292:2500–5.

Hardin, G. (1968). 'The Tragedy of the Commons', *Science*, 162:1243–8.

Harmon, S., and Laurie, G. (2010). '*Yearworth* v. *North Bristol NHS Trust*: Property, Principles, Precedents, and Paradigms', *Cambridge Law Journal*, 69: 476–93.

Harmon, S. (2010). '*Yearworth* v. *North Bristol NHS Trust*: A Property Case of Uncertain Significance', *Medicine, Health Care, and Philosophy*, 13:343–50.

Hawes, C. (2010). 'Property Interests in Body Part: *Yearworth* v. *North Bristol NHS Trust*', *Modern Law Review*, 73:119–40.

Hayden, C. (2007). 'Taking as Giving: Bioscience, Exchange, and the Politics of Benefit-Sharing', *Social Studies of Science*, 37:729–58.

Hoeyer K. et al. (2005). 'The Ethics of Research Using Biobanks: Reason to Question the Importance Attributed to Informed Consent', *Archives of Internal Medicine*, 167:97–100.

Hohfeld, W. (1964). *Fundamental Legal Conceptions as Applied in Judicial Reasoning*. New Haven, CT: Yale University Press.

Homer, N. et al. (2008). 'Resolving Individuals Contributing Trance Amounts of DNA to Highly Complex Mixtures Using High–Density SNP Genotyping Microarrays', *PLoS Genetics*, 4:1–9.

Honoré, A. (1986). *Making Law Bind: Essays legal and Philosophical*. Oxford: Clarendon Press.

Hübner, K. et al. (2003). 'Derivation of Oocytes from Mouse Embryonic Stem Cells', *Science*, 300:1251–6.

Jasanoff, S. (2005). *Designs on Nature: Science and Democracy in Europe and the United States.* Princeton, NJ: Princeton University Press.

Katches, M., Heisel, W., and Campbell, R. (2000). 'Donors Don't Realize They Are Fuelling a Lucrative Business', *Orange County Register*, 16 April, I.D. 1183100, p. H1.

Kennedy, I. (2000). 'Interim Report of The Inquiry into the Management of Care of Children Receiving Complex Heart Surgery at The Bristol Royal Infirmary', May.

Locke, J. (1975). *An Essay Concerning Human Understanding*, edited with an Introduction by P. Nidditch. Oxford: Clarendon Press.

Locke, J. (1988). *Two Treatises of Government*, edited by P. Laslett. Cambridge: Cambridge University Press.

Lyon, D. (2001). *Surveillance Society: Monitoring Everyday Life.* Buckingham: Open University Press.

Macpherson, C. (1962). *The Political Theory of Possessive Individualism: Hobbes to Locke.* Oxford: Oxford University Press.

Morton, O. (1997). 'First Dolly, Now Headless Tadpoles', *Science* 278:798.

National Bioethics Advisory Commission. (1999). 'Research Involving Human Biological Materials: Ethical Issues and Policy Guidance Volume I: Report and Recommendations of the National Bioethics Advisory Commission'. Rockville, MD: NABC.

Nayernia, K. et al. (2006). 'In Vitro-Differentiated Embryonic Stem Cells Give Rise to Male Gametes that Can Generate Offspring Mice', *Developmental Cell*, 11:125–32.

Nelkin, D., and Andrews, L. (1995). 'Homo Economicus: Commercialization of Body Tissue in an Age of Biotechnology', *Hastings Center Report*, 28:30–9.

Northern, K. (1998). 'Procreative Torts: Enhancing the Common-Law Protection for Reproductive Autonomy', *University of Illinois Law Review*, 2:489–546.

Nuffield Council on Bioethics. (1995). *Human Tissue: Ethical and Legal Issues.* London: Nuffield Council of Bioethics.

Office for Protection from Research Risks; Cooperative Oncology Group Chairpersons Meeting, 15 November 1996. 'Exculpatory Language' in Informed Consent. US Department of Health and Human Services; Office for Human Research Protections. Exculpatory Language in Informed Consent Documents.

Priaulx, N. (2010). 'Managing Novel Reproductive Injuries in the Law of Tort: The Curious Case of Destroyed Sperm', *European Journal of Health Law*, 17:81–95.

Porter, R. (2003). *Flesh in the Age of Reason.* London: Alan Lane.

Radin, M. (1996). *Contested Commodities.* Cambridge, MA: Harvard University Press.

Rei, W. (2010). 'Towards a Governance Structure Beyond Informed Consent: A Critical Analysis of the Popularity of Private Cord Blood Banks in Taiwan'. *East Asian Science, Technology, and Society*, 4:53–75.

Retained Organs Commission. (2004). 'Remembering the Past, Looking to the Future. The Final Report of the Retained Organs Commission Including the Summary Accountability Report for 2003/2004', London: Department of Health.

Scott, R. (1981). *The Body as Property.* London: Penguin Books.

Secretariat of the Convention on Biological Diversity, *Bonn Guidelines on Access to Genetic Resources and Fair and Equitable Sharing of the Benefits Arising out of their Utilization* (Montreal: Canada 2002).

Skloot, R. (2006). 'Taking the Least of You', *New York Times*, 16 April.

Sulston, J. (December 2002). 'Heritage of Humanity', *Le Monde diplomatique*, http://mondediplo.com/2002/12/15genome (accessed 21 January 2013).

Sýkoria, P. (2009). 'Altruism in Medical Donations Reconsidered: The Reciprocity Approach', in M. Steinmann, P. Sýkoria, and U. Wiesing (eds), *Altruism Reconsidered: Exploring New Approaches to Property in Human Tissue*. Farnham: Ashgate, 13–49.

The Wellcome Trust and Medical Research Council. (2001). 'Public Perceptions of the Collection of Human Biological Samples', London: The Trustee of the Wellcome Trust and the Medical Research Council.

Thomson, J. J. (1971). 'A Defense of Abortion', *Philosophy and Public Affairs*, 1(1): 47–66.

Tubo, R. (2007). 'Fundamentals of Cell-Based Therapies', in A. Atala et al. (eds), *Principles of Regenerative Medicine*. London: Academic Press, 16–27.

UK Biobank Ethics and Governance Council. (June 2007). 'Revision of the UK Biobank Ethics and Governance Framework: "No Further Use" Withdrawal Option', http://www.egcuk-biobank.org.uk/recentactivity/index.html (accessed 21 January 2013).

Van Diest, P. (2002). 'For and Against: No Consent Should be Needed for Using Leftover Body Materials for Scientific Purposes', *BMJ*, 325: 648.

Wilmut, I., and Paterson, L. (2003). 'Somatic Cell Nuclear Transfer', *Oncology Research Featuring Preclinical and Clinical Cancer Therapeutics*, 13: 303–7.

6.2

Commentary
But Which Body: Body of Labor, or Body of Anatomy?

Kantaro Ohashi

Dr. Capps thoroughly explicated two principal cases of contemporary treatment of the human body and cells in the context of medical and bio-industries. Let me start by admitting that his analyses and criticisms of current medical issues are so persuasive that I have almost nothing to add to them. All I can do is present a frame of thought surrounding these issues from the viewpoint of the history of modern philosophy, which is my specialty. That is, the essence of the problem that Dr. Capps attempted to solve can be reconsidered in the context of modern philosophical thought in order to reveal a general (but supplementary) perspective on these current issues in medicine.

Let me try to explain this by analysing a quotation from John Locke on which Dr. Capps bases his arguments about skill. This Lockean argument is applied to Article 21 of the Explanatory Report, which is referred to in the former section of this report. It says, 'the human body and its parts' are precluded from financial gain 'as such'. Dr. Capps focuses on the phrase 'as such', and offers three possible interpretations of it (Capps 2013): a) relating to the inherent nature of something, b) being exactly the same (i.e. the same nature) or similar to what is mentioned or suggested, and c) being considered alone or by itself. He considers the third interpretation to be the most plausible, while admitting that the first two are also acceptable. And this expression, he concluded, had to rely on the singularity of the subject, that is, the 'human body'. Moreover, he admitted that the preceding two definitions have their own ambiguity, because they invoke the notion of a 'type', that is, a property or properties that can be abstracted from the idea of a human body and ascribed to something else. As a result, interpretations a) and b) encourage us to consider human bodies *in general*, rather than any specific human body.[67] The prudence manifested in Dr. Capps's paper (2013) is worth examining in more detail.

[67] When taking this kind of historical viewpoint, the following question is important: 'which body became the precedent that allowed us to abstract the property "body"'? To address this question fully would require a thorough investigation of cases of Roman law that dominated European culture for over 1,500 years. In particular, we must carefully examine how Roman jurists attempted to introduce Christian tradition into their law system. In his work, *Homo Sacer*, the Italian philosopher Giorgio Agamben discusses the Roman idea of

That there are various interpretations of 'human body' is relevant when considering the body as property. Our body, once regarded as both a subject and an object, becomes not only something of inviolable dignity, but also a material to be operated on. It has a visible wholeness, as well as invisible and intangible parts. From this point of view, it is surprising that the concept of the human body should remain useful; but even when considering medical matters, patients ordinarily understand their conditions in terms of their 'body'. They don't ordinarily view their body in terms of its working as a complicated composition of, for example, a biological information system in the form of DNA. Considering the gap between how the body is treated medically and how it is perceived in an ordinary sense, it is inevitable that our concepts of 'man', 'human', and 'personality' must also undergo a transformation through medical or biological decomposition of the human organism in contemporary practice. Because of this, as a researcher of the seventeenth and eighteenth centuries, I cannot help but have reservations about applying the theories of the classical age to the problems of our time.

As mentioned above, the definition of property that we inherited from John Locke has been, until now, considered the theoretical foundation of property with respect to the human body. To explore this idea, Dr. Capps considered an important passage in Locke's *Two Treatises of Government*:

But the chief matter of property being now not the fruits of the earth, and the beasts that subsist on it, but the earth itself; as that which takes in, and carries with it all the rest; I think it is plain, that property in that too is acquired as the former. As much land as a man tills, plants, improves, cultivates, and can use the product of, so much is his property. He *by his labour does, as it were, enclose it from the common.* Nor will it invalidate his right, to say everybody else has an equal title to it, and therefore he cannot appropriate, he cannot enclose, *without the consent of all his fellow-commoners, all mankind.* (*Two Treatises of Government*, Book II, Chapter V, s. 32; italics added)

This quotation helps us understand why medical scientists or corporations that derive financial gain from participation in scientific research have no right to do so. Locke's concept of property makes it possible to appropriate natural products when doing so is authorized by 'all mankind', typically in circumstances where it is useful to all mankind to give such authorization. In other words, 'mutual benefits' must be respected here. Society accepts the privileges of scientists because scientific progress benefits all. Accordingly, science must be accessible by 'the public' and not monopolized by powerful private enterprises. I wholeheartedly agree with Dr. Capps's view that pure scientific interest and autonomy of all those engaged in scientific inquiry are necessary.

I will now expand on Dr. Capps's view with a longer analysis of a particular phrase by Locke. This analysis is based on a sentence quoted by Dr. Capps: '[the agent] by his labour does, as it were, enclose it from the common'. The key phrase is 'as it were'.

---

homo sacer [sacred person], a citizen who was not only considered a sacred person but also so excluded from the ordinary community that anyone could kill him without this being considered murder. Surveying the issues surrounding DNA and transplanted organs, we could say that the inner property of humans has been also 'exceptional'. They are considered not only as secrets from which emerges the existence of human bodies, but also as information systems or partial goods which can be reduced through specific processes. Human beings' duality, which consists of sacred wholeness and exchangeable goods, might be defined through the eastern historical processes. See Agamben 1998.

Locke's concept of property is widely recognized to have a double meaning: it refers to the right to own materials, as well as to the materials to be owned. It is also widely known that John Locke wrote his *Two Treatises* as a criticism of Robert Filmer's theory of the divine right of kings. Locke argued in support of equal rights for all people, which he called 'natural rights', and considered individuals not to be answerable to 'public-king' power (i.e. that of the privileged). Natural rights protect the territory of individuals by acknowledging their ownership based on their bodies' existence. The term 'property' emphasizes the *non-aggressiveness* of the body. Note a difficulty inherent in Locke's concept of property: this concept did not (and does not) presuppose the notion of the *dividuality* of our body. The body as property can be compared to a person's individuality. Principally, our organs, blood, and other body parts are not distributable objects. According to Lockean arguments, our bodies may not be separated, segmented, or distributed: this acknowledges, at least in principle, our proper ownership of our bodies. Thus, if we think about property rights to our organs, or to our DNA, we must first decide whether these are the sorts of things that may be viewed as property at all, and if so, who are the candidates for being potentially entitled to assert a right to such property. That is, we must demarcate the indeterminate and inherent private goods in order to make them common. Expressions like 'such as' or 'as it were' reveal antecedent assumptions we have about what sorts of things we may consider our property. With this in mind, our right—in terms of our body—to participate in scientific research must be examined carefully, as it concerns the transformation of potential goods into something of actual value.

The second difficulty is related to the idea of potentiality. To appreciate this difficulty we must consider exactly what is involved in Locke's account of property and rights, and its associated ethical ideas. According to Locke, the government is required to reconcile conflicts arising from individual interests, and people must respect their contract with the government not to infringe on the rights of others. In this regard, we can say that Locke's system of natural rights constitutes both political and moral relationships among individuals. Moreover, it is worth noting that Locke's concept of 'right' is, as mentioned above, based on certain assumptions about what sort of things we can consider to be potentially our property. People do not own a natural product *de facto* (in fact) but *de jure* (in law). When people set out to own part of 'nature', their physical movements are transformed into labor, and labor consists in acquiring the natural product using one's living body. What distinguishes labor from mere movement, however, is the situations in which people find themselves: that is, the political system in which they live. The double meaning of 'property' is also derived from this potentiality of human rights: materials are real, whereas rights are invented, and in this sense fictitious. The idea of property strikes a compromise between reality and potentiality, which reflects human values.[68] We must recognize human rights, even though they are a mere invention; that they are an invention is irrelevant. Each concept, such as a contract, property, or even labor, is simply defined as something to be realized; despite being fictitious, they play significant

---

[68] This interpretation of property leads us to the same structure as the Cartesian *cogito* in Locke's empirical system. Does the manifestation of the cogito secretly include ownership of the clear and distinct idea? This complex relationship between understanding and possessing has yet to be resolved. Also analogous is the relationship between science and technology, i.e. between discovery and application. In this sense, this structure might penetrate the problem of our body's property at a deeper level.

roles in Locke's moral-civil system. Morality is nothing more than a set of rules to help people coexist. In classical terms, this relates to 'morals', and not to 'ethics'. Ethics in the traditional sense have no application in the sphere of our mutual understanding of ownership. Philosophers in the seventeenth and eighteenth centuries termed this domain 'moral', designating the statute of our psychology in relation to our physical state. If we focus on ethics, we face questions about our body's potentialities. When it comes to merely potential goods that generate scientific fruits or biogenetic interests, i.e. goods of *real value*, our conceptual tools seem insufficient.

As a philosopher, I wish to consider the question of what are the ethics, and not the morality, of the problem described above. Are the ethics of Locke's time no longer relevant today? In my opinion, the seed of ethics for Locke was already sown in the phrase 'as it were'. Let us recall the key sentence: 'He [the agent] by his labour does, as it were, enclose it from the common.' What Locke implies is that, beyond the potentiality alluded to by the phrase 'as it were', the sphere of 'the common' really exists. His point of view is very close to that of natural theology. For him, constructing a moral system is urgently required in order to secure a system of ethics. Morals and contracts are mortgages for establishing a human-scale system based on the 'body' and its 'labor'. The human body pervasively influences the idea of Lockean property. Furthermore, this sort of ethics lies in, as we saw, the gap between the potentiality (*de jure*) and reality (*de facto*) surrounding our body; to what degree are we responsible for our body's constitution, when all data remains unseen or hidden behind the wall of highly accurate scientific operations?

I conclude with a general comment from a different angle. Nowadays, the human body is finely segmented into, for example, molecular and genetic information systems. In this regard, the concepts of property and labor that are required must also be altered: we need new concepts that reflect these compositions. The question is how we could conceptualize the world and all the relationships between cells, tissues, molecular matters, without doing so solely from the human-scale viewpoint. In this sense, it can be said that we could be *more ethical*, as I believe that all the consideration given to the world system in antiquity, or in the philosophical traditions of China, Japan, and India, still maintain the actualities that each world view has a proper significance closely connected to every mode of the reality of life.

References

Agamben, G. (1998). *Homo Sacer: Sovereign Power and Bare Life*. Stanford, CA: Stanford University Press.

Capps, B. (2014). 'Redefining Property in Human Body Parts: An Ethical Enquiry,' in A. Akabayashi (ed.), *The Future of Bioethics: International Dialogues*. Oxford: Oxford University Press, 235–63.

6.3

Commentary

The Non-Ownership Thesis: A German Perspective

Wilhelm Vossenkuhl

Benjamin Capps argues that human body parts are not commodities to be freely traded like the objects or things people own. The gist of his argument is that we still lack clear-cut rules, which limit the commerce and commodification of human body parts. On the other hand he stresses that human tissue is needed in science and medicine. I fully support his analysis. Capps's discussion focuses—critically—on the Californian case of John Moore (1998) and—more approvingly—on the British Yearworth case (2009). He tries to clarify the ethical grounding of decisions concerning the distribution and commerce of body parts. I shall extend his ethical line of argument. But instead of discussing the above-mentioned cases I shall first consider the German perspective on the ownership of human body parts, as its attitude towards living persons differs crucially from the British one. As the attitude towards dead bodies is similar to the British one I will not discuss it. Secondly, I shall examine the ethical grounding of the German legal attitude towards human body parts.

The idea of a person's ownership of her body or body parts is alien to German law. The reason is that property rights in German law only refer to things, while the body and the body parts of living humans do not count as things. Only the dead body counts as a thing. Therefore, from a legal perspective persons do not stand in an ownership relation either towards their body as a whole or towards any of their body parts as long as they are alive. Nevertheless, in legal terms, humans are in control of their own bodies in a way that comes close to, but isn't, an ownership relation.[69] The consequences of this German peculiarity are immediately obvious from a number of notorious legal bans, which are not always well understood internationally, e.g. the ban on the commodification of organs for transplantation, or the ban on the production of human embryonic stem cells. In order to clarify the motives for this latter ban we may for a moment consider its background. It is not immediately related to questions of ownership but relevant to these questions. The major reason for the ban on the production of

[69] See Ellenberger's comment concerning §90 BGB (short for: Bürgerliches Gesetzbuch) in: Palandt, BGB-Kommentar, 69. Auflage, 2010, München.

human embryonic stem cells is that the human embryo in German law enjoys the same legal protection as the life and dignity of a person. Obviously, this protection rules out all uses that are incompatible with the protection of the life and dignity of an embryo.[70] Nobody is therefore entitled to own a human embryo, not even the couple who contributed to its existence. The freely chosen consent of a female donor, e.g. to offer an ovum for the production of embryonic stem cells, is an offence. The donor's consent is as irrelevant as the otherwise constitutionally guaranteed freedom of scientific research. The life and dignity of the human embryo are overriding. They are as overriding as any natural right or human right. Therefore, any kind of instrumental use of embryos in research is banned. In the same vein any commercial exploitation of the post mortem or live donation of organs is prohibited. Here again the instrumental use of parts of one's own body is banned. One might be amazed to learn that even post mortem donations are exempt from commodification, despite being taken from dead bodies. The primary reason for the respective law regulating the transplantation of organs was to ban any trafficking of post mortem or live donations of organs.

Now, what is true for the human embryo and for the donation of organs is not true in general without further qualification, otherwise we would be at a loss to explain why *in vitro* fertilization with anonymous sperm donors is permitted in Germany. Blood donation is no problem, and the donation of sperm and other bodily substances is allowed under certain legal conditions, which are not always as clear as one might expect. If, e.g., a person wants his sperm preserved for some potential future reproductive use, those sperm are subject to protection. The person's control over his sperm is guaranteed. A doctor who ignored this in a certain case, and destroyed a person's sperm which were entrusted to the doctor's care, was convicted of bodily injury.[71] Obviously, the person's control over the use of his sperm came down to an ownership relation. This is interesting because those sperm were, needless to mention, separated from his body. Following German law, any kind of quasi ownership of human body parts is only possible after these parts are permanently separated from a human body. In the case mentioned, oddly enough the person's sperm did not count as being permanently separated from his body. But even in cases where bodily parts are permanently separated from their donor bodies, it is not at all clear whether doctors, scientists, or labs using and storing these parts may count as their owners. A person's consent for her tissue to be used in research, or her negligent leaving behind of her tissue in some lab, may constitute an ownership on the lab's side. But even in these cases it is far from clear whether an ownership relation is really entailed.[72] One of the questions lurking here concerns the protection of personal data and privacy. Some people are concerned about whether the personal data of donors can really be made anonymous. If not, the rights of privacy and personal rights would not be effectively protected.

---

[70] Whether a human embryo can be ascribed any personal rights as, e.g. a claim to the protection of life and dignity, is heavily debated among ethicists, jurists, and politicians in Germany. I shall not go into any details here concerning this debate, but focus instead on the prevailing legal situation.

[71] The person in the case mentioned had a vasectomy and was therefore unable to repeat his previous donation.

[72] For a discussion of different views concerning the ownership and use of human tissue, see Simon and Robienski 2010.

Obviously, the regulation of the donation and use of human body parts along the lines of the British Human Tissue Act 2004 seems almost impossible in Germany. The British document offers a detailed and most comprehensive account of the rules to be observed in all cases of the removal, storage, and use of human organs and tissue for a restricted number of well defined purposes. Without mentioning the problem of ownership of body parts, the Human Tissue Act indirectly answers questions of ownership on the basis of its again rather detailed account of the consent of authorized persons to a 'scheduled purpose' of using her body parts. Obviously, unlike German civil law, British common law does not exclude human body parts from relations of ownership. There are, of course, a number of laws in Germany regulating the use of human tissue, donated organs, and genetic data, but there is still a lack of norms regulating the donation and use of human body parts for well defined purposes.

Instead of digging further into legal questions concerning the use of human body parts I will now examine the ethical grounding of the non-ownership claim of human body parts. The primary question is whether there are valid arguments denying living humans any ownership of their bodies and body parts. In short, why are bodies and body parts of living humans not *things*, which could be owned like any other personal belongings? Historically, one might go back as far as Roman law in order to see one of the precursors of the German attitude towards human bodies and body parts. And, of course, Christian theology is another possible and most probable source here. But apart from these historical and religious backgrounds, it may still be dubious—from an ethical point of view—why the body parts of living humans are not to be treated as things.

I will try to reconstruct a viable course of argument in order to elucidate and examine the German non-ownership claim. Let us start by considering the claim that living human body parts are not things. Things—as we generally understand them—are objects, which can be owned and ascribed a certain personal, institutional, ritual, or artistic value, or market value as a commodity. Obviously, human organs or other body parts are objects too, but why should these objects be awarded a value beyond commodification, a value even in need of a special legal protection? What makes the body parts of living humans objects with a certain dignity? Even if the meaning of 'dignity' is well understood, it is far from clear what the ascription of dignity to living human bodies and their parts really means, and how it is ethically grounded. The difficulty bothering us is caused by the ascription of an ethical principle—dignity in our case—to a person and her body, to her actual spatio-temporal existence as it were. We easily understand the ascription of personal or market values to things, because we know that these values are contingent and changeable, and that those things exist independently from any possible changing value ascriptions.

Now, as to the ascription of dignity to living human bodies we are puzzled, because that ascription is supposed to be neither contingent nor to be changed at will. We know of similar cases, e.g. the ascription of freedom and integrity to persons. Here again the ascription seems not meant to be contingent. But—*pace* Rawls[73]—it may be an open question whether a person should not be licensed to trade her freedom and integrity

---

[73] J. Rawls in his *Theory of Justice* (1971, 60ff.) takes freedom to be the number one principle of justice, which cannot be traded or substituted by something else.

for any other good she prefers. Why should a person not be entitled to exchange her freedom for slavery or sell her body to customers, e.g. for sexual purposes? There may be libertarians who argue that decisions about these things may be made only by the person involved. But can we really choose not to be free? The libertarian will blithely affirm that we can. Perhaps we can, in the sense of 'we are able to do so if there is no obstacle to hinder us from doing it'. On this understanding of 'can', we can indeed jump off a high-rise building and commit suicide or we can trade our freedom for slavery. Suicide is an example of choosing not to be free, once and forever. This kind of choice is not to be repeated and is therefore self-defeating. It is not the kind of example which may convince us that the ability to choose not to be free is an attractive one. Similarly, trading one's freedom for slavery is a non-starter. It may even be worse than committing suicide if we realize that we cannot escape it once we have chosen it. The meaning and scope of choosing not to be free is neither clear nor attractive. We should therefore consider for a moment what 'can' means with respect to the freedom of choice. This may eventually shed some light on the ascription of dignity to living human bodies and body parts, which is obviously most significant in the German legal system.

We can do a lot of things, but others we cannot do, however much we may want to. A wet and hungry person cannot make himself dry and sated by will alone, and most of us cannot solve Fermat's last theorem. It makes a lot of difference whether the reasons why we can or cannot do things are contingent or not. Some people will necessarily be able to remove an obstacle on their route to enact what they want, others will not. But there are necessities, independent of our will, which hinder us from doing things. Most of these necessities are physical,[74] some are biological,[75] some are social or legal,[76] and some are logical.[77]

Are there any ethical necessities, which are akin to any of the necessities just mentioned? If so, how would they hinder us from doing things we could otherwise choose to do? Let us examine this option with respect to the above-mentioned choice of freedom. Is there any kind of necessity hindering us, e.g. from freely choosing not to be free? The answer is 'yes and no'. No, insofar as we learnt from the examples of committing suicide and trading freedom for slavery, that there is nothing beyond our own will that could hinder us from these deplorable choices. Yes, insofar as we are the only ones who may necessitate (in the sense of coerce) ourselves not to take those choices. But how *can* we do this? The way we can necessitate our own conduct—in ethics and beyond—is by either willing to do so or by introducing and accepting principles of conduct or by consolidating our will and the chosen principle.[78] If we manage to do the latter, will power and principles of conduct may hinder us from choosing to do things that we could otherwise do without much difficulty. But, of course, our will may be thwarted and none of the principles we choose will become part of our physical or biological nature anyway. Principles may be personally or socially binding only if we agree and freely accept them

---

[74] E.g. moving faster than light is physically impossible.
[75] E.g. giving birth as a male is biologically impossible.
[76] E.g. killing somebody we don't like is illegal.
[77] E.g. rationally, honestly, and consciously to assert both 'a' and 'not-a' at the same time is logically impossible.
[78] I ignore meta-ethical doubts concerning this consolidation as offered by Humeans or Act-Utilitarians here.

as laws of behaviour. The principle of freedom alone therefore neither necessitates any physical or mental state or event, nor does it necessarily hinder us from wanting and doing things as long as we are able to do them. It is up to our free choice to accept freedom as a principle that binds us in whatever we are doing. If we do not accept it, some may blame us for our actions, but nobody will sue or prosecute us—as long as we abide by valid laws.[79]

This latter condition—accepting or denying the principle of freedom within some valid legal constraints—casts an interesting light on the choice we have been considering. It disavows, as it were, the principle of freedom and it gives evidence—in Nietzschean terms—of a slavish or at least legalistic mentality too. Making the denial of the principle of freedom contingent upon legal conditions confuses dependent and independent conditions. Principles are meant to work as conditions, which are independent from other conditions. If the choice offered by the principle of freedom is not taken to be fundamental for all other choices, including the choice of abiding by the law, it is not free at all. In short, free choices are only possible within and not beyond the principle of freedom, i.e. only within the domain of this principle are we able to deny it, but we cannot deny it altogether by any kind of choice.

There is an interesting similarity between the ethical necessity we are trying to clarify and the logical one mentioned earlier. Our inability to make free choices beyond the principle of freedom is akin to the law of non-contradiction, i.e. to our logical inability rationally, honestly, and consciously to affirm, e.g., 'a' and 'not-a' at the same time. Whenever we freely choose anything, we cannot—rationally—evade, jump, or avoid the conditions set by the principle of freedom. Therefore, even in denying this principle we move within its scope. There is no alternative to making use of the principle of freedom that we could rationally conceive of, even when we deny this principle and choose not to be free. The principle of freedom leaves us no alternative. The same is true for the law of non-contradiction. Rationality leaves us no alternative, even when we sin against that law. Rationality and freedom are both inescapable; in whatever we say or do we implicitly acknowledge these principles. Is this true for human dignity too?

Before I come back to this latter question I would like to pursue the similarity between freedom and rationality historically for a moment. Kant observed this similarity and congruously argued for a fusion of freedom and rationality in his *Groundwork of the Metaphysics of Morals*. If we take the stance of rationality—let us assume with Kant for a moment that we can—the principle of freedom is inescapable from rational reasons alone, therefore freedom and rationality in his account are two sides of the same coin (see Kant 1968: 421–5). This fusion of freedom and rationality is most elegant but does not work wonders on its own. It does not—as Kant observed—necessitate actions if the agent does not necessitate himself to follow the—self-enacted—moral law. Self-necessitation is Kant's solution to the moral problem, and he names this necessity the 'Categorical Imperative' (see Kant 1968: 423). Obviously, even Kant did not believe that freedom and rationality alone

---

[79] Committing suicide is legally permitted in many countries, including Germany. And although slavery is banned worldwide I don't know of any legal obstacle to trade one's freedom for slavery. Cases of consensual killing or cannibalism of one's own body occasionally cause some legal puzzlement. Obviously, it is not absolutely clear how far one's self-determination may go in legal terms.

necessitate any behaviour to abide by the moral law. We have to command ourselves to follow the moral law—however we shall be able to do that. The gist of this Kantian reminder is
that ethical necessities, like logical ones, are a priori. It would be inconsistent not to observe
them. But this intellectual sin will only be avenged if it happens to be a misdemeanour in
legal terms. Why then should we bother?

Even from a Kantian point of view, the alleged—rational—inescapability of the principles of freedom and rationality is of no immediate practical or real import in human life.
If this is so, the ascription of dignity to a living human body will not make us better off. It
may be inconsistent not to subscribe to the demands of dignity, and all arguments from this
principle may be ethically sound but it nevertheless remains a priori. Human dignity, in
other words, will not in itself necessitate us to behave in any particular way. If this principle
is not part and parcel of constitutional law—as in the German case—it won't be binding
and won't hinder the trafficking of body parts from living humans. From an ethical point of
view, we may conclude that the final step in the application of ethical principles to human
behaviour always remains indeterminate. Ethical necessities, as we saw from considering the
principle of freedom, do not impose themselves as physical or biological necessities do. The
ascription of dignity to a living human body is ethically sound and its consequences may
be well argued in support of the non-ownership thesis. But whether we really subscribe to
demands of dignity seems to be up to us, and if it is up to us it may change just like every
other contingent condition. This seems to be the somewhat sobering penultimate result of
my analysis of the ethical grounding of the non-ownership thesis. But it cannot be the last
word on the standard of dignity as validated in Germany.

As Kant's influence on this standard is presently still valid in the interpretation of the
first article of the German constitution, I may briefly comment on his understanding of
dignity. In his *Groundwork* Kant argues that persons are 'absolute values', that their existence is an end in itself, and that we are bound to acknowledge mankind in one's own
person and in that of everybody else. This latter principle is—as he further argues—to
be realized by 'never using any person', including the person of oneself, 'as a means
alone' but always as an end in itself (Kant 1968: 428–30; my translation). Obviously, these
notorious passages boil down in most ethical or legal accounts to a ban on any instrumental use of persons. But it is far from clear what kind of use is really excluded by the
expression 'never using any person as a means alone'. If any instrumental use is excluded,
regardless of its purpose, the ascription of dignity to living human bodies would rule out
the live donation of organs and of human tissue.[80]

As a matter of fact, human organs and tissue taken from living persons are instrumental for saving the lives of those who enjoy their donation. Therefore, whatever Kant had
in mind, there is no point in taking refuge in a total ban on the instrumental use of living
human body parts. It is nevertheless interesting to remember his notion of dignity in the
analysis of the non-ownership thesis. From a Kantian analysis of dignity it is no surprise
that the body parts of living humans are not things, and are unavailable for any kind of
ownership. Dignity is a value beyond all others, i.e. it is an absolute value, which cannot

---

[80] Rebecca Roache pointed out that Kantians can defend live donations on the ground that a purely instrumental use of the donor can be ruled out if she or he is treated with medical care (personal conversation).
I agree. My point is that it is still not clear how far Kant's ban on the instrumental use of persons really goes.

be balanced or substituted by any kind or amount of other values. The absolute value ascription of dignity to all humans, as found in the first article of the German constitution, is a presupposition of the constitution as a whole and of all laws under its governance. If we accept this unique position of human dignity, we will not have difficulty understanding that it would be incoherent to try and partition dignity into separable bodily parts with lesser value. Dignity is taken to be indivisible. Therefore bodily parts—at least from living humans—are to be treated as if they had dignity too. Not even the person herself is licensed to rule this out. Personal freedom and any liberal-minded notions of self-determination are limited by human dignity.

The ethical grounding of the German non-ownership thesis is based on a principle: human dignity. As J. S. Mill observed, 'questions of ultimate ends do not admit of proof' (Mill 2001: Chapter IV, first sentence). The same is true for fundamental principles too: there are no arguments for the principle of human dignity. Either we take and acknowledge it as valid or we leave it. It is valid without argument.[81] Its validity has to be acknowledged, otherwise it is meaningless and without any real impact on human behaviour. This is the weakness of fundamental principles. And this weakness might eventually contribute to a mitigation of the validity, or even to an abolishment, of the non-ownership thesis altogether.

References

Kant, I. (1968). *Grundlegung zur Metaphysik der Sitten*. Akademieausgabe, Kant Werke IV. Berlin: Walter de Gruyer.

Mill, J. S. (2001). *Utilitarianism*. Indianapolis, IN: Hackett.

Rawls, J. (1971). *A Theory of Justice*. Cambridge, MA: Belknap Press of Harvard University Press.

Simon, J., and Robienski, J. (2010). 'Eigentum an humanem Material in Biobanken und dessen Nutzung', in T. Pottast, B. Herrmann, and U. Müller (eds), *Wem gehört der menschliche Körper?* Paderborn: Mentis, 299–323.

---

[81] I analyse the difference between well argued validities and underived validities, which are not based on argument at all in my 'Geltung' (Neues Handbuch für Philosophie, Freiburg/München 2011, 904–18).

6.4

Commentary
Legal Status of the Human Body and Tissues

Katsunori Kai

1 Introduction

These days, it is very important to discuss the legal status of the human body, its tissues, and their use because we are able to utilize them in various fields of the life sciences. Because the human body consists of many diverse components, it is very difficult to treat them equally from the viewpoint of law and ethics. I therefore find it meaningful that Prof. Benjamin Capps developed his legal theory in connection with the cases of John Moore in the USA (*Moore* v. *Regents of the University of California* (1998) 249 Cal. Rptr. 494; 215 Cal. App. 3d 709; (1990); 271 Cal. Rptr. 146; 793 P. 2d 479; (1991) cert. denied, 111 S.Ct. 1338) and Jonathan Yearworth in the UK (*Yearworth and others* v. *North Bristol NHS Trust* [2009] EWCA Civ 37 [2010] QB 1), because he raised an important question about the future of property law in light of a growing biotechnology industry. The law traditionally does not recognize any property rights to a body, not only in Western jurisdictions, but also in other international ones, including in Japan.

2 Fundamental problems

According to Prof. Capps, reasons that we would expect to protect the integrity of the whole human are no longer persuasive when discussing use of removed body parts. In my opinion, however, we should make a legal safeguard for all aspects of the human body. After all, the question is about to whom the human body belongs. Can we have ownership of our own body or tissues—can these things be our property? What is the legal status of organs and tissues that have been separated from the body? Are they mere things or goods, or something else?

Concerning human organs, the Organ Transplantation Act (1997, revised in 2009) in Japan provides direction for their use. According to this Act, trafficking human organs is a crime (§11, §20) and therefore legally prohibited. Human tissue, however, is not mentioned. Generally speaking, we cannot permit commodification of the human body. However, at the same time we must consider the legal and ethical basis of the prohibition. What should be the legal status of an organ which has been separated from the human body, and has yet to be transplanted in another person? If somebody stole the organ, is it theft or another crime?

Compared to that of organs, the legal status of human tissues is much less clear in Japan. This raises two problems: how to use them for medical research, and how to control their commodification, especially human bodies or tissues derived from either living donors or the dead.

Prof. Jean-Pierre Baud, a legal history specialist, also raised the important issue of the legal status of the human body (Baud 1993). He pointed out the traditional divided-in-two legal system of humans or things in French law, which derived from a case of a severed hand in Roman law. What does 'My body belongs to me' mean? What is the legal status of a body part (e.g. a hand) separated from a body? Is someone who takes it without permission guilty of theft? According to Prof. Baud, such a person is not guilty. Is a person's conduct towards a donor morally acceptable provided that it does not contravene the 'harm principle?' Baud says 'Yes.'

As a rule, body parts may not be sold for profit, but may be donated gratis (as in the case of, e.g., a kidney donated for transplantation). What is the morally relevant difference between these cases? I find that Prof. Capps and Prof. Baud agree on this legal point.

On the other hand, American legal philosopher Prof. Margaret Jane Radin insisted that the human body is not property, but constitutive of personhood (Radin 1982). She felt there is 'human dignity' behind the concept of 'personal property,' and therefore it leads to market inalienability for body parts. Prof. Baud finds the concept of 'human dignity' unhelpful due to its abstraction, an opinion I disagree with. As far as I can ascertain, Prof. Capps has not taken a standpoint on 'human dignity.'

3 Medicine and the use of the human body and its tissues

Nevertheless, human tissues are more complex, especially given the distinction between restorable and unrestorable tissues. In a German case involving the destruction of frozen sperm (Bundesgerichtshof (BGH) 1993), civil liability was recognized due to infringement of 'Persönlichkeitsrecht.' (There are similarities between this case and the Yearworth suit in the UK, which also involved the destruction of sperm.) The Moore case in the USA raised other important questions about ownership: after cutting a nidus for a malignant tumor, cells were separated from the tissue and cultured, cell roots were established, and finally the patent was obtained without the patient's consent. A similar case occurred in Japan at the Jichi Medical School in 2002, where the family of the deceased claimed restoration of some specimens gathered during autopsy and preservation of the body. These new problems derive from the fact that the legal status of human tissues is less clear than that of organs.

There are two main problems relating to tissue. One is how to use it for medical research, and the other is how to control its commodification, especially in the case of human tissues derived from the dead. I believe biomaterials can be divided into four categories: 1) a part of the human body, 2) a separate part of the human body, 3) a corpse, and 4) certain types of human tissues and cells. While we could readily use restorable tissues, unrestorable tissues should only be used under some strict conditions.

4 Conclusion

In the post-genome era, it may be disadvantageous to use laws to regulate the life sciences and medicine too strictly, because this could obstruct progress. Therefore we must search for the best way to use the human body and its tissues for the good of mankind without regarding them as mere property or things.

References

Baud, J.-P. (1993). *L'affaire de la main vole: Une histoire juridique du corps*. Paris: Édition du Seuil.
Radin, M. J. (1982). 'Property and Personhood,' *Stanford Law Review*, 34: 957–1015.

6.5

Response to Commentaries
Does 'Dignity in Property' Tell Us Anything about Dignity and Bioethics?

Benjamin Capps

I am grateful to the three scholars who have taken the time to comment on my paper. I am pleased that all of us are in broad concurrence that the future of bioethics calls for a reassessment of current legal regimes with respect to access to, and use of, human tissues and cells. I think that all of us agree that the law's treatment of such entities in the countries considered (UK, USA, Germany, and Japan) is somewhat deficient; although it is most strongly stated in my own paper, where I argue that current laws, in the UK and USA at least, lack, for the most part, any ethical coherence. Since there is no criticism of the ambitions of my paper,[82] the commentaries are mainly original explorations of topics that I cover to various degrees, and I have structured this response in such a way as to draw together a central theme found in all four works: the ethical consideration of human body parts, as distinct from the body itself, requires careful reflection in terms of commodification and the dignity of the person.

In my paper, the reader will recall that I argued that the archaic reasoning of *Moore* never did provide an ethical solution to the conditions of property in human cells and tissues. My principle err was directed at the curious circumstances in which a person cannot own cells removed from their own body, yet anyone who is capable of modifying them once they are removed, can. I wrote: 'This is because it is now necessary to recognize the implications of routine cell and tissue appropriation *for the source...Moore* has always been justified in terms of the expected utility of commercial interests, and as a justification to subsume individual interests into the "good of science".' I resolved to make the point of consent the telling ethical component in the procurement of cells and tissues for research purposes (and future clinical ones); that is, I argued that society ought to allow the patient to control such transactions *as the owner of removed tissue*, and

---

[82] In the following analysis, I have often taken a critical review of the commentators' works. I hope that I have not been too uncharitable in respect to their insightful comments on my paper; and any misinterpretation on my part should be taken in the spirit of creating a debate on the subject matter, rather than a failing on the part of the commenters, who, after all, were restricted in what they could write by a rather limited word length.

therefore I set out the ethical conditions of them being a donor, or even a vendor, as I did not rule out commodification of body parts in a future market. This is an important argument, as I imagined a future in which hearts, livers, kidneys, or any other body part will be manufactured on a commercial scale and used in clinical treatment.

The rejection of rights of property in human body parts is most clearly articulated in opposition to the possibility of ownership of whole organs (the idea that the living person could be owned, of course, takes a different path in terms of the autonomy of the will—something that by definition cannot be owned).[83] It was noted in my paper, however, that human parts have become 'contested' commodities, torn between the freedom of choice to do with them as we wish (as it were, *as owners of them*) and simultaneously a concern that choices ought to be restricted to protect the integrity of what it means to be a person. In all three commentaries, dignity seemingly denotes the latter idea. Yet, in my paper, I placed dignity *within the idea of consent*, so that all that matters in an ethical transaction is that an agent *agrees* to the transfer of her cells or tissues into the possession of a researcher (I say more about this below). The consideration that 'dignity' calls for restraints upon this waiver of property rights, even though the property in question is a human body part, is therefore inconsequential. Although, I might add, the conditions under which such transfer occurs become far more ethically important.[84]

I can now respond in a little more detail to the three commentaries. Ohashi describes the human body as something of 'inviolable dignity',[85] while also admitting the scientific curiosity in the biological nature of it that drives the desire to pick at, dissect, and understand each and every part in fine detail. Perhaps because contemporary techniques in scientific enquiry allow us to reduce the body to its core bio-mechanical properties, he also writes that 'I cannot help but have reservations about applying the theories of the classical age to the problems of our time' (Ohashi in this chapter). Yet it is exactly because the lasting achievement of the Enlightenment was to ground morality in the immutable agency of persons, rather than any divine or regal law, that the features of ethical rationality persist in modern ethics. I therefore find the systematic rigour of the works of Hobbes, Kant, and Rousseau as persuasive as any contemporary works, and for this reason, I can understand the well-meaning intent to resurrect the prophetic ideas of Locke to explain our relation to property (and as I argued in my paper, this is exactly what happened in the case of *Moore*).

One will also recall that I found the explanation of Lockean property wholly unsatisfactory. I stand by this, despite Ohashi's assertion that Locke was in fact bound by creating the conditions of 'mutual benefits'. In appears to me that the authorization by

---

[83] This assumes that 'What is possessed must under the definition be a thing' (*Regina* v. *Bentham* (Appellant) UKHL 18, (2005), para. 8), and thus the living person cannot be possibly conceptualized as something which can be owned in the way that property is.

[84] I entirely agree with Brownsword on what constitutes and creates the conditions of an ethical community. He describes a community of rights (at least one that adopts a will or choice theory of rights) as one committed to the protection and promotion of individuals' rights, and in which, among other characteristics, one finds that the context that comprises such a community is a fundamental respect for the conditions that include 'elements pertaining to our wellbeing…and our freedom' (Brownsword 2009: 137).

[85] Quotes without an immediate citation should be attributed to the adjacent author's commentary. Where there is a risk of ambiguity, the author's name will appear in brackets immediately after the quote.

'all mankind' that Ohashi expects in terms of distributing property would not in fact be forthcoming, since Locke's claim is actually that property *cannot* be invalidated by proclaiming 'everybody else has an equal title to it'; explicitly, a right to property exists '*without* the consent of all his fellow-commoners' (italics added). Ohashi is quite right to state that Locke's challenge was, in part, to supplant unbounded royal power; but I maintain that Locke's ethics spoke more to the appropriation of the commons by entrepreneurialism, rather than to any distribution in terms of social equality.[86] I admit that this reading of Locke is almost entirely informed by the work of Wilmore Kendall, who argued that the nature and form of Locke's rights depend upon social needs *as defined by society* (Kendall 1941). Kendall's Locke not only rejected any notion that individuals have rights superior to society's demands, but in addition, he found Locke had embraced majoritarianism as the means by which society should order and express its interests and desires. Thus, putting the two together, I argued that the *Two Treatises* directly supports utilitarian-grounded monopolization (but, unlike Kendall, I did not argue that this is necessarily what Locke intended, nor that this is the only proper reading of Locke), and I rather disparagingly concluded that this antiquated idea expresses the kinds of privileges that are afforded to scientists to unjustly exclude patients from transactions today.

Yet such disagreements between Ohashi and myself are trifling, and I find that his later comments are far more valuable in terms of the future of bioethics: the question of the value of 'potential goods', and thus whether and how we convert objects into property. It is here that the terms of defining dignity become particularly important, because among the many conceptions of dignity to be found, one stands out in particular in the property debate: the dignity of the human body and the rejection of its commodification.

Ohashi explains that 'we must first decide whether these are the sorts of things that may be viewed as property at all, and if so, who are the candidates for being potentially entitled to assert a right to such property' (Ohashi in this chapter), and this, I think, indicates the reasons why a disassociation between the body and its parts is often resisted: our bodies exist as discrete entities outside the *invention* of property, with obvious implications for what our bodies can be subjected to, and parts of it are not easily 'reinvented' in terms of ownership. Dignity, therefore, signals the 'visible wholeness, as well as the invisible and intangible parts' of the human being (Ohashi in this chapter). Vossenkuhl likewise explains that German property law 'only refer[s] to things while the body *and* the body parts of living humans do not count as things' (Vossenkuhl in this chapter; italics added), citing that such legal protection concerns the 'life and dignity of the person'. (Kai is also supportive of the idea of 'human dignity' 'behind [grounding?] the concept of "personal property" [and] ...market inalienability' (Kai in this chapter).) Elsewhere, this has been called the *inherent* concept of dignity, but in a peculiar sense it is an exclusive value intrinsic to human beings (Gewirth 1992). This last clause is important because it attaches moral worth to *all* human beings, including non-paradigmatic

---

[86] Cf. 'He gave it to the use of the Industrious and Rational ...not the Fancy or Covetousness of the Quarrelsome and Contentious' (Locke 1988: Second Treatise, Chapter V, s. 34). On the Lockean rights of capitalist accumulation, see Kendall 1941. And on the use of Lockean rights to use 'the moral dignity of labour' to give powerful moral embellishment to the exploitation of peoples, see Dunn (1969: 72).

rights holders, such as human embryos and fetuses. Furthermore, by attaching dignity in this sense to human worth (often in the terms of Kantian morality), one can come to the conclusion that the commercialization of the human body is an affront to dignity (by putting a price on something that is beyond price) (see Brownsword 2003).

But my reservation to such an approach is that dignity now threatens to become a definitional stop, terminating any further discussion on things that Radin calls 'contested commodities'. In my paper I went to great lengths to avoid conflating the human body, organs, and cells (and tissues), and thus I adopted Radin's idea exactly because cases of ownership of body parts (rather than persons) are often contested, and it is plausible that property disputes over the ownership of *parts* is likely to increase as a (likely commercial) industry develops in which organs are produced *entirely* separate from the human body. As far as I am concerned, dignity cannot do the work of regulating such an industry, because it relies on the relationship of such entities with the inviolable self (the human body). A lab-grown heart simply does not have a body from whence it came! Such 'artificial' organs will become instrumental in future health care (what has been called 'regenerative medicine'), and moreover, commercial interests are inevitable in an industry of body part replacement. I suspect, therefore, that it will proceed under the terms of contracts and commodities, which will be rather separate from the practice (and ethics) of donor–recipient organ transplantation.

If there is a point of property, it is to ensure that consent is primary to any transaction between parties.[87] Yet I also wrote that if an object can be properly considered as property, then the kinds of rights attached to it will be determined by an underlying moral principle. My intention in the paper, then, was to show that *Moore*, by entirely bypassing this condition on the grounds that to do so would benefit science and industry, was not only ethically contentious, but because it concluded that ownership of human cells was only possible after they had been modified in some significant way, it relied on a perplexing, and ultimately incoherent, argument that would have significant implications for the future of property in human body parts. The scientific privilege, I argued, came at the expense of the rights of the patient; a conclusion that was informed by the entirely research-unrelated case of *Yearworth*. In that case, the judge argued that ownership of human cells (sperm) was possible regardless of the application of skill (that the patient *could be the owner of products of their body*), and to this extent, the plaintiffs were capable of a claim in tort. I did not intend to show that no benefits should accrue to the industrious researcher that used human tissue (as long as they asked for it!), nor that the patient should dictate the future of any research that she donated tissue to.

However, it is important to note that if consent is not needed then dignity is redundant. I argued that dignity was not inherent, but instead was to be framed within autonomy, or, as Beyleveld and Brownsword argue, dignity in biolaw appeals to an idea of empowerment (Beyleveld and Brownsword 2001). They argue that dignity as empowerment is the basis of legal barriers to pursuing (or inflicting on others) certain goals that are contrary to dignity—it is a theory of rights as positive and negative claims. This

---

[87] Property simply evinces control of an object, that might include (among others) a right to use, right to transfer or sell, and right to exclude others.

concept of rights is also hinted in the judgment in *Yearworth* (without itself using the conceptually troublesome concept of 'dignity') by formulating property in terms of control. Agents, if they can claim to have proper property rights in respect to an object, can also be authors as to its fate (within the bounds of any laws).[88] This means they can not only donate (or even sell) cells or tissue to a researcher upon request, but may also exclude access or further use should they wish to do so. The kind of (mis)appropriation sanctioned by *Moore*, therefore, would be ethically precluded. But, in the same way that one cannot extend control to something they have no ownership rights to, one cannot extend control to an organ that did not originate from their body;[89] and in this respect, an industry-conditioned heart—one created from a genetic 'blank slate', entirely grown *ex vivo*, and without an obvious link to any individual—does not raise the spectre of dignity.

My final comments are on the categorization of body parts. Vossenkuhl writes that some degree of 'permanence' is necessary for body parts to become things (that is, they may become property once the separation from the body is irreversible). Yet the ambiguity of permanence remains a problem, and he indicates (and I concur) that the trepidation in respect to leftover body parts transferring to the ownership of a researcher may lie in the protection of personal data and privacy. Kai broadly agrees with my own conceptual separation of the human body from body parts, placing emphasis on the possibility of commodification of the latter according to its 'restorable' (replaceable?) character. Yet I am already wary of dissociating ownership in terms of what an object is. As I pointed out, for instance, stem cell science has already irrevocably changed the idea of reproductive and non-reproductive tissues (thus, I argued, that narrowing *Yearworth* in respect to its legal applicability to only gametes is naive). I am content to agree with basic separation for the time being, but I see such categorization as becoming redundant as the production of body parts becomes a scaled-up industry.

I am aware that I have not addressed every point raised by the commentators. Any neglect on my part is because the issues they raise demand a more lengthy discussion than can be done here. I want to conclude by expressing my sincere and warm thanks to all three commentators who have taken the time to read my paper and to contribute fair-minded discussions to the debate. In my reply I have certainly not thought that I am saying the last words on any of these weighty issues, and I hope that all four contributions to this book, and my response here, encourage further discussion and an enlightened exchange of ideas on the issues of the future of bioethics.

References

Beyleveld, D., and Brownsword, R. (2000). 'My Body, My Body Parts, My Property?' *Health Care Analysis*, 8: 87–99.

---

[88] For example, the men in *Yearworth* were only permitted to determine the fate of their sperm within the conditions set out in the Human Fertilisation and Embryology Act (at the time of the case, 1998; revised in 2008).

[89] This suggests that one *can* own one's body; see Beyleveld and Brownsword 2000.

Beyleveld, D., and Brownsword, R. (2001). *Human Dignity in Bioethics and Biolaw*. Oxford: Oxford University Press.

Brownsword, R. (2009). 'Regulating Human Enhancement: Things Can Only Get Better?' *Law, Innovation, and Technology*, 1:125–52.

Brownsword, R. (2003). 'Bioethics Today, Bioethics Tomorrow: Stem Cell Research and the 'Dignitarian Alliance." *Notre Dame Journal of Law, Ethics, and Public Policy*, 17:15–51.

Dunn, J. (1969). 'The Politics of Locke in England and America in the Eighteenth Century', in J. Yolton (ed.), *John Locke: Problems and Perspectives: A Collection of New Essays*. Cambridge: Cambridge University Press, 45–80.

Gewirth, A. (1992). 'Human Dignity as the Basis of Rights', in M. Meyer and W. Parent (eds), *The Constitution of Rights: Human Dignity and American Values*. Ithica, NY: Cornell University Press, 10–28.

Kai, K. (2014). 'Legal Status of the Human Body and Tissues', in A. Akabayashi (ed.), *The Future of Bioethics: International Dialogues*. Oxford: Oxford University Press, 275–7.

Kendall, W. (1941). *John Locke and the Doctrine of Majority-Rule*. Urbana, IL: University of Illinois Press.

Locke, J. (1988). *Two Treatises of Government*, edited by P. Laslett, Cambridge: Cambridge University Press.

Ohashi, K. (2014). 'But Which Body: Body of Labor, or Body of Anatomy?' in A. Akabayashi (ed.), *The Future of Bioethics: International Dialogues*. Oxford: Oxford University Press, 264–7.

Vossenkuhl, W. (2014). 'The Non-Ownership Thesis: A German Perspective', in A. Akabayashi (ed.), *The Future of Bioethics: International Dialogues*. Oxford: Oxford University Press, 268–74.

7.1

Primary Topic Article

Genetic Research to Facilitate Personalized Medicine: Ethical and Policy Challenges

Karen J. Maschke

The medical model of genomic-based personalized medicine is based on several expectations: that many genetic variations associated with disease risk will have clinical significance; that genetic risk is meaningfully different from other health risks; that when given their genetic risk information, individuals will make meaningful changes in their diet, exercise, and lifestyle behaviors to mitigate their genetic disease risk; and that physicians will use genetic risk information to guide medical decision-making (Guttmacher and Collins 2003; Burke and Psaty 2007). Many commentators raise concerns that the expectations about the impact of genetics on medicine and health are exaggerated (Evans et al. 2011). However, there is emerging evidence that some genetic information will have an impact on clinical decision-making (Guttmacher and Collins 2003; Burke and Psaty 2007). For instance, genetic risk information about specific cancers and about the metabolism of certain drugs has contributed to the medical care of individual patients (Antoniou et al. 2003; Goldstein, Tate, and Sisodiya 2003). Nonetheless, many hurdles stand in the way of achieving the genomic revolution in medicine that many commentators predict is "just around the corner" (Evans, Kotchetkova, and Langer 2009).

This paper examines two large-scale genetic research initiatives whose ultimate goal is to facilitate the integration of genetic research results into ongoing clinical care: the Coriell Personalized Medicine Collaborative (CPMC) and the ClinSeq project. Of interest here is the "sociotechnical architecture" of these two research initiatives. In her analysis of direct-to-consumer (DTC) genetic tests and breast cancer genetic testing in the US and UK, Shobita Parthasarathy used the concept of sociotechnical architecture to show how "providing access to testing, analyzing genetic material, and conveying test results" influenced the utility of those technologies and "the distribution of expertise in the medical system" (Parthasarathy 2010).

A key "architectural design" of the CPMC and ClinSeq is that they "return" some genetic research results to study participants. With few exceptions, researchers typically have not informed individuals about their genetic test information obtained in the research context. The primary reason for a no-return approach is that most genetic research results have uncertain clinical significance (Ravitsky and Wilfond 2006; Wolf et al. 2012). Yet scientists are discovering that some gene–disease associations have clinical significance, and they expect to uncover additional gene–disease associations as well as gene–environment interactions that could affect a medical diagnosis or the prevention or treatment of a disease (Beskow et al. 2001).

The challenge for the genetic research enterprise is how to shift from the standard no-return approach regarding genetic research results to an approach that facilitates the goals of genomic-based personalized medicine. The CPMC and ClinSeq are testing a conditional-return approach, meaning that some, but not all genetic research results will be offered to research participants. The sociotechnical architecture of the CPMC and ClinSeq reflects an attempt to show that the conditional-return, gatekeeping approach to genetic research results 1) adequately responds to the ethical claims that some results should be offered to individuals whose DNA was analyzed, 2) satisfies individuals' desire "for their own genetic information," and 3) fosters participant and physician use of genetic information to guide personal and medical decision-making, respectively.

Testing the conditional-return approach

The Coriell Personalized Medicine Collaborative

The CPMC is an initiative of the non-profit Coriell Institute for Medical Research in Camden, New Jersey and includes hospital partners Cooper University Hospital in southern New Jersey; Fox Chase Cancer Center in Philadelphia, Pennsylvania; and The Ohio State University Medical Center in Columbus, Ohio. Additional partners include the software and database companies Virtua Health and Helix Health. As a longitudinal, observational study, the CPMC involves three cohorts of adults 18 years and older: a community cohort recruited from the general population; a cancer cohort that comprises individuals with breast and prostate cancer; and a chronic disease cohort composed of individuals with congestive heart failure and hypertension (Keller et al. 2010). Demographic, family history, and lifestyle information is collected from participants, including details about their medical history and use of medications. Participants also complete a short questionnaire that assesses how knowledgeable they are about genetics and genetic risk information. The goals of the CMPC are to determine the best mechanism for providing genetic research results to participants and their physicians, to study how genetic research information is used in a real-world clinical setting, and to find correlations between genetic variants and disease risk using observational data (Corriell Personalized Medicine Collaborative website).

The CPMC consent materials inform prospective participants that the multiple genotyping platforms the project uses will yield a wide array of genetic information, but that they will not receive all of the genetic information obtained from analysis of their DNA (Corriell Personalized Medicine Collaborative website). Instead, they will be offered genetic information that a gatekeeper decides to make available to them. By enrolling in the study, individuals agree to be recontacted to learn what results are available, but have the option not to receive that information. The consent form includes opt-in choices for sharing results with their physician, participating in additional surveys, learning about other studies, releasing their DNA sample and/ or genetic data to other researchers, and releasing their recent medical records to the CPMC. As of April 2010, 4,619 participants were enrolled in the initiative (Gollust et al. 2012).

In early 2011, the CMPC announced that at the Ohio State site research results will be entered into participants' electronic medical records (Coriell Institute Press Release 2011). Up to 35 cardiologists and primary care physicians and 1,800 of their patients diagnosed with congestive heart failure or hypertension will be involved. The goals for this part of the initiative are to learn how likely doctors will use their patients' genetic risk information to guide clinical decision-making, and if they use such information how they do so. An additional goal for returning genetic research results to study participants is to "engage patients to become more actively involved in their own healthcare management" (Coriell Institute Press Release 2011).

The genetic results gatekeeper for the CMPC is the Informed Cohort Oversight Board (ICOB). Research results the ICOB deems returnable are "genetic variants of interest," i.e. variants that are "potentially medically actionable." The CPMC defines potentially medically actionable as a "condition for which the risk is likely to be mitigated by individual action (behavior or lifestyle) or by medical action (screening, preventative treatment or early intervention)" (Keller et al. 2010: 6). "CPMC staff members curate the peer-reviewed scientific and medical literature as well as medical society statements" (Keller et al. 2010: 4) to compile a list of gene–disease associations for the ICOB to review. The minimum criteria for determining which gene–disease associations to place on the list include evidence that a gene variant has "a documented association with the disease in a moderately sized study (defined as having 500 or more subjects) with replication in one or more cohorts of the same race, either replicated within a single peer-reviewed publication or published in a separate study" (Stack et al. 2011: 132).

CPMC staff members present their recommendations to the ICOB, which meets twice a year to review the recommended list and to determine whether "the candidate health conditions are potentially actionable" (Stack et al. 2011: 133). For results the ICOB decides are returnable, CPMC staff members develop risk reports that are offered to study participants who complete a required web-based questionnaire (Keller et al. 2010: 6). As of July 2011, the ICOB approved the release of genetic risk information for 16 complex disease conditions: age-related macular degeneration; breast cancer; bladder cancer; chronic obstructive pulmonary disease; colon cancer; coronary artery disease; inflammatory bowel disease; hemochromatosis; lupus; melanoma; obesity; prostate cancer; rheumatoid arthritis; testicular cancer; type 1 diabetes and type 2 diabetes. The ICOB has also approved the release of results regarding the gene variant associated with response to Clopidogrel (Plavix), a drug used to help prevent blood clots in patients who are at risk for a heart attack or stroke (Christman 2011, no page number).

The ClinSeq project

ClinSeq is a project of the US National Human Genome Research Institute. ClinSeq is designed to develop an infrastructure "to acquire and analyze genome sequence from individual research participants," to pilot a large-scale medical sequence study that will "elucidate the genetic architecture underlying human traits," and to "establish approaches for informed consent and the return of genetic information" (Biesecker et al. 2009: 1665–6). The goal is to enroll up to 1,000 participants. The project's initial approach is to sequence a large set of candidate genes implicated in coronary artery disease, with the long-term goal to sequence the whole genome of every participant (Biesecker et al. 2009). As of June 2011, the project had sequenced the whole exomes of 250 candidate genes in 700 participants, most of whom are healthy volunteers (Heger 2011).

Like the CPMC, ClinSeq uses an opt-in/opt-out consent approach regarding research results: by enrolling in the study, individuals opt in to be informed about what genetic research results are available, but can opt out to receive their results. ClinSeq uses an independent data monitoring board referred to as a "sequence variant review panel" to determine which genetic variants are potentially clinically significant (Biesecker et al. 2009: 1667). Unlike the CPMC, the ClinSeq project has not provided detailed information about the criteria this gatekeeping committee uses to determine what results are returnable.

The CMPC and ClinSeq motivation surveys

The ClinSeq researchers recognize that "the translation of genomics into useful and cost-effective clinical care will require years of translational research" (Facio et al. 2011: 1). Thus, early-phase translational studies like the CPMC and ClinSeq are proof-of-principle studies that examine the "introduction of new technologies to normal volunteers and carefully defined populations" (Facio et al. 2011: 1213). What genetic results participants want, how they interpret and use those results, and whether and how physicians use genetic information about their patients are the key questions these initiatives are designed to investigate. Findings from the first set of surveys each initiative conducted with their participants reveal tensions and contradictions that have implications for the conditional-return approach and the integration of genetic research results into ongoing clinical care.

Both the CPMC and ClinSeq conducted surveys to learn what motivated individuals to participate in these research initiatives. Most of the 305 respondents in the CPMC's motivation study (Gollust et al. 2012) were over 50 years old; over half were women, and nearly half had received graduate or professional school training after obtaining an undergraduate college degree. Nearly 90 percent of the respondents were non-Hispanic whites. When asked whether curiosity about their genes as a motivator for participating was very important, somewhat important or not important, 81 percent said very important, 16 percent said somewhat important, and 3 percent said not important. Using the same response scale, 78 percent of respondents said finding out about diseases for which they were at risk was very important to them and 78 percent also rated finding out what they could do to improve their health as very important. When asked about motivation to participate because they wanted to help others, 56 percent of participants said helping others was an important factor and 39 percent said it was a somewhat important factor; 5 percent of participants said helping others was not an important factor (Gollust et al. 2012).

The sociodemographic characteristics of respondents in ClinSeq's motivation study (Facio et al. 2011) are similar to those of respondents in the CPMC's survey, though the number of men and women in the ClinSeq survey was about even. The ClinSeq survey also collected information about respondents' income level. Sixty-seven percent of the 313 respondents earned more than $100,000 a year. When asked about their reasons for enrolling in the parent study, 56 percent said to get personal health information and 44 percent responded in ways that reflected altruistic reasons (Facio et al. 2011).

Both the CPMC and ClinSeq are studying how participants interpret genetic risk information and how they use the genetic research results the initiatives give them. Although the ClinSeq project has yet to collect this information from its participants, the CPMC motivation survey included questions about what participants planned to do with their genetic research results. Ninety percent of respondents said they would likely share the results with their physicians and fifty-eight percent said they were very likely to do so (Facio et al. 2011). Yet preliminary data from a separate survey conducted six months after 245 participants received some research results revealed that only 15 percent had shared the genetic risk information with their physicians (Gollust et al. 2012).

Genetic research results and the goals of personalized medicine

Given what is known at this time about the CPMC and ClinSeq, there is reason to be cautiously optimistic as well as concerned about the conditional-return approach. Both initiatives succeeded in developing an expert gatekeeping committee that determines what genetic research results will be offered to study participants, though little is known about the criteria and process the ClinSeq project uses to determine what results are deemed returnable. However, at least one commentator has criticized the CPMC for returning only results that meet its definition of "actionable," that involve risk estimates based on only a single genetic variant per disease, and that uses a risk metric of relative rather than absolute risk. According to Daniel MacArthur, the CPMC's conditional-return approach is condescending because it adopts the clinical "need to know" approach to medical information. MacArthur also contends it is "madness" to provide risk estimates for a single genetic variant per disease, and that every DTC genetic testing company aggregates risks across all known disease-associated variants (MacArthur 2011).

The CPMC and ClinSeq also succeeded in showing that many individuals will enroll in genetic research initiatives that use a conditional-return approach. However, given that the "early adopters" of personal genomics who enrolled in these initiatives were overwhelming white, highly educated individuals, it remains to be seen whether individuals from different sociodemographic backgrounds will undergo genetic testing—either in the research or clinical context—to learn about and act on their genetic risk information. Moreover, misperceptions and unrealistic expectations about genetic risk information of some of the highly educated participants in the CPMC survey are also cause for concern. Overall, 32 percent of respondents "expressed unrealistic expectations" about the health benefits of genetic risk information and many, though fewer, conflated genetic testing "for common complex diseases with that for single-gene disorders and reproductive genetics" (Gollust et al. 2012: 28).

Although many participants in the CPMC and ClinSeq expressed altruistic reasons for enrolling in the parent studies, the primary reason for participating was to receive personal health information. Wanting health-related information is not in itself problematic. Yet some individuals who want probabilistic genetic risk information about complex diseases might misconstrue such information as a diagnosis of those conditions. And since the CPMC findings mirror those of other studies showing that few individuals alter their behaviors after receiving genetic information about an increased risk for one or more diseases (Bloss, Schork, and Topol 2011), there is reason for caution in interpreting individuals' desire for "personal genomics" as meaning anything more than information consumption. For the goals of genomic-based personalized medicine to be achieved, information consumption will have to translate into behavioral changes on the part of patients, as well as physicians.

With regard to the return of genetic research results, both initiatives either implicitly (CPMC) or explicitly (ClinSeq) claim that they give participants control over their genetic information. Yet both initiatives minimize the fact that they only give participants control over the information a gatekeeping committee decides to offer them. At least one commentator contends that the gatekeeper approach is paternalistic and fails to satisfy ethics principles of autonomy and respect for persons because research participants do not have access to all of their genetic information obtained from analysis of their DNA (MacArthur 2011). Moreover, several studies indicate that many people want all of their genetic research results even if the results have uncertain clinical significance (Wilson et al. 2010; Bollinger et al. 2012; Harris et al. 2012). As one researcher points out, "most people don't make the distinction between medically actionable and medically not actionable that the medical and research communities keep trying to make" (Couzin-Frankel 2011: 331).

Other genetic research initiatives are using the conditional-return approach, and several consensus groups support returning some, if not all, genetic research results to individual participants (Wolf et al. 2008; Fabsitz et al. 2010; Wolf et al. 2012). What remains to be seen is whether people will continue to enroll in genetic research initiatives like the CPMC and ClinSeq that offer participants only the results a gatekeeper decides are returnable, and whether participants who receive their genetic results use that information to change their behaviors to help prevent disease and improve their health.

References

Antoniou, A. et al. (2003). "Average Risks of Breast and Ovarian Cancer Associated with *BRCA1* or *BRCA2* Mutations Detected in Case Series Unselected for Family History: A Combined Analysis of 22 Studies," *American Journal of Human Genetics*, 72(5): 1117–30.

Morton College Library Cicero, ILL

Beskow, L. M. et al. (2001). "Informed Consent for Population-Based Research Involving Genetics," *Journal of the American Medical Association*, 286(18): 2315–21.

Biesecker, L. G. et al. (2009). "The Clinseq Project: Piloting Large-Scale Genome Sequencing for Research in Genomic Medicine," *Genome Research*, 19:1665–74.

Bloss, C. S., Schork, N. J., and Topol, E. J. (2011). "Effect of Direct-to-Consumer Genomewide Profiling to Assess Disease Risk," *New England Journal Of Medicine*, 364:524–34.

Bollinger, J. M. et al. (2012). "Public Preferences Regarding the Return of Individual Genetic Research Results: Findings from a Qualitative Focus Group Study," *Genetics in Medicine*, 12:451–7.

Burke, W., and Psaty, B. M. (2007). "Personalized Medicine in the Era of Genomics," *JAMA*, 298(14):1682–4.

Christman, M. (2011). "Utility of Genome Information in Clinical Care," *Coriell Personalized Medicine Collaborative*, July 19, http://www.iom.edu/~/media/Files/Activity Files/Research/GenomicBasedResearch/2011-JUL-19/9 ChristmanIOM71911.pdf (accessed January 17, 2013).

Corriell Institute Press Release (2011). "Patients' Genome Information to Be Included in Electronic Medical Records," February 8, 2011, http://www.coriell.org/media-center/press-releases/patients-genomic-information-to-be-included-in-emrs (accessed January 18, 2013).

Corriell Personalized Medicine Collaborative. http://cpmc1.coriell.org/ (accessed December 12, 2012)

Couzin-Frankel, J. (2011). "What Would You Do?" *Science*, 331:662–5.

Evans, J. P. et al. (2011). "Deflating the Genomic Bubble," *Science*, 331:861–2.

Evans, R., Kotchetkova, I., and Langer, S. (2009). "Just Around the Corner: Rhetorics of Progress and Promise in Genetic Research," *Public Understanding of Science*, 18(1): 43–59.

Fabsitz, R. R. et al. (2010). "Ethical and Practical Guidelines for Reporting Genetic Research Results to Study Participants: Updated Guidelines from an NHLBI Working Group," *Circulation Cardiovascular Genetics*, 3:574–80.

Facio, F. M. et al. (2011). "Motivators for Participation in a Whole-Genome Sequencing Study: Implications for Translational Genomics Research," *European Journal of Human Genetics*, 19(12): 1213–17.

Goldstein, D. B., Tate, S. K., and Sisodiya, S. M. (2003). "Pharmacogenetics Goes Genomic," *Nature Reviews Genetics*, 4(12): 937–47.

Gollust, S. E. et al. (2012). "Motivations and Perceptions of Early Adopters of Personalized Genomics: Perspectives from Research Participants," *Public Health Genomics*, 15(1): 22–30.

Guttmacher, A. E., and Collins, F. S. (2003). "Welcome to the Genomic Era," *New England Journal of Medicine*, 349(1): 996–8.

Harris, E. D. et al. (2012). "The Beliefs, Motivations, and Expectations of Parents Who Have Enrolled Their Children in a Genetic Biorepository," *Genetics in Medicine*, 14(3): 330–7.

Heger, M. (2011). "NHGRI's Clinseq Project Moves into Exome, Whole-Genome Sequencing on Illumina GA," Genomeweb, June 8, http://www.genomeweb.com/sequencing/nhgris-clinseq-project-moves-exome-whole-genome-sequencing-illumina-ga (accessed April 9, 2012).

Keller, M. A. et al (2010). "Coriell Personalized Medicine Collaborative: A Prospective Study of the Utility of Personalized Medicine," *Personalized Medicine*, 7(3):301–17.

MacArthur, D. (2011). "When 'Cautious' Means 'Useless'," *Wired Science Blog*, http://www.wired.com/wiredscience/2011/02/when-cautious-means-useless/ (accessed April 5, 2012).

Parthasarathy, S. (2010). "Assessing the Social Impact of Direct-to-Consumer Genetic Testing: Understanding Sociotechnical Architectures," *Genetics in Medicine*, 12(9): 544–7.

Ravitsky, V., and Wilfond, B. S. (2006). "Disclosing Individual Genetic Results to Research Participants," *American Journal of Bioethics*, 6:8–17.

Stack, C. B. et al. (2011). "Genetic Risk Estimation In the Coriell Personalized Medicine Collaborative," *Genetics in Medicine*, 13(2): 131–9.

Wilson, S. E. et al. (2010). "Understanding Preferences for Disclosure of Individual Biomarker Results among Participants in a Longitudinal Birth Cohort," *Journal of Medical Ethics*, 36:736–40.

Wolf, S. M. et al. (2008). "Managing Incidental Findings in Human Subjects Research: Analysis and Recommendations," *Journal of Law Medicine and Ethics*, 36:219–48.

Wolf, S. M. et al. (2012). "Managing Incidental Findings and Research Results in Genomic Research Involving Biobanks and Archived Datasets," *Genetics in Medicine*, 14(4): 361–84.

7.2

Commentary

Genetic Information: Direct to Consumers or Gatekeeping?

Soraj Hongladarom

In her paper, Maschke presents us with a snapshot of two initiatives in the US that collect samples of genetic data from the general population with an eye toward finding solutions that would be useful to clinical care. The main ethical concern she raises is about how this information is going to be used by the consumers. She presents two options, one with the "direct-to-consumer" approach where people can buy their own genetic information which they can use as they see fit and the other with a more conservative approach where "experts" decide which genetic information is most appropriate for the people so that they can make the use of the information for their health purposes. Maschke favors the latter approach, which she calls the "pull" approach as the clinical setting draws upon the genetic information that experts deem relevant and interesting enough. On the contrary the "push" approach favored by companies such as 23andMe and others would seem, according to Maschke, to be offering individualized genetic information to the clinical setting too early.

In this short reply paper, I would like to discuss Maschke's preference of the pull approach and evaluate how this approach fares with the principle of individual autonomy and privacy (Stein 2011). Furthermore, I will also touch upon the question of how individualized or personalized medicine would help or hinder what I believe to be the more pressing problem in the developing world, that of equity in access to medical care. In the context of poorer countries in the developing world, genetic technologies might be of better use when they are tailored, not to individual differences or variations, but in finding possible traits that could occur throughout a group of population. Instead of tailoring medicine to individual *persons*, the technology should be focused on customization at the level of individual groups. This will go further toward reducing the inequity that is still extant in the world today.

Maschke's basic concern with the "push" approach to individual genetic information is that some information that has a minimal role in the clinical setting, or is too early to be of any effective use, might be offered to the health-care provider who does not yet know what to do with it. However, this problem could be solved also by providing the consumer or the general population with adequate knowledge of what their genetic data could do at the moment, or the health-care provider and the company selling genetic data analyses could inform the people what kind of genetic data is useful and what kind is not so useful in the clinical setting. The fact that there are companies that sell results of individual genetic data analyses back to the individuals who might rush the information to the health-care provider should not be used as a basis for preferring the other approach which is much more controlled. Moreover, there are also other reasons beyond health care as to why people send in their tissue samples for genetic analysis. People might want to know their ancestry or their anthropological position within the grand scheme of human genetic relationships, for example.

Maschke also fears that individuals who obtain their own genetic profiling might be scared, if the profiling happens to indicate some chance of their having a disease in the future, that this is an indication that they will actually have the disease. But again this can be solved rather straightforwardly by giving the population a training program where they learn about risks posed by genetic profiling and their probability and the undeniable role of environmental factors. Again there seems to be little reason to do away with the "push" approach. Maschke also notes that commentators have criticized the gate-keeping approach as being "paternalistic" as it takes important decisions away from the individuals whose genetic information is in question. There is nothing wrong with the notion that in some areas the judgments of experts who are genuinely and thoroughly knowledgeable should be respected, but those same experts could also inform people about what kind of their own genetic information is clinically relevant and what kind is not quite relevant. Instead of deciding things on their own, these experts could instead provide basic knowledge about genetic information, susceptibility to diseases, and other relevant topics so that people can make informed choices about their own health and their bodies by themselves.

Perhaps the psychology behind the popularity of companies such as 23andMe is that people naturally want to know something about themselves. This is the same psychology behind the popularity of astrology and horoscopes. People read horoscopes in order to learn what will happen to them in the near future, or what they are like, what their characters are, and so on. In the same vein, people are also attracted to genetic information companies because they would like to know what they are really like, what percentage of this or that ethnicity is in their blood, and so on. There does not seem to be anything inherently wrong about this. It is true that information contained in horoscopes is notoriously unreliable; this is very common knowledge. But what people would need to know, and it is the task of genomics experts to let them know, is that personalized genetic information is in a way not much better than astrological predictions in successfully predicting the future. Certainly there is a certain kind of genetic information that is much more certain, such as the information that one has the gene for thalassemia or Huntington's disease, but most information that people are interested in is not of that kind. Furthermore, there are a lot of environmental factors that can influence whether one's genetic predisposition to get a certain disease might be realized or not. And these environmental factors are very difficult, if not impossible, to control. The uncertainty of one's genetic predisposition to get a disease could be *less* than one's astrological predisposition to get the same disease, but since one almost always treats astrological information with a grain of salt, there is no reason why genetic information should not be treated the same way.

Another topic I would like to cover concerns the role of the technology of personalized medicine in alleviating the problem of inequity in access to health care across the world (Lunshof 2005; Pang 2009). One thing that can be achieved through technology is that genetic traits in a population group could eventually be found that are linked to certain forms of diseases for which methods of treatment could then be found. There are of course many ethical concerns in this attempt, a problem well attested in the literature, such as ones dealing with the Icelandic population. However, if such genetic traits can be found, then the ethical concerns can be overcome if the obtained information is used not as a means toward discrimination but in order to find a way to prevent or treat diseases arising from those conditions. Instead of the group being discriminated against as a result of their possessing some genetic predisposition (if it is actually established that the group does possess the disposition that makes them susceptible), the group should be given priority in resource allocation and other areas so that their conditions are given immediate attention from the policy level downward. In short, instead of focusing resources and effort on narrowing medicine down to the personal level, it might instead be more effective in the context of developing countries to focus at the level of individual groups. And how groups are defined also vary; not only should genetic groups be given attention to, but socio-economic or cultural groups such as the poor, the marginalized, or the underprivileged should also be given priority too. Instead of personalizing medicine to individual persons (many of whom are well-to-do persons in the West), medicine should also be "personalized" to individual groups not only defined by genetics but also by social factors.

References

Lunshof, J. (2005). "Personalized Medicine: How Much Can We Afford? A Bioethics Perspective," *Personalized Medicine*, 2(1): 43–7.

Pang, T. (2009). "Pharmacogenomics and Personalized Medicine for the Developing World— Too Soon or Just-in-Time? A Personal View from the World Health Organization," *Current Pharmacogenomics and Personalized Medicine*, 7(3): 149–57.

Stein, R. A. (2011). "Direct-to-Consumer Genetic Testing," in S. Hongladarom (ed), *Genomics and Bioethics: Interdisciplinary Perspectives, Technologies and Advancements*. Hershey, PA: IGI-Global, 51–84.

7.3

Commentary

The Ethical and Social Aspects of Genetic Information and Personalized Medical Genomics

Koji Ota

Genomics was developed to facilitate biomedical studies and basic life science research, and for use in clinical applications. It involves large-scale genetic investigations, such as the sequencing of thousands of human genomes. Such studies are being conducted by the CPMC and the ClinSeq project. These projects integrate large-scale genetic investigations into clinical applications so that relevant genetic information can be returned to participants and clinicians responsible for participant health. These projects represent pioneering studies in personalized genomic medicine and translational research.

Maschke discusses the ethical and social considerations of such projects. She focuses on how genomic information is conveyed from investigators to participants (whose genetic material is sampled) and clinicians responsible for participant health. Indeed, these two programs have "gatekeepers" who select genetic information to be disclosed to participants and clinicians. This selection is based on the assumption that the returned genetic information will aid participants in health-care decision-making.

The process of genomic information return, as Maschke points out, poses several challenges. First, there may be a disconnect between the genetic information returned to participants and the information they hope to acquire. In particular, it is unclear whether participants understand the distinction between medically significant genetic information and other information. Indeed, they may seek information other than that selected by the gatekeepers. Second, even if participants receive their genetic information, it may not be reflected in their health-care decisions. Consistent with this, only a small proportion (15 percent) of CPMC participants actually shared the results with their physicians, despite the fact that most participants expressed an intention to do so (Gollust et al. 2012). Moreover, participants who underwent a commercial genetic risk assessment test did not exhibit short-term changes in health-care behavior (Bloss, Schork, and Topol 2011).

These discrepancies suggest that the mere development of a procedure for genetic information return, one of the objectives of personalized genomic medicine, may not contribute to the perception of disease risks and alterations in health-care behavior.

The first type of dissociation indicates that participants do not always correctly perceive disease risks upon receiving their genetic information. Even when relevant information is selected for return by the gatekeepers, participants may seek other information irrelevant to disease risks and be content with the mere possession of their own genetic information. The second type of dissociation indicates that the actions of participants do not always reflect the returned genetic information. Even if they correctly perceive disease risks, their behavior is not always altered by such perceptions, suggesting that they lack substantial motivation, or active and practical knowledge, to use the medical information. Thus, although necessary, the return of participant information appears insufficient to achieve the goals of personalized medical genomics.

In light of this, strategies must be developed to incorporate social dimensions into these projects. First, a deeper investigation into participant psychology is required. To develop the social architectural framework of personalized genomic medicine, identifying the conditions that do (or do not) motivate participants to act on their genetic information will be important. This can be carried out in the form of a self-evaluation of health-care behavior as well as social background (e.g. education level), which may determine how participants incorporate genetic knowledge into their behavior. Second, promoting scientific literacy in genetics and medicine may improve the perception of disease risks and enable participants to deal appropriately with the returned information. This would include providing participants a biological perspective of the value of genetic information in disease risk prediction. This type of knowledge is important, as reflected in the fact that two-thirds of surveyed CPMC participants had "unrealistic expectations" of health-related benefits from their genetic information assessment (Gollust et al. 2012).

If the goal of personalized medical genomics is to alter participant health-care behavior as well as biologically explore the genetic basis of diseases, the development of a social architecture cannot be ignored. In reporting the framework of the ClinSeq project, Biesecker et al. (2009) conceptualize large-scale genetics in three dimensions: number of participants, genome breadth, and clinical data. While ideal projects cover all three dimensions, this is impractical at present. Several ongoing projects focus on only one or two of these dimensions. For example, whole-genome sequencing of an individual merely addresses genome breadth. Single-gene studies can investigate numerous participants and their clinical data; however, they lack genome breadth. The "1,000 Genomes Project" involves a large number of participants and provides genome breadth, but lacks clinical data. Biesecker et al. state that the ClinSeq project is designed to be conducted on a substantial scale encompassing all three dimensions, with the possibility of developing into an ideal study. Yet these three dimensions apply to genetic data collection, rather than how the data is used for biological and medical purposes. Additional dimensions, such as a procedure for proper return of genetic data to participants and physicians, and investigations into participant health-care behavior, will need to be addressed in the conceptualization and development of large-scale genetic studies. Moreover, simply exploring these three basic dimensions may lead to biased results. Maschke draws our attention to the existence of specific sociodemographic biases in the investigated participants of CPMC and ClinSeq. Of the 305 respondents in the CPMC project, most are highly educated non-Hispanic whites; ClinSeq participants have a similar profile. These biased distributions may distort the statistics of genetic information and its association with phenotypic traits, including disease risks. Accordingly, more careful examination and considerations must be incorporated into large-scale genetic projects.

While large-scale genetic projects are pursued to achieve the three dimensions described above, genome-wide biological studies face a fundamental obstacle. It is well established that phenotypic traits are not governed by genes working in isolation. Rather, genes constitute an interactive and highly complex network in a cell and an organism. Some genes encode enzymatic proteins that catalyze chemical reactions in complex metabolic networks and body tissues, some encode membrane proteins that are responsible for the interaction between a cell and its external environment, some encode transcriptional regulatory factors that operate on DNA, whereas others encode proteins that modify the activities of other proteins, sometimes constituting signal trans-duction cascades, thereby altering cellular behavior in accordance with transcriptional regulation. Thus, genes work in a highly complex fashion. The phenotypic effects of a gene are heavily dependent on the genetic context and physiological and ecological conditions. Such complexities preclude straightforward scientific exploration of gene–disease associations. To develop comprehensive evidence-based medicine, personalized genomic medicine must involve projects that take such biological complexities into account. Perhaps the mere collection of genetic information encoded in DNA is not sufficient for an ideal study. We will need to investigate how genetic information is transcribed and then translated into functional proteins, and how downstream chemical networks are regulated and maintained in each individual subject. Ideally, personalized medical genomics will incorporate highly integrative genomics, comprising transcrip-tomics, proteomics, and metabolomics, as well as investigations on comprehensive clinical data and motivational/cognitive/socio-psychological behavior of participants. Although it will be long before developments in these dimensions are realized, we must be prepared to deal with any social and ethical problems that arise, as is expected for any novel biomedical technology.

References

Biesecker, L. G. et al. (2009). "The ClinSeq Project: Piloting Large-Scale Genome Sequencing for Research in Genomic Medicine," *Genome Research*, 19:1665–74.

Bloss, C. S., Schork, N. J., and Topol, E. J. (2011). "Effect of Direct-to-Consumer Genomewide Profiling to Assess Disease Risk," *New England Journal of Medicine*, 364:524–34.

Gollust, S. E. et al. (2012). "Motivations and Perceptions of Early Adopters of Personalized Genomics: Perspectives from Research Participants," *Public Health Genomics*, 15:22–30.

7.4

Commentary

Gatekeeping Access to Genetic
Information: A Response to "Genetic Research
to Facilitate Personalized Medicine: Ethical and
Policy Challenges"

Douglas Sipp

In her article, "Genetic Research to Facilitate Personalized Medicine: Ethical and Policy Challenges," Karen J. Maschke outlines the disclosure policies on genetic risk information in two large-scale genetic research initiatives: the CPMC, coordinated by a group of research hospitals, and the ClinSeq project, conducted by the US National Human Genome Research Institute. Both projects are intended to contribute to the development of personalized medicine informed by individual genetic information, and collect and analyze a large amount of such information from volunteer participants in these studies. Both studies inform participants that their ability to opt into accessing genetic information discovered in the research process will be limited to information of possible clinical significance (defined as "potentially medically actionable" in CPMC)—an approach sometimes referred to as "conditional return." Importantly, while the CMPC provides reasonably detailed information during the consent process as to what qualifies as potentially medically actionable, and how this is reviewed and revised, in the ClinSeq this decision-making process is essentially a black box.

Maschke presents arguments that have been made in favor and against the conditional-return approach to disclosure of genetic risk information, and rightly asks what implications it may have on the ability of future human genetics studies to attract volunteer participants.

It seems to me that the question is one of trust, meaning both trust on the part of participants in the experts assigned a gatekeeping function, and trust on the part of the research scientists in the ability of participants to manage, understand, and act on any genetic information they might receive in the course of the study in a responsible and reasonable manner. It also seems that the trust differential in this relationship is large, in that participants in effect permit the scientists conducting the study with unfettered access to the full set of their genetic information (which, admittedly, they would not ordinarily be able to access without the scientists' assistance), while the scientists only commit to returning a subset of that information, specifically that which relates to medical conditions potentially amenable to treatment or lifestyle changes, or which might impact on reproductive decisions.

A case could be made for the line of argument that the need for access to information also differs greatly for the scientists conducting a study and the "healthy" individuals who volunteer to participate; scientists will inevitably acquire individual information that may be of statistical or analytic value when compiled at the level of the cohort or population, but which has no evident informative significance to the individual from whom it was acquired. It is also clear that some participants may make use of genetic information in ways that are considered scientifically unjustifiable, irresponsible, or simply idiosyncratic and benign. Although the rationales behind the access limitations and gatekeeping functions built into the studies described in Maschke's article were not described in detail, it seems that the underlying thought was to minimize such uncontrolled uses of genetic information by individual study participants. There are cases in which this might indeed protect the interests of such individuals from using data garnered in the course of a research study to guide health-care, reproductive, or other decisions beyond the scope determined by experts to be justifiable. Such uses could be risky to individuals, many of whom presumably lack a specialized understanding of medical genetics, if they led to the adoption or avoidance of certain behaviors out of a misunderstanding of the genetic information gained from participation in the study, or of the relationship between such information and health and disease states or outcomes.

A counterargument could also be raised, however, that gatekeeping or otherwise limiting access to an individual's genetic information that has been obtained as a result of that individual's voluntary participation in research is paternalistic. Research participants may not expect to benefit directly from volunteering in a study, but the case could be made that they have (or ought to have) the right to access those sets of data obtained directly as a result of their participation, without restriction. As Maschke correctly notes, putting limits on such access may have a negative effect on the ability of future studies to recruit participants, particularly in the face of potentially increased access to personal genetic testing on a consumer basis.

The custodial approach to genetic risk information may also have the effect of limiting unpredicted, but beneficial, uses of personal genetic information. While many volunteer participants in genetics research studies may lack the expertise to interpret and act on their data, the power of the motivated nonspecialist to contribute to innovation should not be neglected. Full access by individuals to all personal genetic information obtained during the course of research may prove to have positive, as well as negative and neutral, unintended consequences not only for the individual concerned, but for the field.

That said, in the two studies in question, it appears that the terms of access were unequivocally described in the consent process, and as such there does not appear to be any ethical concern within that particular context. The foreseeable continuing evolution of ever faster and cheaper sequencing technologies, however, may make the gatekeeping approach more untenable in the near future, as potential volunteers may have reasonably unlimited access to their own genetic information from other sources, which may have the effect of further limiting the pool of volunteers on which such research depends.

7.5

Response to Commentaries

Karen J. Maschke

The authors who submitted commentary on my chapter, "Genetic Research to Facilitate Personalized Medicine: Ethical and Policy Challenges," identify several issues the chapter raises about translating genomic research information into everyday clinical practice: 1) understanding and misunderstanding genetic risk information; 2) health-related behaviors in response to receiving genetic risk information; 3) overestimation of benefits of genetic-based prevention and treatment interventions; and 4) trust in the genomic research enterprise. My chapter draws attention to these issues by discussing the current debate about whether individuals should have access to their genetic information when their DNA is analyzed in the research context. I point out that while researchers typically have not returned genetic research results to participants in their studies, some researchers, ethics experts, and research participants have criticized the no-return approach. The central focus of the chapter is how one large-scale genetic research initiative—the CPMC—addresses the issue of the return of genetic research results.

The CPMC is one of several new genetic research initiatives that will offer research participants the results of analyses of their DNA that an expert gatekeeping committee deems are "returnable." As Soraj Hongladarom points out, this is "a more conservative approach" than giving research participants all of the genetic information from studies of their DNA. However, Hongladarom may have misinterpreted my analysis of the CMPC and its conditional-return approach. Although I favor that approach over a no-return approach, I did not say that I favor the conditional-return approach over one that returns all results to research participants. Rather, I agree with some of the complaints critics have lodged against the conditional-return approach: that it has a dimension of paternalism to it, that it does not provide research participants with the information they might want, and that it might be the reason why some people decline to participate in genetic research studies or to provide their DNA sample to a research biobank. On the other hand, I am also concerned about research participants interpreting risk information as deterministic, i.e., thinking that having a gene variant means they will get the disease or disorder associated with that variant. Unfortunately, media accounts of genetics—and accounts in the medical and scientific literature—often perpetuate deterministic thinking about genes by referring to the "gene for" some diseases/disorders.

Like many new genetic research initiatives, the CPMC needs large numbers of participants to provide DNA samples for researchers to study. Offering participants some of their genetic research results is an incentive to get people to participate. But the conditional-return approach is not just an incentive. It is key to learning whether and how participants use their genetic information. The genetic research enterprise—and the paradigm of individualized medicine—is based on the assumption that people will use their genetic information to alter their behaviors in ways that minimize their genetic risk for certain diseases/disorders. But as the chapter points out, there is little evidence that when they obtain their genetic information, individuals alter their behavior. Koji Ota suggests that a "deeper investigation into participant psychology is required" in order to understand what motivates people to act on their genetic information. Hongladarom's observation is that the popularity of direct-to-consumer companies like 23andMe may stem from a psychological need that people have to "know something about themselves." Most of us will have many diagnostic tests during our lifetime, yet some of us will likely fail to respond to our results in ways that might improve our health or minimize our risk of illness. That doesn't mean, however, that we should not undergo diagnostic testing, or that physicians should not inform us about the results, even if we do not completely understand the details of an electrocardiogram or a glucose tolerance test. What is important is that physicians disclose test results in such a way that patients understand the information to help guide them in making decisions about current and future preventive or treatment interventions.

The CPMC and other genetic research initiatives are not only based on the assumption that people will use their genetic information to guide their health-related behaviors, but also that physicians will use genetic information to guide their decision-making in everyday clinical practice. This means that a valid evidence base must be in place to support physicians' use of genetic information. As Ota correctly points out, "genes work in a highly complex fashion" and the "phenotypic effects of a gene are heavily dependent on the genetic context and physiological and ecological conditions." A key issue for the CPMC is whether participants understand the complexity of genotype–phenotype relationships, or whether they have unrealistic expectations about the use of genetic information to improve their health and well-being.

As the CPMC and other conditional-return initiatives begin to return genetic research results to their participants, an interesting question will be whether participants are satisfied with receiving only the results cleared by the expert gatekeeping committee. Douglas Sipp notes that for CPMC participants, the "terms of access" to genetic research results were "unequivocally described in the consent process." Thus, he is correct in concluding that with regard to the consent context and the issue of the return of results, "there does not appear to be any ethical concern." But he also acknowledges, as I do in the chapter, that this "consent deal" may be problematic. If potential research participants can get "unlimited access" to their genetic information in other ways—either from direct-to-consumer genetic testing companies or from research initiatives that give them all their genetic information, they may be reluctant to enroll in conditional-return research studies. The architects of the conditional-return studies are aware of this possibility, particularly if the cost of whole-genome sequencing continues to fall and potential research participants want access to their whole genome sequence.

Regardless whether research participants get some or all of their results, both Sipp and I point out that an underlying rationale for limitations on access to genetic research results is the concern that individuals might use their genetic information in ways that could be harmful to them. As Sipp notes, individuals might adopt or avoid "certain behaviors out of a misunderstanding of the genetic information" they obtain from research studies. For example, an individual might engage in risky behaviors she otherwise would not undertake because she misinterpreted genetic risk information as "determinative" of dying at a young age of heart disease.

It is difficult to know how the CPMC and similar research initiatives will play out, and what "success" will mean for these large-scale conditional-return studies. The points the commentators raise in their thoughtful analyses of the challenges of genetic research to facilitate personalized medicine suggest that defining success may not be easy, and that a key feature of success will be whether participants are satisfied with the "terms of engagement" regarding access to their genetic information and whether that genetic information adds value to personal and physician decision-making about prevention and treatment interventions.

8.1

Primary Topic Article
Ethics in Emerging Forms of Global Health Research Collaboration

Michael Parker

1 The growth of collaborative global health research

Although the global burden of disease is disproportionately large in developing countries, only a very small proportion of medical research has historically focused on the problems primarily affecting the world's poorest people (WHO 2010). In recent years, however, there has been a considerable increase in the amount of research being carried out on diseases affecting people in low-income countries—much of this taking the form of collaborations involving partners in developed and developing countries (Global Forum for Health Research 2008). There are a number of reasons why these changes have come about.

In the arena of policy, the International Conference on Health Research for Development (COHRED 1990) and subsequent reports of the Ad Hoc Committee on Health Research (1996) and the Council on Health Research for Development (COHRED 2000) together established something of a consensus on a number of core recommendations for the action needed to move towards a more equitable distribution of medical research resources. These included calls to 'build the capacity of health research systems in developing countries', to 'create international research networks and public–private partnerships', and to 'increase funding for health research by developing countries' (Global Forum for Health Research 2004). These recommendations, together with the United Nations' Millennium Development Goals, which included a commitment to work to eliminate infectious diseases such as malaria, have led to a number of major international collaborative initiatives. Examples include: The Roll Back Malaria Partnership; the Global Alliance for TB Drug Development; and a range of partnerships devoted to addressing HIV/AIDS, including the WHO and UNAIDS '3 by 5 Initiative', and the Global Universal Access campaign.

In addition to these policy developments, the growth in collaborative global health research has also been driven by developments in science and technology. The rapid pace of development in technologies and statistical methods for analysing DNA sequence variation at the level of the whole genome has, for example, made it possible for the first time to contemplate genome-wide analysis of phenotypes relevant to developing country settings such as human resistance to malaria and a wide range of other communicable and non-communicable diseases. The requirement for large sample sets for such studies combined with the importance of cutting-edge sequencing facilities and statistical expertise has led to a number of major funding initiatives to establish research networks that are increasingly bringing together research groups in many countries across both the developed and the developing worlds. Recent examples of such technology-driven initiatives include MalariaGEN—a genomic epidemiology of malaria consortium bringing together more than 30 partners in 21 countries (Malaria Genomic Epidemiology Network 2008)—and H3 Africa, which is an initiative to expand genomic research on the African continent.

2 The ethics of collaborative global health research

Collaborative global health research involving complex partnerships between researchers in developing and developed countries is leading to the parallel emergence of complex ethical issues arising out of the interplay between globalized research and the ways in which such research is manifested locally. These issues are complementary to and interwoven with the well described ethical issues arising out of global health inequalities (Benatar and Singer 2000; Nuffield Council on Bioethics 2002; Pogge 2002; Brock and Wikler 2006; Daniels 2008), informed consent, levels of acceptable risk, the standards of care to be provided to control groups, and post-trial responsibilities to participants (Angell 1997; Lurie and Wolfe 1997), but present qualitatively new challenges.

My aim in this chapter is to attempt to map out the ethical issues that are likely to arise uniquely (or achieve a particular resonance) in collaborative research involving multiple partners whilst recognizing that there will, inevitably, be a great deal of overlap and interplay between the ethics of collaborative research and the issues listed above—with the potential for such well discussed ethical issues, e.g. consent, to emerge in new and different ways in this new globalized research context.

In what follows I outline eight ways in which the ethical issues arising in collaborative global health research, that is, research involving large numbers of partners in many developed and developing countries, can be different from those arising in other, more bilateral collaborations between researchers in developed counties and those in developing countries.

2.1 Ethical issues will arise across multiple, diverse, but interconnected locations

Collaborative global health research of the kind described above brings partners in many different settings in both developing and developed countries together in the same project. The scale and diversity of these collaborations are of a different order from most previous biomedical research. The Malaria Genomic Epidemiology Network, for example, involves 30 partner institutions in more than 20 countries and has collected samples and associated phenotype data from approximately 100,000 people. This is medical research with a scale and reach beyond those of most previous forms of medical science collaboration. Given this, it is highly likely that views about what is ethically problematic and about what constitutes ethical research are going to vary considerably across these collaborative international research partnerships. This diversity might manifest itself in a number of different ways.

(i) *Different ethical worries in different places* It will sometimes be the case that the ethical concerns about a research project in one partner setting will be very different from those in another, or in several others. For example, an ethics committee in one place might be concerned about a project because they think it may be difficult to obtain valid consent or refusal given the complexity of the research and the difficulty of the concepts used in the participant information sheet. In another setting, the consent processes—in the same project—may be judged to be acceptable, but the ethics committee may have concerns about the fairness of the project's proposed arrangements for benefit sharing or capacity building.

(ii) *Different views about a shared ethical concern* In other cases, what is ostensibly the 'same' issue will be understood in different and possibly conflicting ways by partners across the collaboration. In one setting, for example, the export of archived biological samples may be a concern because of worries about ownership and about the importance of securing an appropriate share of the benefits of any potential commercial exploitation of such samples for the community or the local research institute. In another setting, there might be a concern that the proposed use of samples goes beyond the remit of the original consent, e.g. there may be uncertainty about whether consent given for previous 'genetic research into malaria' should be interpreted as constituting consent for 'genomic research into malaria'. These differences can lead to conflict between the judgements of different ethics committees or partners across the collaboration. In the export of archived samples case, for example, those who are primarily concerned to ensure appropriate benefits for the community may be less worried about the precise interpretation of consent and vice versa.

(iii) *Differences about acceptable solutions to ethical problems* Sometimes, even where the perceived ethical problem is both shared and understood in similar ways by all stakeholders, differences may still emerge about the acceptability of proposed solutions. An example of this might be where there are different views about what constitutes appropriate approaches to informed consent. A good example of this was reported in *Science* in 2002 (Mfutso-Bengo and Taylor 2002). This case concerned a difference of opinion between research committees in Malawi and in the United States about the information to be provided to research participants in a research project on severe malaria in childhood. The research involved carrying out autopsies on children who were thought to have died of malaria to determine the actual causes of death. As part of the autopsy process, the eyes of deceased children were to be removed and replaced with prostheses. Parents of the children were to be provided with information about the need for an

autopsy and reassured about the 'appearance' of the child after the process was completed, but were not going to be informed explicitly about the removal of the child's
eyes. The research was considered to be ethically acceptable by the local ethics committee, and was approved and thought by them to be an appropriately sensitive approach to
discussing the implications of the research with recently bereaved parents. However, the
US ethics committee would not approve the study unless parents were 'fully informed'
about the removal of the child's eyes.

Given the potential for these three kinds of difference, an important practical ethical challenge within many scientific collaborations is going to be how best to go about
identifying, addressing, and reaching agreement about the emerging ethical issues. These
differences are of practical ethical importance because they are differences between the
views and practices of partners and institutions who or which are all part of the 'same project'. This means that they are differences that cannot be avoided and, in practical terms,
this means that within a single collaboration, there is going to have to be an ongoing
engagement with multiple institutional review boards (IRBs), communities, and partner
institutions, each of which may have different, legitimate demands to establish what is
going to count as 'good practice'. This is going to involve complex work across multiple
settings. What counts as right or wrong is likely, at least sometimes, to be very different in
different places and this raises the issue of moral relativism not as a theoretical, philosophical problem but as a problem in practical ethics and project management. When, if ever,
is it acceptable to adopt different ethical solutions in different settings? And, when, if ever,
is it going to be important to work across the collaboration to find shared solutions? It is
likely that in any enduring large-scale collaboration some combination of the two will
be necessary. This suggests that negotiation across different moral domains is going to be
called for on at least some occasions—which will inevitably generate new ethical problems of its own. It may, for example, raise issues of fairness and trust in the collaboration.

2.2 Ethical issues will arise and need to be resolved at multiple levels of analysis

The fact that partners are all part of the same project means that these 'local' ethical
problems are all interconnected. And this raises the question of what the responsibilities
are of the project as a whole, that is, at the global level in the context of such diversity.

This is an important question for a number of different but related reasons:

(i) Accountability at the level of the project

There will be occasions on which the project 'as a whole' will be called upon to give
an account or justification of its practices and of how it addresses ethical issues across
the whole range of its activities. This might be at the point of obtaining ethics approval
in the sponsor country, in the application for funding, or perhaps in the submission of
papers for publication about the collaboration on which, perhaps, there are multiple
authors.

(ii) The practical and methodological limitations of moral diversity

Sometimes the need to think about ethics at the level of the project will arise for practical, methodological, or even moral reasons. Examples of practical or methodological

constraints on thinking locally might be where effective and methodologically rigorous sample management or the systematic collection and management of phenotype data calls for universal systems to be in place across the collaboration as a whole. Examples of moral constraints might include situations where there is a perceived need for consent forms, information leaflets, and other documentation across the collaboration to have at least some shared essential information, or where the adoption of different solutions would have significant implications for resources or an impact on the progress of the research.

(iii) The shared nature of moral responsibility

Another limitation on the scope for radically different approaches in different settings, in the context of a collaborative partnership across many countries, is that partners may have an ethical interest in what happens in sites other than their own. They may find some proposed solutions elsewhere unacceptable and feel that their own reputation or sense of moral integrity is at stake in decisions made in other local settings. Local partners may also take the view that they are responsible to at least some degree for the practices of the project as a whole.

Together, these three considerations mean that against a backdrop of significant diversity, solutions to ethical problems will sometimes need to be found at the level of the collaboration (the 'project') as a whole as well as at the level of the individual partner 'sites'. This means that there are likely to be occasions when the variety of potential answers to ethical problems in particular settings across the collaboration will be in practical tension not only with each other but also with the need to develop network-wide policies on key issues such as consent or with the need for scientists to be able to provide coherent and methodologically sound accounts of the initiative as a whole. And this will present important questions in practice about the extent to which it is acceptable to have different solutions to ethical problems across the same project. What are the limits to this? What are the limits of the tension between the importance of respect for local values and practices on the one hand and maintaining internationally credible standards of practice across the project as a whole on the other?

2.3 Research will involve communities (or a community) in many different and disparate locations

'Collaborative partnership' and 'social value' have been proposed as 'benchmarks' against which the ethics of clinical research in developing countries should be assessed (Emanuel et al. 2004; Lavery et al. 2007). The achievement of these benchmarks is only possible in the context of effective community engagement and accountability (CIOMS 2002; Quinn 2004; Nuffield Council on Bioethics 2005; Tindana et al. 2007; Marsh et al. 2008, 2010; Lavery et al. 2010). Despite the growing emphasis on the importance of these benchmarks and of community engagement, there is relatively little published experience of community engagement in practice and there have been a number of recent calls for further research (Foster, Eisenbraun, and Carter 1997; Diallo et al. 2005; Marsh et al. 2008).

Successful and appropriate community engagement presents a number of practical and ethical problems in the context of collaborative research. Some of these relate to the question of how the relevant community is to be identified (Marsh et al. 2008; Cheah et al. 2010; Nyika et al. 2010) in diverse settings across a collaboration. Others concern the question of identifying and establishing procedures, principles, and mechanisms of engagement that are effective, fair, inclusive of different groups within communities (for example by gender, age, and ethnicity), accountable, and appropriate (Chokshi, Parker, and Kwiatkowski 2006; Daniels 2008; Marsh et al. 2008; Shubis et al. 2009; Cheah et al. 2010). Whilst problematic enough in the context of well established research institutions in relatively stable populations (Marsh et al. 2008), community engagement can be particularly difficult in situations where research is carried out with refugees or migrating populations (Cheah et al. 2010), in emergency situations (Calain et al. 2009), or with groups that may be particularly hard to reach. A related set of issues concerns the relationship between community engagement and consent. Real challenges are presented for both engagement and consent, for example, by some large-scale collaborative studies in which even many of the scientific partners may not understand specialized aspects of research (such as statistical analysis of genomic data) being carried out by other partners, and very few may understand the collaborative enterprise as a scientific whole. Collaborative research also presents problems for community engagement arising out of the complexity of concepts and practices such as data sharing (Lowrence and Collins 2007) and in particular types of research, such as genomics (Chokshi, Parker, and Kwiatkowski 2006; Chokshi et al. 2007), or public health research (Garnett and Baggaley 2009). Furthermore, in this context, a key ethical and practical issue arising for international scientific collaborations with a commitment to community engagement is how to achieve an appropriate balance between shared good practice in community engagement across the collaboration on the one hand and sensitivity to important local variation on the other (Parker and Bull 2009).

Against this diverse background, discussion about the responsibilities of researchers, funders, and research institutions to research populations attains a new level of complexity. It has been argued that clinical research in developing countries should have 'social value', that there should be 'fair selection of study populations', that there should be a 'favourable risk–benefit ratio', and that such research should 'show respect for recruited participants and study communities' (Emanuel et al. 2004; Lavery et al. 2007). The debate about the ethics of research has also emphasized the importance of the fair sharing of benefits. International debate about the regulation of research also addresses key obligations arising in research in developing countries and, in particular, the 'standards of care' appropriate during research and the obligations of researchers to communities and participants when the research is completed (Nuffield Council on Bioethics 2005; Declaration of Helsinki 2008; Vallely et al. 2009; CIOMS 2002).

Inevitably, this presents questions about the acceptability of different solutions, i.e. different accounts of the responsibilities of researchers to research populations, in different settings across the collaboration. And it raises issues too about fairness and about comparisons between how these responsibilities are defined and met across the range of settings. If attractive benefit-sharing arrangements are available in one setting, why should they not be available everywhere? The commitment to 'collaborative partnership' and 'community engagement' suggests that the resolution of these challenges ought to involve discussion and the genuine engagement of the communities themselves. And this raises another interesting set of questions relating to the question of when it is going to be right to think of the collaboration involving research with multiple communities in diverse settings (in which community engagement might be with individual communities) and when (if at all) it is sometimes going to be necessary, or right, to think of the research project as engaging with a single distributed and very diverse community. And if so, what might engagement with *this* community look like?

2.4 Ethical issues will arise in relation to the nature and form of research collaboration

The large and diverse multinational scientific networks required for collaborative global health research will require the development and maintenance of partnerships involving a range of diverse yet interdependent forms of expertise such as: epidemiologists; geneticists, statisticians, specialists in IT, database managers; health professionals; fieldworkers; cutting-edge sequencing facilities; multiple funding agencies; and communities. Such research also brings together diverse institutions in both developed and developing countries such as government agencies, e.g. ministries of health, research institutions, funders, etc., which may in other respects be in competition both for scientific prestige and for resources, or have competing or only partially overlapping interests and concerns. The dependence of science upon such partnerships means that the building and maintenance of the relationships, shared values and practices underpinning collaborative science, and the mechanisms for working in the context of different ethical values and commitments are going to be particularly important.

In addition to, but interwoven with, the other ethical issues discussed above, variations in power and interests between actors in collaborative global health research generate a number of ethical issues 'internal' to such collaborations relating to sharing of data and samples, the development of scientific capacity across the network, the allocation of scientific resources and setting of scientific priorities, decisions about authorship and ownership of intellectual property. This suggests that the building of sustainable relationships, shared practices and values, and ways of working within the broader diversity of practice and values is going to be essential to successful and appropriate science.

A key challenge presented by the development of collaborative global health research is the need to develop appropriate mechanisms for the oversight of data release and data sharing. This is an especially pressing issue in the context of the pressures for open access, and in relation to the responsibility for such consortia to protect the emerging scientific capacity in developing countries, and in particular that of their partners (Parker et al. 2009). If the data produced by the network on the basis of samples and phenotype descriptions collected by partners in developing countries is exploited by institutions in the north at the expense of emergent capacity in the south, for example, this has the potential to undermine long-term trust and may also undermine the emergence of the kind of networked science that is currently seen to be essential to understanding disease and addressing the health-care needs of the poorest people. Capacity building is likely to be an important consideration in any collaboration, given the discrepancies in power and resources between partners. To what extent is capacity building a moral obligation in the context of such collaborations? This is a question about which partners in a collaboration—and, potentially, the ethics committees which oversee them—are likely to have different and even competing views.

This suggests the possibility of an internal ethical politics in such collaborations and the need to look carefully at relational or procedural issues such as fairness, transparency, accountability, trust, and so on.

2.5 There will be a need to develop practical ethical solutions in the context of multiple, ambiguous, and sometimes conflicting forms of guidance and regulation

The governance environment within which collaborative research takes place is highly complex (OHRP 2010). Not only are researchers sometimes faced with applying multiple and conflicting forms of guidance; some documents, such as the Declaration of Helsinki, have also been criticized as being internally inconsistent (Forster, Emanuel, and Grady 2001). Given the volume of guidance and regulation currently available, it is important for collaborative international research consortia to develop rigorous and transparent procedures to inform the movement from theory to practice when determining best practice in conducting research at specific sites.

It is widely accepted that decisions about the appropriate conduct of research require independent, competent, and transparent ethical review (NBAC 2001a; NBAC 2001b; CIOMS 2002; Nuffield Council on Bioethics 2002; EGE 2003; Emanuel et al. 2004; Lavery et al. 2007; Declaration of Helsinki 2008). In practice, however, the effective and appropriate functioning of research ethics review in developing country settings is frequently undermined not only by the complexity of the guidance but also by inadequate training and resources (Milford, Wassenaar, and Slack 2006; Effa, Massougbodji, and Ntoumi 2007; Kass et al. 2007; Berkley 2009; Gisselquist 2009; Nyika et al. 2009; Office of Inspector General 2010; Mabeya, Singer, and Ezezika 2010) and such review is altogether non-existent in some research settings (Nuffield Council on Bioethics 2005). In response to variable ethical review capacity in Africa, a number of collaborative groups have been established, such as the Strategic Initiative for Developing Capacity in Ethical Review (SIDCER), the South African Research Ethics Initiative (SARETI), the International Research Ethics Network for Southern Africa (IRENSA), the Training and Resources in Research Ethics Evaluation (TRREE), and the African Malaria Network Trust (AMANET)—all working to enhance ethics review capacity. Nevertheless, ethics review remains patchy, and against this background of partial and stretched capacity, the emergence of collaborative forms of often highly sophisticated global health research presents significant governance challenges and raises problems about the moral obligations of researchers working in settings when regulatory structures and oversight are suboptimal.

Against this backdrop, collaborative global health research presents a range of important new governance challenges. Some of these challenges emerge out of the distribution of scientific and technological expertise across the diverse and multiple sites of 'the project' in developed and developing countries. This can present challenges for research ethics committees because the nature of the research enterprise only makes sense in the context of activities going on in a number of distant socially, technologically, and scientifically diverse locations. Reviewing such research often requires expertise not available locally, suggesting, perhaps, the need for networked forms of ethics review where the ethics committees involved in reviewing the activities of scientific networks are linked, or trained together, and in which good practice is shared. There is some evidence of the emergence of networked ethics support and advice in the spaces created by 'ethics support' within networks such as MalariaGEN.

If governance is to be effective and evidence based, in the context of a highly complex governance environment, it will be necessary for researchers to develop methods for moving from theory to practice on a case-by-case basis in particular settings in, for example, the development of consent processes. This suggests the need for the development and evaluation of the effectiveness of such models and for the sharing of expertise (Macklin 1999; Molyneux, Peshu, and Marsh 2004; Marsh et al. 2008; Tekola et al. 2009).

2.6 Change will be a pervasive feature of the ethical landscape

One of the implications of the scale, diversity, geographical distribution, and institutional complexity of many scientific collaborations is that change will almost inevitably be a pervasive feature of the contexts within which most research of this kind is carried out. In the context of enduring research networks such as the Malaria Genomic Epidemiology Network, which brings together 30 partners in 21 countries, it is highly likely that change will occur in guidelines, regulations, the views of research partners and research ethics committees, and in public and community attitudes on a fairly frequent basis through the life of the project, with ramifications for the research and for the consideration of ethical issues and policies across the network as a whole. One reason why this kind of change will be important in this kind of research arises out of the rapid development in technologies such as sequencing which may mean that researchers will need to return to research ethics committees for the approval of amendments to their protocols several times during the course of their research project. Furthermore, it is also likely that each time the researchers approach an ethics committee the membership and hence also potentially attitudes towards the research will have changed. The existence of change of each of these interrelated kinds suggests that scientists involved in such collaborations may need to have ready access to ethics support and advice.

2.7 There will be a need for 'priority setting' in ethics

It will be apparent from the preceding discussion that over the course of its existence any multi-partner global health research collaboration is likely to generate a very large number and broad range of complex and changing ethical issues. Some of these issues may perhaps need to be addressed locally, others will need to be thought through at the level of the collaboration. It is likely in practice, on at least some occasions, that there will be more ethical issues to consider than there are resources to deal with them—situations in which there may be insufficient ethics resources to identify and address all of the relevant ethical issues. This suggests that there will be cases (perhaps many) in which it is no longer going to be viable to identify, analyse, and address all of the ethical issues presented by a research project, and this implies that decisions are going to have to be made about which ethical issues are going to be prioritized for attention—there will be, that is, a need for priority setting in ethics. How should decisions be made about which ethical issues to focus on? Who should be making such decisions? This suggests the need for something like an ethics of ethics.

This also suggests that a key role in ethics in such collaborative research projects is going to have to be played by complementary empirical social research to begin to make it possible to understand the complexities of and differences between ethics as it emerges and is played out across the distributed and diverse institutions and activities across the collaboration. This suggests the need for interdisciplinary work involving social scientists, ethicists, scientists, and others to identify and understand the signifi-cance of the relevant ethical issues and make decisions about how to set priorities in the context of ethics. It is likely that in these decisions too there will be significant differ-ences of opinion across the various partners.

2.8 Issues of global justice and inequality are inevitably foregrounded

Finally, research collaborations which involve partnerships distributed across low- and high-income countries and include within their membership and research settings wide disparities in power and resources are inevitably going to have to engage with questions about fairness, inequality, and justice both in relation to their research activi-ties with participants in low-income countries but also in their interactions with and responsibilities towards each other as partners with access to different levels of resources. The collaboration is likely to raise issues of fairness and justice, for example, in ques-tions about the responsibilities of better-resourced partners in developing countries to build the capacity of those in developing countries. To what extent is capacity building a responsibility in all collaborations between partners in developed and developing coun-tries? If it is, what form or form(s) might such capacity building take? And how, and by whom, should it be funded?

3 Conclusions and implications for ways of thinking about and doing ethics

I have argued that new and emerging forms of collaborative global health research net-works have the potential to generate ethical issues not previously found in combina-tion in biomedical research, even in bilateral research carried out by developed-world scientists in developing-country settings. I have attempted to describe some of the key ways in which such ethical problems might arise in the future as such global collabora-tions proliferate. I have argued that the scope, scale, and complexity of emerging forms of research collaborations mean that:

- Ethical issues will arise differently across multiple, diverse, but interconnected locations.
- Ethical issues will arise and need to be resolved at multiple levels of analysis—particularly at both the global and local levels.
- Ethical issues will arise out of the fact that collaborative research involves com-munities in many different and disparate locations.

- Ethical issues will arise in relation to the nature and form of research collaboration.
- There will be a need to develop practical ethical solutions in the context of multiple, ambiguous, and sometimes competing forms of governance and regulation.
- Change will be a more common feature of the ethical landscape than in other forms of research.
- There will be a need for priority setting in ethics.
- Issues of global justice and fairness will be more likely to be foregrounded.

There is a need for more research on these questions. What is also clear, however, is that these new forms of biomedical research are not only going to generate new ethical issues but are also going to call for new ways of doing ethics, that is, for the development of new research methodologies in ethics. What might an ethics of collaborative global health research networks look like? Firstly, it is likely that this will be a form of ethics research which involves, or is at least complemented by, empirical social science research investigating the ways in which ethics and values are played out in local (and global) settings and exploring ways of understanding collaborative global health research. Secondly, it suggests that an ethics of collaborative, multi-sited scientific research will itself have an important multi-sited and collaborative aspect, perhaps itself involving partnerships between ethics research groups in many settings. Thirdly, it is likely that an ethics capable of engaging with the ethical dimensions of collaborative global health research will be an ethics that is both nimble and dynamic—able to move swiftly between sites and levels of analysis in both responsive and proactive modes. Penultimately, such an ethics is going to need to be capable of using ethical analysis and deliberation across the variety of settings to ensure that the range of arguments, reasons, values are identified, engaged with, and subjected to critical reflection across the collaboration. And, finally, all of this suggests that an ethics of collaborative global health research is going to have a strong procedural element, that is an emphasis on working towards a better understanding of the moral implications of the various ways in which ethical issues should be identified, deliberated, and decided upon in the context of globalized research collaborations.

References

Ad Hoc Committee on Health Research Relating to Future Intervention Options. (1996). *Investing in Health Research and Development*. Geneva: World Health Organization.

Angell, M. (1997). 'The Ethics of Clinical Research in the Third World', *New England Journal of Medicine*, 337(12): 847–9.

Benatar, S., and Singer, P. (2000). 'A New Look at International Research Ethics', *BMJ*, 321: 824–6.

Berkley, S. (2009). 'Thorny Issues in the Ethics of AIDS Vaccine Trials', *Lancet*, 362(9388): 992.

Brock, D., and Wikler, D. (2006). 'Ethical Issues in Resource Allocation and New Product Development', in D. T. Jamieson et al. (eds). *Disease Control Priorities in Developing Countries*. 2nd edition. Washington, DC: World Bank, 259–70.

Calain, P. et al. (2009). 'Research Ethics and International Epidemic Response: The Case of Ebola and Marburg Hemorrhagic Fevers', *Public Health Ethics*, 2(1): 7–29.

Cheah, P. Y. et al. (2010). 'Community Engagement on the Thai-Burmese Border: Rationale, Experience and Lessons Learnt', *International Health*, 2(2): 123–9.

Chokshi, D., Parker, M., and Kwiatkowski, D. P. (2006). 'Data Sharing and Intellectual Property in a Genomic Epidemiology Network: Policies for Large-Scale Research Collaboration', *Bulletin of the World Health Organization*, 84(5): 382–7.

Chokshi, D. et al. (2007). 'Valid Consent for Genomic Epidemiology in Developing Countries', *PLoS Medicine*, 4(4): e95.

Council for International Organizations of Medical Sciences (CIOMS). (2002). *International Ethical Guidelines for Biomedical Research Involving Human Subjects*. Geneva: CIOMS.

Council on Health Research for Development (COHRED). (1990). *Commission's Report-Health Research: Essential Link to Equity in Development*. New York: Oxford University Press.

Council on Health Research for Development (COHRED). (2000). *International Conference on Health Research for Development*, Bangkok, http://www.cohred.org/publications/library-and-archive/international_confer_1_236/ (accessed 15 April 2010).

Daniels, N. (2008). *Just Health: Meeting Health Needs Fairly*. Cambridge: Cambridge University Press.

Diallo, D. A. et al. (2005). 'Community Permission for Medical Research in Developing Countries', *Clinical Infectious Diseases*, 41(2): 255–9.

Effa, P., Massougbodji, A., and Ntoumi, F. (2007). 'Ethics Committees in Western and Central Africa: Concrete Foundations', *Developing World Bioethics*, 7: 136–42.

Emanuel, E. J. et al. (2004). 'What Makes Clinical Research in Developing Countries Ethical? The Benchmarks of Ethical Research', *Journal of Infectious Diseases*, 189: 930–7.

European Group on Ethics in Science and New Technologies to the European Commission (EGE). (2003). *Opinion Nr 17 on Ethical Aspects of Clinical Research in Developing Countries*. Brussels: EGE.

Forster, H. P., Emanuel, E., and Grady, C. (2001). 'The 2000 Revision of the Declaration of Helsinki: A Step Forward or More Confusion?' *Lancet*, 358(9291): 1449–53.

Foster, M. W., Eisenbraun, A. J., and Carter, T. H. (1997). 'Communal Discourse as a Supplement to Informed Consent for Genetic Research', *Nature Genetics*, 17(3): 277–9.

Garnett, G. P., and Baggaley, R. F. (2009). 'Treating our Way out of the HIV Pandemic: Could We, Would We, Should We?' *Lancet*, 373(9657): 9–11.

Gisselquist, D. (2009). 'Double Standards in Research Ethics, Health-Care Safety, and Scientific Rigour Allowed Africa's HIV/AIDS Epidemic Disasters', *International Journal of STD and AIDS*, 20(12): 839–45.

Global Forum for Health Research. (2004). *10/90 Report on Health Research 2003–2004*. Geneva: Global Forum for Health Research.

Global Forum for Health Research. (2008). *Equitable Access: Research Challenges for Health in Developing Countries*. Geneva: Global Forum for Health Research.

Helsinki, Declaration of ([1964], revisions 1975, 1983, 1989, 1996, 2000, 2002, 2004, 2008). World Medical Association, http://www.wma.net/e/policy/b3.htm (accessed 16 November 2010).

Kass, N. E. et al. (2007). 'The Structure and Function of Research Ethics Committees in Africa: A Case Study', *PLoS Medicine*, 4(1): e3.

Lavery, J. et al. (2010). 'Towards a Framework for Community Engagement in Global Health Research', *Trends in Parasitology*, 26(6): 279–83.

Lavery, J. V. et al. (eds). (2007). *Ethical Issues in International Biomedical Research: A Casebook.* Oxford: Oxford University Press.

Lowrence, W.W., and Collins, F. S. (2007). 'Identifiability in Genomic Research', *Science*, 317: 600–2.

Lurie, P., and Wolfe, S. M. (1997). 'Unethical Trials of Interventions to Reduce Perinatal Transmission of the Human Immunodeficiency Virus in Developing Countries', *New England Journal of Medicine*, 337(12): 853–6.

Mabeya, J., Singer, P., and Ezezika, O. (2010). 'The Role of Trust Building in the Development of Biosafety Regulations in Kenya', *Law, Environment and Development Journal*, 6(2): 216–27.

Macklin, R. (1999). *Against Relativism: Cultural Diversity and the Search for Ethical Universals in Medicine.* New York: Oxford University Press.

Malaria Genomic Epidemiology Network. (2008). 'A Global Network for Investigating the Genomic Epidemiology of Malaria', *Nature*, 456(7223): 732–7.

Marsh, V. et al. (2008). 'Beginning Community Engagement at a Busy Biomedical Research Programme: Experiences from the KEMRI CGMRC-Wellcome Trust Research Programme, Kilifi, Kenya', *Social Science and Medicine*, 67(5): 721–33.

Marsh, V. M. et al. (2010). 'Experiences with Community Engagement and Informed Consent in a Genetic Cohort Study of Severe Childhood Diseases in Kenya', *BMC Medical Ethics*, 11:13.

Mfutso-Bengo, J. M., and Taylor, T. E. (2002). 'Ethical Jurisdictions in Biomedical Research', *Trends in Parasitology*, 18(5): 231–4.

Milford, C., Wassenaar, D., and Slack, C. (2006). 'Resources and Needs of Research Ethics Committees in Africa: Preparations for HIV Vaccine Trials', *IRB*, 28(2): 51–9.

Molyneux, S., Peshu, N., and Marsh, K. (2004). 'Understanding of Informed Consent in a Low-Income Setting: Three Case Studies from the Kenyan Coast', *Social Science and Medicine*, 59(12): 2547–59.

National Bioethics Advisory Commission (United States) (NBAC). (2001a). *Ethical and Policy Issues in International Research: Clinical Trials in Developing Countries.* Volume 1: Report and Recommendations of the National Bioethics Advisory Commission. Bethesda, MD: National Bioethics Advisory Commission.

National Bioethics Advisory Commission (United States) (NBAC). (2001b). *Ethical and Policy Issues in International Research: Clinical Trials in Developing Countries.* Volume 11: Commissioned papers and staff analysis. Bethesda, MD: National Bioethics Advisory Commission.

Nuffield Council on Bioethics (NCOB). (2002). *The Ethics of Research Related to Healthcare in Developing Countries.* London: Nuffield Council on Bioethics.

Nuffield Council on Bioethics (NCOB). (2005). *The Ethics of Research Related to Healthcare in Developing Countries: A Follow-up Discussion Paper.* London: Nuffield Council on Bioethics.

Nyika, A. et al. (2009). 'Composition, Training Needs and Independence of Ethics Review Committees across Africa: Are the Gate-Keepers Rising to the Emerging Challenges?' *Journal of Medical Ethics*, 35: 189–93.

Nyika, A, et al. (2010). 'Engaging Diverse Communities Participating in Clinical Trials: Case Examples from across Africa', *Malaria Journal*, 9:86.

Office for Human Research Protections (OHRP). (2010). *International Compilation of Human Research Protections.* U.S. Department of Health and Human Services.

Office of Inspector General. (2010). 'Challenges to FDA's Ability to Monitor and Inspect Foreign Clinical Trials', Department of Health and Human Services, OEI-01-08-00510, http://www.oig.hhs.gov/oei/reports/oei-01-08-00510.pdf (accessed 17 January 2013).

Parker, M. et al. (2009). 'Ethical Data-Release in Genome-Wide Association Studies in Developing Countries', *PLoS Medicine*, 6(11): e1000143.

Parker, M., and Bull, S. (2009). 'Ethics in Collaborative Global Health Research Networks', *Clinical Ethics*, 4:165–8.

Pogge, T. W. (2002). *World Poverty and Human Rights: Cosmopolitan Responsibilities and Reforms.* Cambridge: Polity Press.

Quinn, S. C. (2004). 'Ethics in Public Health Research: Protecting Human Subjects: The Role of Community Advisory Boards', *American Journal of Public Health*, 94(6): 918–22.

Shubis, K. et al. (2009). 'Challenges of Establishing a Community Advisory Board (CAB) in a Low-Income, Low-Resource Setting: Experiences from Bagamoyo, Tanzania', *Health Research Policy and Systems*, 7:16.

Tekola, F. et al. (2009). 'Tailoring Consent to Context: Designing an Appropriate Consent Process for a Biomedical Study in a Low Income Setting', *PLOS Neglected Tropical Diseases* 3: e482.

Tindana, P. O. et al. (2007). 'Grand Challenges in Global Health: Community Engagement in Research in Developing Countries', *PLoS Medicine*, 4(9): e273.

Vallely, A. et al. (2009). 'Microbicides Development Programme: Engaging the Community in the Standard of Care Debate in a Vaginal Microbicide Trial in Mwanza, Tanzania', *BMC Medical Ethics*, 10:17.

World Health Organization (WHO). (2010). *WHO's Role and Responsibilities in Health Research: Draft WHO Strategy on Research for Health*, A63/22 25 March 2010.

Acknowledgements

Professor Michael Parker's research on global health bioethics is support by a Wellcome Trust Strategic Award (096527)

8.2

Commentary
Reconciliation between Universality and Diversity

Zhaocheng Wang

Professor Michael Parker in his paper, 'Ethics in Emerging Forms of Global Health Research Collaboration', provides a comprehensive and detailed account of ethical issues surrounding global health research collaborations, and shares his first-hand experiences of research on projects including the Malaria Genomic Epidemiology Network.

In recent years the amount of health research all over the world has increased considerably, with a huge number of research projects extending across many developing and developed countries. In China, more and more international collaborations are being launched, and grant funding keeps increasing. In 2011, for example, the National Natural Science Foundation of China (NSFC) alone has funded 63 major international collaborative research programs (NSFC 2010). Collectively the grants amount to about USD 2 billion, an average of CNY 2.01 million for each program. It was estimated that in 2011 the support would increase to average 3 million for each major international collaborative research program. Furthermore, due to the booming trends of international collaborative research, abundant resources, and prosperous markets, China may gradually become one of the largest pharmaceutical markets in the world, as well as one of the largest experimental sites.

1 Ethical issues in applying international guidelines and ethical relativism

Before considering the practical and detailed questions relating to the global health research collaboration, Parker pointed out that those ethical issues would arise across multiple, diverse, but interconnected countries and regions because of different ethical worries embedded within different cultures. The issue appears not just as a theoretical,

* This article was written under the directorship of Professor Xiaomei Zhai, to whom I am very much obliged

philosophical problem of moral relativism that may challenge the fundamental premise of the collaboration, but also as a problem in practice that would raise ethical difficulties and affect project management. Moreover, in Parker's article, he notes the importance of developing practical ethical solutions against a background of multiple, ambiguous, and sometimes conflicting forms of guidance and regulation. In considering this issue he focuses mainly on the method of weighing and balancing within different guidance and regulations. Therefore, inspired by the two issues described above, our first discussion will focus on ethical issues in applying international guidelines, i.e. on the tensions between international guidelines and native cultures, and against ethical relativism.

Many countries accept that in biomedical research, international guidelines can be seen as a universal baseline or common ground that provides the foundation for international collaborations. In China, the main rationales of international guidelines, such as the Helsinki Declaration and CIOMS/WHO International Ethical Guidelines on Biomedical Research Involving Human Subjects, have been incorporated into the national regulations. But on the other hand, the value system of Chinese native resources has its own characteristics that may include elements like collectivism (priority given to collective interests over individual interests), emphasis on harmony over disagreement, emphasis on proprieties, etc. Furthermore, in China even today laws and regulations are greatly influenced by tradition and native culture, and may be modeled on the basis of traditional norms, well accepted state laws, common laws, village rules, community rules, civil conventions, business rules, religious rules, etc.

So how can universal and native values be integrated? This question can be posed in relation to China and, of course, other countries too. When international guidelines are embedded in national regulations, there should be a presumption that all of us have shared values. However, this presumption of shared values faces the following challenges, to which we will try to respond.

1.1. One might claim that there is no such thing as universal values, and that Asian values are very different from Western values. To reply to this challenge, we say that if someone recognizes Asian values, he or she must accept there are universal values. For in Asia there is a wide diversity of cultures, including Confucianism, Daoism, Buddhism, Hinduism, Christianity, Islam, and many other aboriginal cultures. If these different cultures all share common features in virtue of which they can be deemed Asian values, then in the same vein, we can expect there to be common features among Asian values, European values, African values, etc., in virtue of which they can all be deemed universal values. Moreover, since universal values exist and can be seen as the intersection of various value systems, we cannot conclude that Asian values have nothing in common with other value systems. And whilst there could be some features of Asian values that are not found in other value systems, the existence of such unique features hardly shows that there are no shared values. It is relevant here to recall Confucius's teaching: 'By nature people are similar; they diverge as a result of practice' (Confucius 2003: 17.2).

1.2. Another argument against universal values claims that all these international ethical guidelines are Western, and that China should have Confucian guidelines to guide its ethical judgments. It is, however, difficult to defend the claim that all international ethical guidelines are Western, because many of them were developed with the participation of representatives from a variety of cultures and countries, including China. Furthermore, Confucianism does not provide precise and specific guidance on how to address issues arising in the context of modern biomedical research collaborations.

1.3. One may question whether certain proposed universal values such as democracy, liberty and human rights really are universal, rather than Western. This position does not deny the in-principle possibility of universal values; rather, it questions whether those values generally taken to be universal really are so. Most cultures (including Chinese culture) recognize that there are some basic values underlying these international guidelines, such as non-maleficence/beneficence, respect for persons, and justice. I will not attempt to provide a list of values that ground international guidelines here; however, a remark by Premier Wen gives an indication of how universal values are identified: 'Science, democracy, legal system, freedom and human rights are ...common values pursued by mankind in the long historical process and they are fruit of human civilization created by mankind' (Wen 2007).

Indeed, the precise implementation of international guidelines does not simply follow deductively from the content of these guidelines. Additional premises are required. When applying guidelines to real cases, which are embedded in local culture and carry with them certain socio-cultural characteristics, there may be various possible ways of proceeding. The tension between international guidelines and native cultures means that we have to take the cultural context into account when implementing the guidelines, but this gives us no reason to reject their general applicability. The basic values mentioned above such as non-maleficence/beneficence, respect for persons, and justice are recognized by almost all cultures, and these universal values may constitute the core of any international guidelines in that they must be adhered to, and cannot be compromised across cultures. Non-core aspects of the guidelines, however, may be flexible and variable depending on specific cultural context. This periphery part reflects the different values and beliefs among different cultures, which should be respected.

2 Community engagement in informed consent in China

Parker remarks that '[s]uccessful and appropriate community engagement presents a number of practical and ethical problems in the context of collaborative research...The commitment to "collaborative partnership" and "community engagement" suggests that the resolution of these challenges ought to involve discussion and the genuine engagement of the communities themselves.' Having discussed the theoretical issue of how to combine international guidelines with local values, we will turn to the practical issue of community engagement in informed consent, especially against the background of Chinese culture (Zhai 2009).

Consent in medical practice and research can be defined as the acceptance of a physician-proposed therapeutic intervention, or of an investigator's invitation to participate in research or clinical practice, by a prospective patient or human research participant. Obtaining consent from patients and research participants is now routine practice in China.

In China, however, the concept of 'person' does not have the same connotations of independence as it does in the West, since in China family and community ties and traditional culture are much stronger influences on people's lives. In particular, Confucius has a great influence on Chinese secular ethics, and the Confucian idea of personhood is monistic, gradualist, and relational. On the relational view, Confucians do not think of personhood as confined to the individual; on the contrary, human beings are distinguishable from animals because of their relational or social capacity. A person is never seen as an isolated individual, but is always conceived of as part of a network of relations. The self-cultivation of an individual person to become a fully developed, moral person is a process that is carried out in and through the social context, and for the purpose of fulfilling social responsibility rather than self-actualization per se. When an individual lives relatively closely with his or her family and/or community, he or she is a person 'in relation'. This can be illustrated in the clinical context: a patient's family provides him/her with care and emotional support, as well as with financial support. So the family, or sometimes the community, is often involved in the process of informed consent. And when the research is conducted in rural areas, the family/community is usually involved in the process of informed consent. In these cases, the relevant form of consent is sometimes called 'family consent' or 'community consent'.

However, the community involvement in the informed consent process may be distorted or misunderstood as the imbalance of power in a community, or the prevailing paternalism may run against the wishes of the individual members of the community. This violates their autonomy and deprives them of their freedom of choice.

To reply to this challenge, the jurisdiction of this kind of 'family consent' or 'community consent' should be limited under certain specific conditions. In fact, the community engagement does not mean that the community leader or family head has the power to decide which member should participate in the research. The decision of whether or not to participate in the research must be made by the individual member. It seems the terms 'family consent' and 'community consent' are misleading. The type of consent in question might be better expressed as 'informed consent with the guidance of family or community'.

Broadly speaking, community engagement in research or clinical practice is the process of working collaboratively with people in the community to address issues affecting the well-being of those community members who may be patients or candidates for research participants. The aim of this community engagement is to safeguard the people's best interests.

This engagement encourages the community or family to organize itself in managing its research or clinical practice. Within the engagement, the head of the community or family may recognize the cultural differences between the community and the investigators or physicians, who may not be familiar with the local context. This engagement may also enhance the quality of individual informed consent and the level of active engagement in the research, and it protects members of a community from agreeing to participate in research without being informed of possible harmful consequences for the community. When the project becomes the community's self-project as opposed to an outsider's project, the informed consent process launched by investigators will be smoothly and successfully achieved with the help of the community members and their leaders.

Also, community engagement encourages researchers to be aware of the local context, having an obligation to take certain community views and interests into account, and to recognize that community input can be essential to conducting research ethically. Moreover, it expands research constraints by adding the obligation to protect vulnerable communities from significant harms and to respect their integrity.

References

Confucius. (2003). *Confucius Analects: With Selection from Traditional Commentaries*, translated by Edward S. Indianapolis, IN: Hackett.

Editorial Board, National Natural Science Foundation of China. (2010). *Type Introduction of International (regional) Joint and Cooperation Project*, http://www.nsfc.gov.cn/nsfc/cen/xmzn/2011xmzn/10/01.html (accessed 20 December 2012).

Qiu, R. Z. (2010). 'Promoting Responsible Research and Making the Results of Scientific Research to Serve People', *Chinese Medical Ethics*, 2: 3–6.

Wen, J. (2007). 'Our Historical Tasks at the Primary Stage of Socialism and Several Issues Concerning China's Foreign Policy', *China Daily*, 5 March. http://www.bjreview.com.cn/document/txt/2007-03/12/content_58927_5.htm (accessed 12 December 2012).

Zhai, X. M. (2009). 'Informed Consent in the Non-Western Cultural Context and the Implementation of Universal Declaration of Bioethics and Human Rights', *Asian Bioethics Review*, 1(4): 5–16.

8.3

Commentary

Research Ethics Governance in Korea: How and Why Does a Nation Adopt an Ethical Perspective into Research Oversight?

Ilhak Lee

1 Introduction

Professor Michael Parker's article raised an agenda of global, joint research ethics oversight, especially in the case of projects involving researchers from diverse backgrounds. The topic of global governance of research ethics is also of international academic interest. For example, the UNESCO International Bioethics Committee (IBC) has long been trying to provide guidelines for domestic and international genetic research. But global research oversight requires common ground on which to build and enforce the necessary regulations. We are diverse not only in terms of religion and culture, but also in terms of economic, socio-political circumstances. Politely we refer to cultural differences, but many of those differences are actually due to economic disparity between nations and different perspectives of different socio-political arrangements. It may not be appropriate to raise this issue in the context of bioethics, for bioethics should not be confused with politics. But how can we resolve ethical difficulties without tackling reality?

Parker's initiative on 'globalized health research' is a remarkable endeavor to address this issue from the bioethicist's side. He tried to show that once human society started to pay attention to fellow human beings, the search began for a working solution not only by intervention, but also by empowerment. Some of the collaborations really symbolize the recognition of the helping parties that aid cannot be the solution, and that capacity building is needed.

While human rights advocates worry about the possible exploitation of research participants in developing countries, some of the international collaborations definitely benefit people directly or indirectly. But even in the case of research with good intentions, we find ethical problems typical of medical research. These include problems of informed consent, the concept of acceptable risk, and justice issues.

But Parker pointed out that there are other problems inherent to international collaborations. They are related to an increase in the number of research locations, structural complexities from the diversity of participating researchers and research subjects; and resulting confusion about the locus of responsibility, and how to take cultural and social issues into consideration. Parker argues that ethicists should be more flexible in their approach to real ethical issues, and that the new ethical perspective has to deal with priority setting in ethical deliberation. Meanwhile, it seems that he did not lose sight of the problem of injustice or inequality that is deep seated in some political environments.

This broad and insightful perspective may be the fruit of Parker's commitment to ethical health research in which beneficial intentions are not distracted by neglecting ethical aspects of the research, especially in less advantaged countries. I deeply sympathize with his point that a new approach is needed for ethics governance: for empirical social science research, partnership between ethics research groups in different settings, responsive and proactive modes of ethical analysis, and focus on procedures. I want to point out that we need to be aware of the political situation, and to be realistic about the limits of doing ethics in harsh reality. In developing countries, there are political instability and corruption, severe shortage of (human and material) resources, and culturally incompatible conventions and understandings. Ethical oversight should be guided by the people who will be affected by the research, and this means international collaboration should focus on empowering the locals. Bioethics itself is unprepared for this reality: it lacks the proper methodologies. This may be due to the nature of philosophical bioethics, which focuses on argumentation rather than on consensus building and finding practicable solutions. The interdisciplinary approach reflects the efforts of bioethicists to handle this weakness, but the result is hardly integrated into one practical norm. Whilst bioethics has contributed to the development of human rights protection, we need to think about how ethics can be applied in countries where ethics is a new or foreign concept. Korean experiences of incorporating ethical norms into standards of medical practice may be instructive here. I will refer to this incorporation of ethical norms as 'adopting bioethics'.

2 Ethics as theory and ethics as practice

'Being ethical' has different implications in different locations. Sometimes it means being considerate of others and willing to resign one's share for the sake of another. And sometimes ethics implies something about blame and punishment rather than prevention or fair resolution of conflict. Sometimes raising ethical questions about convention is regarded as threatening the harmony of some community such as family, the local people, or a professional body. And ethics is easily misunderstood as placing values in conflict with (economic or academic) flourishing: people erroneously view being ethical as denying one's achievement. In 2005, when renowned stem cell scientist W. S. Hwang's research fraud was discovered (and possible oocyte selling became a subject of public debate), those who defended Dr. Hwang argued that so-called bioethics is not applicable to Korean society. This argument was based on the shared consensus that ethics is a Western idea, and that Hwang's behavior should be judged in the light of Korean norms. They also argued that sacrificing oneself for the good of society and one's own research team comes before any other value. However, the Korean government and scientists' society established standards for ethical research that met international requirements. Now Korean scientists are quite familiar with ethics guidelines, legal provisions, and institutional review boards.

As a medical ethicist working in Korea, I found it difficult to convince medical practitioners and researchers of the importance of ethics for their activities. There can be several reasons for this difficulty, but the most prominent one is that ethics is unfamiliar to most Korean people. In Korea, law and ethics are inseparably related, and people naturally are more concerned about legal provisions than ethical principles. For Korean ethicists, ethics is hard to enforce without legislation. (This may explain the poor progress in clinical ethics compared to that in research ethics. Medical research is regulated by laws, but clinical practices are generally regulated only by ethical resolution, not by law. So researchers are more concerned about ethical issues than practitioners. And some innovative researchers can evade strict ethical monitoring by trying to classify their research as treatment.)

The scandal and aftermath of the Hwang scandal taught us that when there is no recognition of ethics among those who are supposed to be guided by it, it will be extremely difficult to ensure that an ethical practice is fully adopted; although it is possible to change the behavior of scientists. To many scientists, being ethical means complying with a process imposed on them by someone else, rather than identifying, deliberating, and deciding moral problems through collaboration. But this could be a hopeful sign: ethics is part of their practice, even if they do not enter fully into its spirit.

In Korea, the adoption of ethics into research practice was implemented by researchers rather than ethicists. One reason for this is that there were not enough experts on the ethical regulation of research; but I wonder whether there exists a certain pressure to be ethical. I think the following examples illustrate that there are instrumental reasons to be ethical:

2.1 Accreditation from Joint Commission International for medical practice

Even though the Korean government provides an accreditation program for hospitals, highly renowned tertiary hospitals applied for Joint Commission International (JCI) accreditation, which is based on US standards. Among the motivations for this application was promotion to medical consumers. Fortunately, there are patients' rights provisions in JCI criteria, and hospital administrations noted the importance of ethics in patient care. Hospitals set up hospital ethics committees, revised patient informed consent forms, and began to provide in-patients with patients' rights brochures. The motive may not be ethical, and the goal was to satisfy given criteria, but it resulted in some progress in the ethics of patient care. The hospitals in question did not develop their own ethical standards or principles, but adopted given procedures.

2.2 Accreditation from FERCAP or AAHRPP

Because new drug trials were thought to add value to the hospitals conducting them, research hospitals as well as the government invested resources in drug trials. To enable them to host drug trials, research hospitals applied for research ethics accreditation from foreign organizations, such as the Forum for Ethical Review Committees in the Asian Western Pacific Region (FERCAP) or the Association for the Accreditation of Human Research Participants Program (AAHRPP), as proof of their preparedness. More than 40 percent of tertiary hospitals are now recognized by these bodies (Han and Yim 2010).

Whilst not treating the goal of becoming more ethical as an end in itself, institutions and practitioners adopted ethical standards in their work. In the context of globalized health research, we can expect that ethical requirements are adopted for similarly instrumental reasons, to recruit foreign health research programs, especially when those programs satisfy health-care needs. For those who view adopting ethics as a qualification, ethics would not mean theoretical justification but practical guidance of action.

3 Ethics as practice

To view ethics in the context of practice, we must turn our attention away from theoretical concerns and focus on the concerns of practitioners. Practitioners see the issues from the field; their ethics are not matters of the ideal world (Rawls 2003: 6–10). They try to decide whether a research proposal is acceptable under given conditions. Even though they accept some ethical imperatives, they try to take an 'all things considered' view. They are ready to accept exceptions, the unexpected, and inabilities. All ethicists are thought to be experts at discerning, but unfortunately some are not equipped with the relevant ability and experience. They may rather be regarded as ethical theorists; but the type of ethicists that interest me here are practitioners, dealing with everyday problems, revising earlier decisions, gathering information from the field, and facilitating consensus on the principles to apply. Since these activities are part of practice, the emphasis is on applying theory in real situations. As medical practitioners constantly change their current therapies, ethical practitioners must be open to making changes to currently accepted ethical practices. This does not entail that all ethics should be subject to the strict scrutiny of a reality test; but such an attitude is sometimes needed from ethicists working under certain conditions, such as those found within medical practice.

I think it would be instructive to develop a casuistry of research ethics. Casuistry is the method of testing moral principles by applying them to particular, often novel, cases. In the globalized context, an ethicist should be adept at assimilating diverse perspectives, sympathetically analyzing them, and comparing them with his/her own. He/she should deal honestly with the available evidence and the intuitions used to analyze it, and exercise integrity. This approach aims at more than merely ensuring compliance from researchers. It asks them, in addition, to be more flexible about their own ethical theories.

4 Questions to be answered

Some questions must be addressed before this approach to ethics of globalized health research can be made more practicable. It would be bioethicists' task to address these questions in the beginning. These questions are: (1) What will be the content of glo-balized research ethics? (2) How can we ensure compliance from participants? (3) What is the purpose of imposing ethics on researchers from either side? (4) How should ethics be done in research practice? and (5) What should be included in ethical deliberation about global health research? The purpose of answering these questions is to enhance the applicability of globalized ethics, not to doubt or deny its value.

4.1 What will be the content of globalized research ethics?

We have to provide ethical grounds for guiding actions. Some mention Belmont's Report or Beauchamp and Childress's four principles, and others mention human rights. Each proposal has its merits as well as weakness. I hope we can develop some initial principles of globalized research ethics, but we must bear in mind that they may need to be revised.

4.2 How can we ensure compliance from participants?

The idea of globalized research ethics as practice raises the problem of how to imple-ment the principles in practice. There are elaborate procedures to guarantee the quality of oversight, not only the compliance. However, we all know that the standard operating procedure does not solve anything without the willingness and capacity to apply it.

4.3 What is the purpose of imposing ethics on researchers from either side?

Research ethics is concerned with procedures, not with the contents that arise from those procedures. But those procedures exist to help clarify what would otherwise be obscure data, not to enable those participating to exercise their capabilities. Imposing ethics should be regarded as an extension of capacity building, not the solution. Capacity building, rather than focusing on short-term ethical improvements in situations, should be the goal of globalized research ethics. This requires asking funding institutions to be more responsive to situations, difficulties, and considerations, from the agenda setting to evaluating the results.

4.4 How should ethics be done in research practice?

Ethical practice should focus on developing those aspects of practice that effectively and efficiently improve the research practice. Researchers should be assured that ethical research is good for them, not only for the participants. The requirement to behave ethi-cally should not be viewed as a threat to cut down the budget or to cancel publications. It should be more fundamental. As long as ethics is regarded as a possible hindrance to scientific progress, it can work only through threats.

4.5 What should be included in ethical deliberation about global health research?

We have to consider justice the most important matter in global health problems. Domestic and international injustice and inequality make this difficult issue all the more problematic. Ethics alone cannot properly address the situation, the causes, and possible initiatives to rectify it. As global health research is interdisciplinary in nature, its ethics should reflect this. We might need some mechanism to ensure ethical decision-making in interdisciplinary research.

5 Conclusion

Globalized heath research presents difficult ethical challenges, but also presents a very important opportunity to ensure that its contribution to human development is ethical. To make the most of this opportunity, ethics should be about more than merely ensuring compliance with ethical standards. It should begin with identifying ethical norms that must have binding force, and assessing their applicability by taking account of diverse perspectives, conducting sympathetic analysis of these perspectives, and making comparisons between them to enable revision and acceptance.

References

Han, S., and Yim, D. (2010). 'Current State of Clinical Trials in Korea,' *Journal of the Korean Medical Association*, 53(9): 745–52.

Rawls, J. (2003). *A Theory of Justice*. Revised ed. Cambridge, MA: Belknap Press of Harvard University Press.

8.4

Response to Commentaries
Some Reflections

Michael Parker

In my chapter, 'Ethics in Emerging Forms of Global Health Research Collaboration', I attempted to map out some of the ethical issues arising out of the recent and ongoing increase in the number and size of global health research collaborations. The chapter attempted to articulate some of the many ways in which well known and important questions in research ethics are being transformed by the emergence of these new forms of scientific collaboration and to highlight the ways in which new ethical issues are being produced. The chapter drew on my experience of leading the ethics programme of the Malaria Genomic Epidemiology Network (MalariaGEN) but also included reflection on the growth of scientific collaborations involving partners in both high- and low-income countries more generally.

I am really very grateful to Zhaocheng Wang and Ilhak Lee for their perceptive and thought-provoking comments on my chapter. My initial motivation for writing the chapter was to explore the extent to which it might be possible to map out a research agenda relating to the ethics of international research collaboration. In writing the chapter, I came to the conclusion that there were indeed some new issues to be investigated. In their commentaries, Zhaocheng Wang and Ilhak Lee have some sympathy for this argument but have both also suggested a number of ways in which this research agenda might be enriched and expanded, and have made it clear that there is much more work to be done on these issues.

In her commentary, Zhaocheng Wang investigates two important sets of practical and theoretical problems. The first of these is the set of ethical issues that arise in the 'application' of international guidelines in particular contexts and the related question of whether and to what extent moral values are to be seen as context specific or universal. It is clear from her commentary that the investigation of the implications of these questions will need to be central to any consideration of the ethics of collaborative global health research. She argues that whilst there are increasingly a number of international guidelines and regulation that command widespread agreement, such as the Declaration of Helsinki—despite the ongoing controversies about standards of care and responsibilities at the end of research—there are also strong critical voices calling for a more situated ethics. In her commentary, Zhaocheng Wang gives the example of calls for a more collectivism-oriented approach to research ethics in China. Against this backdrop, Zhaocheng Wang argues that one of the key questions for the future in international research bioethics is going to be how universal values can be integrated with native resources. That is, how can and should research collaborations, governance bodies, and local ethics committees manage in practice to take these two fundamentally different positions into account in deciding what is to count as good practice? She gives a number of arguments why such decisions cannot always come down on the side of a localized, contextual approach to ethics. She criticizes the idea of an 'Asian bioethics' which might stand in opposition to a 'Western bioethics' on a number of grounds, including by emphasizing the diversity of Asian values and cultures and by highlighting the many overlaps and shared values. Zhaocheng Wang also reminds us that the development of many international guidelines, such as the Declaration of Helsinki, involved significant Asian contributions. Finally, she highlights the fact that there are important voices in China emphasizing and calling for a greater emphasis on human rights, and the fact that these and other important, ethical values are often mistakenly seen as only 'Western' when in fact they have a much wider and more diverse constituency of support.

The second important set of issues raised by Zhaocheng Wang in her commentary are those relating to consent, community engagement, and the role of the family in China. Using the example of the relational model of the person which lies at the heart of much Chinese thinking about ethics and the idea of respect for 'informed consent with the guidance of family or community', she illustrates some of the challenges faced by any research collaboration carrying out research in many different places and yet attempting to develop a shared model of good practice in relation to consent across the collaboration as a whole. What this example shows very nicely is that any approach to consent and respect for the interests of research participants which takes the local very seriously is going to need to be able to find ways of balancing the tensions between the local and the global in ways that are reasonable, transparent, and accountable.

In his commentary too, Ilhak Lee highlights the key importance of the potential tensions between global health governance on the one hand and the taking seriously of local or national contexts on the other in considerations about what is to count as good practice in international research collaborations. Using a number of practical examples from Korea, including the case of Dr Hwang, Ilhak Lee makes a powerful case for the argument that identifying, analysing, and addressing these issues is going to call for the development of new models of bioethics and that such models will only be effective if they are integrated into daily scientific practice. And one thing that struck me as I read this over was the implication that such models might themselves need to be international, even global, collaborative partnerships between ethicists and others—and, interestingly, that scientists might themselves need to be involved in ethics as well as ethicists being involved in science.

In addition to the areas in which there was a significant amount of overlap between the commentaries of Ilhak Lee and Zhaocheng Wang, such as those related to the tensions between the global and local in ethics, Ilhak Lee also highlighted the importance of thinking carefully about the complementary roles of ethics regulation, ethics education, and the role of ethicists themselves in ensuring high ethical standards in science.

He rightly reminds us of the key role of ethics education in scientific training and of the moral motivation of scientists themselves in ensuring ethical science. Not everything can be achieved through the development of laws, regulation, and oversight. Laws and principles require interpretation and judgement, and laws can be ambiguous and even contradictory. Against this background, ethical practice is going to rely upon the ethical awareness and moral motivation and judgement of scientists. This, Ilhak Lee believes, is another way in which the development of global health research collaborations is going to present new challenges to ethics and ethical thinking. Ilhak Lee concludes his commentary by setting out a number of key questions that any approach to the ethical aspects of collaborative global health research is going to need to address. These include clarifying the form and content of global health bioethics and the development of models of good ethical practice and approaches to the provision of ethics support and advice that have the potential to actually change practice.

When I began to think about the question of whether there was anything ethically special about the new forms of collaborative global health science, I was not convinced that the kinds of ethical issues they presented would be significantly different from those arising in other more traditional forms of medical research. As the writing of the chapter progressed, however, I did begin to come to the conclusion that there is something interesting and difficult about these forms of research collaboration and that thinking carefully about them might also be productive for bioethics. It might require bioethics to develop new methods and, in particular, to find ways of—itself—collaborating globally in ways that are sensitive to the interplay between the global and the local. The two fascinating and helpfully critical commentaries on the chapter by Zhaocheng Wang and Ilhak Lee have convinced me that there is a lot more to be done on this topic and that there is the potential for this to be a productive and novel area of bioethics research.

SECTION D
Synthetic Biology and Chimera

9.1

Primary Topic Article
The Ethical Issues of Synthetic Biology

Gregory Kaebnick

Introduction

Synthetic biology, a technology that seeks to bring the principles of engineering to bear on the field of biology and make possible the design and construction of organisms, may have very significant benefits, but also poses a variety of questions that will be a challenge to evaluate fully and to address in public policy. The questions go beyond "What is the right balance of risks and potential benefits?" They include: "How should we *think about* the risks and benefits? Is the synthesis of organisms *intrinsically* troubling, and should any concerns about the synthesis of organisms affect public policy? How do we—indeed, how can we—ensure that the changes wrought by the field are just and environmentally beneficial?"

This paper will outline the growth of the field of synthetic biology, develop some of the questions that arise in it, and attempt to point out a way forward on some of them. The strategy for developing these questions will be to set out, in somewhat greater detail, a particular category of research within synthetic biology—research aimed at developing organisms that can produce fuel. This research provides a "case study" of sorts for articulating and examining the questions that synthetic biology raises. Three kinds of questions will be explored.

The state of the science

With synthetic biology, scientists hope to build biological systems from the ground up, eliminating some of the complexity and unpredictability of naturally occurring biological systems and producing systems that will function like computers or factories—safely producing the products we want, when we want, in the amounts we want. Industrial analogies are inescapable when talking about this work, and while they do not appropriately capture the "living" element of synthetic biology, they do exemplify the field's central goal: to make biology easier to engineer.

In principle, then, synthetic biology is not defined in terms of and not limited to any particular kind or category of organism. In practice, however, although some work is being done in mammalian systems (Aubel and Fussenegger 2010), the main lines of work in synthetic biology are currently on microorganisms.

Exactly which aspects of biology the term "synthetic biology" refers to is contested (Brent 2004), and various taxonomies can be found to explain the term (Presidential Commission 2010: 45), but one or more of three broad lines of work are usually in mind when it is used. One line, and arguably the line that aims most directly at the grand vision of integrating biology and engineering, is what Maureen O'Malley et al. have called "DNA-based device construction" (O'Malley et al. 2008). It is exemplified by the construction of "biobricks," made from DNA and other molecules, that can function as standardized and interchangeable parts or tools to perform very specific functions— turning gene production on or off, say, or measuring the concentration of a particular gene product. Assembled in sequences and installed in "platform" organisms, these parts would, as proponents describe it, turn that organism into a very specialized tool of sorts. The parts would also be well characterized and available to the public in catalogues (BioBricks Foundation, http://biobricks.org). Drew Endy, a civil engineer by trade, is the leading figure in this line (Endy 2005).

In a second line of research, Craig Venter and colleagues at the J. Craig Venter Institute are engaged in what O'Malley et al. have called genome-driven cell engineering. For example, they hope to use synthetic DNA to build a "minimal genome" that contains only the genetic material needed to sustain bacterial life (Gibson et al. 2008). Such a minimal genome might provide a standardized platform that could then be equipped as desired with biological sequences (such as biobricks). In May 2010, researchers at the J. Craig Venter Institute announced that they had taken a step toward creating a minimal genome by successfully synthesizing the entire genome of the bacterium *Mycoplasma mycoides* (Gibson et al. 2010). To prove that the synthesis was successful, they inserted the genome into a cell of a closely related species, *Mycoplasma capricolum*, resulting in what was to all appearances fully functioning *M. mycoides*. The researchers described the resulting cell as a "synthetic cell," the first ever created by human beings, and said that it represented a new species, which they dubbed *Mycoplasma mycoides JCVI-syn1.0*. Thus the announcement seemed tantamount to a "synthetic life form."

A third line might be cobbled together from what are really distinct lines of research, but are united in that they seek to reinvent the basic mechanisms and materials found in living things. For example, in what is known as minimal cell creation or protocell creation (also the creation of "chemical cells," or "chells"), the goal is to design and build organisms from the ground up, first identifying the basic functions necessary for the simplest forms of life (for example, mechanisms for metabolism, for control, for replication, for organization) and then constructing them from basic parts (Forster and Church 2006). The new cells might use chemicals not found in naturally occurring organisms (Ball 2004). In principle, the development of protocells could lead to an entirely new biochemistry—a nonorganic biochemistry, in that it need not be carbon based. Additionally, mechanisms for control and replication need not depend on DNA.

The case of synthetic organisms to produce biofuels

The ethical questions raised by synthetic biology are varied and complex, and they are most effectively studied by examining the applications. Production of fuels, one of the most commonly cited potential applications, offers something like a "base case" for considering outcomes. There are, however, multiple lines of research under way simultaneously, posing somewhat different ethical considerations.

Even within this one "case," a taxonomy of sorts is necessary, as research is under way on different fronts, using different organisms and aiming at the production of different kinds of fuel. First, there is research on the development of organisms that can process substrates found in biomass, typically crops such as corn, into biofuels such as ethanol. The organisms considered candidates for ethanol production include *Saccharomyces cerevisiae* (yeast) and *Zymomonas mobilis*, which naturally produce ethanol out of glucose fairly efficiently, and *Escherichia coli*, which naturally produces only a small amount of ethanol but can process a broader variety of substrates (Jang et al. 2012). The work conducted on them is aimed to make them produce ethanol more efficiently, eliminate metabolic pathways that compete with ethanol production, make them tolerate higher levels of ethanol, and broaden the range of substrates that they can process. An organism that could process cellulose would allow for biofuel production processes that employed easily produced and minimally processed feedstocks, such as switchgrass or wood chips. The genetic manipulations include the introduction of foreign genes and the elimination of native ones.

Another target biofuel is butanol, which has several advantages over ethanol—it has a higher energy density, leading to better gas mileage, and its properties are very similar to gasoline, allowing it to be used as a direct replacement in engines and in the industrial systems for storing and transporting gasoline. Some strains of *Clostridium* are natural butanol producers, and strains have been produced (through random mutagenesis and the disruption of competing metabolic pathways) that are more efficient. Genetic manipulation of these strains has proven difficult, however, leading researchers to work on *E. coli* as an alternative host organism, with clostridial genes introduced to impart butanol production.

Research is also under way on the development of organisms that produce alkanes (which, depending on the number of carbon atoms, can be used either as gasoline or as diesel or aviation fuel), isoprenoids, and hydrogen (which has an extremely high energy density and produces only water when it burns).

Another set of research is on organisms—algae and cyanobacteria (also called blue-green algae)—that could produce some of these same kinds of fuel photosynthetically. Biomass from feedstocks would not be necessary; the inputs would be carbon dioxide, water, and sunlight. In the dream scenario, then, not only would this method of producing fuel avoid or limit the environmental harms of drilling and transporting oil and of growing feedstocks to produce biomass, but it would also, because it is itself carbon fixing, help offset the environmental costs of burning fuel. Of course, the process is not without its own costs: some methods of producing fuels this way would require a lot of equipment—greenhouses, in effect, to protect the algae and promote photosynthesis—and others would require construction of vast acres of open ponds.

The research is a focus of academic, corporate, and government effort, including the Joint BioEnergy Institute (a public–private research partnership that brings together Lawrence Berkeley, Sandia, and Lawrence Livermore national laboratories along with the University of California campuses of Berkeley and Davis and the Carnegie Institution for Science), the J. Craig Venter Institute (with $600 million in funding from ExxonMobil Corporation), Amyris Biotechnologies (with funding from Crystalsev, a large Brazilian ethanol distributor), and an assortment of start-ups and smaller biotechnology companies. Some methods are expected to be commercially viable in the next few years; others are longer-term propositions (Presidential Commission 2010: 59, 61).

It is worth noting that none of these lines of work illustrates the more sensationalistic claims about what synthetic biology can achieve—the "creation of life," the development of platform organisms that can be outfitted with interchangeable genetic parts, or the integration of biology with engineering so that the work can be performed by nonexperts in the kitchen. Many, actually, start with the identification of wild-type strains that already produce biofuel, followed by random mutagenesis and isolation of the best strains, and many of the genetic interventions then conducted on them aim not to transform them into fundamentally new biological processes but to tweak them so that they do some one thing as well as possible. For this kind of work, arguably, the label "synthetic biology" is a bit overblown, if that term suggests (as I think it does) the construction of organisms. More apt might be the term "metabolic engineering"—the study and alteration (including by genetic manipulation) of metabolic processes within existing organisms (Nielsen and Kiesling 2011). The work also resembles "traditional" genetic engineering in that it is essentially gene transfer, differing chiefly in that it can now be done faster, on a larger scale, potentially combining genetic sequences from three or more organisms, and with more information about the genetic sequences and the organism into which they are put, and therefore with greater ability to design the resulting organism. (Given the links and differences with gene transfer, critics sometimes refer to it as "extreme genetic engineering" (The ETC Group 2007)). None of this is to belittle the field, but only to try to get clear on the facts about it.

Concerns about consequences

The high-profile concerns about synthetic biology are about the potential for deliberate misuse, accidental threats to public health, and environmental hazards. The development of organisms to produce fuel appears to steer clear of the first two problems, except to the extent that work on these applications also leads to advances elsewhere in synthetic biology that raise such questions. More serious are concerns about environmental hazards, although the severity of the threat is uncertain. Even in commercial production mode, many of the organisms under development to produce fuel would be confined to bioreactors or contained facilities. Also, organisms that produce excess quantities of hydrocarbons are likely to be at an evolutionary disadvantage if they escape into the field, and fail-safe mechanisms could be implemented to hamper their survival in the field. Indeed, some in the field have argued that the organisms separated from the environment may be more important for protecting the organisms than for protecting the environment.

These considerations have not quelled concern, however. One reason for continued caution is that synthetic biology involves a high level of unpredictability. The possibility must be considered that organisms developed to have one set of characteristics in a highly controlled setting might turn out to display other characteristics if they escaped into the environment. Micro-organisms can also evolve rapidly and can exchange genes laterally with each other, leaving open the further possibilities that escaped microorganisms might either acquire new properties or transfer genes to a wild-type microorganism, giving it new properties.

It is also true that once organisms invade new environments, they can be extremely difficult to eradicate, and microbes would presumably be ineradicable. Environmental contamination by living organisms would be very different in this respect from contamination by a chemical spill (Snow 2010).

At the outset, then, extremely careful analyses are needed of the organisms proposed for commercial application. In testimony to the Presidential Commission for the Study of Bioethical Issues, ecologist Allison Snow offered the following recommendations for thinking about the risks posed by synthetic algae designed to produce fuel: "a good start for micro algae would be to publish professional monographs dealing with the biology and ecology of each species and its close relatives including information about how they reproduce, how they spread, whether they exchange genes with other strains, whether they have been bred to be suicidal, whether they could become more abundant or might die out, and whether they produce any kinds of toxins or other side effects" (Snow 2010).

We should also give some thought to the underlying philosophical and psychological questions about the perception and weighing of risk. Evaluating a technology involves both factual claims and value claims—claims about both potential outcomes and their likelihood and magnitude, and claims about the significance of those scenarios. Bringing out these values is what "evaluating" outcomes means. Among these value considerations are questions about what *counts* as a risk, a cost, or a benefit, how heavily to weigh it, how much to discount a risk or potential benefit that is low probability or would occur only many years later, and how much more heavily to weigh a potentially catastrophic impact.

The tools used to evaluate outcomes, such as risk assessment and cost–benefit analysis, make assumptions about these issues. Unfortunately, though, the assumptions are often buried and unexamined. Also, risk assessments and economic evaluations frequently focus on outcomes that can be measured easily, which may not adequately reflect what we care about most (Stone 2011). In short, evaluating outcomes requires value assumptions that often go unexamined. One result is that people may feel that important values have been ignored or suppressed. Public discourse and public policy could therefore benefit from a thorough interdisciplinary inquiry into the role of values in evaluating the potential outcomes of synthetic biology.

In its report on synthetic biology issued at the end of 2010, the Presidential Commission recommended that policy toward emerging biotechnologies, including synthetic biology, should be based on a principle of "responsible stewardship" toward collective human well-being and the environment, which in turn "calls for prudent vigilance" (Presidential Commission 2010: 124). The content of this recommendation remains ambiguous, however. Although the notions of "responsibility" and "prudent vigilance" suggest some degree of precaution, the commission did not attempt to fit its recommendations into the existing literature on the precautionary principle, and though it said that evaluation of the technology should be "ongoing," it did not explain which evaluation processes are appropriate. Since it also did not call for any particular constraints on synthetic biology, critics were left with the impression that the commission had not called for any substantive policy changes.

Intrinsic objections to synthetic biology

One of these concerns is whether the very idea of creating organisms is intrinsically morally troubling. (I say "morally troubling" in order to capture a broader set of possible positions than would be captured if we were thinking only about permissibility—that is, about what is not just morally troubling but morally wrong.) This concern is a recurrent topic for synthetic biology and is probably the most controversial and philosophically difficult of the ethical issues of synthetic biology. Many feel that the alteration of nature should have limits of some sort; the opposition to genetically modified organisms is connected to this feeling, and more than a little of the concern about the environment is rooted in it.

Perhaps the classic way of articulating concerns about synthetic biology suggests a religious or metaphysical point, not just a moral point. For example, one might worry that synthetic biology puts human beings into a role in the cosmos properly held by God. This would be the explicit way of understanding the complaint that scientists are "playing God," as people say. This would be an inappropriate elevation of human beings. Alternatively, one might hold that synthetic biology constitutes an inappropriate degradation of the religious or metaphysical category of life (Boldt and Muller 2008).

One problem with this way of advancing the moral argument is that if the religious or metaphysical claims are robust, then one needs buy-in on them, and the more robust they are, the less likely they are to be widely shared and the less traction they will have in public debate (and the more problematic it will be to invoke them in order to formulate public policy). Another problem is that the argument treats "life" as a very general moral category, comprising a variety of different kinds of living things—complex animals (such as mammals), microorganisms, plants, and fungi. But people mostly do not aggregate all living things together in this way (Evans n.d.). Instead, moral distinctions between different kinds are common. Vegetarians can use antibacterial soap and vaccines, after all. Thus sacredness might be attributed to some but not to all living things.

How might the concern be advanced just as a moral point? The comparison to concerns about the protection of endangered species and "wilderness" areas suggests one route. Bruce Jennings, a scholar at the Center for Humans and Nature and a participant in a two-year research project at The Hastings Center on the ethical issues of synthetic biology, formulates the general moral concern as a choice between two kinds of discourses that might govern the relationship between humans and nature—two competing moral ideals to guide that relationship. One discourse is that of "altering nature to meet human demands"; the other is that of "adjusting human demands to accommodate nature" (Jennings 2010). The former holds that nature is no more than stuff to be put to use—to be pumped out of the ground, cut down, burned, turned to waste, and disposed of as needed. The latter calls on us to cherish the natural world as it is and limit the harm humans are wreaking on it—not just in order to keep the planet habitable for humans as long as possible, but because the planet, with its diversity of life, is valued in its own right.

If we focus on synthetic biology's grand, abstract mission of integrating biology and engineering, then the field looks like the nonpareil example of the former ideal, and stands starkly at odds with the ideal of cherishing the natural world. If we focus, however, on the concrete forms the field takes—what it actually accomplishes—then it looks less threatening. In the case of creating synthetic organisms to make fuel, for example, two things stand out. First, the field is aimed not at altering life, but at developing specialized microorganisms. Second, those organisms would be put to a use in which the discourse of altering nature is already dominant. If cyanobacteria can be modified to produce gasoline, for example, the question is whether that would really be a more dramatic way of adapting nature to human ends than drilling for oil, processing it in huge refineries, and shipping it around the world. Arguably, they could also be characterized as a way of adapting human ends to nature, since they might have some beneficial environmental effects. However, this way of formulating the question leaves open the possibility that, if synthetic biology turns out to be harmful for the environment, it might be morally troubling *even if* it appears to be beneficial for human well-being.

Justice

Another kind of concern has to do with the social distribution of the benefits and harms. In a nutshell, the worry is that the benefits of synthetic biology will accrue to wealthy nations, and especially to those who have secured patents on the relevant technical technological developments, while those in poorer, undeveloped nations are either excluded from the benefits or are actively exploited and harmed, in terms both of the economic effects of synthetic biology and of damage to the environment or public health.

The production of biofuel with synthetic organisms illustrates these concerns sharply. Methods that rely on the processing of substrates collected from biomass would require the cultivation of vast acreages of feedstock crops, possibly with harmful effects in places where these crops might be grown. The feedstocks might replace crops that produce food for humans, for example. "The most productive and accessible biomass," writes a civil society organization called the ETC Group, "is in the global South—exactly where, by 2050, there may be another 2 billion mouths to feed on lands that (thanks to climate chaos) may yield 20–50% less" (The ETC Group 2010, iii). Industrial-scale production of the feedstocks might also have ramifications for land ownership, water use, and soil quality, all of which are already often under pressure in undeveloped countries

(The ETC Group 2007, 31). Giving land over to production of feedstocks might also have bad environmental consequences.

Finally, there is a debate about the environmental benefits of producing fuel from raw materials harvested from plants, since growing the plants itself requires a lot of energy. Synthetic biology aims to make the process fuel much more efficient, notably by turning to more common raw materials and more easily grown feedstocks, but the outcome of this work is still in doubt. Reliance on photosynthetic techniques, though it avoids the feedstock issue, would nonetheless also probably be resource intensive; in particular, the techniques would require a huge supply of water. If the production of fuel through photosynthesis were conducted in arid locations (which often have plentiful sunlight— another resource requirement), then providing water might exacerbate water supply problems.

The Presidential Commission suggested that synthetic biology might well avoid exacerbating social disparities. Indeed, it declared, "Much of the optimism surrounding synthetic biology stems directly from its potential to address some of the longstanding, significant problems associated with these disparities. Synthetic biology offers potential applications that may be particularly beneficial to less-advantaged populations, including improved quality and access to vaccines against infectious diseases, medications, and fuel sources" (Presidential Commission 2010: 165). Remediation of long-term environmental harms, such as climate change—on the assumption that synthetic biology can help address these problems—would clearly benefit less-advantaged populations, since it is likely that those populations will be disproportionately harmed by those problems.

But how can we achieve this vision? We are left with some outstanding questions that need more study: First, how much constraint does the goal of achieving just outcomes justify? That is, is the goal of just outcomes an ideal that ought to be achieved to the extent possible, or is it a requirement of some sort—a condition of receiving public funding, or (at the extreme end) a condition for existence? As a corollary of this question, we should consider what sorts of policy mechanisms might appropriately be employed to advance this goal. Two much-discussed kinds of options include funding decisions, which can influence the directions in which the field advances and therefore the kinds of commercial enterprises it makes possible, and intellectual property policy, which determines control over and access to new developments in the field, and may therefore influence the direction in which the field advances both by affecting the incentive structure for conducting research in the field and by affecting access to the fruits of others' research.

Second, how do we deliberate publicly about what distributions of which outcomes are deemed acceptable? Unsurprisingly, there are starkly different visions of justice at play in synthetic biology. Some in the field would undoubtedly assert that justice grants the liberty to experiment with the technology in whatever direction one likes, to the extent permitted by public safety. Some would also hold that in any adequate understanding of justice, those who have worked to advance the field should benefit disproportionately. Some would also hold that if the financial rewards are curtailed, none of the benefits will be realized. Moreover, the challenge is not just the abstract problem of determining the content of justice, but that abstract problem concretely instantiated in the practical issue of deliberating publicly, even globally, about justice.

Third, who bears responsibility? Only those working on lines of business that emerge from publicly funded research? Or is it a broader obligation, borne by anyone who might profit from synthetic biology? The Presidential Commission has suggested a broader rendering: "Manufacturers and others seeking to use synthetic biology for commercial activities should ensure that risks and potential benefits to communities and the environment are assessed and managed so that the most serious risks, including long-term impacts, are not unfairly or unnecessarily borne by certain individuals, subgroups, or populations. These efforts should also aim to ensure that the important advances that may result from this research reach those individuals and populations who could most benefit from them" (Presidential Commission 2010: 164).

Conclusion

In one way, these questions about the ethics of synthetic biology are timeless. They are questions about how to figure well-being, about how humans may treat the natural world, and about justice. They are questions that people have been thinking about for millennia, and questions that arise for previous biotechnologies as much as for synthetic biology. At the same time, they are new questions. Asking about the consequences of synthetic biology may lead toward a reassessment of conventional risk assessment and cost–benefit strategies, for example: they ask us to reconsider the weight we assign to risks. What weight should we assign to a low-likelihood but high-impact risk? Concerns about justice are not new, but it is novel to raise them in advance of a technological development and ask that the technology be shaped or implemented in a way that allays those concerns. We are to some extent, then, not only witnessing new scientific work, but breaking new moral ground.

References

Aubel, D., and Fussenegger, M. (2010). "Mammalian Synthetic Biology: From Tools to Therapies," *Bioessays*, 32:332–45.

Ball, P. (2004). "Synthetic Biology: Starting from Scratch," *Nature*, 431:624–6.

Boldt, J., and Muller, O. (2008). "Newtons of the Leaves of Grass," *Nature Biotechnology*, 26:387–9.

Brent, R. (2004). "A Partnership between Biology and Engineering," *Nature Biotechnology*, 22(10): 1211–14.

Endy, D. (2005). "Foundations for Engineering Biology," *Nature*, 438:449–53.

Evans, J. H. (n.d.). "Evaluating 'Teaching Humanness' Claims in Synthetic Biology and Public Policy Bioethics," unpublished paper produced for the Hastings Center research project, "Ethical Issues in Synthetic Biology" (funded by the Alfred P. Sloan Foundation).

Forster, A. C., and Church, G. M. (2006). "Towards Synthesis of a Minimal Cell," *Molecular Systems Biology*, 2: 45.

Gibson, D. G. et al. (2008). "Complete Chemical Synthesis, Assembly, and Cloning of a Mycoplasma Genitalium Genome," *Science*, 319:1215–20.

Gibson, D. G. et al. (2010). "Creation of a Bacterial Cell Controlled by a Chemically Synthesized Genome," *Science*, 329:52–6.

Jang, Y.-S. et al., (2012). "Engineering of Microorganisms for the Production of Biofuels and Perspectives Based on Systems Metabolic Engineering Approaches," *Biotechnology Advances*, 30(5): 989–1000.

Jennings, B. (2010). "Toward an Ecological Political Economy: Accommodating Nature in a New Discourse of Public Philosophy and Policy Analysis," *Critical Policy Studies*, 4(1): 77–85.

Nielsen, J., and Kiesling J. (2011). "Synergies between Synthetic Biology and Metabolic Engineering," *Nature Biotechnology*, 29(8): 693–5.

O'Malley, M. A. et al. (2008). "Knowledge-Making Distinctions in Synthetic Biology," *Bioinformatics*, 30:57–65.

Presidential Commission for the Study of Bioethics Issues. (2010). *New Directions: The Ethics of Synthetic Biology and Emerging Technologies*. Washington, DC: Government Printing Office.

Snow, A. (2010). *Testimony to the Presidential Commission for the Study of Bioethical Issues*, July 8–9, Washington, DC, http://bioethics.gov/cms/meeting-one-transcripts (accessed December 20, 2012).

Stone, D. (2011). *Policy Paradox: The Art of Political Reason*. 3rd ed. New York: W. W. Norton.

The ETC Group. (2007). "Extreme Genetic Engineering: An Introduction to Synthetic Biology," Ottawa, ON: The ETC Group.

The ETC Group, "Groups Criticize Presidential Commission's Recommendations on Synthetic Biology: 'Business as Usual' Wins Out Over Precaution," http://www.etcgroup.org/content/groups-criticize-presidential-commission%E2%80%99s-recommendations-synthetic-biology; December 16, 2010 (accessed 15 April 2013).

The ETC Group. (2010). "The New Biomassters: Synthetic Biology and the Next Assault on Biodiversity and Livelihoods," Ottawa, ON: The ETC Group.

9.2

Commentary
Synthetic Biology, Intellectual Property, and Buddhism

Soraj Hongladarom

Greg Kaebnick has presented a wonderful account of the various ethical implications that synthetic biology has raised. His main concern is with the roles that synthetic biology is going to play in the near future, and he seems to have an overall positive view on synthetic biology, believing that it can create benefits to humankind in various ways, such as eliminating toxic waste and altering available chemical compounds into fuel. The ability of synthetic biology to help us survive in the twenty-first century underscores Kaebnick's emphasis in the paper on the relationship between human beings and nature. On the one hand, there is the view that nature is there to be used and exploited. According to this view synthetic biology would seem to be a clear reflection of how humans exploit nature through creating life itself according to the demands that fulfill humans' insatiable and egoistic desires. On the other hand, there is another view that there should be limits on what humans can do to the natural world. Kaebnick argues in the paper that there could be a role for synthetic biology in the second option. Products of synthetic biology could be used, for instance, in creating fuel out of other organic compounds that are already abundant. The question is what kind of humans' relationship to nature is reflected by this kind of synthetic biology. Kaebnick points out an option where artificially developed algae could produce fuel for us, perhaps eventually freeing us from the need to keep on searching for the elusive fossil fuels. The environment does not have to be sacrificed by taking this route of synthetic biology.

This is all fine and good. However, in this paper I would like to focus on another aspect of the ethics of synthetic biology, one that is discussed tangentially in Kaebnick. The issue concerns intellectual property rights and their role in helping alleviate the disparity between the developed and the developing countries (Boyle 2008; Himma 2008; Johns 2009). This is the issue that is bound to take place when the technology of synthetic biology becomes viable on an industrial scale. The main question is: What kind of justification could be offered for claiming ownership of synthetic biological products? Knowing how to answer this question is necessary for the further discussion of how to realize the benefits of synthetic biology, benefits that Kaebnick is so eloquent about in his paper. In this short reply paper, it is obviously not possible for me to provide the justification in any detail. So a sketch will be offered, a research program that could perhaps be a starting point for further discussion and studies. The discussion on intellectual property here will tie in with Kaebnick's paper through his discussion of justice.

It is quite well known that there are strong arguments against claiming intellectual property rights over living organisms. Pharmaceutical companies that go to rainforests in developing countries looking for local plants that might contain novel compounds for development of new drugs are accused of "bioprospecting" or "biopiracy," primarily because they do not recognize the rights of the locals who own the land on which the plant grows (Bhat 1996; Fenwick 1998; Tedlock 2006). Moreover, multinational corporations are also accused of appropriating the knowledge of indigenous people without giving the latter credits. The idea behind this is that claims of intellectual property rights should not be confined only to those who have the sophisticated capacity of developing the local plant into new drugs, but the protection should also be expanded to cover the local people who have acted as the "guardians" of the plant in question and who might have indigenous knowledge which could be highly beneficial to the world.

In synthetic biology, however, there is no such concern with the local, indigenous people. The technology is highly advanced and sophisticated; it is no longer a matter of finding organisms from the tropical forests or from any other parts of the environment and extracting useful compounds from them. It is instead a matter of creating organisms from scratch or altering existing ones to serve particular purposes, such as creating fuels cheaply. The developing world does not seem to have any role at all to play in this type of enterprise. The developing world may lay claim to the organisms that are taken from forests in their areas and demand their share when new techniques developed from the organisms prove to be profitable and useful. With synthetic biology, however, no such possibility exists. Everything from the beginning to the end of synthetic biology engineering is highly infused with very advanced knowledge and technology. If left unchecked, it is conceivable that this progress would widen the gap between the developing and the developed world further. Synthetic biology is here a clear example of the knowledge economy, where the key for economic progress is no longer in manufacturing per se, but in infusing sophisticated knowledge into economic production. Given the likely possibility that the synthesized algae will be powerful enough to turn common organic compounds into usable fuel, the economic impact will be enormous. The countries that hold the key to the technology will surely maintain their dominance far into the future. However, without an effective benefit-sharing scheme among the countries of the world, it is also quite likely that the growing disparity will generate more conflicts and instability. Thus the principle of global justice demands that an effective benefit-sharing scheme be in place.

Such a scheme will have to depend on a massive rethinking of the whole idea of intellectual property rights. What I have in mind is that the principle should be supplemented by the idea, derived from Buddhism, that the very existence of the idea of personal property depends on the usefulness of the idea on survival and flourishing of individuals having the property. This in Buddhism has to be accompanied by the idea of interdependence, the realization that nothing stands alone in the world and everything owes its very existence through connection with other things (Siderits 2007). There is not enough room in this paper to explicate the Buddhist concept in detail, but the outline is clear enough. Personal property is useful in maintaining the survival of an individual. One needs a portion of the material world to survive: one needs to eat, to find clothing and shelter, and so on. The ultimate goal of being a Buddhist is to perfect oneself thoroughly so that one achieves final liberation from the bonds of samsara, or the world that is full of suffering. Translated into ordinary language, this means that the goal is to create a perfectly peaceful world for oneself and others through changing *oneself* rather than the outer world. This is only possible when oneself and others are essentially interconnected. The idea is that perfecting oneself in this way would not be possible at all without some dependence on the material world. Hence Buddhism in general is not opposed to the idea of personal property, and as intellectual property is an offshoot of personal property Buddhism does not have anything in principle against the former either.

Individuals' dependence on the material world, nonetheless, also needs to be complemented by the fact that individuals live together in groups and communities and cannot even survive without depending on others. This fact according to Buddhism dictates that acquisition of private property cannot be used solely for one's own purposes alone, but the property needs to be shared or given back to the community as a concrete realization of everyone's dependence on one another. In today's terms this means that those who have put effort into creating and developing something beneficial should share it with others. There is nothing wrong with getting some return from one's investment in the form of material benefits back to oneself. The principle of justice requires that too; otherwise that would be nothing more than exploiting the inventor for his effort while he gets nothing back in return. But the return should not be such that the others, those who make use of the invention, are exploited instead, such as by having to pay a very high price. If everyone strongly subscribes to the principle of interdependence of everyone on one another and of everything on everything else, then a workable solution can always be found when there is a conflict arising from the problem of distribution.

So we are now in a position to provide a sketch of an answer to the main question raised before. Justification for holding rights to *intellectual* property in the case of synthetic biology would need also to include the notion that all things are interdependent and thus everyone in a sense has a role to play in creating the intellectual property in question, which would mean that the claim to intellectual property rights cannot be exclusive to any individuals or groups. Apart from the problem of whether creating life from scratch or from existing "biobricks" is right or wrong in itself, products created through this technology, as well as the technology itself, need to be shared equitably among the population of the world. Even though it seems at first sight that synthetic biology does not need any involvement from the developing world at all, further consideration shows that in fact such involvement cannot be avoided. Globalization is entirely pervasive and the livelihood of those in the West has been dependent on input in various forms from the East through export and import of goods and material as well as continual movement of students, researchers, and professors across the boundary. The Buddhist principle of interdependence implies that one does not achieve one's own flourishing and realization of one's ultimate goal if one does not give back to others; this principle would then imply that the fruits of the labor in synthetic biology, such as the creation of fuel-creating synthetic algae, should be shared equitably with the world.

The upshot, then, is that the whole concept of intellectual property, as an offshoot of more tangible personal property, needs to be reconsidered. Perhaps one difference between the old concept of property and that of intellectual property is that one physically needs some kind of personal property to survive. The food one eats, for example, is one's personal property in a very real sense. However, with intellectual property, physical survival does not seem to be at stake. Instead it is used more by business corporations to protect their interests. One might look at the survival of the corporations themselves if their intellectual property rights are taken away; that could be the case, but it seems a far cry from the older scenario of a person on the verge of death when they are deprived of food. Consequently, the tie between personal property and intellectual property should be loosened. Instead of treating intellectual property as a kind of personal property (belonging either to an individual or to a corporation functioning as a juristic person), it should be treated as a distinct type in its own right, a special kind of property loosely connected to the old concept of personal property but not wholly so. Intellectual property should be understood as a tool for maintaining the interests of the inventors who created the property only for a certain period of time; it should not be considered as fully personal property belonging to the inventor, but something that ultimately belongs to humankind as a whole.

The way this works, for example in the case of synthetic biological products, is that the technique behind the creation of the fuel-producing algae and other synthetic biological inventions should in all cases be made open to the public. Business interests should not cloud the mindset of those involved to such an extent that they are blind to the ultimate benefits that the opening up will bring to humankind as a whole, which in the end will benefit themselves too. Here the Buddhist would emphasize that what is going on in someone's mind is of the utmost importance. What need to be changed the most are the beliefs and mentalities of those involved so that they become less dominated by their own narrow personal, selfish interests and begin to see the real benefits that opening up knowledge and techniques to the world community would bring. Intellectual property is not personal in the sense that it can be used up and consumed by an individual or a group thereof; on the contrary, it can be copied to all those who are interested, thereby benefiting everyone. Here would be a clear illustration of the Buddhist notion of interdependence.

Conclusion

The fear that synthetic biology will create new life forms that could harm our environment is perhaps overblown. The level of technological progress today does not enable us to do that. Instead what scientists have been doing is to engineer the building blocks of life in order to accomplish various engineering tasks, or to design what could be regarded as "life" using other forms of chemicals not found in normal life forms. Either way the likelihood that a monster will be created that threatens our environment or our existence is remote. As the current state of the technology goes, one should regard synthetic biology as of now more as an engineering project rather than a fully biological one. The life forms that will be created (if indeed they can be classified in that way) will function more like chemical compounds than living microbes. If the public understands this point, then the fear might be diminished.

Nevertheless, the fear is perhaps not founded solely on inadequate awareness of the technical content. Even though one understands that synthetic biology now is only at an embryonic stage of development, one might not be able to stop thinking that some day in the future scientists will be able to create and manipulate advanced life forms at will, and the possibility emerges that some evil scientists might use that ability for their own purposes. This, however, is true for all other kinds of technology. Nuclear technology is a very powerful example of how destructive a new form of technology can become. Hence an effective regulatory scheme at the international level that is robust enough to ensure public safety must be in place, and it is now time to design and implement such a scheme while synthetic biology is just beginning to be developed.

Furthermore, I have argued in the paper that a new way of thinking about intellectual property rights should be adopted, one that loosens the existing bind between the familiar conception of *personal* property and intellectual property. Based on Buddhist teaching, a way can be found so that the notion of intellectual property rights can act as a facilitator of global justice and equity instead of its enemy (Pogge 2008).[1]

References

Bhat, M. G. (1996). "Trade-Related Intellectual Property Rights to Biological Resources: Socioeconomic Implications for Developing Countries," *Ecological Economics*, 19(3): 205–17.

Boyle, J. (2008). *The Public Domain: Enclosing the Commons of the Mind*. New Haven, CT: Yale University Press.

Fenwick, S. (1998). "Bioprospecting or Biopiracy?" *Drug Discovery Today*, 3(9): 399–402.

Himma, K. (2008). "The Justification of Intellectual Property: Contemporary Philosophical Disputes," *Journal of the American Society for Information Science and Technology*, 59(7): 1143–61.

Johns, A. (2009). *Piracy: The Intellectual Property Wars from Gutenberg to Gates*. Chicago. IL: University of Chicago Press.

Pogge, T. (2008). *World Poverty and Human Rights*. 2nd ed. Cambridge: Polity Press.

Siderits, M. (2007). *Buddhism as Philosophy: An Introduction*. Aldershot: Ashgate.

Tedlock, B. (2006). "Indigenous Heritage and Biopiracy in the Age of Intellectual Property Rights," *Explore*, 2(3): 256–9.

[1] Research for this paper has been supported partially by a grant from the Thailand Research Fund, grant no. BRG5380009.

9.3

Commentary
Before the Dawn of Ethics in Synthetic Biology

Osamu Kanamori

I General

Based on Gregory E. Kaebnick's "The Ethical Issues of Synthetic Biology," in this short essay I will evaluate synthetic biology research from philosophical and social perspectives.

Before I tackle synthetic biology, I would like to consider a more general problem. In general, human beings do not live in a perfectly harmonious, integrated relationship with the world. Even if people were to live quietly in the mountains, a time would come when they would need to abandon their dwellings, such as when a wildfire occurs because of, say, a lightning strike. Have we not just recently witnessed scenes in which people's homes are destroyed by a great earthquake and tsunami? In this world, human beings live side by side with obstacles and dangers.

Let us then conduct a thought experiment. Suppose we have a special device that generates extremely strong winds with the power to level hundreds of ordinary wooden houses to the ground. We will refer to this device as Device W. Meanwhile, as is well known, large-scale tornadoes frequently occur in the central and southern regions of the United States, and in some cases there is massive damage to houses. Now suppose there occurs an extremely dangerous tornado, one of the largest among all such natural tornadoes, and we name it Tornado T. Here we can pose a question. At a certain time, Tornado T strikes naturally and destroys 500 houses, causing dozens of casualties. We compare this case (Case A) to another in which a certain person creates Device W and generates strong winds that cause great damage to 500 houses (Case B). Although both cases appear to be similar in that they are both disasters caused by strong winds, there is a critical difference. There is no man-made element whatsoever in the case of Tornado T, which occurred for some natural reason. In contrast, Device W is created by the work of people at every stage, including its conception, design, construction, and operation. Although Case A and Case B are both calamities, beneath the outward appearance of similarity is an important difference. Case A is natural, while Case B is man-made. In this case, Case B is clearly the more problematic of the two, as there is no justification for the voluntary and active creation of a disaster in a world already awash with various obstacles, disasters, and calamities.

The implications of this rather primitive thought experiment are not trivial. An analogy can be drawn with the case of synthetic biology. This world is already teeming with life forms that live functionally and adeptly in their environments. Whilst the last century has seen much environmental destruction and reduction of biodiversity, on the whole the biosphere boasts a harmony and richness that are unique. Nature itself tends towards exquisite balance. Intentionally introducing a man-made factor and jeopardizing this balance can hardly be deemed appropriate. Just as extraordinarily strong justifications should be required for producing Device W, it is natural that extraordinary strong justifications should be demanded for advancing synthetic biology.

Let us recall that immediately after the introduction of recombinant DNA technology, nightmares such as *Escherichia coli* that produce deadly poisons entered the minds of biologists. Owing to ensuing discussions and the enhancement of safety designs, no such risks have yet materialized, and biotechnology has continued to develop rapidly. However, in some ways, synthetic biology research can be said to bring the potentially dangerous scenarios accompanying the introduction of recombinant DNA closer to reality. Whether carrying out special procedures on existing microorganisms or creating uniquely designed synthetic bacteria without mimicking nature, it is easy to see how frightening possibilities could unfold if such technology becomes applied to military purposes, for instance. If in the future synthetic biology research as a whole were to increase in related fields, and to that extent had the potential to bring disaster, we will likely end up having to hold a Second Asilomar Conference to devise comprehensive regulations for such research.

Indeed, as in the case of biological weapons, non-military research in which hazardousness is the direct objective is nearly inconceivable. In this context, what is more important and highly probable is a scenario in which a synthetic organism, despite being developed with good intentions, ultimately causes a disaster when released into the environment (intentionally or not). Kaebnick has introduced the optimistic argument that even in such cases the synthetic organism will be weeded out by natural organisms, which ought to be stronger. However, this is nothing more than wishful thinking. How the natural world will respond is entirely unpredictable. Akin to saying that Device W is more difficult to justify than Tornado T, we will likely need to be cautious about large-scale advancement of synthetic bacteria as well, in the absence of some extraordinary reason.

However, a supplementary point needs to be borne in mind when considering how cautious we should be about synthetic biology research at the micro level (e.g. on synthetic bacteria or viruses) because of its high unpredictability and uncontrollability. Artificially transforming life forms based on a certain type of purposive rationality is something that we have already been doing in various fields, such as livestock, vegetables, and flowering/ornamental plants. That the human species modifies the surrounding environment for its own convenience may even be said to be one of its essential characteristics. Therefore, it would not be surprising if humans modified other life forms too. Humans have long domesticated other animals, and will likely continue to do so. Should we be as cautious about the modification of large organisms like livestock, which are visible and hence are much more controllable, as we are about the modification of microscopic organisms?

There are reasons for answering both "yes" and "no." On the one hand, research subjects that are subtly different, at least from those of current synthetic biology, ought to become primary subjects. Research on subjects such as pigs with livers that are as close as possible to a human liver, fish that grow at twice the normal speed, and silkworms that spin silk of enhanced quality will likely continue in the future. I reiterate that their relative controllability ought to be greater, with the caveat that the comparison is strictly with synthetic bacteria. However, on the other hand, among the examples just given, rapidly growing fish will also become uncontrollable if released into the ocean; hence, we may encounter a problem similar to that of synthetic bacteria. Whilst these examples may appear similar, they are in fact quite different. Yet they are all life forms transformed by purposive rationality. Consistent with the history of livestock development, the biology of modification in the broader sense can be predicted to advance in the future in tandem with the ever-sharper incisiveness of modern biology.

If we return again to the potential problems posed by the development of synthetic biology, we could perhaps make the following judgments. At least for the moment, it is premature to discuss "an *ethics* of synthetic biology." To begin, research in this area has not advanced to any considerable degree. Furthermore, it remains unclear whether synthetic biology will raise unique ethical issues, or whether—as seems more likely—it can be viewed as a subgroup of biotechnology, raising ethical issues that are familiar from other applications of biotechnology.

There will undoubtedly be some readers who will be suspicious, having just been told that the biology of modification in general is not a problem of ethics. However, there is no contradiction here. The ethics I mention within the context of biological modification in general, and the ethics I mention in the context of synthetic biology are in fact quite different. It is well known that bioethics does not merely delve into individual perspectives on life or ethical norms, but instead encompasses the entirety of political regulations and procedural guidelines regarding behaviors in fields such as advanced medicine. What I mean by the expression "ethics of synthetic biology" is something similar to bioethics. Theoretically, an ethics of synthetic biology in this sense can be established. However, we currently find ourselves at the dawn, where even the possibility of an independent field of ethics is unclear.

2 Specific

I have made some general observations, inspired by Kaebnick's thesis. Now, based on these premises, I wish to touch upon his article in greater detail; however, after the general considerations above, there is in fact not much left to mention. As I have argued up to this point, it is still too early to discuss an ethics of synthetic biology. Moreover, the main topic in this area is biofuel development, which is more about metabolic engineering than synthetic biology, as noted by the author himself. This is a topic that could fit perfectly into the discussion of biotechnology ethics.

Furthermore, in this case, regarding considerations of risks and social justice, the problems of synthetic biology closely resemble those arising from biotechnology in general. Therefore Kaebnick's thesis, in fact, is not particularly related to synthetic biology, and is much less an example of the ethics of synthetic biology (although I am not saying it is no good for this reason).

At any rate, if we return to the biofuels issue with which he deals, the primary problem here, as he rightly notes, is likely to be one involving justice. This not only includes the issue of the increasing gap between developed and developing nations, but also the more biopolitical issue of using as fuel materials normally used for food. In the future, as a further population explosion is predicted worldwide, there is no doubt that the issue of determining the relative priorities of fuel production and a survival infrastructure (i.e. securing food for human beings) will present as an enormous problem. As Kaebnick notes as well, the outlook of the American President's committee is indeed overly optimistic and is not very helpful.

Conversely, we cannot help but think that the central point of discussion is far from that of synthetic biology itself. This only serves to highlight anew what I have been stating up to this point, which is that it would be premature to attempt to address an ethics of synthetic biology at this point.

9.4

Response to Commentaries

Gregory Kaebnick

The commentaries by Soraj Hongladarom and Osamu Kanamori highlight important questions in thinking about the ethical issues of synthetic biology. Both also raise questions that I did not touch upon in my essay, and for giving me an opportunity to clarify my views about these issues I am very grateful. Hongladarom raises questions about the appropriate intellectual property framework for synthetic biology, and Kanamori raises questions about the appropriate moral framework for synthetic biology.

Before I address the specifics of these essays, however, I would like to register a more general point about the overall tone or thrust of my essay. Both Hongladarom and Kanamori suggest that I am generally in favor of synthetic biology, Hongladarom writes that I present "an overall positive view on synthetic biology," and Kanamori describes me as introducing "the optimistic argument" that organisms developed using synthetic biology would pose little risk to the environment, if they accidentally escaped, because they would be too weak to compete against the organisms naturally occurring there. In fact, I sought to outline a more complicated position. I registered several kinds of concerns one might have about synthetic biology—concerns about risks and potential benefits, concerns that "synthetic organisms" raise the level of human alteration of the natural world in intrinsically undesirable ways, and concerns about justice—and I argued that concerns about outcomes—about risks and potential benefits and about the possibly unjust distribution of risks and potential benefits—are the most important considerations for synthetic biology. I do not think the possible outcomes tell generally in favor of synthetic biology or generally against it. Instead, I think we need to consider the development and use of synthetic biology on a case-by-case basis. In making those assessments, I would favor a somewhat more cautious approach than was described by the US President's Commission for the Study of Bioethical Issues. I would not favor a complete moratorium on development or use of synthetic biology, but I think good arguments could be mounted for moratoria on some kinds of applications.

Kanamori groups together applications that involve two kinds of environmental release—those that are released intentionally, and those that are not—and suggests that I think the organisms in both kinds of releases would quickly succumb to wild-type competitors. I would distinguish these applications. Organisms developed for deliberate environmental release would presumably have to be designed to survive more effectively in the wild; it is only those that are designed to be confined, separated from the environment, that one might expect (and all the qualifications are important here) to quickly die out in the wild. Applications involving intentional environmental release would be good candidates for a moratorium. If the moratorium on these applications is instituted, then at the very least, the particular applications should not proceed until more is known about the type of organism that has been engineered—how it would interact with the environment, for example, how quickly that organism can be expected to evolve, and how easily it might exchange genes with other microorganisms in the environment (Dana et al. 2012).

The main thrust of Hongladarom's commentary is to explore what intellectual property framework would be most appropriate for synthetic biology. Hongladarom is right to raise this question, for while I did not address it in my chapter, it is a large and hotly contested question in the field of synthetic biology. The J. Craig Venter Institute has applied for several patents on processes involved in the production of a synthetic genome, and critics have charged that the patent applications are overly broad and might give the Institute considerable control over the creation of synthetic genomes. Those arguing for a more open intellectual property scheme—one that would likely accord with Hongladarom's suggestions—include some within synthetic biology, who argued that a more open scheme is necessary in order for the field to flourish and in particular in order to make the field an engineering discipline, accessible to many people, rather than an arcane science that can be undertaken only in well-funded laboratories led by very specially educated people.

Hongladarom's discussion of the proper intellectual property (IP) framework for synthetic biology is in one way narrower than it might be, and in one way a bit broader than might be helpful. It is narrower in that Hongladarom probably distinguishes too sharply between the IP issues of synthetic biology and those that have been raised in discussions of "bioprospecting" by pharmaceutical companies. Hongladarom writes that synthetic biology does not involve bioprospecting because it does not require travelling to tropical forests in the developing world to find organisms that produce useful novel compounds. "It is instead a matter of creating organisms from scratch or altering existing ones to serve particular purposes." It can, however, involve a search for organisms that have useful genetic sequences, as illustrated by one of the examples of a near-term application for synthetic biology, the engineering of organisms that produce artemisinic acid, from which the very effective antimalarial treatment artemisinin can be produced. The engineered organisms incorporate genes from sweet wormwood, a plant that originated in Asia. One can certainly imagine that other synthetic biology applications would employ genes located in plants or animals found only in developing countries. Whatever objections might be lodged against bioprospecting would presumably also apply to these applications.

Hongladarom's discussion is exceptionally broad in that, as he notes, his concerns about intellectual property are grounded ultimately not in claims unique to synthetic biology or to genetic technologies more generally, but in claims about the idea of intellectual property overall—indeed, in claims about the idea of any kind of property.

"Buddhism dictates that acquisition of private property cannot be used solely for one's own purposes alone, but the property needs to be shared or given back to the community as a concrete realization of everyone's dependence on one another." I am sympathetic to the spirit of this position. However, it is a very large claim and would require some very strong arguments to get it accepted and established internationally.

The main thrust of Kanamori's commentary is to consider what sort of conceptual framework is best suited for assessing synthetic biology. Kanamori argues that, at least for the time being, "it is still too early to discuss an ethics of synthetic biology." I quite agree, at least if I understand Kanamori's position correctly.

On the one hand, if by "ethics of synthetic biology" we mean simply "the ethical issues raised by synthetic biology," then I believe it is not at all too early to discuss the most important ones. (The one which, though important in some other contexts, I would largely set aside for synthetic biology as the field currently stands—namely, the concern about whether engineering microorganisms is intrinsically morally undesirable—is probably a Rubicon we have already crossed.) Indeed, it is vitally important that we have that discussion now, so that we do not mistakenly accept an overly optimistic or pessimistic risk–benefit calculus.

On the other hand, if "ethics of synthetic biology" refers to a possible special field of ethics, a subfield of bioethics, then I believe Kanamori is quite right. And I think this meaning is what Kanamori has in mind; his argument appears to be that the ethical issues raised by the field do not appear to be unique. Synthetic biology applications have much in common with other biotechnologies, and some of the ethical issues connected to them are issues that are not at all unique to synthetic biology. Thus Kanamori joins with my colleagues at The Hastings Center in lamenting the balkanization of bioethics into a handful of supposedly separate domains (Parens et al. 2008)—"gen-ethics," "nano-ethics," and now perhaps "synth-ethics" (Synth-Ethics 2012).

I might, in fact, go just a little further and argue that not only is it still too early to say that there is "an ethics of synthetic biology," but it will always be too early to say that it exists. There are no brand new ethical questions in synthetic biology, nor is there any synthetic-biology-specific way of addressing those questions. The ethical issues raised by synthetic biology are the same, in general form, as those raised by earlier waves of technologies, and indeed by many other kinds of human endeavors. These issues have to do with how they may advance or impair human well-being, with the intrinsic value of limiting human intrusion into nature (aside from any questions about benefits and harms), and with the implications for equality and justice. The most that can be said in favor of their uniqueness is that, while familiar in broad outline, they sometimes take particularly interesting and challenging forms with synthetic biology. The potential benefits and harms are uncommonly great, for example, and the issue of human intrusion into nature amounts, with synthetic biology, to concerns about the very idea of synthesizing living organisms. Nonetheless, we will approach these questions most fruitfully if we do not regard them as matters of "first impression," as one might say in the law, but rather connect them with other ethical discussions and try to extend our ethical deliberations from the earlier precedents to the emerging technology.

References

Dana, G.V. et al. (2012). "Four Steps to Avoid a Synthetic-Biology Disaster," *Nature,* 483:29.

Parens, E., Johnston, J., and Moses, J. (2008). "Do We Need 'Synthetic Bioethics?'" *Science,* 321:1449.

Synth-Ethics. (2012). "Synth-Ethics: Ethical and Regulatory Issues Raised by Synthetic Biology," http://www.synthethics.eu/ (accessed April 9, 2012).

10.1

Primary Topic Article
Why Would It Be Morally Wrong to Create a Human–Animal Chimera?

Stuart J. Youngner

Those who would defend human dignity in the face of science's relentless march towards "discovery" are once again under attack. Senators Sam Brownback (R-KS) and Mary Landrieu (D-LA) are making headlines for introducing controversial legislation that would ban the American scientific community from developing embryos that contain both human and animal material. Dubbed the Human-Animal Hybrid Prohibition Act of 2009, the bill upholds the unique dignity of the human species and condemns human-animal hybrids as "grossly unethical because they blur the line between human and animal, male and female, parent and child, and one individual and another individual."

(Connor 2012)

Senator Brownback is clearly concerned about crossing or blurring boundaries between humans and animals, species, sexes, and individuals. In fact, disagreements about the acceptability of crossing these boundaries has become not only of interest to bioethics but has also become the fodder for a bitter "culture war" in the United States that is deeply influencing our political system. In this essay I will ask and try to answer the following questions:

- By what authority and methodology are boundaries created, identified, and defended?
- Once identified, how do we distinguish between moral and other types of boundaries?
- What could motivate one to cross a boundary?
- What could motivate one to protect a moral boundary?

Examples of moral boundaries of interest to bioethics include: human–animal; male–female; life–death; killing–allowing to die; human–machine; and natural–unnatural, among others. After reviewing some characteristics of boundaries, I will focus on developments in biomedicine and society that some would call progress and others would decry as moral abominations. I will argue here that the rhetoric of moral repugnance is merely that and has little to contribute to our pluralistic society's efforts to cope with social change and technological development. I will suggest that Jeffrey Stout, in his book *Ethics After Babel* (Stout 1988) offers a deeper and more helpful understanding of our society's moral framework. I will conclude that in modern, pluralistic society, religious dictates, the so-called "wisdom of repugnance" and simple tradition that resists change must be taken into account in the political sphere. Too often, however, they stand unnecessarily in the way of human progress.

How do we identify boundaries?

The term boundary initially calls to mind a geographical line on a map that separates two physical or political entities—countries, counties, properties, etc. Such boundaries can be created or changed by various political or legal entities, and once fixed, can be identified by survey instruments or, in modern times, a global positioning system (GPS). Before we can decide not to cross a boundary or to cross one, we have to know where it is. In bioethics, important boundaries can be drawn and identified by quite different "methodologies," and although some of these may be useful at times, none is without problems.

In addition to its more "objective" virtues, modern society looks to and trusts *science* as a powerful explanatory model. We often use science to mark distinct boundaries between species, sexes, races, and life and death. But science is not entirely definitive (Charo 1999). Genetically speaking, many species are much more similar than they are different. For example, human individuals' DNA may differ by only 0.1 percent. Humans and chimpanzees differ by 1.2–1.6 percent (Robert and Baylis 2003). As Robert and Baylis point out:

There is, however, no one authoritative definition of species. Biologists typically make do with a plurality of species concepts, invoking one or the other depending on the particular explanatory or investigative context. (2003: 4)

Surely, science can identify the line between life and death. The modern intensive care unit, where many life functions can be maintained while others have been irreversibly lost, has challenged that assumption. There is a substantive literature that that claims the task is philosophical. Only philosophy can answer the question "Which life function is so essential that its loss marks the moment of death?" Not until philosophy has completed its task can medical science try to identify the anatomical locations and tests necessary to demonstrate the loss (Bernat, Culver, and Gert 1981). Still others claim that death is a social construct (Arnold and Youngner 1993; Youngner and Arnold 2001).

Analytic philosophy is the primary methodology for drawing another important bioethics boundary, the one between killing and letting die. However, there are competing philosophical arguments about exactly where to draw this line, and it is highly unlikely that any one of these arguments will ever prevail.

Another powerful force in drawing boundaries is *religion,* where judgments are not subject to modification by evidence or logic. Here, religious texts or priests draw boundaries. It is rare, however, for ancient religious texts to contain specific or definitive opinions about modern bioethics dilemmas. Instead, religious edicts usually grow from interpretation by theologians and priests, leading to the same inconsistency that characterizes philosophical arguments. Furthermore, in pluralistic societies, no one religious view predominates, leaving the problem of finding a way to have a useful discussion or debate in which everyone can join in.

Sometimes, boundaries are drawn by *blind trust of authority*, including parents and political leaders. One should not overlook the power of *tradition*: boundaries are unconditionally accepted because they have "always" been there, often reinforced by authority figures.

Recently, there has been discussion of the role of emotional intuition in identifying boundaries, what some call "the wisdom of repugnance." In its more moderate form, this line of argument merely suggests that emotions *may* flush out immoral behavior but can be trusted only after careful moral reasoning.

What could motivate us to cross or blur a boundary?

Humans are inquisitive creatures and sometimes will explore or cross boundaries out of simple *curiosity.* People will also cross boundaries for *personal advantage.* For example, in the eighteenth and nineteenth centuries, women posed as men in order to seek employment that was restricted to men. Some famous women authors are examples. The 1982 movie *Tootsie* portrayed an unemployed man who posed as a woman to secure a secretarial job (IMDB 2012).

Another reason for crossing boundaries is *personal fulfillment.* Examples here include homosexuals and transsexuals, individuals who often feel they must cross boundaries in order to find happiness by realizing their full potential as human beings.

The goals of medicine and biomedical research are to heal and to cure. These goals can become powerful *personal and social necessities.* Current examples include using embryonic stem cells to treat Parkinson's disease or diabetes and the chimera research that has offended the moral sensibility of Senator Brownback. Such controversy is not new to science. For centuries, the utilitarian promise of scientific "progress" has provoked moral outrage by crossing boundaries. For example, in Europe and the United States, the use of cadavers for dissection was considered a moral abomination for centuries. In England, the only legal dissection was done in public as a further punishment to prisoners who had been executed for particularly heinous crimes. Over time, however, the utilitarian value of dissection became apparent—it allowed surgeons to learn anatomy. Tellingly, the objections faded away (Richardson 1987).

Why should boundaries be defended?

Sometimes, boundaries are defended to *protect personal or economic advantage*, for example, men over women or upper over lower classes. Boundaries may also be defended because of personal or social necessity. Here, we see arguments that crossing boundaries will lead to *individual or societal dissolution or destruction*. Finally, boundaries are often defended because crossing them would in and of itself constitute a *moral violation*. One common way of avoiding this dilemma is conceptual gerrymandering—i.e. simply moving a boundary to avoid a moral dilemma. For example, the definition of death has been changed to facilitate organ procurement without violating the dead donor rule (Youngner and Arnold 2001).

Reactions to crossing or blurring boundaries

The crossing of boundaries can result in a variety of feelings including: *excitement, fear, anger, disgust and moral outrage*. If the outrage is sufficiently strong, a boundary crossing may be viewed as an *abomination*, which the dictionary defines as "a thing that causes disgust or hatred" (Oxford English Dictionary 2012). In eighteenth-century England, failed suicides were executed. In some countries, homosexual acts are punishable by death, even today.

According to Talcott Parsons (Parsons 1979), societies have developed explanatory models to deal with boundary crossings or what he calls social "deviations." These models not only attempt to explain the origins of the deviation but provide a route for the deviant to return to the fold. Two of the models assume the free will of the deviant. The first, religion, sees deviant behavior as *sin*, a chosen act against God (or the gods). Sometimes, sins have been punished by death—as in the Inquisition. More often, those who stray are given the opportunity for forgiveness. Confession in the Catholic Church is an example.

Second is the criminal model. Here, deviant behavior (again considered a matter of choice) is viewed as a *crime* against the state. Punishment means physical separation from society in prison until the criminal is rehabilitated and ready to join his or her fellow citizens. It is interesting to note that Senator Brownback's Bill has chosen the criminal model to deal with human–animal hybrid research. If the Bill had been passed into law (which it has not despite repeated attempts), scientists doing this research would face up to ten years in prison.

The third Parsonian category is the medical model. Here the deviation is considered an *illness* or *disease* and free will is not at play. The *sick* person is not responsible for his or her sickness. But, there is a responsibility to seek medical attention and follow medical advice. If a person misses work because they are sick, it is acceptable, as long as they seek medical attention and follow the physician's instructions about how to get well. Employing this model, some have argued that homosexuals should seek the care of psychiatrists to "cure" their deviance and *all* people who seek the assistance of a physician in dying should instead seek mental health treatment.

Homosexuality and suicide are great examples of boundary crossings where society has, over the years, chosen all three models—the religious, the criminal, and the medical—to deal with the "problem." Some would argue that none of the three models should be applied to homosexuality and selected cases of suicide. Homosexuality is no more a moral choice or illness than heterosexuality. A desire to die rather than face the prolonged suffering of a debilitating illness can be an entirely rational one rather than always being the product of depression (Sullivan and Youngner 1994).

The wisdom of repugnance

I will address the work of two scholars: Leon Kass and Mary Midgley. The term "wisdom of repugnance" was coined by Leon Kass in his seminal article by that title arguing the immorality of human cloning (Kass 1997). Kass takes mainstream bioethics to task for a narrow approach that emphasizes judgments based on notions of autonomy, beneficence, and utility.[1] He calls these the "thin gruel" of bioethics (Kass 1997: 18). In place of this "gruel" he prefers "the wisdom of repugnance" as a method for examining the moral aspects of what he calls "the big human questions." For example, he writes:

Today, one must even apologize for voicing opinions that twenty-five years ago were nearly universally regarded as the core of our culture's wisdom on these matters. In a world whose once-given natural boundaries are blurred by technological change and whose moral boundaries are seemingly up for grabs, it is much more difficult to make persuasive the still compelling case against cloning human beings. (Kass 1997: 18)

He says that "In crucial cases…repugnance is the emotional expression of deep wisdom, beyond reason's power fully to articulate it" (Kass 1997: 20). He never seems to address the fact that extreme racists, sexists, and homophobes throughout history have justified their deeply felt opinions in exactly the same way. He specifically cites abortion, the pill, and reproductive rights of single women, homosexuals, and lesbians as examples of violations of "universally regarded" opinions (Kass 1997: 18).

Kass is an excellent rhetorician. His work reads well. But it is, ultimately, superficial. Ruth Macklin characterizes Kass's arguments as "metaphors and slogans as substitutes for empirical evidence and reasoned arguments" (Macklin 2006).

Kass's generalizations are often painfully overdrawn and devoid of context. For example, he asks if we can indeed find moral arguments "fully adequate to the horror…of eating human flesh" (Kass 1997: 20). The book *Alive* describes the plight of a group of young athletes and their families trapped high in the Andes Mountains after their plane crashed (Read 1974). On the verge of starvation, they ate their dead companions. Were these acts of eating human flesh unjustifiable because of the horror? Again we must resort to the thin gruel of bioethics. First, no one was forced to eat human flesh. It was an autonomous choice. Second, survivors' motive for cannibalism was to live and return to their homes and communities. Interestingly, they coped by turning meals into the Catholic ritual of communion.

---

[1] He does not include social justice in his list of superficial reasons for making judgments, but since he never seems to write about social justice, he would most likely do so. In fact, Kass criticizes bioethics (its analytic philosophers at least) as having succumbed to "routinization and professionalization." He further accuses bioethics of "rubber-stamping all technical innovation, in the mistaken belief that all other goods must bow down before the gods of better health and scientific advance." It is noteworthy that neither here, nor anywhere else that I am aware, does Kass make a much more telling critique of bioethicists, namely, their failure to adequately take on the issues of lack of access to health care and the influence of big corporations on the institutions that employ them.

In her article "Monstrosity: Why We Should Pay Attention to the Yuk Factor," Mary Midgley echoes Kass in her style (Midgley 2000). While briefly acknowledging that feelings of repugnance should serve as a stimulus for more analytic reflection, she launches into slogan slinging. In arguing for the respect of species boundaries and against the rise of biotechnology, she makes an entirely circular argument:

It is interesting to notice that some consequences are not just a matter of chance. Acts that are wrong in themselves can be expected to have bad effects of a particular kind that is not accidental. Their badness follows from what is wrong in the act itself, so that there is rational, conceptual line between them and their results. The consequences are a sign of what was wrong in the act in the first place ... Hubris calls for nemesis and in one form or another it's going to get it. (Midgley 2000: 8)

She is not talking here about the fact that science is a two-edged sword; that the application of new technology almost always has the potential for good or evil—depending on how it is used. She is claiming that when deontological rules or natural boundaries are crossed, punishment is forthcoming. She gives historical examples, one being slavery. Like Kass, she makes broad claims that have little basis in historical fact. "In a most intelligible phrase," she says, "those who institute slavery *get what they are asking for*" (Midgley 2000: 8; italics in the original). Slavery in the Western world went on for centuries. True, many slave owners in the pre bellum South of the United States were sometimes devastated by the Civil War, but not all, and their fathers and grandfathers certainly were not. Nor did generations of slaveholders throughout the world "get what they [were] asking for."

Midgley's main example of scientific hubris is the propagation of mad cow disease by feeding sheep brains to cows (mixed in with other things). Was the resulting danger to humans nemesis or simply the result of imprudent behavior? Was it sin or stupidity?

The rhetoric of Kass and Midgley has little to offer our understanding of difficult questions about science policy. Both give the impression that *their* repugnance is not merely correct but is also more reliable than those of their political opponents. It is tempting to conclude that their categorical pronouncements spring from deep religious beliefs that they are unwilling or unable to articulate. When all is said and done, analysis of the best evidence available and a reliance on the thin gruel of bioethics are still the best bets for heading off science disasters.

Jeffrey Stout and moral abominations

In his book *Ethics after Babel*, Jeffrey Stout gives an anthropological perspective[2] to understanding moral abominations (Stout 1988). His analysis is a nice complement to the work of Talcott Parsons mentioned earlier. Stout insists we must look at a given abomination as "a transgressor across boundaries that guard cosmic and social order" (Stout 1988: 150). An abomination, he writes, is "anomalous or ambiguous with respect to some system of concepts" (Stout 1988: 148). "And," he adds, "the repugnance it causes

---

[2] He acknowledges his debt to the work of anthropologist Mary Douglas.

depends on such factors as the presence, sharpness, and social significance of conceptual distinctions" (Stout 1988: 148). Whatever the social order, an object, event, or act that "seems to pose, or becomes symbolic of a threat to the established cosmological or social order" (Stout 1988: 149) is branded as abominable. Acts like cannibalism and bestiality blur the line between humans and beasts. He points out that homosexuality is much more likely to be considered an abomination in a society that draws sharp lines between the roles (dress, work, behavior, rules of inheritance) of men and women. Stout writes:

We can understand these responses if we set them in their context—the network of cosmological and social categories relative to which some phenomena are bound to seem anomalous or ambiguous. We see at once that the responses are hardly a matter of blind emotion. They are thoroughly informed by cognitive categories, the categories of a moral language infused with cosmological and sociological assumptions. Nor are the responses incorrigible. Change the relevant network of categories enough, and you will alter the list of abominable acts while redirecting the corresponding sense of revulsion. (Stout 1988: 157)

Leon Kass seems to be informed by categories of a previous culture or rules set down by ancient books. Certainly, many people in the United States share his views and revulsions. A shocking percentage of Americans believe in a literal interpretation of the Book of Genesis and reject Darwinism out of hand (I am not suggesting that Kass and Midgley share *this* view). Kass's proud but unexamined revulsion has a pre-Enlightenment flavor. He belittles an ethical analysis that depends on autonomy, beneficence, utility, and regulation (and rationality) to temper our emotional intuitions. He offers nothing much to replace them, at least nothing that can contribute to a reasoned discussion about what science should and should not do.

Unfortunately, the language of abomination has entered our political discourse. It is disquieting that a recent Harris poll found that 24 percent of Republicans in the United States thought that President Obama might be the "Antichrist" (LiveScience Staff 2012). Perhaps citizens with these views will ultimately win the culture wars and will indeed be in a position to remake the network of relevant categories. It is not clear how the rest of us will react to such a rearrangement of *our* ethical boundaries.

References

Arnold, R. M., and Youngner, S. J. (1993). "The Dead Donor Rule: Should We Stretch It, Bend It, Or Abandon It?" *Kennedy Institute of Ethics Journal*, 3(2): 263–78.

Bernat, J. L., Culver, C. M., and Gert, B. (1981). "On the Definition and Criterion of Death," *Annals of Internal Medicine*, 94(3): 389–94.

Charo, A. (1999). "Dusk, Dawn, and Defining Death: Legal Classifications and Biological Categories," in S. J. Youngner, R. M. Arnold, and R. Schapiro (eds), *The Definition of Death: Contemporary Controversies*. Baltimore, MD: Johns Hopkins University Press, 277–92.

Connor, K. (2012). "Frankenstein's Folly," http://www.renewamerica.com/columns/connor/090801 (accessed May 16, 2012).

Oxford English Dictionary. (2012). "abomination," http://oxforddictionaries.com/us/definition/american_english/abomination?q=abomination (accessed May 16, 2012).

IMDB. (2012). http://www.imdb.com/title/tt0084805/ (accessed May 16, 2012).

Kass, L. (1997). "The Wisdom of Repugnance," *New Republic*, 216(2): 17–26.

Macklin, R. (2006). "The New Conservatives in Bioethics: Who Are They and What Do They Seek?" *Hastings Center Report*, 36(1): 34–43.

Midgley, M. (2000). "Biotechnology and Monstrosity: Why We Should Pay Attention to the 'Yuk Factor,'" *Hastings Center Report*, 30(5): 7–15.

LiveScience Staff. (2012). "Quarter of Republicans Think Obama May Be the Anti-Christ," http://www.livescience.com/8160-quarter-republicans-obama-anti-christ.html   (accessed May 16, 2012).

Parsons, T. (1979). "Definition of Health and Illness in Light of American Values and Social Structures," in E. G. Jaco (ed), *Patients, Physicians, and Illness*. New York: Free Press: 120–44.

Read, P. (1974). *Alive*. New York, Harper.

Richardson, R. (1987). *Death, Dissection, and the Destitute*. London: Routledge and Kegan Paul.

Robert, J. S., and Baylis, F. (2003). "Crossing Species Boundaries," *American Journal of Bioethics*, 3(3): 1–13.

Stout, J. (1988). *Ethics after Babel: The Languages of Morals and Their Discontents*. Boston: Beacon Press.

Sullivan, M. D., and Youngner, S. J. (1994). "Depression, Competence, and the Right to Refuse Lifesaving Medical Treatment," *American Journal of Psychiatry*, 151(7): 971–8.

Objective

Youngner, S. J. and Arnold R. M. (2001). "Philosophical Debates about the Definition of Death: Who Cares?" *Journal of Medicine and Philosophy*, 26(5): 527–37.

10.2

Commentary
In Defence of Repugnance

Catherine Mills

Professor Youngner's paper takes its lead from attempts in 2009 in the United States Senate to introduce legislation to prevent the production of human-animal chimeric embryos for the purposes of research on the basis that such practices threaten fundamental moral boundaries. He discusses two points raised by this attempt—the first regarding the creation and crossing of boundaries and the second regarding the so-called "wisdom of repugnance"—and draws the conclusion that while religion, feeling, and traditionalism must be taken into account in the political sphere in modern pluralistic societies, they often stand unnecessarily in the way of human progress. While there is much in Youngner's paper that warrants response, in this commentary I will focus on the second of his two main points before addressing the conclusion.

1 Boundary making and unmaking

In the first section of his paper, Youngner lays out a brief analysis of the identification, function, and maintenance of moral boundaries. He argues that moral boundaries are identified through science, analytic philosophy, religion and tradition, and, arguably, through emotional response, and specifically that of repugnance. Of course, repugnance does not have to be elicited by the crossing of moral boundaries. But recent ethical discussions of it have linked it with the transgression of moral boundaries such as that between humans and animals in chimera research, between species in transgenic research, and most generally a transgression of the very notion of human nature in the possibility of human reproductive cloning.

2 Repugnance and the role of emotion in ethics

It is these recent discussions that occupy Youngner, especially the contributions of Leon Kass (1997) and Mary Midgley (2000). The key claim that Youngner wants to make is that "the rhetoric of moral repugnance is merely that and has little to contribute to our pluralistic society's efforts to cope with social change and technological development." The first part of this claim interests me most in this section, for it suggests that rather than being an expression of deeply felt sentiment, claims about repugnance are *merely* rhetorical.

This clause could be taken to mean that such claims are made simply for effect, and perhaps specifically to manipulate the emotive responses of the reader or listener, without any real basis in the emotive experience of the speaker. This is not really what Youngner means, though; instead, his idea is that rather than offering reasonable argumentation for their positions, defenders of the "wisdom of repugnance" or the "yuk factor" too quickly resort to slogans and generalizations that add little to real bioethical debate about biotechnology. It is certainly true that both public and philosophical debates about biotechnology are replete with rhetoric—and this is in no way limited to critics of biotechnology. Indeed, I would go so far as to say that every discourse or argument has its own rhetorics, even the most stridently rationalistic of them. It is also true that Leon Kass is a master rhetorician. But to simply dismiss claims about the moral significance of repugnance on this basis is altogether too hasty.

The underlying issue that Youngner fails to address in any convincing way is that of the proper role that emotion plays, or should play, in individual ethics and public policy formation. It would be difficult to argue that emotion plays no role in ethics. Sympathy, after all, can convincingly be seen as fundamental, if not constitutive of ethics. It is a concern for others, felt in sympathy, which motivates ethical concern and behaviour. Moreover, it can be argued that emotive responses such as compassion do and indeed should play a role in public policy formation. In Australia, critics of refugee policy that includes offshore processing and mandatory detention of children often couch their claims in terms of the need for a more compassionate response. Demands for increased foreign aid and charitable responses after natural disasters are also often motivated by emotions such as compassion and sympathy.

If we accept that emotions such as sympathy and compassion play a role in individual and public ethics, then it behoves us to ask what is specific about repugnance, and whether that specificity should exclude repugnance from being a morally significant emotion. In its contemporary usage, repugnance simply means a "strong dislike, distaste, antipathy, or aversion (to or against a thing)" (*Oxford English Dictionary*). There is nothing obvious in that definition that suggests that repugnance could not be a morally serious emotion. Further, it is not hard to think of examples where repugnance seems to play a significant role in motivating moral and political practice. For instance, the repugnance that I feel at state-sanctioned torture may motivate me to write against that practice. Or the repugnance that many feel at capital punishment may motivate them to political and legal campaigning against it.

Note that I am saying that emotions such as sympathy and repugnance may *motivate* ethical concern. In other words, I am suggesting that while they can yield an interest in moral reflection and moral behaviour, they do not necessarily justify any particular behaviour, course of action, or principle in themselves. This admittedly sketchy distinction between moral motivation and moral justification points toward an important difference between Kass and Midgley to which Youngner pays little attention.

In a much-cited sentence, Kass claims that repugnance entails a wisdom that is deeper than "reason's power to articulate it." He goes on to ask: "[W]ould anyone's failure to give full rational justification for his or her revulsion at these practices [of incest, bestiality, and cannibalism] make that revulsion ethically suspect? Not at all…we intuit and feel, immediately and without argument, the violation of things we rightfully hold dear" (Kass 1997: 20). Thus, Kass holds that the feeling of repugnance is enough in itself to show that a practice is morally wrong. Repugnance both motivates and *justifies* a certain moral response. In the course of making this argument, Kass moves very quickly from examples such as bestiality and cannibalism to human cloning and other social and technological changes wrought in the field of human reproduction and relationships in recent decades. In this, he does the case for a "wisdom of repugnance" a disservice. Nevertheless, later I will suggest that there is a grain of truth to found amongst Kass's rhetoric.

For now, let me note that Midgley holds a more moderate and obviously defensible position. She explicitly argues that while emotions are indispensible to ethics, they are not sufficient in themselves to justify any given position. She writes:

Feeling is an essential part of our moral life, though of course not the whole of it...Whenever we seriously judge something to be wrong, strong feeling necessarily accompanies the judge-ment...someone who has merely a theoretical interest in morals, who doesn't feel any indignation or disgust or outrage...has missed the point of morals altogether...Of course we know these feel-ings are not an infallible guide...we need to supplement them by thought, analysing their mean-ing and articulating them in a way that gives us coherent and usable standards. (Midgley 2000: 9)

This kind of rational articulation of feelings and moral intuitions is, I think, precise-ly what many moral philosophers, including from competing traditions of thought, actually do.

This is also just what Midgley attempts to do in her article, a point that seems to be missed in Youngner's response, giving rise to several misunderstandings or misreadings. For instance, when Midgley claims that "hubris calls for nemesis, and in one way or another it's going to get it," she is attempting to articulate a popular sense that human actions that grossly transgress against the moral standing of other humans, or the species nature of other animals, have their consequences. This is not as a matter of strict causal law; rather, these consequences are "effects that anyone who acts in this way invites and is committed to accepting" (Midgley 2000: 8). Midgley is not herself committed to this form of reasoning at this point; she is merely drawing attention to it as a form of reason-ing adopted by others. Furthermore, in regards to the example of Creutzfeld-Jacobs dis-ease that Midgley uses, she is not claiming that this is a punishment for "sin" as Youngner suggests. She herself writes that it is a more a matter of stupidity—or rather, "the moral obtuseness that goes with greed" (Midgley 2000: 8). Her point of reference in this dis-cussion is not Christianity, or even monotheism, but Ancient Greek mythology, specifi-cally the goddess Nemesis, avenger of hubris.

3 Public morality and progress

This leads me to my final point, regarding the conclusion Youngner draws that the "wis-dom of repugnance" has little to contribute to a pluralistic society's attempts to cope with social and technological change, and unnecessarily hinders human progress. This can be understood to mean that emotion plays no constructive role in democratic deliberation and consensus building. Rather, as the examples that Youngner cites throughout imply, its impact is pernicious and perhaps inherently conservative or reactionary. This is a fairly straightforward liberal position of urging rational debate and deliberation as a means of achieving moral consensus on technological changes. But I think it is wrong, both in its view of how public debate currently happens, and how it should happen. In short, there is no such thing as wholly rational debate, and this is a good thing too.

To return to Kass's point about the moral immediacy of emotion, being a citizen of a pluralistic polity involves in a deep way that persons not only know something to be wrong, but feel it as such. Belonging to a political and moral community involves a kind of ethics of the self whereby moral precepts are internalized and expressed in feeling, rather than solely as consciously articulated and articulable rational arguments. For example, there is little community debate about whether acts such as the brutal abuse and murder of young children are morally wrong. In advanced liberal democracies, as in most contemporary and historical societies, it is taken for granted that such acts are wrong, and it would be subjectively peculiar if a person required argumentation so as to be convinced of that. This is not to say that all persons do necessarily feel this to be so—but those that do not are typically seen as sociopathic or criminally insane.

Of course, not all, and indeed, perhaps few, moral questions facing a polity fall into this category of what might be called the pre-discursive. For most, an ongoing agonism and negotiation of values and regulatory frameworks are more appropriate. Nor does this mean that all expressions of repugnance are to be taken equally seriously, or accepted without question. As with other emotions, repugnance can be subject to various prejudices or shortfalls in understanding or sympathy, which are properly challenged. Moreover, our sense of repugnance is often deeply guided by social norms, the effects of which are difficult to make fully conscious to ourselves. But the point is that the key rhetorical and argumentative task of Kass's essay is its attempts to place intuitions about cloning and other reproductive technologies in the category of the pre-discursive moral intuition. Thus, following a brief discussion of examples such as bestiality and cannibalism, he claims that "the repugnance at human cloning belongs in this category" (Kass 1997: 20). About this, he may well be wrong (and I believe he is, though this is not the place to argue it). But he is nevertheless right in general to suggest that in some sense, some moral intuitions are beyond debate.

At this point, it may be worth considering the rhetorical effects of Youngner's own essay. In the final paragraphs, he suggests a broad analogy between arguments that draw on a sense of repugnance in bioethics and the more extreme politico-religious views of those opposed to the presidency of Barack Obama. The implication of this is that there is a kind of outlandishness to claims of moral repugnance—they are both dangerous and hardly creditable—such that they should be dismissed from public debate. We allow them to play a part in debate at our own peril, in particular the peril of irrationality and radical social revision. However, this obscures the necessary role that repugnance plays in individual ethics and public policy, and presents a one-sided view of repugnance that largely ignores the positive contribution of this moral emotion, for instance, to the historical development of more expansive conceptions of social belonging.

To conclude, then, there is much that I disagree with in the arguments of Midgley and Kass. But to dismiss the idea that repugnance in particular, and emotion in general, has something to contribute to moral debate on contemporary technological developments on the basis that it is mere rhetoric is overly hasty. In taking this position, Youngner comes dangerously close to that of which he accuses Kass and Midgley, that is, of relying on rhetoric to make his argument for him.

References

Kass, L. (1997). "The Wisdom of Repugnance," *New Republic*, 216(2): 17–26.

Midgley, M. (2000). "Biotechnology and Monstrosity: Why We should Pay Attention to the 'Yuk Factor'", *Hastings Center Report*, 30(5): 7–15.

10.3

Commentary

On Crossing the Line between Human and Nonhuman: Human Dignity Reconsidered

Takashi Ikeda

1 Reconsidering the line between human and nonhuman

In his essay "Why Would It Be Morally Wrong to Create a Human-Animal Chimera?" Stuart J. Youngner focuses on the current state of this topic in the United States, both in legal debate and popular literature: those who defend *human dignity* tend to regard scientific attempts at creating human-animal chimeras or hybrids as *unethical* or *immoral*. As Youngner suggests, such negative reactions should not be treated as a single issue, for they are connected to the broader theme of boundaries in bioethics. The most specific question here is: Is it morally wrong to cross the line between human and nonhuman?

To address this issue, Youngner refers to Jeffery Stout's analysis of moral abominations. Stout states that we must look at a given abomination as a transgression across boundaries that guard the cosmic and social order. From the perspectives of authors such as Stout, popular negative reactions to the creation of human-animal chimeras are not based on moral intuition, but are rather informed by cosmological and social categories, such as those found in the Bible. Importantly, these categories are not immutable; thus, it is not conceptually impossible to rearrange our ethical boundaries.

Youngner's essay provides persuasive explanations for why those who defend human dignity react negatively to technologies that blur the line between human and nonhuman. Unfortunately, we cannot find a positive, normative argument in favor of the ideas and praxis that cross this line.

In my view, the attempt to provide positive arguments is not extraneous to Youngner's concern, so long as the leading question in his essay is: Is it *wrong* to create human-animal chimeras? A theoretical answer or solution to such a question involves the choice between right or wrong. We can assume that those who consider it right believe that creating human-animal chimeras is (at least partially) a good thing. It is also widely accepted that ethical sentences that include the term good or bad do not merely describe the state of matter in the world, but also conceptually dictate whether or not one should perform a particular action, such as crossing the line between human and nonhuman.

Admittedly, Youngner is not inclined to state that crossing this line is wrong, as those who hold human-animal chimeras in abomination do. He apparently leans more toward a negative answer to the question of whether it is wrong to create human-animal chimeras and nearer to the claim that to do so is (at least partially) good. In that case, we may not have a choice but to try and provide a positive, normative argument for why we should cross the line between human and nonhuman.

I entirely concur with Stout's basic idea that negative responses to crossing boundaries are not morally intuited, but are rather unreflectively based on old cosmological and social categories. In the following sections, I argue that there are good reasons for crossing the line, but, importantly, without losing the central meaning of the concept of human dignity. By showing this, I intend to prevent the debate from being separated into two extremes, i.e. the extreme conservatism that uncritically rests on old traditional notions and will not accept a new moral language, and the extreme liberalism that barely casts a critical eye on emerging situations that have not existed in human history.

2 Utilitarianism as a moral principle

Let me first take up the *utilitarian* argument that speaks against the old notion of human dignity and for the idea of crossing the line between human and nonhuman. In the history of contemporary ethics, the leading utilitarian theorist P. Singer has opened the way to a wider discussion on animal ethics. Since the publication of his book *Animal Liberation* (Singer 1975), it is not at all self-evident that only entities belonging to the human species are members of our moral community. Some animals, if they can feel pain, are also considered entities that deserve moral treatment. Thus, the line between humans and animals is crossed.

It is also important to note that Singer's utilitarian approach to crossing the line between humans and animals led to the definition of a line between persons and non-persons within the human species. J. McMahan takes over Singer's criticism against speciesism and argues that privileging species membership is equivalent to a virulent nationalism. According to anti-speciesism, not only should some animals be treated in a morally appropriate way, but "a congenitally severely retarded human being having cognitive capacities comparative to those of a dog" should be regarded as a non-person who would have neither a fortunate nor unfortunate life (McMahan 2002: 146). McMahan says:

While our sense of kinship with the severely retarded moves us to treat them with great solicitude, our perception of animals as radically "other" numbs…when one compares the relatively small number of severely retarded human beings who benefit from our solicitude with the vast number of animals who suffer at our hands, it is impossible to avoid the conclusion that the good effects of our species-based partiality are greatly outweighed by the bad. (McMahan 2002: 221)

In my view, the utilitarian view that leads to such a conclusion cannot provide a satisfactory rearrangement of moral language categories that are infused with cosmological and social assumptions.

It is noteworthy that, despite its claim, the anti-speciesism of McMahan's utilitarian thinking is in itself equivalent to a virulent nationalism. As E. Kittay points out in her criticism of McMahan, historically, pernicious nationalism or racism has not always been related to the claim of group membership, giving priority to one's own group. Rather, what make racism and pernicious nationalism moral evils are their attribution of desirable properties to humans and their exclusion of those who lack these properties. In Nazism,

> Germans were deemed to be Aryans by an elaborate enumeration of the special properties possessed by Aryans. The elimination of those Germans who lacked those properties, and the assurance through sterilization that Germans would in the future not have the unwanted properties, were paramount to the Nazis. (Kittay 2005: 120)

The way McMahan seeks the intrinsic properties that sort individuals into those who belong to "us" and those who do not is basically equivalent to virulent nationalism. Drawing the line between those who have desirable properties and those who lack them is an abomination to society. It seems impossible to deny that traditionally inherited cosmological and social assumptions are accepted without examination when only certain properties are considered desirable. However, what ethical considerations should critically focus on are exactly these assumptions.

3 Re-evaluating the concept of human dignity

To critically examine cosmological and social assumptions on the basis of which the old notion of human dignity seems to be considered self-evident, I would like to take up another debate regarding the problem of crossing the line between human and nonhuman. Today, it is technologically possible not only to create human-animal chimeras, but also *cyborgs*, which are human-machine chimeras or hybrids. This kind of chimera also elicits negative reactions. For example, those whose lives depend on a mechanical ventilator might be regarded as a type of cyborg. It is often claimed that a life totally dependent on technological devices is "unnatural" and contrary to "death with dignity." Once again, we encounter the concept of human dignity, which draws a line between human and nonhuman, or strictly speaking, persons and nonpersons within the human species.

Here, we should recall Kittay's point in her criticism against the utilitarian view: anti-speciesism, which seeks intrinsic properties or desirable capacities that sort individuals into those who are a part of "us" and those who are not, is basically equivalent to a virulent nationalism. If ethical considerations are biased by traditionally inherited assumptions, one cannot assume that desirable properties are *intrinsic* to humans.

To be critical, I raise the following question: How can the so-called "cognitive capacities," through which properties are attributed to individuals, be measured? This question, related to the *concept of capacity*, seems to be the most significant for evaluating utilitarian anti-speciesism. It maintains that if some animals have the capacity to feel pain, they should be treated appropriately, and that if some human beings lack certain capacities, they cannot be members of our moral community.

Singer typically discusses cognitive abilities or disabilities by referring to scientific observations of biological or psychological functions (Singer 2010). However, with the possibility of creating human–animal or human–machine hybrids in today's technologically advanced world, "capacity" is not recognized by merely observing biological or psychological functions. "Capacity" changes according to what individuals can achieve with scientific technology. In my view, the concept of *capability* proposed by A. Sen and M. Nussbaum offers an insight into the "capacity" of human beings in the modern technological world.

Capability reflects a person's ability to achieve a given functioning. In other words, it signifies "an achievement of a person: what she or he manages to do or be" (Sen 1999: 7). Functioning comprises a wide range of activities, such as moving around. The capability approach emphasizes that the achievement of a functioning not only depends on personal factors, but also on instrumental goods and social factors. In the case of a disabled or severely sick individual, a functioning (e.g. moving around or breathing) is achievable only with a given bundle of commodities (e.g. wheelchair, ramp, lift, oxygen tank, or mechanical ventilator). However, mere availability of these commodities does not guarantee the achievement of a certain functioning. Rather, the achievement of a functioning with given commodities depends on a range of personal and social factors, including body size, age, gender, activity level, health, knowledge and education, human support, and economic conditions (see Sen 1999: 17). (Note: The list of personal and social factors is arranged by the author.)

While much can be said about the concept of capability, for the purpose of this piece, I wish only to emphasize one implication of the capability approach: a person's ability, defined as capability, cannot be measured merely by observing his or her personal features. According to Nussbaum, "functionings are beings and doings that are the outgrowths or realizations of capability" (Nussbaum 2011: 25). Capability is not to be observed, but to be developed and realized. In this respect, the fact that some individuals' lives are unsustainable without technological devices or other people's constant support does not immediately imply that they lack the abilities to live a worthy life. The central question here is: What can be done to promote their capabilities socially, economically, and politically?

In this context, Nussbaum emphasizes the significance of human dignity, which differentiates her version of the capability approach from that of Sen. As seen before, dignity is a vague notion used to designate certain ways of life as hopelessly unworthy. However, in Nussbaum's view, the central sense of dignity is in fact exactly opposed to such a use of the word:

The basic idea is that some living conditions deliver to people a life that is worthy of the human dignity that they possess, and others do not. In the latter cases, they retain dignity, but it is like a promissory note whose claims have not been met. (Nussbaum 2011: 30)

Surely, it makes sense to say that there is, on the one hand, a life worthy of human dignity and, on the other hand, a life that is not. However, this does not lead to a conclusion that the latter way of life is not worthy of living. To say that a life is not worthy of human dignity rather means that an ample threshold of central capabilities is required. If there are individuals whose capacities are "comparative to those of a dog" in McMahan's expression, what should be done is to not exclude them from the human moral community, but promote their capabilities socially, economically, and politically so that their life is worthy of human dignity.

4 Dignity of nonhuman animals

In moral language, the notion of human dignity is often considered an obstacle to blurring the line between human and nonhuman animals. Nussbaum would argue that while her capability approach begins from the notion of human dignity and a life worthy of it, the idea of dignity can be extended to nonhuman animals.

The capability approach relates to the dignity of a way of life that possesses both deep needs and abilities. Its basic goal is to address the need for a rich plurality of life activities. This basic concern and goal should not be restricted to human species, because our ways of life enormously influence the lives of animals. Therefore, the human–animal relationship is also discussed in Nussbaum's approach:

> The general aim of the capabilities approach in charting political principles to shape the human-animal relationship would be, following the intuitive ideas of the theory, that no animal should be cut off from the chance at a flourishing life and that all animals should enjoy certain positive opportunities to flourish. (Nussbaum 2004: 307)

A noteworthy point about Nussbaum's idea is that extension of the concept of dignity to nonhuman animals requires an acknowledgement of the differentiation between human and nonhuman species. Surely, as supporters of utilitarianism point out, capacities that are seemingly possessed only by humans are in fact widely found in nature. However, such facts do not directly lead to the conclusion that species membership is morally and politically irrelevant.

> For a child born with Down syndrome, it is crucial that the political culture in which he lives make a big effort to extend to him the fullest benefits of citizenship he can attain, through health benefits, education, and the reeducation of the public culture. That is so because he can only flourish as a human being. He has no option of flourishing as a happy chimpanzee. For a chimpanzee, on the other hand, it seems to me that expensive efforts to teach language, while interesting and revealing, are not matters of basic justice. A chimpanzee flourishes in its own way, communicating with its own community in a perfectly adequate manner that has gone on for ages. (Nussbaum 2004: 310)

Differentiation between humans and nonhuman animals does not preclude the extension of the concept of "life that is worthy of dignity" to nonhuman animals. Rather, differentiation is required for the appropriate extension of this concept. Even if a child born with Down syndrome and a chimpanzee are comparable with respect to observable capacities, there is still a great difference between providing educational opportunities to such a human child and teaching language to a chimpanzee. The act of teaching human language to a chimpanzee does not designate its life as worthy of dignity, but rather prevents it from developing capabilities that are derived from interacting with its own community.

In conclusion, there are morally good reasons for crossing the line between humans and nonhuman animals. However, importantly, the crossing should be achieved not by depriving the concept of dignity of its central meaning, but rather by making central use of this concept.

References

Kittay, E. F. (2005). "At the Margins of Moral Personhood," *Ethics*, 116:100–31.

McMahan, J. (2002). *The Ethics of Killing: Problems at the Margins of Life*. New York: Oxford University Press.

Nussbaum, M. C. (2004). "Beyond 'Compassion and Humanity': Justice for Nonhuman Animals," in R. S. Cass, and C. N. Martha (eds), *Animal Rights: Current Debates and New Directions*. New York: Oxford University Press, 299–320.

Nussbaum, M. C. (2011). *Creating Capabilities: The Human Development Approach*. Cambridge, MA: Harvard University Press.

Sen, A. (1999). *Commodities and Capabilities*. New Delhi: Oxford University Press.

Singer, P. (1975). *Animal Liberation: A New Ethics for Our Treatment of Animals*. New York: Random House.

Singer, P. (2010). "Speceisism and Moral Status," in E. F. Kittay, and L. Carlson (eds), *Cognitive Disability and its Challenge to Moral Philosophy*. Chichester/Malden, MA: Wiley-Blackwell, 331–44.

10.4

Response to Commentaries

Stuart J. Youngner

Catherine Mills

Catherine Mills makes a good point when she notes that I do not address in "any convincing way" the proper role of emotions in moral deliberation. Certainly, this issue is important. Neuroscience has hinted that in the functioning of the brain emotion precedes rational thought, which may be, as Freudians suggested long ago, mere flotsam and jetsam, bobbing on the sea of our instincts. Mills, however, does not seem interested in neuroscience, and, in any case, neuroscience has little to offer in discovering the "proper" as opposed to actual role of emotion.

I did address the *improper* role of emotion in the arguments of moral philosophers in their role as teachers and scholars. By granting wisdom to their own emotions, they abandon scholarship to become advocates (political or religious) pushing some cause or another. In this endeavor, objective analysis too often becomes inconvenient. Unfortunately, Dr. Mills's criticism of my essay puts her in into the category of advocate.

Mills points out that "emotive responses such as compassion" play a role in individual and public policy formation. What she does not mention is that hate and fear have also played more than a minor role in the history of humankind—and they still do.

Dr. Mills gives us no way of deciding which emotions should be given prominence. When she touts her own favorite form of repugnance without argument, she abandons her role as scholar. She praises the role of the repugnance *she* feels against state-sanctioned torture and capital punishment. But Mills fails to give a reason why this repugnance is a wiser moral guide than the repugnance that less "wise" others feel toward suspected terrorists and murderers—the "intuitive morality" that leads *them* to advocate torture and execution. She gives no argument for privileging *her* repugnance. Like Leon Kass, she seems to be saying that her moral repugnance is morally serious simply because it is *hers*, or, perhaps, shared by her friends and political allies.

Dr. Mills has a similar problem when she talks about "pre-discursive" moral intuitions, some of which are "beyond debate." Should this pre-discursive status make them immune from discussion and analysis? Does it make them morally wise? Homophobia and a servile role for women have certainly been pre-discursive intuitions in our own society. But scholars, among others, insisted on examining what was beyond debate and have rejected the wisdom of the repugnance felt by homophobes and sexists to justify their policies. Did moral arguments by these scholars have anything to do with our society's dawning acceptance of women and homosexuals? I hope so. I believe it is a duty of moral philosophers to ask tough questions about deeply "felt" repugnancies, including their own.

In her role as *advocate*, Dr. Mills pleases me (as a fellow advocate) by endorsing the repugnancies I share with her. But surely Dr. Mills is capable of using some of the "thin gruel" of bioethics—such as respect for persons, human flourishing, non-maleficence, etc.—to defend them. Here, she has come up short.

Takashi Ikeda

Takashi Ikeda has taken on the sticky wickets of dignity and speciesism. I have a few questions about his analysis and would like to point out a problem or two.

Peter Singer, notes Ikeda, has crossed the boundary between humans and animals by situating both in a moral community. Ikeda goes on to criticize McMahan's claim that "privileging species membership is equivalent to a virulent nationalism."

McMahan says that the good effects of such speciesism, i.e. treating severely compromised human beings well, are outweighed by the bad effects of treating animals cruelly. Ikeda seems to infer from this statement that McMahan thinks we should treat certain animals well and certain humans badly. Another interpretation is that we should treat both well.

Ikeda next argues (quoting Kittay) that "pernicious nationalism or racism has not always been related to the claim of group membership." For example, Nazis did not respect the dignity or values of all Germans, just Aryans. But is this not simply a matter of categories, in this case race versus nationality? Seeking intrinsic properties as a way of assigning moral worth—for example, cognition or the ability to suffer and feel pain, is certainly a risky business but so is speciesism without any moral consideration of intrinsic properties.

I am also concerned with Ikeda's use of Down syndrome on two counts. First, he seems to equate the mental capacities of persons with Down syndrome with those of dogs or chimpanzees. This is simply inaccurate. Persons with Down syndrome are not only capable of love and suffering, but of complex social roles, including holding jobs. Second, there are much better examples of mental limitation that would challenge our notions of speciesism—for example, anencephalic newborns (born with no cerebral hemispheres) or persons reliably diagnosed as in persistent vegetative state. Unlike Down syndrome, people suffering from these conditions afford us no opportunity to "promote their capabilities, socially, economically, and politically." They have no such capabilities. Kinship offers the only argument to treat them as members of our moral community, those who have a promissory note, as Nussbaum says, "whose claims have not been met." Does a dog or chimpanzee have less of a promissory note because they are not members of our species? I would like to hear more about this from Ikeda.

Finally, Ikeda seems to say that a robust critique of speciesism means that our obligation to educate a child with Down syndrome is equivalent to our obligation to teach language to a chimpanzee. If this is indeed what he is saying he has surely gone too far.

Singer, for example, would agree than we should not conduct painful, unwanted medical experimentation on either people with Down syndrome or chimpanzees. A duty to provide a formal education is another matter.

Taking animal rights seriously has opened a Pandora's Box where we will struggle to get our moral obligations and behavioral boundaries straight for some time to come.

11.1

Primary Topic Article
Chimera in Bioethics and Biopolitics

Jonathan D. Moreno

Introduction

In this paper I explore the bioethical issues concerned with the creation of the laboratory animal model known as a chimera. I argue that these issues need to be placed within the context of the politics of biology, or biopolitics. One can view biopolitics not only as a problem of discipline over bodies and populations, as Michel Foucault observed, but in light of the new biology, the new biopolitics involves control over body parts, such as cells.[1] For Foucault biopolitics is a consequence and manifestation of biopower, the management of bodies and the collections of bodies that we call populations. Key to understanding this idea of biopower is suspending the standard modern tendency to think of the state as the main or even the principal locus of power. Rather, as the philosopher Jason Robert has observed, Foucault's focus is on those powers among people who have certain key positions in the knowledge economy: "bureaucrats, administrators, public health nurses, teachers, physicians, genetic counselors, psychotherapists, statisticians, economists. The political government of individuals is effected through special competence and disciplinary credentials...Foucault documents a new power over life, distinct from the right of the sovereign" (Jason 1996).

Prior to the Enlightenment, Foucault argued, traditional sovereigns exercised sovereign power over life with the threat of death. With the rise of rationality as a criterion of acceptable sovereignty, the modern state asserts control not merely over life and death but over ways of living. The justification for the exercise of this biopower is the need to regulate labor, punishment, public health, reproduction, and various other core cultural habits for the sake of social well-being. Biotechnology may now be added to the list. In the words of one writer on Foucault and biopower, "[g]enetic engineering and genetic-based pharmaceuticals, among other biotechnological pursuits, share an

---

[1] A number of Foucault's works illustrate his view of biopolitics and biopower, including: *The Order of Things*. New York: Vintage Books, 1970; *Discipline and Punish: The Birth of the Prison*. Trans. Alan Sheridan. New York: Vintage Books, 1977; and *The History of Sexuality*, volume 1: An introduction. Trans. Robert Hurley. New York: Vintage Books, 1978.

approach aimed at identifying and engineering what are seen as the most basic components of life" (Majia 2008).

The chimera

In Greek mythology the chimera was a fire-breathing monster, a combination of parts of a lion, a snake, and a goat. Now the word is used by scientists to describe creatures containing cells from two or more genetically distinct sources. Some human beings are chimera. For instance, when two embryos merge *in utero*, they yield one person with two cell types and, perhaps, two blood types. Once a woman has been pregnant she herself is a chimera, carrying cells from her fetus, apparently for the rest of her life. Chimera can also cross species boundaries (Robert and Baylis 2003), as when an adult human is surgically implanted with a heart valve from a pig.

Sometimes the word chimera is used to connote an illusion, but these lab animals are quite real. Chimera of various kinds have also been used in important medical research for decades. In addition to heart valves, pig skin grafts are used to minimize scarring in severe burn cases, and cow arterial grafts are used by vascular surgeons as alternatives to synthetics during arterial reconstruction. Moreover, chimera are being used to build a foundation in stem cell regenerative science, the study of the ability of stem cells to hone to and replace damaged tissue. For instance, in models of neurological disorders, human-primate and human-rat brain chimera have been used to test the feasibility of future neural stem cell treatment of Parkinson's disease (Bjugstad et al. 2005) and stroke[2] (Chu et al. 2005). In addition to being used as model organisms, human-animal chimera are a fundamental part of understanding the basic biology of cellular development and of viral disease. Human-mouse bone marrow transplants have occurred since the 1980s and have been used to study human AIDS (Namikawa et al. 1988) and leukemias (Kamel-Reid et al. 1989).

These examples should suggest that the word chimera is more exotic than it is descriptive. The word's very strangeness imparts a distracting mystery to the animal models to which it applies, which are not combinations of body parts like those of a lion, a snake, and a goat. No doubt the scientist who first applied the term innocently aspired to align these valuable creatures with an aura of poetry, but the net effect is to sustain long-standing cultural anxieties about monsters. In the ancient world the sighting of a chimera was quite literally a bad sign. Now add the modern laboratory environment, itself a black box to most people, along with the widely held notion that scientists are either eccentric or too damn smart and ambitious or all of the above. Words like these can be setbacks for science in the public mind and they cohere all too comfortably with the legacy of Dr. Frankenstein.

Concerns about the creation and use of chimera generally fall into three headings: the inadvertent creation of transgenic viruses that may be a public health menace; the undermining of human dignity; and the violation of the order of nature. I take up

---

[2] Another investigation into the use of neural stem cells to improve brain function in stroke model.

each of these concerns and conclude that none of them is compelling as a unique objection to chimera.

The politics of chimera

In 2005 I gave a talk about stem cells and chimera to a group of United States congressional staff members. Afterwards I was approached by an experienced legislative aide to a senior senator. He asked me if I could send him a list of "normal-sounding" chimera. Perhaps his concern was partly motivated by a question that had been raised by a distinguished Stanford University scientist a few months before: What are the ethical issues that would be raised when doing experiments that involve putting human brain cells into mice? The purpose of these experiments is to gain a better understanding of diseases like brain cancer, but some would be discomfited by the possibility, however remote, that some human properties could arise in a mouse whose brain was composed mainly of human neural cells. Thus arose the inquiry by the senator's staffer.

Chimera are often confused with hybrids, a subset of chimera that goes one step further, containing genetic material from two or more species within a single cell. A mule is a hybrid, the sterile offspring of a male donkey and a female horse. Conservative bioethicists have worried about hybrids between humans and nonhuman animals. For example, an embryo resulting from a human egg fertilized by a nonhuman sperm would be a hybrid, as would an embryo created by inserting the nucleus of a fully human cell into an enucleated egg from a nonhuman species (since egg cells contain maternal DNA outside the nucleus). The latter has already been the subject of research in the United Kingdom, where the government body that regulates human embryonic research has permitted studies to create embryos by inserting human nuclei into cow eggs that have had their nuclei removed, due to a severe shortage of human eggs for research.[3] The products of these procedures would not be permitted to develop beyond a few days in the laboratory, and they certainly wouldn't be able to produce some sort of science fiction version of a humanized cow. But they can provide important insights into human fertility and genetics and will be important in training embryologists.

Control over the production chimera and hybrid research has already been a point of contention in US politics. When he was a senator, Governor Sam Brownback of Kansas crusaded against human–nonhuman organisms. His latest attempt, the Human–Animal Hybrid Prohibition Act of 2009, would have prohibited the creation of a whole range of human–nonhuman organisms, most—but not all—of which are hybrids. The Bill includes findings that human–nonhuman hybrids are "grossly unethical" because they "blur the line between human and animal, male and female, parent and child, and one individual and another individual." Brownback also emphasizes that human–nonhuman hybrids are a threat to human dignity and to "the integrity of the human species."

---

[3] See Human Fertilisation and Embryology Authority, Press Release: HFEA Statement on licensing of applications to carry out research using human-animal cytoplasmic hybrid embryos, http://www.hfea.gov.uk/418.html (accessed January 17, 2008).

Supporting Senator Brownback's efforts, in his 2006 State of the Union address President Bush asked for legislation to prevent the creation of human-animal hybrids.

An important if unstated motivation for this kind of political action on the part of bioconservatives is the now-familiar suspicion of scientists' moral compass, as well as larger worries about the direction of science itself. According to some etymologists—and this view is controversial—the words hybrid and hubris derive from the same Greek word, denoting a wanton act, an outrage, a mongrel; in effect, a crime against nature. Whether the etymology is accurate or not, the association of the two words goes to the heart of Brownback's concern and those of others like him, that crossing species boundaries undermines or calls into question what it means to be *human*. Species identification here is elevated to moral necessity. The politics of biology often reduces to worries over our place in the natural order, or what one historian has called the "great chain of being." I will return to this idea later.

Brownback was especially worried that chimera and hybrids can blur species boundaries. The idea of a species is actually a fairly complex one, subject to various definitions, and scientific research has called into question whether the concept of species can, in fact, be fixed. Some would say that species are distinct if they don't interbreed, but such a "definition" is suspiciously circular. Humans are of course also defined by species membership. In biopolitical discourse what counts about these concepts is not their precise scientific justification but the fact that they represent a certain moral dimension, one that has to do with a certain status in the natural order. But, as we've seen before, the great chain of being isn't what it used to be. Deciding what the links are in the new chain of being and where we human beings fit will be a battleground of biopolitics.

This focus on species membership can be seen in familiar battles over abortion, where opponents have long argued that membership in the human species is sufficient to trigger the full panoply of legal rights. It is easy to see why blurring seemingly fixed species boundaries would therefore be a threat to the values these anti-abortion advocates hold dear. Debates over chimera and hybrids thus build on old divides, but extend them into new contexts and against new ends. In this iteration, opponents of chimera making cast themselves as protectors of the "human genome," although the "human genome" is a statistical construct at best.

Another notable aspect of both Brownback's Bill and the state laws is their focus on the inviolability of the human brain. A similar Bill up for consideration in the Arizona state legislature defines "human-animal hybrid" to include any combining of human cells and "non-human" life forms that involves an embryo and a "non-human life form engineered so that it contains a human brain." It is noteworthy that although these Bills are justified partly by public health worries about dangerous novel viruses that could leap from the chimera to humans, brain-based chimera are the focus and not those having to do with the "humanization" of other laboratory animals. In this legislation the human brain is given a special legal status above other vital organs, perhaps because for many moderns the brain is viewed as the seat of the soul, rather than other historical candidates for such status as the liver or the heart.

Brownback emphasized that his new Bill sought to prohibit only hybrids, leaving space for medically useful chimera creation, such as the use of pig heart valves. This is all to the good. But the terms of his draft Bill would have prohibited certain kinds of non-hybrid chimera as well. Most broadly, the Bill would have banned "a human embryo into which a non-human cell or cells (or the component parts thereof) have been introduced to render the embryo's membership in the species *Homo sapiens* uncertain." Mixing human and nonhuman cells in a single *embryo* yields a chimera, not a hybrid. Hybrids comprise only those organisms that incorporate two or more distinct genomes in a *single cell*. This slippage is telling, and it threatens to hobble critical research. How many human cells can a chimera or hybrid organism have before its membership in the human species is "uncertain"? And what relevance ought we attach to the developmental stage (embryo, fetus, born organism) of such organisms?

Although the Brownback Bill never got out of committee, at the state level there has been some success on this track. In 2009 Louisiana governor Bobby Jindal signed into law a Bill that was similar to Brownback's, prohibiting human–nonhuman hybrids. The Arizona Bill would forbid the intentional creation of a human embryo by any means other than fertilization of a human egg by a human sperm, as well as "A nonhuman life form engineered so that it contains a human brain or a brain derived wholly or predominantly from human neural tissues" (HB 2652 2010). If it goes into effect, violation of the law would be considered a felony. So far the governor has not taken a position on the Bill. Other states with strong bioconservative movements are attempting to impose bans on these kinds of organisms. A Bill passed by the Ohio senate lists eight kinds of "human-animal hybrid" that would be outlawed, including normal human embryos into which animal cells are inserted, zygotes formed of one human and one animal gamete (for instance a human egg fertilised by animal sperm), animal eggs with an implanted human nucleus and any "nonhuman life form engineered such that it contains a human brain or a brain derived wholly from human neural tissues" (SB 243 2009–1010). One supposes that, having been elected as governor of Kansas in 2010, Mr. Brownback will put forward a similar Bill in that state.

The new ladder of nature

Chimera challenge certain deeply entrenched ontological views. Consider our understanding of nature in its most general sense. Besides the growth of knowledge itself, the momentum behind the new politics of biology will be fed by a variety of factors, including the burgeoning global nature of science; the rapid growth of widely distributed expertise that globalized scientific cooperation generates; competition between countries for control of the knowledge and its applications; jockeying between governments and private companies for access to information that will generate new wealth and power; and, especially salient in the new politics of biology, the central political proposition whether certain aspects of the science should be pursued at all because of the possibilities for fundamentally altering society, human beings, and indeed the more or less established array of all living things.

Formerly philosophers and theologians spoke of a "natural ladder," or in the language of intellectual historian Arthur Lovejoy, a "great chain of being." This chain was conceived as a divinely created hierarchical spire in which all entities had a unique place, as in steps on a ladder. At the top is God, then the angels, then man, the other creatures, and finally earth. The chain is a Platonic passage from the most perfected, pure spirit, down to the least perfect, mere matter. Even earthly matter can be viewed as a hierarchy from precious metals at the top to dirt at the bottom. Thus is order given to the universe in which everything has a place, fulfilling the Greek vision of a cosmos. What is unclear is whether according to this ontology man can add links to the chain, or whether in doing so he upsets the natural order. Do physics and chemistry upset this comforting cosmological scheme by introducing new elements to the periodic table, for example, or are these accomplishments only applications of the divine spirit in man? In creating new life forms, modern biology provides still more disconcerting counterexamples to entities once thought to have been excluded from creation, In fact, if the "chain of being" metaphor any longer has any resonance at all, it lies in one of the most satisfying aesthetic ironies in the history of ideas: the double helix of the DNA molecule. Less than 50 years after the decoding of the structure of DNA, the controversy about a rather mechanical set of laboratory techniques often referred to as "cloning"[4] and human embryonic stem cell research was a transformative episode that brought the control of biology to the political foreground on an international scale.

Social institutions will have to prove that they are legitimate stewards of the new biopower. At this early stage no institution has met that standard; mistrust abounds. As a result, the biopolitics now unfolding is in some respects a version of what Jürgen Habermas calls a "legitimation crisis." For German philosopher Habermas a legitimation crisis occurs with the impotence of government oversight and subsequent loss of public confidence in government's ability to manage public affairs. The legitimation crisis that is even now energizing the new biopolitics is an accelerating crisis of public trust not only in government's ability to manage the science, but also the public's persistent ambivalence about the goals, power, and values of science and scientists. This problem is aggravated by the widespread sense that science is sometimes oversold, that promises are made that cannot be kept—the promise of the genome or the payoffs from stem cell research are common examples—or that contradictory assertions pop up, especially with regard to subjects of universal concern such as nutrition.

Moderns tend first to look to government for control of new technologies and their effects. Competent oversight of potential threats to personal security and well-being is one measure of public confidence in government, but if it succeeds too well government may also be an object of suspicion due to worries about excessive state control over and appropriation of science. Government agencies like the US Food and Drug Administration that seek to impose their jurisdiction over emerging science for the public interest may be accused both of over-regulating and thus discouraging innovation and of "knowing too much" about proprietary matters. On the other hand, conspiracy theorists and some human rights advocates fear that these agencies' missions arrogate too much information into the hands of shadowy bureaucrats. Less noticed, there

---

[4] Even the name of this technology has been a matter of intense political debate. From the biologists' point of view cloning is an imperfect term for the maneuvers in question because it refers to so many laboratory techniques. They prefer the more descriptive "somatic cell nuclear transfer," but the use of that phrase has been challenged by opponents of the research as too neutral for most people to understand the stakes involved in this particular type of cloning.

is also the competing prospect of private control over basic knowledge about life, as in the case of genetic testing companies that market analysis of one's genome and in the process are collecting vast amounts of genetic information.

Neither government nor industry is immune from the life sciences' legitimation crisis, nor are scientists themselves, for government and the private sector are not the only players. A joker in the deck is the role of the scientific community in the direction of science. As early as 1624, Francis Bacon's *New Atlantis* described a utopia in which a clique of scientists ensure an enlightened society through the continuous study and application of new knowledge. In doing so they keep their powerful discoveries close to their chests, having judged them too dangerous to share with those not in the fraternity. Secret societies are nothing new, including the ancient medical cult named for Hippocrates, whose members swore an oath of loyalty to their colleagues and teachers and that they would keep their knowledge within the fraternal circle. Although their intentions may be benign, the fact that these in-groups often identify themselves with some special knowledge makes those not among the elect nervous, especially if that knowledge is regarded as a key to great power that conflicts with the natural order.

At the very outset of the Enlightenment, Bacon's vision set a pattern of joyous and unlimited discovery for the sake of human flourishing along with a narrative of special insight and control by scientists. Evidently Bacon's governing scientists did not provoke suspicion among the other residents of the New Atlantis, or if they did we didn't hear about it. The same is not always true of the often ambivalent relationship between modern scientists and their lay countrymen. In our own time scientists are admired for their acumen and the improvements to which their work may lead are much desired, but their increasingly technical and highly specialized vocabulary makes their discourse inevitably somewhat exclusive. Scientists' very ways of thinking and perceiving as they dig into underlying and invisible processes are different from the ways we approach the obvious world of everyday experience.

Sigmund Freud's idea of the uncanny, a situation that is both familiar and disconcertingly unfamiliar, applies well to the fruits of the thinking of modern scientists, who routinely transform understanding of the seemingly familiar—"solid" objects, fixed species—making them uneasily unfamiliar, as though we've never really seen them at all. Scientists are of course not the only sources of the uncanny. There are false conjurers, alchemists, writers of fiction, poets, and painters who often brilliantly challenge our sense of the familiar. But those who subject their observations to the crucible of experiment and demonstration, whose revisions of the world lead to nuclear weapons, genetically modified rodents, and even the (so far) beloved and ubiquitous WorldWide Web, may understandably elicit special scrutiny. (Remember when we found "webs" creepy?) They present fertile ground for accusations of hubristic overreaching, aggravated by the fact that, like all experts, they seem to talk in code. All the transparency in the world may not easily enable many of us to understand what a geneticist or microbiologist or stem cell biologist or computer scientist is talking about when they talk to each other.[5] Even if we are inclined to trust their good

---

[5] The problem is not limited to scientists in relation to non-scientists. We have reached a point at which highly specialized scientists who are formally in the same field or academic department, or even working on closely related problems, do not necessarily understand their colleagues' work.

intentions (as many are not), we may wonder who is keeping track of what they're doing and where it's all heading. The noted anti-technology activist Jeremy Rifkin has said of the creation of chimera, "One doesn't have to be religious or into animal rights to think this doesn't make sense. It's the scientists who want to do this. They've now gone over the edge into the pathological domain" (Mott 2005).

Biopolitics

The biopolitics of chimera is only one example of problems stimulated by the new experimental biology. Biopolitical issues are volatile "wedge" issues in our politics because they raise appeal to uncertainties about how to apply values. These uncertainties are especially clear when human dignity seems to be threatened, as critics charge is the case for embryo-related research. In 2005 the Johns Hopkins University-affiliated Genetics and Public Policy Center found that three-quarters of Americans opposed human embryo cloning for research (Javitt, Suthers, and Hudson 2005). A 2008 survey sponsored by the conservative Ethics and Public Policy Center found that, when the question of embryonic stem cell research is put in terms of curing disease most favored it, but when described as destroying embryos a small majority opposed it (Levin 2008).[6] Five polls by the Pew Center on Religion and Public Life from 2004 to 2007 found that a small majority agreed that it was "more important to continue stem cell research that might produce new medical cures than to avoid destroying the human embryos used in the research," but during that period the number declined (Pew Forum on Religion and Public Life 2008), perhaps as a consequence of the moral and cultural stresses that came with the intense political debate about embryonic stem cell research. Deep-seated worries about science that are as old as the Enlightenment itself were being poured into bottles made new by the experiences of the twentieth century.

The role of biological issues in politics is not new; witness the ongoing debates about abortion. The ethical and social questions stimulated by the life sciences, and the subsequent debates about biology in politics, will surely persist. However, as reactions to the applications of biology reach a certain level of public fervor, one may perceive a transition from biology in politics to the politics of biology. In this second sense the term biopolitics refers to the ways that society attempts to gain control over the power of the life sciences. Although instances of the politics of biology can be found at the earliest stages of Western philosophy, biopolitics may become far more prominent in public life as the power of the modern life sciences becomes ever more obvious to the public at large. And while the old politics of biology operated in the dark about the underlying mechanisms of biology, the new politics of biology arises in the midst of rapidly growing understanding of basic life processes, with seemingly limitless opportunities to use it to direct individual and social change. Simply put, in the modern politics of biology the stakes are about as great as they can get.

---

[6] Arguably the wording of the relevant question was rather loaded: "It is unethical to destroy human embryos for the purposes of research because doing so destroys human embryos that are human beings and could otherwise have developed and grown like every other human being."

The modern abortion controversy has elements of both biology in politics and the politics of biology, especially as it has been a recurrent theme in the United States since the 1970s. As an example of biology in politics, the positions taken by pro-life and pro-choice forces have served as organizing principles. In an example of the politics of biology, each side attempts to manage the power behind the decision whether to continue a pregnancy or not. But the binary simplicity of the abortion decision (i.e. to abort or not), and the relative straightforwardness of the positions one may take on this issue in its strictly political sense will be vastly outstripped by the scenarios forced upon us by the new biology. As biological knowledge grows and as its applications become available, vastly more complicated and subtle new issues of biopower will emerge.

Thus we have entered the era of the new biopolitics. Rather than power over bodies and populations per se, the new biopolitics has to do with control over the tissues, systems, and information that are the basis and manifestation of life in its various forms. This new political struggle is vastly more subtle and in some ways potentially more powerful than more familiar examples such as the ability to terminate a pregnancy or certain gross efforts to manage heredity, and many more parties will be in a position to compete with the state for biopower than in the past. Whether the new biology actually achieves the Promethean power that is often touted, the symbolism alone invites struggles for control. Neither government, the private sector, nor the scientific community will be immune from the risk of a grave loss of confidence in their ability to manage the emerging forces. If only some of the predictions made of the new biopower bear fruit, the new biology will challenge everything in its path, from our understanding of ourselves as living creatures, the ways we live, our relationship to the world, to our social arrangements and values, and our political systems.

References

Bjugstad, K. B. et al. (2005). "Neural Stem Cells Implanted into MPTP-Treated Monkeys Increase the Size of Endogenous Tyrosine Hydroxylase-Positive Cells Found in the Striatum: A Return to Control Measures," *Cell Transplantation*, 14(4): 183–92.

Chu, K. et al. (2005). "Combined Treatment of Vascular Endothelial Growth Factor and Human Neural Stem Cells in Experimental Focal Cerebral Ischemia," *Neuroscience Research*, 53(4): 384–90.

HB 2652. (2010). *State of Arizona House of Representatives*, Forty-ninth Legislature, Second Regular Session, http://www.azleg.gov/legtext/49leg/2r/bills/hb2652p.htm (accessed December 20, 2012).

Jason, R. (1996). "Biotechnologies of the Self: The Human Genome Project and Modern Subjectivity," M.A. thesis (McMaster University, Hamilton, ON).

Javitt, G. H., Suthers, K., and Hudson, K. (2005). "Cloning: A policy Analysis," Washington, DC: Genetics and Public Policy Center. http://www.dnapolicy.org/images/reportpdfs/Cloning_A_Policy_Analysis_Revised.pdf (accessed December 20, 2012).

Kamel-Reid, S. et al. (1989). "A Model of Human Acute Lymphoblastic Leukemia in Immune-Deficient SCID Mice," *Science*, 246(4937): 1597–600.

Levin, Y. (2008). "Public Opinion and the Embryo Debates," *New Atlantis*, No. 20: 47–62. http://www.thenewatlantis.com/publications/public-opinion-and-the-embryo-debates (accessed December 20, 2012).

Majia, H. N. (2008). *Governmentality, Biopower, and Everyday Life.* New York: Routledge

Mott, M. (2005). "Animal-Human Hybrids Spark Controversy," *National Geographic News*, January 5, http://news.nationalgeographic.com/news/2005/01/0125_050125_chimeras.html (accessed December 20, 2012).

Namikawa, R. et al. (1988). "Infection of the SCID-hu Mouse by HIV-1," *Science*, 242(4886): 1684–6.

Pew Forum on Religion and Public Life. (2008). *Declining Majority of Americans Favor Embryonic Stem Cell Research.* http://www.pewforum.org/Science-and-Bioethics/Declining-Majority-of-Americans-Favor-Embryonic-Stem-Cell-Research.aspx (accessed December 20, 2012).

Robert, J.S., and Baylis, F. (2003). "Crossing Species Boundaries," *American Journal of Bioethics*, 3(3): 1–13.

SB 243. (2009–10). State of Ohio Senate, 128th General Assembly, http://www.legislature.state.oh.us/bills.cfm?ID=128_SB_243 (accessed December 20, 2012).

11.2

Commentary
The Question of the Family in the Biopolitics of Chimeras

Tomoko Sato

In his recent works, Professor Jonathan Moreno has made penetrating remarks on political issues associated with the production of chimeras, with references to Congressional
debates (see, for example, Moreno 2006). His paper "Chimera in Bioethics and
Biopolitics" is of particular interest in that it puts forward the point of view of "biopolitics" more forcefully than he has ever done before. In doing so it highlights the
importance of a more comprehensive or elaborate analysis of questions related to the
production of chimeras. My commentary situates itself in the perspective thus opened
by Moreno, with focus on his remarks about the use of the term "species" in different
discourses on chimeras. It aims to introduce some terms that may open the way to a cultural and sociological analysis of discourse—in particular, "family" and "family membership"—and to use them to formulate hypotheses which I hope are useful for further
exploration of the biopolitics of chimeras.

"Species" as a political notion

Moreno's article draws our attention to how and at what moment the notion of "species" intervenes in discussions about chimeras. Moreno notes that the term "chimera"
is used in biology to signify "creatures containing cells from two or more genetically
distinct sources" (see Moreno's article; Kuře 2009). It can cover quite a wide range of
entities, such as a person treated with pig skin grafts for severe burns as well as a mouse
with a brain containing human cells. The notion of species also frames Congressional
debates about the production of chimeras. As comments by Senator Sam Brownback
reveal, the motive for the debate about the regulation of work involving chimeras can
be expressed in terms of the defense of human dignity and the integrity of the "human
species." However, these motives are not clearly explicated. We should bear in mind
that the concept of "species" itself is insufficiently defined for scientists whose activities
would be affected in the regulations (see remark mentioned above by Moreno; Meier
and Wheeler 2000). More precisely, Michael Bader (2009) argues that the concept is

especially problematic with respect to the question of chimeras. Most textbooks, he observes, feature the definition of species as "all the individual organisms of a natural population that generally interbreed at maturity in the wild and whose interbreeding produces fertile offspring" (Bader 2009: 6). According to him, this definition causes few problems in cases of "normal breeding mammals," but proves inadequate "as soon as hybrids or chimeras are considered," and "in particular, in the rare cases of fertile inter-species hybrids, and when one asks to which species a mixed embryo belongs, the term [species] is useless" (Bader 2009: 6).

It is clear, then, that the notion of species has a doubly political significance. First, it is used to identify what is at stake, and tends therefore to define from the outset, to some extent, the course and direction of the discussions that follow. Second, the ambiguity of the notion of species introduces scope for political considerations to influence how we delimit a "human species." Thus Moreno, examining plans to introduce a Bill banning "a human embryo into which a non-human cell or cells (or the component parts thereof) have been introduced" resulting in its "membership in the species *Homo sapiens*" becoming "uncertain" (Brownback 2009), asks how few human cells a chimera organism could have before its membership in the human species is "uncertain."

Membership in the human species; or the problem of demarcation

Let us consider some of Moreno's observations about the role that the notion of species plays in debate about chimeras.

Whilst the debate draws its terminology from the language of scientists, it has been inattentive to relevant terminological questions and has shown disregard for the precision usually expected of scientific statements. Moreno notes that this is especially true of the distinction—important for scientists—between "chimera" and "hybrid," which has not always been made clearly and accurately in Congressional discourse.

In examining debates on public interest using the concept of species, we should follow Moreno in counting this concept among those which often represent a certain moral dimension. The abortion controversy sparked in the US during the 1970s saw debate which used the concept in a similar way (Ogino 2001: 207). Moreno looks at an argument often used by anti-abortion advocates, according to which membership of the human species is sufficient to trigger the full panoply of legal rights. Taking this debate into account is, it seems to me, crucially important in appreciating the historical, sociological, and cultural context in which the current question of chimeras is inscribed.

The assertion that "membership of the human species" begins along with "life" at the moment of conception marks out and delimits for "pro-lifers" what is to be saved from abortion. It is most likely that they defend only what seems to them worthy of this membership. It is, then, interesting to wonder whether the designation "pro-life" suffices to convey their moral position. We could perhaps get a clearer and more nuanced characterization if we examine the underlying values inherent in the formulation "membership in the human species," and consider how these values might be situated in relation to the position named "pro-choice." Also relevant here is another application of the notion "species" that Moreno identifies in discussions about the production of chimeras: one that anchors it in a conception of nature and the universe, placing it within the "natural order" or "great chain of being."This use of "species" calls to mind the cultural continuity that dates back far before the forming of the notion in question; or more precisely, creates a long tradition leading up to the present use of this notion. In accordance with that, reproduction bringing into being a life that should in its turn be capable of the reproduction of a similar life form—or, to put it another way, reproduction deemed to be in the service of saving and preserving the integrity of a "species"—is seen as valuing the natural order. In contrast, the production of chimeras is taken as contrary to this order, or even as threatening its destruction.

The question of the family: a hypothesis for the deconstruction of a political paradigm

The notion of "biopolitics" is said to date from the first decade of the twentieth century (Esposito 2008[2004]: 16). Nowadays it is likely most strongly associated with the name of Michel Foucault; yet in fact he only used the term rarely, and in a restricted sense. Foucault is aware of the problems posed to governmental practice by phenomena such as health, hygiene, birthrate, life expectancy, race, and so forth. He declares on at least one occasion that he uses the term "biopolitics" to circumscribe relatively well defined or restricted concerns: concerns about these phenomena insofar as they relate to a "population," and about the way the "rationaliz[ation]" of the problems posed has historically been attempted (2008[2004]: 317; see also 1990[1976], 2003[1997]). The notion has evolved, especially since the 1990s, with works that use it to analyze a longer period of history, in some specialized fields and on specific subjects. We might wonder if this evolution is to be explained by the structure of the notion itself (Kanamori 2010: 4).

Moreno's argument, too, makes use of this notion. It discerns contexts in which the question of chimeras has been posed: the scientific literature, Congressional debates and, more widely, contexts that require historical, cultural, and sociological analysis. His argument takes a biopolitical view that is transcontextual without losing sight of these contexts. It permits us to reveal what works deterministically on the administration of populations, or even of our lives, in each of these contexts and, furthermore, in correlation with them. One can thus identify philosophical traditions or cultural values inherent in the terms "chimera" and "natural ladder" that influence the biopolitics of chimeras, public health interests central to Congressional discussions, and diverse interests associated with research in genetic engineering.

The hypothesis that I would like to propose here identifies another factor which may be obscured by the use of the term "species." I suggest that insistence on "species membership" in certain political debates can be partly analyzed in terms of "family membership," which affirms the form of family centered on reproduction as normal or as the natural model. By attending to the concept of family, we make possible a more nuanced cultural and sociological analysis of the way decisions about the boundary of an embryo's membership in *Homo sapiens* are made when nonhuman cells are introduced to it. My hypothesis is inspired partly by a historical philosophical study of Giorgio

Agamben, which tried to draw fundamentally important biopolitical consequences from the exclusion of "simple natural life" from the polis in the strict sense and confining it, as merely reproductive life, to the sphere of the *oikos* or "home" (1998[1995]: 9). My hypothesis is nonetheless founded on the indications given by Moreno in his article concerning the effects of the intervention of the notion of "species," and, as such, it can enable us to take a new view of the historical context. To this end, it would be interesting to seek out, by analyzing the biopolitics of chimeras, factors that indicate the limits of the schematic representation of pro-life versus pro-choice opposition, and justify the interpretation of this representation as a complex of representations involving diverse cultural and sociological values.

References

Agamben, G. (1998)[1995]. *Homo Sacer: Sovereign Power and Bare Life*, translated by D. Heller-Roazen. California, CA: Stanford University Press.

Bader, M. (2009). "Problems with Terminology and Definitions," in J. Taupitz, and M. Weschka (eds), *Chimbrids: Chimeras and Hybrids in Comparative European and International Research. Scientific, Ethical, Philosophical, and Legal Aspects*, Berlin: Springer, 5–6.

Brownback, S. (2009). Text of S. 1435 [111th]: Human-Animal Hybrid Prohibition Act of 2009. http://www.govtrack.us/congress/bills/111/s1435/text (accessed December 20, 2012).

Esposito, R. (2008)[2004]. *Bíos: Biopolitics and Philosophy*, translated by T. Campbell. Minneapolis, MN: University of Minnesota Press.

Foucault, M. (1990)[1976]. *The History of Sexuality Volume 1: An introduction*, translated by R. Hurley. New York: Vintage Books.

Foucault, M. (2003)[1997]. *Society must be Defended. Lectures at the Collège de France 1975–76*, translated by D. Macey. New York: Picador.

Foucault, M. (2008)[2004]. *The Birth of Biopolitics. Lectures at the Collège de France 1978–79*, translated by G. Burchell. Basingstoke: Palgrave Macmillan.

Kanamori. O. (2010), *Seiseiji no Tetsugaku [The Philosophy of Biopolitics]*, Kyoto: Minerva Syobo.

Kuře, J. (2009). "Etymological Background and Further Clarifying Remarks Concerning Chimeras and Hybrids," in J. Taupitz, and M. Weschka (eds), *op. cit.*, 7–20.

Meier, R., and Wheeler, Q. (eds). (2000). *Species Concepts and Phylogenetic Theory*. New York: Columbia University Press.

Moreno, J. D. (2006). "Congress's Hybrid Problem," *Hastings Center Report*, 36(4): 12–13.

Ogino, M. (2001). *Chuzetsu Ronso to America Shakai—Shintai wo Meguru Senso, [Abortion Controversy and American Society—Battles over bodies]*, Tokyo: Iwanami Shoten.

11.3

Commentary

The Biopolitics and Bioethics Surrounding Chimeric Embryo Research in Japan: A Comment on Jonathan Moreno's "Chimera in Bioethics and Biopolitics"

Satoshi Kodama and Kyoko Takashima

According to Professor Jonathan D. Moreno, the fundamental concerns raised by chimera research are not the typical ethical problems of safety and human dignity. Instead, he suggests that the politics of biology, or biopolitics, which "refers to the ways that society attempts to gain control over the power of the life sciences," has become a central issue. In this commentary, we will focus on the following two points in order to characterize the Japanese perspective on chimeras:

1. The definition and use of chimeras in Japan are explained in the context of current national regulations, and we will highlight the usage of the unfamiliar terms "aggregated embryo" (*shūgō-hai*) and "specified embryo" (*tokutei-hai*).
2. Ethical arguments about chimeras are discussed, with emphasis on the considerably different perspectives between the United States and Japan.

1 Japanese regulations concerning chimeric embryo research

In his article, Professor Moreno defined chimeras as "creatures containing cells from two or more genetically distinct sources." Is there a corresponding definition in Japanese laws and government guidelines concerning research ethics?

As of 2012, policies most closely related to this topic are the Act on Regulation of Human Cloning Techniques (hereafter referred to as the Cloning Regulation Act) (2000), and the Guidelines for Handling of a Specified Embryo (2001, revised in 2009) developed by the Ministry of Education, Culture, Sports, Science, and Technology.[1] The term "chimera" or "chimeric embryo" is not explicitly used in these laws; instead, embryos subject to the regulations are collectively referred to as "specified embryos" (*tokutei-hai*) and classified into the following nine groups based on their production processes:[2]

- human split embryo;
- human embryonic nuclear transfer embryo;
- human somatic cell nuclear transfer embryo;
- human-human chimeric embryo;
- human-animal hybrid embryo;
- human-animal clone embryo;
- human-animal chimeric embryo;
- animal-human clone embryo;
- animal-human chimeric embryo.

Transplantation of human somatic cell nuclear transfer embryos, human–animal hybrid embryos, human-animal clone embryos, and human–animal chimeric embryos into human or animal wombs is prohibited by the Cloning Regulation Act. Transplantation of the other specified embryos is also prohibited for the time being by the Guidelines for Handling of a Specified Embryo. Only the creation of animal-human chimeric embryos and human somatic cell nuclear transfer embryos for scientific purposes is approved by the aforementioned guidelines.[3] However, the creation of an individual by chimeric embryo transplantation into the womb is prohibited in Japan.

These regulations raise two points regarding terminology. The first is that the various artificially created embryos are referred to as "specified embryos" (*tokutei-hai*) in laws and government guidelines. The term was previously non-existent in Japanese vocabulary, and its origin is unclear to the best of our knowledge and requires further investigation. In any case, "specified embryos" must have been an unfamiliar term for researchers that handled cloning, let alone laypeople.

The second point is that although the term "chimeric embryo" appears in the English translation of the Cloning Regulation Act, a corresponding term does not appear in Japanese; *shūgō-hai* is used instead. The literal translation of *shūgō-hai* is "aggregated embryo," a phrase entirely incapable of evoking the word "chimera." According to

---

[1] Act on Regulation of Human Cloning Techniques (Act No. 146 of 2000), http://www.cas.go.jp/jp/seisaku/hourei/data/htc_2.pdf (accessed December 20, 2012).
The Guidelines for Handling of a Specified Embryo (2001). http://www.lifescience.mext.go.jp/files/pdf/30_82.pdf (accessed December 20, 2012).
The revised version (2009) (in Japanese). http://www.lifescience.mext.go.jp/files/pdf/30_226.pdf (accessed December 20, 2012).

[2] Article 2 of the Cloning Regulation Act.

[3] Creation of human somatic cell nuclear transfer embryos for research purposes was approved in the 2009 guideline revisions.

Japanese bioethicist Shohei Yonemoto, hybrid embryos and chimeric embryos were translated as *yūgō-hai* (fusion embryos) and *shūgō-hai* (aggregated embryos), respectively, when the Cloning Regulation Act was drafted (Yonemoto 2006: 163–4). According to Yonemoto, such unusual and unfamiliar terms were used due to restrictions on expressions used in Japanese legislation (Yonemoto 2006: 164)[4].

We have thus described current regulations for chimeric embryo research in Japan, as well as use of the terms "specified embryos" for manipulated embryos in general and "aggregated embryos" for chimeric embryos in particular.

2 Ethical issues surrounding chimeras

In his article, Professor Moreno noted that although the purpose of creating chimeric mice is to conduct research on diseases such as brain tumors, citizens may nevertheless fear that a mouse-human hybrid (i.e. humanized mice) could result. He suggested that the term "chimera" has contributed to negative impressions of this research in the United States, reminding people of Dr. Frankenstein's monster. Professor Moreno also stated that Americans are worried that genetic manipulation could destroy the natural order, or "the ladder of nature," and that the government and scientists may not have enough control over such research. Could the same be said for Japan?

As mentioned above, the word "chimera" does not appear in Japanese legislation. Professor Moreno mentioned in his article that it originally described a monster in Greek mythology—a combination of parts of a lion, a snake, and a goat. Japanese citizens, however, may be unfamiliar with the term as well as the negative image it evokes. Given this circumstance and the unfamiliar terms used in the Cloning Regulation Act and the ensuing guidelines, it may have been difficult for the Japanese public to understand what is at issue with the research involving chimeric embryos. This might partly explain why government surveys have been conducted on public attitudes toward cloning but not on chimeras.[5] It would therefore seem that the foundation for public debates on this topic is lacking in Japan.

Professor Moreno characterized the main ethical issues regarding chimeras as 1) the inadvertent creation of transgenic viruses, 2) the undermining of human dignity, and 3) the violation of the order of nature. In addition, he pointed out that a bioconservative senator in the United States attempted to submit legislation prohibiting the creation of human-nonhuman organisms using the argument that "the integrity of the

---

[4] In a report titled "Fundamental Policy on Human Embryo Research Focused Primarily on Human Embryonic Stem Cells," produced by the subcommittee on Human Embryo Research in 2000, the chimeric embryo was defined as "an embryo containing cells from two or more distinct embryos," and the term was used in the report throughout. The term, however, does not appear in the Cloning Regulation Act and other government guidelines, as explained by Yonemoto. As for the report, see http://www.mext.go.jp/b_menu/shingi/kagaku/rinri/kio0306.htm (in Japanese). (accessed December 20, 2012).

[5] The National Survey on Human Embryo Research (Cabinet Office 2002, in Japanese) was conducted by the government to measure public awareness of and interest in human embryo research and its terminology (human embryos, regenerative medicine, cloning techniques, and use of cloned embryos). A national survey has never been conducted on chimeric research.

human species" would be lost (i.e. the dividing line between humans and animals would become blurred).

What ethical concerns regarding chimeras have developed in Japan? Although there have been various debates on the creation of human clones and destruction of human embryos (see Kodama and Akabayashi 2010), the propriety of chimeric embryos or specified embryos has not been discussed to the same degree. Violation of human dignity (devaluing individual uniqueness and dehumanizing the creation of life), disruption of the social order, and safety issues have been mentioned regarding the creation of human somatic cell nuclear transfer embryos.[6] However, these issues referred to cloning techniques in general and not particularly to the creation of chimeric embryos. Deliberations in the Diet to establish cloning legislation did note that "an individual organism, neither human nor animal, could be created from an embryo born of technology to fuse or aggregate human and animal cells (i.e. specified fusion/aggregation technology), which may affect human dignity at least as gravely as cloning techniques."[7] This point was later reflected in Article 1 of the Cloning Regulation Act. To the best of our knowledge, however, issues that do not exist for human clones but may arise for chimeras (i.e. problems caused by "mixing" humans and animals) never became an independent point of discussion in public debates in Japan.

Finally, we would like to comment on why the debate on chimeras has been intense in the United States but not in Japan. There are two potential reasons. The first is the culturally relativistic explanation that Japan does not share a Christian background with the United States that sharply distinguishes between humans and animals. The second is the linguistic explanation that while the mythological Greek chimera is widely known in the United States, its image is not as pervasive in Japan; moreover, regulation on chimeras was debated with unfamiliar terms such as "specified embryos" and "aggregated embryos." We support the second possibility. If Japanese citizens associated the word "chimera" with negative images as in the United States and understood the research content to some degree, what might have happened? Debates similar to those in the United States might have occurred, or the differences in Eastern and Western values might have still prevented controversy. Yet this is a speculation and it would appear that a debate on the creation of chimeric embryos did not occur this time due to terminology issues, rather than a difference of values.

Yonemoto asserted that the term "specified embryo" has contributed to an understanding of the human embryo as comparable to an object (Yonemoto 2006: 165–6). As is true with "chimera," the images citizens have of certain aspects of science and technology will differ depending on word usage. Consequently, the involvement of citizens and the intensity of debates could be affected by something as simple as language. This situation is clearly at work in Japan, where terminology may have prevented citizens from participating in the debate on chimeric research propriety. Such considerations are

---

[6] From the "'Act on Regulations of Human Cloning Techniques' Reference Materials," Office of Bioethics and Safety, Research Promotion Bureau, Ministry of Education, Culture, Sports, Science, and Technology (in Japanese).

[7] The 6th Science and Technology Committee of the 147th Diet Session (May 18, 2000) (in Japanese).

likely to become important in the future when the politics of biology, or biopolitics as defined by Professor Moreno, becomes a greater issue.

References

Kodama, S., and Akabayashi, A. (2010). "Neither a 'Person' nor a 'Thing': The Controversy concerning the Moral and Legal Status of Human Embryos in Japan," in B. J. Capps, and A. V. Campbell (eds), *Contested Cells: Global Perspectives on the Stem Cell Debate*, London: Imperial College Press, 421–39.

Yonemoto, S. (2006). *Biopolitics*. Tokyo: Chukoshinsho. (in Japanese)

11.4

Response to Commentaries

Jonathan D. Moreno

I am very grateful to Satoshi Kodama and Kyoko Takashima and to Tomoko Sato for their illuminating remarks on my paper.

For me, the core point made in Tomoko Sato's commentary is this:

> I suggest that insistence on "species membership" in certain political debates can be partly analyzed in terms of "family membership," which affirms the form of family centered on reproduction as normal or as the natural model. By attending to the concept of family, we make possible a more nuanced cultural and sociological analysis of the way decisions about the boundary of an embryo's membership in *Homo sapiens* are made when nonhuman cells are introduced to it.

In *The Body Politic* I suggest that the notion of species membership is one of those comforting, convenient, and familiar categories that modern biology is undermining. No wonder, then, that so many people find biology threatening, so much so that arcane laboratory technologies like those involving the manipulation of human and animal cells have become objects of political activism. Tomoko Sato's suggestion is an heroic attempt to rescue the notion of species membership from the operations of modern biology by associating it with the idea of family membership. With its hint of family resemblances and pragmatism, this suggestion is very much in the spirit of two of my favorite philosophers, Ludwig Wittgenstein and William James.

But the findings of evolutionary biology itself complicate matters. Consider the idea of *Homo sapiens*, which many of us might want to think of as one big (if not always happy) family. Recent work suggests that modern human DNA often includes some small percentage of DNA from Neanderthals, perhaps 1–4 percent. Suppose those findings are correct. In that case modern humans and Neanderthals coexisted from the British Isles to Asia up to about 30,000 years ago. The disappearance of Neanderthals is commonly attributed to ecological pressures: a period of rapid swings in temperature defeated the Neanderthals' lifestyle, and they were not clever enough to adapt.

How then to account for the DNA admixture, which is evidence that there was some cross-breeding? The dominant view is that these were cases of rape, but a minority of evolutionary geneticists believe that there might have been rather frequent, voluntary mating and that the Neanderthal genome gradually drifted into and was overcome by the modern human genome. Obviously these hypotheses are to some degree compatible.

This prehistoric story is fascinating in its own right. But for the purposes of this exchange, here is the important point: Neanderthals are sometimes regarded as a sub-species of *Homo sapiens*, and sometimes as a separate species. In either case, how are we to decide whether they are in the family or not? And of course the very suggestion that so many of us are descended from another species, even in a very small measure, will be intolerable to cultural conservatives for whom species membership is a non-negotiable value and which figures so strongly in the their estimation of the value of a human embryo.

The comments of Satoshi Kodama and Kyoko Takashima demonstrate the usefulness of comparative bioethics. For example, there is no corresponding typology in US policy to the nine items in Japan's Act and the Guidelines that they cite. The 2005 National Research Council (NRC) *Guidelines for Human Embryonic Stem Cell Research* state that:

All research involving the introduction of hES [human embryonic stem] cells into nonhuman animals at any stage of embryonic, fetal, or postnatal development should be reviewed by the [Embryonic Stem Cell Research Oversight committee. Particular attention should be paid to the probable pattern and effects of differentiation and integration of the human cells into the nonhuman animal tissues.

The NRC Guidelines also state that these forms of research should not be permitted at this time:

Research in which hES cells are introduced into nonhuman primate blastocysts or in which any embryonic stem cells are introduced into human blastocysts.
No animal into which hES cells have been introduced at any stage of development should be allowed to breed.

These guidelines appear to cover the last five items mentioned in the Japan laws (i.e., human–animal hybrid embryo, human–animal clone embryo, human–animal chimeric embryo, animal–human clone embryo, and animal–human chimeric embryo). They permit creation of animal–human chimeric embryos (but only following review by a special committee and never in nonhuman primate blastocysts), and human somatic cell nuclear transfer embryos for scientific purposes (and again only with committee review). Although these US guidelines are voluntary and do not have the force of law (except in California, where they have largely been adopted in state law), they became the *de facto* professional standards as soon as they were announced by the National Research Council.

The language problems are striking. In the US the main difficulty has been the inherent ambiguity in the term "chimera," which refers equally to an embryo or fetus with cells from another individual, to a person with a porcine heart valve, to a woman who has once been pregnant and has circulating fetal cells, to a mythological creature. Often in the public discourse there is poor understanding of the difference between a chimera of any sort and a "hybrid." Perhaps what this demonstrates is that even if one already has the terminology in one's language, when there are technical applications of the terms there is still need for public education.

I agree with the authors' analysis of why the chimeric embryo debate has been particular to the US and not Japan. But I would add that the influence of conservative cultural views of the human embryo and its "inviolability," even for medical science, is a distinct factor, in addition to the sharp delineation that they mention between human and nonhuman species.

One final note about the way the language issue has been prominent in the United States. Opponents of somatic cell nuclear transfer (SCNT) have insisted that the term "cloning" be used to describe SCNT, arguing that the general public does not understand the meaning of a technical term like SCNT. On the other hand, defenders of SCNT for research argue that "cloning" is too general and is inherently misleading. So in other ways biopolitics can be tied up with language, even if the terminology is in principle available.

Here I am reminded of a remark by George Orwell in his 1946 essay, "Politics and the English Language":

Most people who bother with the matter at all would admit that the English language is in a bad way, but it is generally assumed that we cannot by conscious action do anything about it.

Let us hope that, in English and in Japanese, we may yet prove Orwell wrong.

References

National Research Council (2005). *Guidelines for Human Embryonic Stem Cell Research*.Washington, DC: National Academies Press.

Orwell, G. (1946). "Politics and the English Language," *Horizon*, 13:252–65.

PART II

Globalization and Bioethics

SECTION A

Organ Transplant

12.1

Primary Topic Article
Trafficking and Markets in Kidneys: Two Poor Solutions to a Pressing Problem

Arthur L. Caplan

The harsh reality of markets involving the poor: trafficking

Levy Izhak Rosenbaum, an Orthodox Jewish Rabbi in Brooklyn, New York called himself a "matchmaker." However, he was not arranging dates for his congregants. Rosenbaum was one of five rabbis indicted on July 23, 2009 in New Jersey for broker-ing the sale of black-market kidneys (and in a few cases lobes of livers). He apparently found poor, vulnerable Syrian Jews, newly immigrated to Israel, and allegedly paid each of them $10,000 to travel to the US to sell a kidney to patients in various US transplant centers. Rosenbaum was quite a businessman. He pocketed as much as $160,000 per organ for serving as the middleman in his organ-trafficking scheme while charging the sellers of kidneys for their transportation and room and board.

Rosenbaum's scheme constitutes trafficking in persons for the purpose of obtaining organs. Those involved were compelled by poverty to think about kidney sale. The mid-dlemen then took advantage of their poverty and illiteracy, duping them into thinking that they would earn a large sum of money free and clear by selling a kidney. Sadly, in most of the world a market or allowing financial incentives in kidneys means that traf-ficking, exploiting, and often harming the sellers of kidneys, are the reality.

Trafficking is an all-too-real phenomenon in the world of transplantation. It can take many forms. Sometimes people are brought to hospitals against their will or with no true informed consent to sell their kidneys. Sometimes would-be patients travel to hospitals where they will meet someone found by a broker to whom they have been assigned to sell a kidney. And, in some instances, the organs themselves are sold or sim-ply forcefully removed and then sent to waiting patients. Properly preserved kidneys remain transplantable for a few hours. Some studies estimate that nearly 10 percent of all kidneys transplanted around the world are trafficked in one of these ways (Caplan et al. 2009).

The New Jersey indictments represent the first known instance of trafficked human organs reaching patients in the United States. But, as numerous reports have documented, there are many examples of organ markets that are essentially trafficking occurring in many locations around the globe.

In the past few years wealthy persons needing transplants have traveled from the United Arab Emirates to Sri Lanka, from the United States to Azerbaijan, and from many nations around the world to Pakistan, Egypt, China, and Iraq to receive kidneys sold by desperately poor, ill-informed, uneducated persons. The sellers of these organs are only of interest to those trafficking them as sources of income. Once a kid... is removed the seller's fate in terms of follow-up care is of no concern to traffickers.

For example, a 64-year-old American underwent kidney transplantation in Baku, Azerbaijan at the end of May 2009. The seller was a 31-year-old poor Ukrainian unknown to the recipient. Individuals outside Azerbaijan arranged the transplant but it was performed in Azerbaijan by an Israeli transplant surgeon. Post the transplant, the seller was left to fend for himself, including finding the means to return home. The details of this incident were reported to the Israeli and Azeri authorities by the physician who cared for the patient upon his return to the United States post surgery (Postrel 2009).

Patients from the United Arab Emirates, Kuwait, Oman, Australia, the Netherlands, Turkey, Kosovo, and India have undergone transplantation at the Kidney Center of Rawalpindi and the Aadil Hospital of Lahore, Pakistan. It appears trafficked organs, that is organs obtained from very poor, often illiterate individuals with little capacity for true informed consent, were used (Robertson 2009; Zubeida 2009).

Not all trafficking involves crossing national borders. The television network Al Jazeera reported on July 20, 2009 that organ brokers were arranging for poor Iraqis to sell their kidneys at the Al-Khakal hospital in Baghdad (Al Jazeera 2009). And, according to numerous press accounts, despite government condemnation, there continues to be a brisk market in organs in India (Fearon 2007).

Sales can lead to behavior that goes beyond simply taking advantage of poverty to obtain a kidney. The Associated Press reported on July 20, 2009 that a Saudi Arabian man married a Filipino woman as a cover for buying her kidney, trying to circumvent a recent law prohibiting foreigners from undergoing transplantation in the Philippines. The patient was ultimately denied access to transplantation in the Philippines (*Daily Mail* reporter 2009).

There are few defenders of trafficking as a solution to organ shortage. Forcing, coercing, or duping adults or removing a kidney from a child is inconsistent not only with international human rights conventions prohibiting exploitation but violates the ethical norms of the professional transplant community. Trafficked persons, meaning those who by definition are duped, forced, coerced, or deceived, are simply being exploited by middlemen. No one looks out for their interests or health once a kidney has been removed. Trafficking has rightly been condemned by all international bodies that have examined the problem (Caplan et al. 2009).

Trafficking is seen as a reprehensible response to scarcity by those suffering from kidney failure desperate to find some way to save their lives. So why does trafficking persist? And is it possible to create systems using financial incentives to obtain kidneys that would not degenerate into trafficking? And are there other ideas or strategies which might alleviate the shortage of transplantable kidneys?

Scarcity creates trafficking

Every day dozens of people die around the world while waiting for transplants. Many more await bone, cornea, dural matter, tendon, and other tissue transplants—suffering severe disability while they wait. These deaths and lives with disabilities are especially tragic since many might be prevented if more organs and tissues were available for transplantation.

Scarcity means that hard choices have to be made about who will live and who will die. With more than 100,000 people on waiting lists for kidneys, hearts, livers, lungs, and intestines just in North America alone, the pressure to distribute the scarce supply of organs fairly and to minimize rationing by finding ways to increase the worldwide supply of organs, tissues, and transplantable cells is enormous.

Kidneys are paired organs. There is data to show that in carefully screened donors, living with one kidney is generally not dangerous (Ibrahim et al 2009: 459–69). Also the surgery to remove a kidney in competent hands is not hugely risky. So obtaining kidneys from living persons has been one strategy to meeting the mounting demand for them.

Kidneys are usually donated by family members or friends or those with emotional ties to those in need. In a few instances strangers offer to donate a kidney to someone in need (Zink et al. 2005: 581–5). For the first time in the United States in 2005 donated kidneys from living persons constituted a larger source of transplanted kidneys than did those obtained from cadaver sources (McCurdle et al. 2005: 605–6).

Scarcity is growing worse every year. Waiting lists are growing faster than the supply of organs. Physicians are becoming more adept at dealing with harder cases. Aging populations in many nations increase the demand for kidneys. And increases in the rates of obesity, diabetes, and hypertension are driving up the demand for more kidney transplants as well. The capacity to do transplants is spreading to many nations around the globe, increasing the demand for organs worldwide.

Scarcity is actually a worse problem than it appears to be from published data on demand. Demand for transplants is actually underestimated from that shown on public waiting lists in Canada, the US, Europe, Asia, the Middle East, and South America. If there were greater access to primary health care more people might be identified as needing an organ or tissue transplant before becoming too sick to survive a transplant. And if transplant centers were to relax their current admissions standards to include more people—such as those who lack money or insurance, have severe intellectual disabilities, older persons, prisoners, and foreigners who cannot get transplants in their own countries due to a lack of transplant centers and surgeons—then the lists of those waiting in rich nations could easily triple or quadruple (Quinn et al. 2007: 1362–7).

Those who care for persons dying of renal failure know the terrible toll the shortage of transplantable kidneys takes. That is why trafficking flourishes. Some doctors and nurses are, apparently, willing to remain ignorant of the source of kidneys out of the belief that their sole ethical duty is to their dying patients.

But transplant teams have an ethical duty to protect donor interests as well as to help those in need of transplants. Intentional ignorance about the fact that a person or an organ has been trafficked is not an acceptable ethical stance on the part of transplant teams and hospitals. These teams are obligated to protect the interests and health of the sources of kidneys as well as recipients. Ultimately, transplant teams and hospitals must be held accountable for knowing the origin and source, or provenance, of the kidneys and any other organs they transplant (Caplan et al. 2009). Trafficking flourishes not because anyone has made a convincing case that it is morally or legally defensible but in part due to the willful ignorance of transplant centers eager to help their patients and to turn a profit doing transplants tolerating trafficking.

If trafficking is an unacceptable response to scarcity then what? In order for policy makers to consider the merits of new proposals for inducing people to donate or sell organs, tissues, and cells, it is necessary to fully understand the bioethical framework that has guided organ and tissue donation in nearly every part of the globe since kidney transplant's inception in the 1950s (Caplan and Coehlo 1999).

The prevailing ethical framework for obtaining organs and tissues

The existing bioethical framework for obtaining organs and tissues is grounded on four key values—respect for persons, the autonomy of the individual, consent, and altruism. The notion that organs or tissues can be removed from a body for the purposes of transplantation, living or dead, without voluntary consent has not been accepted in any nation except in highly unusual circumstances (i.e. unclaimed bodies at morgues under a coroner's jurisdiction, Indiana state law code IC 36-2-14-19 2009; Bagheri 2005: 4159–62). Persons and their families are recognized in law and ethics as having a controlling interest over the disposition of the body upon death. Deceased and living persons are to be treated with dignity and not merely used to serve the needs of others.

Even though someone might well benefit from obtaining my liver or having bone marrow from my body, these organs and tissues ought not be removed from me, whether I am alive or newly dead, without my permission or that of a surrogate family member or guardian. To do so is to commit a battery or assault upon a living person and to desecrate the body of a newly deceased person. The act of treating persons with dignity is exemplified by affording them control over the disposition of their body and its parts in life and upon death (Santiago 1997: 1625–8; IOM 2006).

Another core element of the existing bioethical framework governing the procurement of organs and tissues is that the body and its parts not be made the object of commerce. Prohibitions against slavery and trafficking of persons for prostitution are based upon the bioethical principle that human beings ought not be bought and sold as objects (UN human rights, Council of Europe human rights). The transplant community has incorporated this view into a prohibition against trading in body parts for profit. In part, this position reflects the fundamental dignity of persons, which is to say they ought not be enslaved, bought, or sold. Altruism as reflected in the use of the term "donation" for obtaining organs signals the notion of human dignity is created by putting sale off limits and only permitting gifts (Cohen 2002: 47–64).

In order to obtain organs and tissues from the living there is agreement that ethically one must have a competent person who is fully informed and who can make a voluntary, uncoerced choice about donation. In the situation where organs and tissues are sought from the recently deceased, the notion of voluntary consent has been extended, in many nations, to the recognition of donor cards as adequate to direct a donation, permitting family consent if the deceased is not known to have any objection or, for those not wishing to donate, registration of objections in computer-based registries. Variants of policies about who bears the duty to consent exist around the world but from a bioethical perspective it is voluntary, informed consent that is crucial in making organ and tissue procurement ethical (Sperling 2009: 299–306).

Proposals to increase the supply of organs must be very carefully weighed against this prevailing bioethical framework that has long served to adequately protect the interests of prospective donors. Changes in these values might well alienate the public, who have grown used to the prevailing ethical framework. Major religious groups who support this bioethical framework or health-care workers, the majority of whom believe that the current bioethical framework is the appropriate one to govern organ, tissue, and cell procurement for transplantation purposes, could react very negatively to any major shift in the ethical infrastructure of organ and tissue procurement (Henegan 2008).

Increasing the supply

A number of steps have been taken over the years in many nations to try to increase the supply of organs. An early effort in the 1970s was to enact laws permitting the use of organ donor cards that allowed family consent to donate a deceased relative's organs (Caplan and Coehlo 1999). Some nations began requiring hospitals to ask all patients' families about organ and tissue donation upon death—so-called required request laws (Caplan 1986: 49–5; Caplan 1988: 34–7; 6). Most recently, some countries require hospitals to honor a patient's donor card even when a family member opposes donation.

These policies were somewhat effective but the gap between supply and demand continued to increase. Therefore, some now argue for a shift away from a reliance on voluntary altruism in organ donation toward a paid market or system that uses financial incentives (Satel 2009).

Organ markets

Two basic strategies have been proposed to provide incentives for people to sell their organs upon their death. One strategy is simply to permit organ sale by allowing persons to broker contracts while alive with persons interested in selling at prices mutually agreed upon by both parties (Radcliffe-Richards et al. 1998: 1950–2; Satel 2006: 20). Markets already exist on the Internet between potential live sellers and people in need of organs (Barclay 2004; Caplan 2004).

The other strategy is a "regulated" market in which the government would act as the purchaser of organs—setting a fixed price and enforcing conditions of sale (Harris and Erin 2002: 114–15; Matas 2004: 2007–17). Iran appears to have such a market in operation although reports on how it is actually being implemented and how well it functions in terms of protecting sellers are not encouraging (Griffin 2007: 502–5).

Both proposals have drawn heated ethical criticism. One criticism is that only the poor and desperate will want to sell their body parts. If you need money, you might sell your kidney to try and feed your family or to pay back a debt. This may be a "rational" decision, but that does not make it a matter of free, voluntary choice (Caplan 2007: 431–4; Hughes 2010).

Watching your child go hungry when you have no job and a wealthy person waves a wad of bills in your face is not exactly a scenario that inspires confidence in the "choice" made by those with few options to sell vital body parts. Talk of individual rights and autonomy is hollow if those with no options must "choose" to sell their organs to purchase life's basic necessities. Choice requires information, options, and some degree of freedom, as well as the ability to reason about risks without being blinded by the prospect of short-term gain (Feinberg 1986; Beauchamp and Childress 2008).

It is hard to imagine many people in wealthy countries eager to sell their organs either while alive or upon their death. In fact, even if compensation is relatively high, few will agree to sell (Rid et al. 2009: 558–64). That has been the experience with markets in human eggs for research purposes and with paid surrogacy in the United States—prices have escalated, but there are still relatively few sellers (Baylis and McLeon 2007: 726–31).

Moreover, markets if successful only have an impact on kidneys. It is not clear what the impact would be of allowing the creation of a market in kidneys from living or deceased persons on the willingness of people to altruistically donate hearts, lungs, and corneas, for which a market would not be tolerated. The risk of alienating altruistic donors of hearts, lungs, faces, limbs, and livers by creating a narrow market is a huge one to take given the potential loss of life involved.

Selling organs, even in a tightly regulated market, violates the existing bioethical framework of respect for persons since the sale is clearly being driven by profit. It also violates, in the case of living persons, the ethics of medicine itself.

The core ethical norm of the medical profession is the principle, "Do no harm." The only way that removing an organ from someone seems morally defensible is if the donor chooses to undergo the harm of surgery solely to help another, not to make money. The creation of commerce in body parts puts medicine in the position of removing body parts from people solely to abet those people's interest in securing compensation as well as to let middlemen profit (Rothman and Rothman 2006: 1524–8).

Is this a role that the health professions can ethically countenance? In a market—even a regulated one—doctors and nurses still would be using their skills to help living people harm themselves solely for money. In a cadaver market they would risk making families and patients uncertain about the degree to which appropriate care was being offered and continued if a person might be "worth more dead than alive." The resulting distrust and loss of professional standards are a high price to pay to gamble on the hope that a market may secure more organs and tissues for those in need (Harmon and Delmonico 2006: 1146–7).

Presumed consent

There is another option for increasing the organ supply that has been tried in Spain, Italy, Austria, and Belgium. These nations have enacted laws that create presumed consent. In such a system, the presumption is that a deceased person wants to be an organ donor upon their death—basically an ethical default to the desirability of donation (Caplan 1983: 23–32; Caplan 1994: 1708–9). People who do not want to be organ donors have to say so while alive by carrying a card indicating their objection or by registering their objection in a computerized registry, or both. They may also tell their loved ones and rely on them to object should procurement present itself as an opportunity (Caplan April 2012).

What is remarkable about this legislation is that it has worked (Abadie and Gay 2006: 599–620; Gil-Diaz 2009: 256–61). Unlike the hypothetical but unsupported assertions of advocates of financial incentives and markets, presumed consent has produced results without creating any problems or difficulties in the nations that have enacted such legislation and without any significant increase beyond the costs of education and training in the overall cost of transplantation.

What is important about this strategy from a bioethical perspective is that it is completely consistent with the existing bioethical framework governing organ and tissue procurement. Respect for persons and voluntary altruistic consent remain the moral foundation for making organs available. The main ethical objections to presumed consent are fear of mistakes in which there is the presumption that someone consented when, in fact, either the individual had failed to indicate opposition or the record of that opposition was lost, and some resistance to the notion of presuming anyone's consent. A more felicitous description of presumed consent might be "default to donation." Individuals are familiar with such defaults in a way that might make them far more comfortable with this strategy for obtaining more organs (Thaler and Sunstein 2008).

Conclusion

The worldwide shortage of transplantable organs has led to a significant degree of trafficking in kidneys. Some of the groups involved in this illicit trafficking are also linked to trafficking in women and children for prostitution.

Shortage has led some to call for policies that would legitimize the sale of kidneys. But it is difficult to believe that in most parts of the world sufficient oversight and government authority exist to regulate markets and that they would not quickly deteriorate into trafficking. Even in nations that might be able to regulate a market in kidneys it is not evident that this would lead to an increase in the overall supply. There is no empirical evidence that money is a key factor in guiding decisions about making kidneys available for transplant. Nor is it likely that any but the most desperately poor or disadvantaged would be drawn to kidney sale, making a mockery of the entire notion of autonomous, free choice to sell a body part. Markets would also create an untenable situation for health-care workers, asking them to use their skills to harm patients solely for the purpose of allowing those patients a one-time chance to earn money.

There are alternatives to creating markets. Greater efforts can be made to secure all organs, including kidneys, by enacting presumed consent legislation. This has been done in some nations with notable results. With sufficient training and educational resources, presumed consent policies are known to boost the supply of all organs for transplantation. And by outlawing financial systems, those nations which have made no effort to build procurement systems using cadaver organs will be led to do so, thereby decreasing the pressures that contribute to exploitative and immoral organ trafficking.

References

Abadie, A., and Gay, S. (2006). "The Impact of Presumed Consent Legislation on Cadaveric Organ Donation: A Cross-Country Study," *Journal of Health Economics*, 25(4): 599–620.

Al Jazeera. (2009). "Poverty Drives Iraq Organ Trade," *Al Jazeera*, July 20, http://english.aljazeera.net/news/middleeast/2009/07/200972052636416787.html (accessed December 20, 2012).

Bagheri, A. (2005). "Organ Transplantation Laws in Asian Countries: A Comparative Study," *Transplantation Proceedings*, 37(10): 4159–62.

Barclay, L. (2004). *Medscape*, http://www.medscape.com/viewarticle/491837 (accessed December 20, 2012).

Baylis, F., and McLeon, C. (2007). "The Stem Cell Debate Continues: The Buying and Selling of Eggs for Research," *Journal of Medical Ethics*, 33(12): 726–31.

Beauchamp, T. L., and Childress, J. F. (2008). *Principles of Biomedical Ethics*. 6th edition. Oxford: Oxford University Press.

Caplan, A. L. (1983). "Organ Transplants: The Costs of Success," *Hastings Center Report*, 6: 23–32.

Caplan, A. L. (1986). "Requests, Gifts, and Obligations: The Ethics of Organ Procurement," *Transplantation Proceedings*, 18(3): 49–56.

Caplan, A. L. (1988). "Professional Arrogance and Public Misunderstanding," *Hastings Center Report*, 18(2): 34–7.

Caplan, A. L. (1994). "Current Ethical Issues in Organ Procurement and Transplantation," *JAMA*, 272:1708–9.

Caplan, A. L. (2004). "Organs.com: New Commercially Brokered Organ Transfers Raise Questions," *Hastings Center Report*, 34(6): 8.

Caplan, A. L. (2007). "Do No Harm: The Case Against Organ Sales from Living Persons," in H. P. Tan, A. Marcos, and R. Shapiro (eds), *Living Donor Organ Transplantation*. New York: Informa, 431–4.

Caplan, A. L. (April 2012). "Bioethics of Organ Transplantation," *eLS* [online encyclopedia], http://onlinelibrary.wiley.com/doi/10.1002/9780470015902.a0003481.pub2/full, DOI:10.1002/9780470015902.a0003481.pub2 (accessed January 19, 2013).

Caplan, A. L., and Coehlo, D. (eds). (1999). *The Ethics of Organ Transplants*, Buffalo, NY: Prometheus.

Caplan, A. L. et al. (2009). "Trafficking in Organs, Tissues, and Cells and Trafficking in Human Beings for the Purpose of the Removal of Organs," *Joint Council of Europe/United Nations Study*. Strasbourg: Directorate General of Human Rights and Legal Affairs, Council of Europe.

Daily Mail reporter. (2009). "Saudi Man Marries Filipino as Cover to Buy One of Her Kidneys," *Mail Online,* July 21, http://www.dailymail.co.uk/news/article-1200926/ Saudi-man-marries-Filipino-cover-buy-kidneys.html (accessed January 19, 2013).

Cohen, C. (2002). "Public Policy and the Sale of Human Organs," *Kennedy Institute of Ethics Journal*, 12(1): 47–64.

Fearon, P. (2007). "Kidney Sales Brisk on India's Black Market," *Newser,* May 9, http://www.newser.com/story/2038/kidney-sales-brisk-on-indias-black-market.html (accessed December 20, 2012).

Feinberg, J. (1986). *Harm to Self.* New York: Oxford University Press.

Gil-Diaz, C. (2009). "Spain's Record Organ Donations: Mining Moral Conviction," *Cambridge Quarterly of Healthcare Ethics*, 18(3): 256–61.

Griffin, A (2007). "Kidneys on Demand," *BMJ*, 7592:502–5.

Harmon, W., and Delmonico, F. (2006). "Payment for Kidneys: A Government-Regulated System Is Not Ethically Achievable," *Clinical Journal of the American Society of Nephrology*, 1(6): 1146–7.

Harris, J., and Erin, C. (2002). "An Ethically Defensible Market in Organs," *BMJ*, 325:114–15.

Henegan, T. (2008). "Pope Slams Human Organ Trade, Warns on Transplants," *Reuters,* November 7, http://www.reuters.com/article/idUSTRE4A658820081107 (accessed December 20, 2012).

Hughes, P. M. (2010). "Ambivalence, Autonomy, and Organ Sales," *Southern Journal of Philosophy*, 44(2): 237–51.

Ibrahim, H. N., et al., (2009). "Long Term Consequences of Kidney Donation," *New England Journal of Medicine*, 360:459–69.

Institute of Medicine (IOM), (2006). *Organ Donation: Opportunities for Action.* Washington, DC: National Academies Press.

Matas, A. J. (2004). "The Case for Living Kidney Sales: Rationale, Objections and Concerns," *American Journal of Transplantation*, 4:2007–17.

McCurdle, F. J. et al. (2005). "Outcome of Assessment of Potential Donors for Live Donor Kidney Transplants," *Transplantation Proceedings*, 37(2): 605–6.

Postrel, V. (2009). "…With Functioning Kidneys for All," *Atlantic Magazine,* July, http://www.theatlantic.com/doc/200907u/kidney-donation (accessed December 20, 2012).

Quinn, R. R., Manns, B. J., and McLaughlin, K. M. (2007). "Restricting Cadaveric Kidney Transplantation Based on Age: The Impact on Efficiency and Equity," *Transplantation Proceedings*, 39(5): 1362–7.

Radcliffe-Richards, J. et al. (1998). "The Case for Allowing Kidney Sales," *Lancet*, 351: 1950–2.

Rid, A. et al. (2009). "Would You Sell a Kidney in a Regulated Market System? Results of an Exploratory Study," *Journal of Medical Ethics*, 35(9): 558–64.

Robertson, N. (2009). "Man Must Choose between Selling Kidney or Child," *CNN.com,* July 16, http://edition.cnn.com/2009/WORLD/asiapcf/07/16/pakistan.organ.selling.index.html?iref=mpstoryview (accessed December 20, 2012).

Rothman, D., and Rothman, S. (2006). "The Hidden Cost of Organ Sale," *American Journal of Transplantation*, 6:1524–8.

Santiago, C. (1997). "Family and Personal Consent to Donation," *Transplantation Proceedings*, 29(1–2): 1625–8.

Satel, S. (2006). "The Kindness of Strangers and the Cruelty of Some Medical Ethicists," *Weekly Standard*, 11: 20.

Satel, S. (2009). "The Case for Paying Organ Donors," *Wall Street Journal,* October 18, http://online.wsj.com/article/SB10001424052748704322004574477840120222788.html   (accessed December 20, 2012).

Sperling, D. (2009). "Israel's New Brain-Respiratory Death Act," *Reviews in the Neurosciences,* 20(3–4): 299–306.

Thaler, R. H., and Sunstein, C. (2008). *Nudge: Improving Decisions about Health, Health, and Happiness.* New Haven, CT: Yale University Press.

Zink, S. et al. (2005). "Living Donation: Focus on Public Concerns," *Clinical Transplantation,* 19(5): 581–5.

Zubeida, M. (2009). "Mr Shahbaz Sharif, Please Act," *Technology News, Free Wallpapers, Download Icons, News, NewsPapers, Inspiration, Jung, Ummat, Dawn, Jazba, Nawa e Waqt, Jasarat: Urdu Newspapers,* June 17, http://urdunews.wordpress.com/2009/06/17/mr-shahbaz-sharif-please-act/ (accessed December 20, 2012).

12.2

Commentary
Against Organ Markets but Be Cautious in Adopting Presumed Consent

Daniel Fu-Chang Tsai

Caplan's paper has rightly argued against organ trafficking, organ markets, and using financial incentives to increase organ supply, since these violate four key bioethical values: "respect for persons," "the autonomy of the individual," "consent," and "altruism."

Markets in organs and tissues will also exploit the poor, decrease public trust, compromise social altruism, and endanger medical professionalism. Despite there being always some arguments for a free and regulated market for organs (Harris and Erin 2002: 114–15; Meckler 2007), all international professional guidelines and national laws are opposed to commercialization of organ transplants. Such a position is made very clear in the "Statement on Human Organ and Tissue Donation and Transplantation" by the World Medical Association (WMA) (2006): "In the case of living donors, special efforts should be made to ensure that the choice about donation is free of coercion. Financial incentives for providing or obtaining organs for transplantation can be coercive and should be prohibited." "Payment for organs for donation and transplantation must be prohibited. A financial incentive compromises the voluntariness of the choice and the altruistic basis for organ donation. Furthermore, access to needed medical treatment based on ability to pay is inconsistent with the principles of justice. Organs suspected to have been obtained through commercial transaction must not be accepted for transplantation. In addition, the advertisement of organs in exchange for money should be prohibited." "Physicians who are asked to transplant an organ that has been obtained through a commercial transaction should refuse to do so and should explain to the patient why such a medical act would be unethical: because the person who provided the organ risked his or her future health for financial rather than altruistic motives, and because such transactions are contrary to the principle of justice in the allocation of organs for transplantation" (World Medical Association 2006).

At this part, the author has no disagreement with Caplan's position and would like to comment on how in his country professional efforts have been made to prohibit overseas organ purchases. Taiwan has the highest incidence and prevalence rate of end-stage renal disease (ESRD) and dialysis in the world (United States Renal Data System 2009). In 2010, there were about 65,000 persons receiving dialysis therapy (the population of Taiwan is 23 million), which cost more than 10 percent of the country's yearly health-care expenditure. However, the cadaveric organ donation rate is only about one-third to one-fifth of that in Western developed countries. The living organ donation rate is similarly low. The shortage of transplant organs and the escalating dialysis expenses are a major health and financial problem for the country's health-care system. Potential recipients on the waiting list are just desperate and helpless in their waiting. Consequently, transplant tourism from Taiwan to China has developed fervently in the past decade. There were about 1,900 domestic renal transplant cases, but about 2,300 overseas renal transplant cases from 1998 to 2007 (Tsai 2010). Evidence showed many overseas organ transplantations were arranged or conducted with doctors' participation and cooperation. As organ trade is in violation of fundamental bioethical principles, and doctors' involvement in such transactions is certainly against medical ethics. Therefore the Medical Ethics Committee of the Department of Health in April 2006 discussed and concluded that doctors and health-care professionals, if involved with (1) introducing patients to a broker agency without receiving payment, (2) introducing patients to a broker agency and receiving payment, (3) personal involvement with brokering, and (4) bringing patients overseas and performing transplant surgery and receiving payment, would be considered to be participating in medical practices violating medical ethics under the Physician's Act, article 25, item 4, which could incur punishment including a warning, compulsory education programs, termination of medical practice, or revoking of medical licenses. Such regulations made an explicit prohibition for doctors participating in organ tourism. At about the same time, the National Taiwan University Center for Ethics, Law and Society in Biomedicine and Technology also launched an "Asian Task Force on Organ Trafficking: Battling Organ Trafficking Across Borders in Asia," and in 2008 announced the "Taipei recommendation on the prohibition, prevention, and elimination of organ trafficking in Asia," which "urge[s] Asian countries to achieve a national self-sufficiency in organ donation and transplantation;" "call[s] on countries in which the buying and selling of organs [are] outlawed to prohibit activities that perpetrate the illegal practices in other countries, such as the travel abroad of their citizens in order to obtain the same or similar services outside their own national territories," and "encourage[s] countries to limit organ procurement to the recipient with the same nationality as the donor" (Asian Task Force on Organ Trafficking 2008).

Caplan's paper then advocated a "presumed consent" model, which means the presumption of a person wanting to be an organ donor upon their death unless he chooses to opt out. Such a model has proved to be effective in many countries. The most successful and famous one is in Spain, which reached the donation rate of 34 per million population (pmp) by 2010. Other countries which adopted presumed consent also have more satisfactory results, for example Portugal (26.7 pmp), Belgium (25.61 pmp), France (25.31 pmp), Austria (20.72 pmp), and Norway (20.42 pmp). In contrast, countries which adopt "informed consent" (the opt-in model), generally have lower donation rates, for example the Netherlands (12.8 pmp), Germany (14.59 pmp), the

UK (14.7 pmp), Denmark (11.82 pmp), and Canada (14.59 pmp).[1] Although presumed consent has a better organ procurement outcome, its acceptance in Asian countries seems less.

Singapore adopted this model in 2004 to expand their organ pool. However, an incident showed that such a policy might be recklessly enforced and cause serious harm to families. In February 2008, a 43-year-old Singaporean, Mr. Sim, was declared to be brain-dead due to a stroke. "Sim's family had no objection to his organs being used for transplants but wanted doctors to wait one more day before turning off the life-support machine. But as Sim's 68-year-old mother and about 20 other relatives knelt weeping before the doctors, begging them to wait, nine police officers entered the ward and restrained the distraught family while Sim's body was quickly whisked away." "The hospital staff were running as they wheeled him out of the back door of the room. They were behaving like robbers," said Sim's elder sister (Berger 2007; Koh 2007). This event triggered waves of public outcry and protest. Critics have challenged that the law was inadequate because the definition of death is debatable, life support might be turned off prematurely, and people might be unaware of the opt-out option. Some doctors urged amending the law and giving families the right to veto (Berger 2007). And it is unfair for the opt-out system to take advantage of those who failed or were unable to opt out.

The acceptance of presumed consent seems low in Taiwan too. According to the commentator's survey for health-care professionals' opinions on organ procurement policy (314 respondents) in 2007, 56.4 percent are for an informed consent/opt-in model, 28.8 percent are for a mandated choice/required request model, and only 8.2 percent are for a presumed consent/opt-out model. Another telephone survey of 1,117 citizens' opinions for organ procurement models conducted in November 2010 showed 43.7 percent are for an informed consent/opt-in model, 50.5 percent are for a mandated choice/required request model, and only 2.7 percent are for a presumed consent/opt-out model. The reason why the acceptance of a presumed consent/opt-out model is so low in the general public in Taiwan is a worthwhile question for the government, policy makers, and researchers to explore if this model actually leads to a better procurement rate. However, it is clear that if the society does not discuss thoroughly the reason and rationale of making legislation based on a deliberated public consensus, the implementation and practice of a presumed consent model will surely incur controversy and rebuttal.

The WMA statement supports informed donor choice. "National Medical Associations in countries that have adopted or are considering a policy of 'presumed consent'…or 'mandated choice'…should make every effort to ensure that these policies do not diminish informed donor choice, including the patient's right to refuse to donate" (World Medical Association 2006).

In 2008, a UK report also maintained "that an opt-out system should not be introduced in the UK at the present time. The taskforce concluded that such a system has the potential to undermine the concept of donation as a gift; to erode trust in NHS

---

[1] Transplant Procurement Management at http://www.tpm.org/ (accessed December 20, 2012).

professionals and the government; and negatively impact on organ donation numbers. It would distract attention away from essential improvements to systems and infrastructure and from the urgent need to improve public awareness and understanding of organ donations. Furthermore, it would be challenging and costly to implement successfully. Most compelling of all, we found no convincing evidence that it would deliver significant increases in the number of donated organs" (Organ Donation Taskforce 2008).

In adopting "presumed consent," we must consider whether we are trying to take advantage of people's indifference or lack of interest in social/medical policy. If so, is it ethical to harm a few in order to benefit many? Therefore, despite the better outcome that "presumed consent/opt-out" can achieve, the commentator's advice is that the "mandated choice/required request" model is preferable in many Asian country contexts.

References

Asian Task Force on Organ Trafficking. (2008). "Recommendation on the Prohibition, Prevention, and Elimination of Organ Trafficking in Asia," January, http://www.law.ntu.edu. tw/center/ntucels/admin/UserFiles/File/Taipei-Rcommendations(Summary).pdf (accessed December 20, 2012).

Berger, S. (2007). "Singapore's Compulsory Organ Transplants," *Telegraph,* March 2, http://www. telegraph.co.uk/news/1544379/Singapores-compulsory-organ-transplants.html (accessed December 20, 2012).

Harris, J., and Erin, C. (2002). "An Ethically Defensible Market in Organs," *BMJ,* 325: 114–15.

Koh, G. Q. (2007). "Scuffle for Organs Sparks Donor Debate in Singapore," *Reuters,* February 28, http://www.reuters.com/article/2007/02/28/us-singapore-organs-idUSSIN17324120070228 (accessed December 20, 2012).

Meckler, L. (2007). "Kidney Shortage Inspires A Radical Idea: Organ Sales," *Wall Street Journal,* November 13, http://online.wsj.com/article/SB119490273908090431.html   (accessed December 20, 2012).

Organ Donation Taskforce. (2008). "The Potential Impact of an Opt Out System for Organ Donation in the UK: An Independent Report From the Organ Donation Taskforce," http:// www.dh.gov.uk/prod_consum_dh/groups/dh_digitalassets/@dh/@en/documents/digital-asset/dh_090303.pdf (accessed December 20, 2012).

Tsai, D. F.-C, (2010). "Transplant Tourism from Taiwan to China: Some Reflection on Professional Ethics and Regulation," *American Journal of Bioethics,* 10(2): 22–4.

United States Renal Data System. (2009). *USRDS 2009 Annual Data Report, 2009,* Vol. 2: *Atlas of End-Stage Renal Disease,* 343–54.

World Medical Association. (2006). "WMA Statement on Human Organ Donation and Transplantation," http://www.wma.net/en/30publications/10policies/t7/ (accessed December 20, 2012).

12.3

Commentary
Can a Presumed Consent System Stop Organ Trafficking?

Takahiro Nakajima

Two approaches to decrease organ scarcity

It is noteworthy that Dr. Caplan's paper takes a clear stand against organ trafficking, especially kidney trafficking, from a bioethical viewpoint. He states that "[f]orcing, coercing, or duping adults or removing a kidney from a child is inconsistent not only with international human rights conventions prohibiting exploitation but violates the ethical norms of the professional transplant community" (Caplan 2014: 408). He then analyzes the history of organ trafficking, and underscores organ scarcity as well as poverty and lack of information on the part of trafficked persons as primary causes. If this analysis is correct, organ trafficking will cease when the organ scarcity is resolved or when the situation of those vulnerable to organ trafficking is changed through education and economic development. Dr. Caplan emphasizes the former solution (addressing the scarcity of organs) by presenting two possible approaches.

The first approach is to increase the supply of organs through "a paid market or system that uses financial incentives" (Caplan 2014: 411). However, Dr. Caplan criticizes this approach as follows:

Selling organs, even in a tightly regulated market, violates the existing bioethical framework of respect for persons since the sale is clearly being driven by profit. It also violates, in the case of living persons, the ethics of medicine itself. (Caplan 2014: 412)

His criticism seems convincing, not only because it considers the sale of organs as contradicting norms of bio- and medical ethics, but also because it emphasizes that selling organs as commodities shares the same economic framework as organ trafficking.

This leads us to a further question. How can we increase the organ supply while somehow avoiding this economic framework? Dr. Caplan proposes another approach: a system of presumed consent for organ donation.[2]

There is another option for increasing the organ supply that has been tried in Spain, Italy, Austria, and Belgium. These nations have enacted laws that create presumed consent. In such a system, the presumption is that a deceased person wants to be an organ donor upon their death—basically an ethical default to the desirability of donation. (Caplan 2014: 413)

He evaluates this legislation of presumed consent on the basis that it does not create "any problems or difficulties" and that it is "completely consistent with the existing bioethical framework governing organ and tissue procurement" (Caplan 2014: 413). There are, nevertheless, some ethical objections to presumed consent.

Ethical objections to presumed consent 1: fear of mistakes and the representation of will

The first objection is what Dr. Caplan introduces as "fear of mistakes," which is defined as a misunderstanding of one's will to oppose a donation. He regards this as one of "the main ethical objections to presumed consent" (Caplan 2014: 413). This is clearly a serious ethical concern.

It may seem that such a "fear of mistakes" could be avoided if one receives sufficient and adequate information on presumed consent and the right to indicate opposition to donation. Although this might work for adults who still have reason enough to judge their situation, it becomes difficult when considering the case of an infant.

Assuming that presumed consent is applied consistently, a deceased infant's organs will automatically be donated because he/she cannot express opposition to donation. To regulate this process, we could appeal to the family's right to express opposition on the infant's behalf. However, what does it mean ethically or legally to represent the infant's opposition to donation? If there are unintentional "mistakes" in the process of representation, how and to whom can we assign ethical and legal responsibility?

The worst-case scenario is that a family member with a covert intent to traffic organs from this child[3] could realize it at the moment of the infant's death without the infant's intentional expression of the will to donate organs. This not only demonstrates the ethico-legal limitations of presumed consent, but also indicates that presumed consent might enable a new type of organ trafficking as a crime of omission.

---

[2] As for the need of the concept of "presumed consent," see Cohen 1992: 2168–70.

[3] While there are many arguments concerning a family's consent to donate their child's organs, what is newly accepted in the recent Japanese law, Revised Act on Organ Transplantation (2009), is a family's voluntary expression of organ donation by their child. If there are family members who intentionally misunderstand the will of children, it seems difficult to condemn them within the framework of this revised law.

Ethical objections to presumed consent 2: violation of voluntary consent

The second ethical objection is related to the idea of "voluntary." Does not presumed consent violate the basic ethical norm of voluntary consent or altruism with respect to organ donation? In this regard, Dr. Mitsuyasu Kurosu argues as follows:

> The concept of informed consent is to respect an individual's autonomy. This is emphasized in the Declaration of Helsinki (WMA) and the Universal Declaration on Bioethics and Human Rights (UNESCO). To compel a patient to express his/her will, will be violation of an individual autonomy and an outrage against informed consent.
>
> Compelling patients is unethical. Donations should not be forced but should be voluntary. The presumed consent system is not adopted in the Human Tissue Act 2004 in the UK and in the "Research Involving Human Biological Materials," which is a report of [the] National Bioethics Advisory Commission in the USA. (Kurosu 2008: 78)

The main point of his argument is that informed consent as the basis of current bioethics becomes void when the presumed consent system is legitimized because the idea of "voluntary" is dismissed.

A counterargument to this position would emphasize that efforts to obtain informed consent for donation and refusal would continue to be made in the presumed consent system. However, this will lead to an ironic and unexpected result. In order to grant donors sufficient information for informed consent about presumed consent, the cost will be similar to that of the present system based upon voluntary donation.

Ethical objections to presumed consent 3: fear of health-care refusal

The third ethical objection focuses on patient fears of diminution or refusal of health care. For example, the Japanese National Cancer Center (NCC) has adopted a system of presumed consent for use of patient materials in research. According to Dr. Kurosu, patients at the NCC not only fear being refused health care, but also do not receive medical records if they object to the use of their biological material (Kurosu 2008: 79). His judgment of presumed consent at NCC is severe:

> Thus, the author regards the presumed consent system at the NCC to be an abuse of the patient's position, which is already weak since he/she is unwell and anxious to consult a physician. This presumed consent system is unethical because it compels patients to express their will and the patients are apprehensive that the physician may refuse health care. (Kurosu 2008: 80)

Considering that the NCC might be an exceptional case, or that the center might have a different view than Dr. Kurosu, the presumed consent system may not always provoke fear of diminution or refusal of health care. However, it is necessary to devise a procedure that avoids such an objection.

Can the presumed consent system stop organ trafficking?

Last but not least, we must consider the efficacy of the presumed consent system. The scenario for presumed consent described by Dr. Caplan is based upon the following argument:

1   Scarcity creates organ trafficking.
2   A system of presumed consent can supply enough organs to resolve scarcity.[4]
3   Presumed consent helps stop organ trafficking.

This argument becomes convincing if the first assumption (1) is true. The most essential question is whether or not scarcity creates organ trafficking and, if so, what form of scarcity creates it.

Scarcity as a key term in economics is always expressed in the framework of supply and demand. When goods in demand are scarce, their price increases until a sufficient supply is available. In this framework, every good has to be regarded as a commodity. However, human organs are not something we should regard as commodities. They must be excluded from the economy of supply and demand. From this rigorous perspective, it is not adequate to use the concept of "scarcity" for human organs.

Nonetheless, we are obliged to think about human organs in terms of supply and demand because this problem is part and parcel of bio-techno capitalism. In this economic structure, we confront the *invented* scarcity of human organs. Our demands or needs are aroused by bio-techno capitalistic discourse. In this respect, the "scarcity" of human organs defined here is nothing but the most typical economic phenomenon in the capitalistic world. As long as our desire for human organs is intensified by the structure of bio-techno capitalism, the "scarcity" becomes increasingly severe.[5] From the rigorous perspective described above, an alternative to the bio-techno capitalistic structure would stop this process, but it is hardly a simple matter to implement it.

I argue that organ trafficking is not only due to scarcity in the number of available organs, but also to scarcity in their order of priority. Even if a system of presumed consent were to cover the entire world and organs were to become "free goods" in volume, organ trafficking would never cease because a scarcity in the order of priority would still remain. For example, following the Fukushima nuclear crisis in March 2011, the Japanese suddenly confronted a "scarcity" of mineral water. In fact, there were adequate stocks of mineral water, but a kind of panic spread as demand for mineral water was amplified through the media. Those who were rich enough to buy it in Tokyo felt that mineral water had become a top priority, and thus they wanted to buy it as quickly as possible and at any cost. Meanwhile, those who lived in Fukushima gave it up because they were not rich enough to buy mineral water except for daily needs. This incident shows, by analogy, that as long as there remains scarcity in the order of priority, there

---

[4] Singapore has legislated presumed consent. However, the number of organ donors has not dramatically increased. See Kwek et al. (2009). The countries adopting presumed consent are listed here: Abadie and Gay 2006: 617–19.

[5] For an objection against scarcity of organs in terms of volume, see Scheper-Hughes (2002: 67).

will always be room for organ trafficking. Even when a system of presumed consent is wholly realized, organ trafficking will continue unless we give sufficient attention to prioritizing recipients (who first?).

As mentioned above, parents who intend to sell their children's organs will be able to contribute to organ trafficking without any legal condemnation under the first condition of presumed consent. If so, a shrewd organization for organ trafficking could invent subtle means to escape legal condemnation at every step in the process. This is truly a nightmare, but it has already been realized in the literary imagination. In *Never Let Me Go*, Kazuo Ishiguro describes a situation in which children are born as cloned humans to donate their organs. They are obliged to accept their "fate" without any informed consent. Even when Madame Marie-Claude, the director of a school for these children in Hailsham, tries to improve the atmosphere in which they grow up and to treat them as human beings with souls, she never allows teachers or guardians to grant the children the right of informed consent. However, in the last part of this story, Madame recalls a memory of the young Kathy H., one of children in Hailsham, who danced while singing a song called "Never Let Me Go." She says:

I was weeping for an altogether different reason. When I watched you dancing that day, I saw something else. I saw a new world coming rapidly. More scientific, efficient, yes. More cures for the old sickness. Very good. But a harsh, cruel world. And I saw a little girl, her eyes tightly closed, holding to her breast the old kind world, one that she knew in her heart could not remain, and she was holding it and pleading, never to let her go. That is what I saw. It wasn't really you, what you were doing, I know that. But I saw you and it broke my heart. And I've never forgotten. (Ishiguro 2005: 266–7)

How can we completely avoid organ trafficking in any form in this "new world"? Although the idea of presumed consent that Dr. Caplan proposes is worth considering, many problems still remain to be discussed.

References

Abadie, A., and Gay, S. (2006). "The Impact of Presumed Consent Legislation on Cadaveric Organ Donation: A Cross-Country Study," *Journal of Health Economics*, 25:599–620.

Caplan, A. (2014). "Trafficking and Markets in Kidneys: Two Poor Solutions to a Pressing Problem," in A. Akabayashi (ed.), *The Future of Bioethics: International Dialogues*. Oxford: Oxford University Press, 407–16.

Cohen, C. (1992). "The Case for Presumed Consent to Transplant Human Organs After Death," *Transplantation Proceedings*, 24(5): 2168–70.

Ishiguro, K. (2005) *Never Let Me Go*. London: Faber and Faber.

Kurosu, M. (2008). "Ethical Issues of Presumed Consent in the Use of Patient Materials for Medical Research and the Organ Donation for Transplantation," *Journal of Philosophy and Ethics in Health Care and Medicine*, 3:64–85.

Kwek, T. K. et al. (2009). "The Transplantable Organ Shortage in Singapore: Has Implementation of Presumed Consent to Organ Donation Made a Difference?" *Annals Academy of Medicine*, 38(4): 346–53.

Scheper-Hughes, N. (2002). "The Ends of the Body: Commodity Fetishism and the Global Traffic in Organs," *SAIS Review*, 22(1): 61–80.

12.4

Commentary

Presuming Minor Consent and Allowing Family Veto: Two Moral Concerns about Organ Procurement Policy

Hitoshi Arima

In his new article "Trafficking and Markets in Kidneys: Two Poor Solutions to a Pressing Problem," Dr. Arthur Caplan expresses his concern over the recent prosperity of the international organ trafficking business. Besides the economic disparity among those countries that produce organs and those purchasing them, Dr. Caplan finds the scarcity of organs domestically available within the wealthier countries as a major cause of international trafficking. He thus urges that policy makers should make efforts to build an infrastructure that will increase the domestic supply of transplantable organs without violating basic bioethical principles. It is then concluded that countries currently relying on expressed consent legislation for organ procurement should replace it with a presumed consent system.

However, presumed consent is not always considered perfectly effective or innocuous. In this paper, I shall first briefly review why some commentators are wary of the idea of presuming people's willingness to donate organs in general. Then I discuss two more worries that are also often raised against the legislation. Both of these worries are related to rather pragmatic questions that policy makers should face when they consider implementing the policy in concrete terms: namely, whether we should allow children to donate organs by assuming their consent, and whether we should allow family members to make the final decision in the absence of a brain-dead patient's expressed wish. Consideration of these questions will reveal that our task to justify presumed consent legislation is more complicated and difficult than Dr. Caplan's rather brief discussion on this subject may indicate.

Japan revised its organ transplantation law in 2009. The revision was part of the country's effort to increase domestic organ supply and thereby to prevent people from going abroad in seeking organs. In the last section of this short paper, I shall also briefly describe how Japanese legislators answered these two questions.

* I would like to thank my former colleague, Dr. Yusuke Inoue, for providing me with helpful information about minor brain-dead patients' status in presumed consent countries.

1 Effects and ethics of presumed consent

Dr. Caplan maintains that in order to prevent international organ trafficking, policy makers should try to increase the domestic supply of transplantable organs in ways that are ethically acceptable. Dr. Caplan is not alone in making this claim. In May 2008, the Transplantation Society issued its Istanbul Declaration to call on each country for their cooperation to extirpate transplant tourism and organ trafficking. Besides urging each country to ban various practices related to the promotion of transplantation commercialism, the declaration also recommends each country to make efforts to create an infrastructure that increases the number of cadaveric organ donors (Participants in the Istanbul Summit 2008).[6] Dr. Caplan is here taking a step further along this line of proposal by being more specific about the nature of a desirable infrastructure and about the moral framework within which the infrastructure should be developed. In particular, Dr. Caplan asserts that an organ procurement policy is morally justifiable only when it is compatible with the following four key values which comprise such a moral framework: namely, respect for persons, autonomy of the individual, informed consent, and altruism (Caplan in this chapter). The article concludes with a recommendation that presumed consent legislation be adopted on the grounds that the legislation is "completely consistent" with this framework (Caplan in this chapter).

However, presumed consent is not always considered effective in increasing organ supply or perfectly innocuous. First, as far as I am aware, people still disagree over whether presumed consent will really increase the number of usable organs. To be sure, on average, countries adopting presumed consent enjoy higher rate of cadaveric organ donations as compared to countries relying on expressed consent. However, many other factors are also known to influence the rate of organ donation, notable examples including the number of deaths caused by automobile accidents, governmental campaigns and education, public trust in medical professions, and the frequency with which brain-dead patients' families refuse donation (I shall come back to this last point shortly). It follows that it is difficult to ascertain that the differences in donation rates are really generated by the different types of legislation. In fact, the US, basically an expressed consent country, surpasses most presumed consent countries by the number of cadaveric organ donations per population size. Some commentators doubt that, given its current success, the US would produce more organs if it switches to presumed consent (see Baily 2010).[7]

Secondly, the moral status of presumed consent can also be questioned. As Dr. Caplan also mentions, an often raised worry is that the legislation may erroneously presume a brain-dead patient's willingness to donate organs when in fact she had merely failed to express opposition. *Pace* Dr. Caplan, I suspect that we cannot eliminate people's worry simply by calling it "default to donation" instead of "presumed consent." It seems clear

---

[6] Similar statements can be found in the "Recommendations on the Prohibition, Prevention, and Elimination of Organ Trafficking in Asia" drafted by Asian Task Force on Organ Trafficking (2008). See also Dr. Tsai's article in this volume for more details about the recommendations (Tsai 2013).

[7] Dr. Caplan once held the same belief about the policy's effect before he changed his view. See Caplan (1994).

to me that if in fact a significant proportion of the population in a society feels uncomfortable with donating organs, it would be morally problematic to change the default from refusal to agreement without making the effort to give sufficient publicity to the change. In other words, default to donation would be morally acceptable only if we can make sure that (a) people are well informed of the relevant facts, (b) the majority of people either prefer donation or are indifferent about donation, and (c) those who opt for refusal know how to do so. Unless these requirements are fulfilled, there is a fear that presumed consent will increase organ supply more by violating the rights of those who abhor donation than by saving those preferring donation the trouble of signing a donor card.

2   Presuming children's consent

What I stated now is a worry that is generally applicable to the very idea of presuming people's consent to donation. In the rest of this paper I would like to mention two more worries in relation to the same policy. Both of them are concerned with a more pragmatic question that we should face when considering the implementation of presumed consent policy in concrete terms. One of these questions is whether we should allow children to donate organs by presuming their consent. The other is whether we should allow the family of a brain-dead patient to make the final decision in the absence of the patient's expressed wish.

The first question is already addressed in Dr. Takahiro Nakajima's article in this volume (Nakajima 2013). I also discussed the question extensively elsewhere (Arima 2009), so I shall be brief here. Minor organ recipients typically need organs of smaller sizes, thereby requiring minor organ donors. The problem here is that children may still lack the cognitive faculties needed to understand the relevant facts and rules about brain death and organ transplantation. In such cases it hardly seems justifiable to presume that their silence on the matter indicates their real wish to donate organs. If we are to take seriously Dr. Caplan's claim that procurement policy must be grounded in the value of respect for autonomy and altruism, we should exclude younger children from being potential donors, otherwise we need a very different sort of argument (for example, by appealing to the idea that very young children are not even capable of taking an interest in the issue and therefore we should only consider the benefit to organ recipients) to justify such a policy.[8]

3   Family's veto

The other question is about the family's veto under the presumed consent legislation, and this I would like to discuss in a little more depth. In most countries, regardless of whether the country uses presumed consent or expressed consent, the family of a

---

[8] Some presumed countries, for example, Singapore and France, do allow minors to donate organs except when their family refuse to provide consent. In another paper (Arima 2009), I have critically examined five different arguments that may be offered in defense of such a policy.

brain-dead patient is allowed to have a final say over the donation decision, and even to override the patient's expressed wishes. Medical providers or transplant professionals in such presumed consent countries as Spain, France, and Bulgaria routinely ask for the family's consent before procuring organs. What justification can be given to this practice is an urgent question, given the fact that not a few families refuse donation in the absence of the patient's expressed wish (Siminoff et al. 2001; Frutos et al. 2002; Merchant et al. 2008), and that this may possibly be frustrating a sincere but unexpressed wish of a large number of brain-dead patients. Space does not allow me to discuss this question thoroughly, but I shall attempt to shed new light on the issue by considering some recent works of medical economists.

To repeat, in most countries, whether the country employs a presumed consent or an expressed consent policy, the policy is rarely enforced in its "pure" form in practice and family consent is always required before organs are procured. In addition, studies indicate that many families do refuse donation under either legislation. This is in fact a major reason why commentators often hypothesize that presumed consent will not produce a significantly higher number of organs than expressed consent. Recently, however, two economists, Alberto Abadie and Sebastien Gay, challenged this hypothesis (2006).

Their argument is based on an insight taken from analyses done by other economists. Eric Johnson and Daniel Goldstein maintained that once such other factors as educational level, religion, and transplant infrastructure are controlled, it can be demonstrated that switching from expressed consent to presumed consent would increase organ supply by up to 56 percent. They also hypothesized that it makes this difference, not merely because most people are indifferent about the issue, but because the types of legislation themselves influence individuals' choices (especially when people do not have a strong preference on the issue in advance) (Johnson and Goldstein 2003: 1338–9). Thus it is suggested that people might believe that donation is recommended by policy makers when it is made the default, or that it might be stressful or unpleasant for many people to make an active decision about donation and therefore they tend to stay with the default (Johnson and Goldstein 2003: 1338).[9] Now, Abadie and Gay's claim is that such influence of the types of legislation will not only be exerted upon the potential donors, but will also be extended to their family members.

Abadie and Gay first observe that the family of a brain-dead patient is less likely to have a clear knowledge about the patient's real wish on donation (Abadie and Gay 2006: 603). While it is possible that a patient had communicated her preference regarding organ donation directly to her family members in advance, surveys suggest a widespread reluctance to discuss organ donation issues with family members.[10] Thus, when the patient did not sign a donor card, family members usually have to decide based on limited information about the patient's real preference. Abadie and Gay's claim is that

---

[9] A similar analysis was also given by J. Verheijde and his colleagues (2009). Richard Thaler and Cass Sunstein argue that it is morally justifiable that policy makers exert such influence upon the choice of potential donors on the basis that it does not violate potential donors' freedom as well as benefiting organ recipients (2008).

[10] Here Abadie and Gay refer to a survey conducted by the Gallup Organization (1993). Some other studies that interviewed brain-dead patients' families also suggest that the patients' wishes are often unknown to the family members (Martinez et al. 2001: 412; Rodrigue et al. 2006: 193).

in such situations, they are more inclined to think that the patient had a preference for donation under presumed consent than under expressed consent. The very fact that the patient had kept silent under presumed consent legislation hints to the family that the patient had preferred donation (Abadie and Gay 2006: 605). Dr. Caplan in fact quotes just these economists' analyses in support of his conviction that presumed consent should increase organ donation (Caplan in this chapter).

Abadie and Gay's analysis, if it is correct, shows that the presumed consent legislation produces more organs principally because the legislation itself influences the family's understandings as to what the potential donor would have wanted. To be more specific, under presumed consent legislation, family members tend to think that the potential donor had a wish to donate organs when in fact they do not know much about her preference on the particular subject. Now I am worried that the manner in which presumed consent increases organ supply (as explained by Abadie and Gay) may be incompatible with the basic bioethical framework advocated by Dr. Caplan.

My worry may be best articulated in the following terms. As above mentioned, a major criticism against presumed consent legislation is that it may sometimes erroneously presume that a brain-dead patient is willing to donate when in fact she was not. In response to this criticism, it may be argued that transplant professionals' customary practice of asking for the family's consent must be understood as a safeguard against such errors. The idea is that the family should know the patient's values and character best and therefore may interrupt with procurement when it is in fact incongruent with the patient's values and character. It must be clear that the same argument can also be employed for the purpose of defending the family's veto power against the above-mentioned complaint that it violates the principle of respect for autonomy by allowing the family to override the potential donor's autonomous choice.

However, if Abadie and Gay's analysis is correct, the family is not suitable to assume such a role. For the family's decision is influenced by the very choice of the policy makers, i.e. the choice to adopt presumed consent legislation, whose principal aim is to increase the organ supply. In particular, under presumed consent legislation, when a potential donor merely failed to express her opposition to donation in advance, her family is likely to take this fact as an indication that she wanted to donate. Hence the family consent will not function as a safeguard in such cases, and the worry remains that many organs are being procured on an erroneous basis.

The point is not merely that the family cannot work as a safeguard if it is true that their decisions are influenced by the procurement policy. Abadie and Gay's claim is that presumed consent produces more organs than expressed consent principally because of its influence upon the family's decision as such. If this is true, then what I show in the previous paragraph will amount to saying that if presumed consent in fact increases organ supply, there is a fear that it does so to a large degree by way of violating the rights of those who prefer non-donation.

This conclusion also poses a difficult question regarding the moral status of a family's veto power. Given the fact that not a few families refuse donation under presumed consent, and that this may possibly be frustrating a sincere but unexpressed wish of brain-dead patients, their veto power as such apparently needs justification. As said above, a most straightforward way of giving such justification would be by pointing out that it may function as a safeguard against the error of taking organs from those who abhor donation. However, if in fact most family members do not know a brain-dead patient's real wish on the particular issue, and their decision is more likely to be influenced by the legislation, such justification would fail. What this means is that if (as most of the presumed consent countries currently do) we are to continue to give the family a veto power, we would probably need a very different type of argument in order to justify it. For example, we may need to appeal to the fact that families often feel distressed when they learn that their loved one's organs are extracted after death, and then justify the family's veto power by saying that it protects their own (not the brain-dead patient's) interest. While I am not sure if such an argument is still compatible with the moral framework advocated by Dr. Caplan, it seems certain that incorporating such an argument will make the framework more complicated than it initially appeared.

4 Revision of Japanese organ transplantation law

In any surveys Japan has been ranked lowest for the number of cadaveric organ donation per population size. Wealthy Japanese go abroad to seek organs. When transplant tourism became a target of criticism in the international community, a phenomenon which was made especially visible by the publication of the Istanbul Declaration in 2008, Japan was quick to act on its recommendations. In the spring of 2009, the Japanese Diet started to discuss revision of organ transplantation law. The new law was passed in July of the same year, and was implemented a year later. The revision was understood to be a part of the country's effort to increase domestic organ supply and thereby to prevent people from going abroad in seeking organs (Yomiuri Newspaper 2009).

Before the revision, Japan was an expressed consent country. But the revised organ transplantation law maintains that organs may be procured from minors of all ages (including infants and newborns) provided that (i) they had not explicitly refused donation in advance and (ii) their families provide consent. To both of the two questions discussed above, Japanese law provided a positive answer. It allowed children to donate organs by presuming their consent, and allowed family members to make the decision in the absence of an expressed wish of the brain-dead patient.[11] Thus far it appears that

---

[11] Japanese law differs from other presumed consent countries in that its text explicitly requires the family's consent for organ donation. To be more specific, the family of a brain-dead patient can do the following: (1) override the patient's documented wish to donate organs, and (2) decide whether to donate organs when the patient did not leave a wish (Japanese Law on Organ Transplantation, Article 6, Section 1 and 3, as amended by No. 86, 2009). However, (3) the family does not have the right to overturn the patient's will in case the patient had explicitly refused donation. It may be arguable that Japanese law, as such, is not a presumed consent system, since its text does require an explicit consent from the family. The underlying thought may be that the family is here allowed to make the decision only as a surrogate, and as long as the family provides consent, this means that we have an expressed consent from the potential donor as well. Alternatively, it may be thought that the patient's organs belong to the family and the family has the right to self-determination on these organs. However, I do not know if these ways of thinking can really justify the above legal rules; the first thought is apparently in contradiction of the rule which allows the family to override the patient's documented wish to donate organs (1), and the latter also seems to contradict the rule which stipulates that the family may not overturn the patient's expressed wish to refuse donation (3).

the policy change has proved to be effective in increasing the number of cadaveric organ donations.[12] However, justifications for these rules (especially in terms of whether they are compatible with the value of donor's self-determination) were scarcely discussed in the Diet.[13] Given the complexity of the moral problems regarding these pragmatic questions, a concern may be raised that Japanese legislators have been too hasty in providing their answers.

The present paper reviewed some of the major worries that have been raised against presumed consent legislation. In general, for it to be morally acceptable, it is at least required that the majority of people in a society either prefer donation or are indifferent about the choice after bing sufficiently informed of the problem, and that those who have a strong preference for refusal know how to opt out. If these requirements are not met, there is a fear that presumed consent will increase organ supply more by violating the rights of those who abhor donation than by saving those who prefer donation the trouble of signing a donor card.

Now, some may argue that we can alleviate this worry by requiring the family's consent so they can safeguard against such violation. The idea is that the family should know the patient's values and character best and therefore may interrupt with procurement when it is in fact incongruent with the patient's values and character. However, some recent studies in medical economics suggest that the family may not be suitable for assuming such a role. Family members usually do not know a brain-dead patient's real wish on the particular issue, and their decision is more likely to be influenced by the legislation itself. Given that in other cases families may also make decisions against a known wish of brain-dead patients, this fact further poses a serious question with regard to the justifiability of family's veto power.

In addition, I have also maintained that the case of minor organ donors incurs a special problem. The problem here is that children may still lack the cognitive faculties needed to understand the relevant facts and rules about brain death and organ transplantation. In such cases it hardly seems justifiable to presume that their silence on the matter indicates their real wish to donate organs. Thus justification of minor organ procurement requires something other than the principle of autonomy and voluntary altruism. Considerations of these pragmatic questions show that the moral framework within which organ procurement policy should be developed may well need to be more complicated than Dr. Caplan advocates.

References

Abadie, A., and Gay, S. (2006). "The Impact of Presumed Consent Legislation on Cadaveric Organ Donation: A Cross-Country Study," *Journal of Health Economics*, 22:599–620.

---

[12] In the past 13 years before the law revision (1997–2009), only 6.5 brain-dead patients donated their organs a year on average in Japan. After the revision, 29 cadaveric organ donations took place in the first six months (from July 17 to December 31, 2011).

[13] Indeed, the House of Councillors took only two days to discuss the Bills (Mainichi Newspaper 2009).

Arima, H. (2009). "Children as Organ Donors: Is Japan's New Policy on Organ Procurement in Minors Justifiable?" *Asian Bioethics Review*, 1(4): 354–66.

Asian Task Force on Organ Trafficking. (2008). "Recommendations on Prohibition, Prevention, and Abolishment of Organ Trafficking in Asia," http://www.law.ntu.edu.tw/center/wto/04research.asp?tb_index=403 (accessed June 30, 2011).

Baily, Mary Ann. (2010). "This Is Very Bad Idea," *New York Times*, May 2, published online http://roomfordebate.blogs.nytimes.com/2010/05/02/should-laws-encourage-organ-donation/#maryann (accessed 15 April 2012).

Caplan, A. (1994). "Current Ethical Issues in Organ Procurement and Transplantation," *JAMA*, 272:1708–9.

Caplan, A. (2014). "Trafficking and Markets in Kidneys: Two Poor Solutions to a Pressing Problem," in A. Akabayashi (ed.), *The Future of Bioethics: International Dialogues*. Oxford: Oxford University Press, 407–16.

Frutos, M. A. et al. (2002). "Family Refusal in Organ Donation: Analysis of Three Patterns," *Transplantation Proceedings*, 34:2513–14.

Gallup Organization. (1993). *American Public's Attitudes Toward Organ Donation and Transplantation*. Conducted for the Partnership for Organ Donation, Boston.

Japanese Law on Organ Transplantation [Zoki no isyoku ni kansuru horitsu], as amended by No. 86, 2009. http://law.e-gov.go.jp/htmldata/H09/H09HO104.html (in Japanese) (accessed June 30, 2011).

Johnson, E., and Goldstein, D. (2003). "Do Defaults Save Lives?" *Science*, 302:1338–9.

Mainichi Newspaper. (2009). "Hito no shi: giron hukamarazu [Human's Death: Discussions Were Not Deepened]," July 10, Morning Edition (in Japanese).

Martinez, J. et al. (2001). "Organ Donation and Family Decision-Making within the Spanish Donation System," *Social Science and Medicine* 53:405–21.

Merchant Shaila, J. et al. (2008). "Exploring the Psychological Effects of Deceased Organ Donation on the Families of the Organ Donors," *Clinical Transplantation*, 22:341–7.

Nakajima, T. (2014). "Can a Presumed Consent System Stop Organ Trafficking?" in A. Akabayashi (ed.), *The Future of Bioethics: International Dialogues*. Oxford: Oxford University Press, 421–5.

Participants in the International Summit on Transplant Tourism and Organ Trafficking Convened by the Transplantation Society and International Society of Nephrology in Istanbul, Turkey, April 30–May 2, 2008 (Participants in the Istanbul Summit). (2008). "The Declaration of Istanbul on Organ Trafficking and Transplant Tourism," http://www.multivu.prnewswire.com/mnr/transplantationsociety/33914/docs/33914-Declaration_of_Istanbul-Lancet.pdf (accessed June 30, 2011).

Rodrigue, J. R., Cornell, D. L., and Howard, R. J. (2005). "Organ Donation Decision: Comparison of Donor and Nondonor Families," *American Journal of Transplantation*, 6:190–8.

Siminoff, L. A. et al. (2001). "Factors Influencing Families' Consent for Donation of Solid Organs for Transplantation," *JAMA*, 286:71–7.

Thaler, R. H., and Sunstein, C. (2008). *Nudge: Improving Decisions about Health, Health, and Happiness*. New Haven, CT: Yale University Press.

Tsai, D. F.-C. (2014). "Against Organ Markets but Be Cautious in Adopting Presumed Consent," in A. Akabayashi (ed.), *The Future of Bioethics: International Dialogues*. Oxford: Oxford University Press, 417–20.

Verheijde, J. et al. (2009). "Enforcement of Presumed-Consent Policy and Willingness to Donate Organs as Identified in the European Union Survey: The Role of Legislation in Reinforcing Ideology in Pluralistic Societies," *Health Policy*, 90: 26–31.

Yomiuri Newspaper. (2009). "Kiso kara wakaru noshi to zoki-isyoku [Basics of brain death and organ transplantation]," May 14, Morning Edition, 13 (in Japanese).

12.5

Commentary

Organ Donation and Social Amelioration: A Two-Pronged Approach to Organ Trafficking

Leonardo D. de Castro and Peter A. Sy

This paper explores a model for reciprocating the contribution of organ donors to a health-care system characterized by inadequate resources and faced with the challenge of trying innovative ways of providing much-needed health care. A conceptual framework is proposed that recognizes a soft altruism being manifested in the contributions made by people who donate in the context of a social amelioration scheme. In order to bring out some of the characteristic features, a comparison is made with a presumed consent regime, which, while focused on cadaver organs, would appear to take advantage of the vulnerabilities of the poor when implemented in economically disadvantaged countries.

The model makes it possible for people to make their organs available for transplant while receiving benefits under a social amelioration program. The aim is to enable poor organ donors to emerge from the transactions in better health than otherwise, without loss of dignity, and having taken part in a collective undertaking that promotes the interests of organ donors and recipients alike.

An alternative model is offered that could be compared to better known methods for encouraging more people to donate organs for transplantation. Its merits can be seen in the following: (1) compared to other proposals based on the provision of incentives, it is less likely to be seen to regard human organs as mere commodities or to legitimize market transactions; (2) it involves a system for monitoring behavior of organ donors after transplant, ensuring post-transplant health care; (3) it offers a set of benefits that are already part of a social amelioration program in countries around the world; (4) rather than merely providing incentives, it seeks to ameliorate the conditions of the donors on a sustained basis; and most importantly, (5) it seeks to remove the donors from the exploitative conditions that have encouraged the poor to participate in human organ trade as vendors.

The socio-economic context

The context assumed in this paper is one where there are many gaps in the public health care system as well as in the socio-economic support system so that many basic services are not readily available. In developing countries where kidney trade has been a problem, the public health insurance system is not comprehensive in scope. A similar situation is presumed to prevail in the discussion here. Health care is either too expensive or inadequate for many poor people. Private health insurance is beyond the reach of the poor. In a country like the Philippines, emergency health care for the poor is available only through public hospitals, which are already operating beyond capacity. In many instances, hospital clerks, interns, and residents have to provide medicine and medical supplies out of their own pocket so that necessary procedures can be carried out on patients assigned to them.

Although it costs less than protracted renal dialysis, organ transplantation is unaffordable for patients in developing countries who belong to the economic classes that many organ vendors are coming from. Thus we have a terribly asymmetrical situation where the sources of organs for transplant are always the poor and the beneficiaries of the transplants are always the rich.

Another area of disparity can be found in the foreigner–local citizens divide. A medical tourism program that caters more to foreign than local transplant patients has supported the activities of transplant centers. Despite current bans on organ selling, foreigners are attracted not only to relatively cheap organs but also to the relative ease of procurement through a network of organ brokers. Medical tourism has become a flagship program not only of private hospitals but also of governments as it provides them an opportunity to boost income and to promote other related services.

The system of governance is likely to be relatively weak and inefficient. As a result, a centralized waiting list is difficult to maintain. Transplant centers are left to devise their own procedures for matching ESRD patients with available kidney donors or cadaveric organs.

Will presumed consent work?

Against this backdrop, it is difficult to see that presumed consent can serve as a viable and just option to improve transplantation rates. The establishment of a presumed consent or opt-in system for organ donation has been tried in many countries as a means of increasing the number of available organs for transplant. While its implementation may have resulted in an increase in donations, it is not certain that the success could be attributed directly to the removal of the need to opt in since other intervening factors come into play (Mossialos 2008; Gil-Diaz 2009: 260). Moreover, it would be risky to implement a presumed consent or opt-in system in developing countries where relevant governing institutions are not run efficiently and where the dissemination of information is not fully reliable. Many developing countries are also plagued by rampant corruption. Many countries where we would probably want a presumed consent system to succeed are also countries where the above-mentioned barriers to effective governance exist. We can accept that presumed consent has had a positive impact on donation rates, but that that impact has not been due directly to the legalization of taking organs without the consent of families because in practice such consent has been sought, as in the case of Spain. Probably more important is the development of greater awareness among the public as a result of the intensive campaign among the relatives of the recently dead. But this intensive campaign does not necessarily have to take place in the context of presumed consent. It is also dangerous to implement presumed consent systems in developing and not efficiently managed countries where information dissemination cannot be fully relied upon and the poor and ignorant could be taken advantage of, even after death.

Persistent organ trade

While organ selling has been prohibited, ESRD patients have continued to explore the resources available in an underground market, which has apparently flourished. Administrators of a leading hospital in the Philippines say that vendors have been roaming their premises, playing hide and seek with hospital guards who have had to chase them away. Out of 311 respondents to a survey of organ vendors conducted in the Philippines in 2007, 43 (13.8 percent) indicated the National Kidney and Transplant Institute as the site center where their nephrectomy was done. This represents a very significant number of cases that should not have taken place had authorities been more effective in their implementation of pertinent regulations. The situation reflects the economic desperation that has gripped organ sellers. The situation partly explains why the practice of organ selling has proven to be difficult to contain and control. It also illustrates a context where there has hardly been an opportunity for organ sellers to be altruistic in attitude. Obviously, organ sellers are being lured into the practice by the material incentives. An organ "donation" is often cast primarily as a straightforwardly monetary transaction. Given their tight economic situation, prospective organ vendors are ready to jump at any opportunity to make money in order to provide for their family's needs. The focus is on the material gain and in what purportedly is beneficial in the transaction for them. The transaction is not situated in a context where an opportunity for altruistic contribution could be offered or where an altruistic attitude could be cultivated. This is evident in the particular reasons given by people for selling their kidneys—"feed one's family," "cancel a debt," "buy land," "improve the family shack," "buy a pedicab," having no better money-earning options, being tricked, being forcefully trafficked, and to purchase consumer items (Zargooshi 2001: 1790–9; Awaya, et al. 2009: 140; Mendoza 2010: 259). These studies also confirm some of the characteristics often attached to organ vendors—poverty, ignorance, and desperation.

Altruism

In the context described above, one would think that there is no room for altruistic organ donation. Since material compensation is a primary consideration, any talk of altruism would seem to be incompatible. However, the view is offered here that it makes sense to speak of altruism in a "soft" sense of the organ donor having the willingness to accept something of lesser value in exchange for the organ to be transplanted. In contrast, a "hard" form of altruism involves a willingness to give up an organ as part of a system of exchange where compensation is not expected (or is even forbidden) and is not regarded as a necessary condition for the donation of an organ.

In the soft sense, then, it is possible for an organ donor to receive compensation and still be regarded as altruistic. Because the organ that is being offered ordinarily has much greater value than the payment exchanged for it, the vendor can be regarded as altruistic, at least in the soft sense. There is a level of exchange value that the organ donor is sacrificing. A kidney has "incalculable" worth, at least to the extent that it has the potential to extend the life of a person indefinitely. Money or material concessions paid to an organ provider or donor cannot match the value of that life.

Closely related to this point is the view that those who accept compensation for their transplanted organs cannot truly be regarded as donors. One cannot be a donor and at the same time accept compensation for one's donation. When certain people speak of "organ donation" in this context, it is merely as a euphemism for "organ trading." For them, "organ donor" is a mere euphemism for "organ trader" or organ vendor.

This view is rejected here for failing to give due recognition to the contribution a person makes by making an organ available for transplant, regardless of whether that contribution is rewarded with monetary compensation or not. Moreover, the value of having a functioning kidney for an ESRD patient is so much higher than the money or materials usually paid to an organ seller. To refuse to recognize the organ seller as a donor is grossly to underestimate the value of the contribution being made to the organ recipient. (It is actually difficult to say that the amount given under the circumstances should be regarded as a payment for the kidney itself. Perhaps more acceptable is the interpretation that it is an incentive for the donor to part with a kidney.)

Moreover, the view that the organ seller cannot be a donor is inconsistent with the ordinary understanding of donors. Many donations are subjected to self-serving conditions. To take an example one encounters with academic research projects, a donor country might insist that only equipment sold by companies based in that country may be bought with the use of money it has donated.

The soft conception of altruism does not make a reference to an attitude toward another person. What it does involve is a readiness to accept an exchange in which one ends up with something of less value than that which is transferred. The organ donor is being altruistic by accepting compensation that is not at least equal in value to the kidney itself. One can see that this phenomenon is also related to the exploitation that often takes place in these settings. The kidney seller is exploited by not being given compensation proportionate to the value of the organ.

Giving recognition to soft altruism is significant in that it does not make altruistic giving an exclusive option for those who have the economic means to live a life that is comfortable enough. By accepting that even the poor and underprivileged can be altruistic, society signals its appreciation of what this group can contribute to society and of their productivity in terms of such a valuable input to the health-care pie.

Indeed, the contribution is so valuable that it would be exploitative to allow contributors to continue suffering because they themselves do not have adequate access to basic portions of that pie. The situation is patently unjust when people who contribute so significantly to the health-care pie (or to any other service pie) are systematically prevented from getting a fair share when they are the ones in need. Instead of being systematically prevented, they should be helped to access certain services as they themselves require as citizens of the same state. So this is not saying that they should necessarily be paid for the benefits that they bring into the pie. The idea is to assist them to get what they are entitled to as citizens because they are being good citizens by playing their role as contributors to the system.

Avoiding exploitation through a social amelioration program

The experience in developing countries shows that legislation or public pressure to prevent people from accepting compensation for organs has not worked. In countries like the Philippines and India, regulations prohibiting the sale of organs for transplant have not stopped the practice. The regulations have merely served to drive the practice underground. The practice has resulted in greater exploitation of organ donors since many are not given adequate information about the procedures and concomitant risks, proper preoperative and postoperative care, psychological guidance and counseling, or other information and services that are essential for their safety and well-being.

Prohibitions have also tended to leave the vulnerable poor disempowered and exposed to medical risks when they sell their organs anyway. In developing countries like the Philippines and India, bans on organ trade not only lack force but also tend to punish sellers and cause them more shame. Brokers and recipients have the means to run away. Poor donors hardly receive postoperative care and counseling, whether they received compensation or not. The health risks generally associated with organ trade might even be worse on the donors, as they stay away from "legal" health services for fear of being caught having done an illegal trade.

A successful compensation package must be able to explain how it can deal with the ways in which exploitation could arise. For example, the ignorance of organ donors tends to undermine their capability to make a well balanced decision on the basis of all relevant information—the risks and their likelihood, the proportion of risks to benefits, the anticipated benefits for the donor and the recipient, the impact of particular benefits on the life of the donor, the appropriateness of the specific benefits to the donor's life goals, etc.

The poverty of organ donors constitutes a multidimensional barrier to their ability to make a balanced decision. Hence, it is also necessary to show how the poverty can be dealt with. Poverty puts individuals in a relative position of dependence or captivity associated with material or non-material indebtedness. A compensation scheme must be able to minimize (at least) the inhibiting effects of such indebtedness.

A social amelioration package for organ donors

A social amelioration package for organ donors must be proportionate to the contribution they make to the exchange system. The level of compensation one receives may be considered proportionate to the contribution one makes when it matches the benefits that one ought to expect from a hypothetical health-care and social security system to which it contributes. That system must be fair and responsive to the needs of the population. In the same way that the organ recipient is able to gain benefits from the transaction that are not provided in the existing health-care system, the organ donor must be able to expect benefits that ought to be part of, but are not yet provided by, that system.

One example of a compensation package could consist mainly of the elements of the Conditional Cash Transfer Program (CCTP) being implemented in the Philippines following models that had been tried in a number of countries earlier on. The program is aimed at bootstrapping people from vicious cycles of poverty by dangling incentives for people to achieve certain desirable outcomes in health, education, and nutrition. In what is known as the "Pantawid Pamilyang Pilipino Program" (Dizon 2010; Philippine Information Agency 2011), the poor are methodically enrolled to keep their children in school, meet nutritional goals, and, as parents, receive training to engage in livelihood projects. Similar programs in many parts of the world have achieved desired health and educational outcomes (Gertler 2004; Son 2008). The program could provide an organizing structure for multi-stakeholder "buy-in" for concrete, measurable outcomes in health, education, and economic productivity and could well take in energies from business, non-government organizations, and other civil society groups.

In addition to the elements of the CCTP, the package should perhaps include the following items that are crucial for non-exploitative organ donation: life and medical insurance, psychological counseling, and livelihood assistance and/or job placement.

Medical insurance is an obviously necessary component of a social amelioration package. Since organ donors are providing something that contributes to the health status of the transplant recipients, it makes good sense to help ensure that they can be given reasonable health care. They will then be contributing to a health insurance system that they also derive benefits from. It will be ironic if, after having contributed to overall health within their community, they were to be excluded from receiving benefits similar, or comparable to those that they will have contributed.

Life insurance ought to be a part of the package because the donor's family also assumes certain risks arising from the donor's involvement. The wife or husband and the children are part of the exercise and should not be left out of the calculations.

Psychological counseling is another need of organ donors that is not usually available in the black market. Studies have shown that organ sellers report various symptoms that are not usually expected of well informed donors. While some of them may actually have a reason to complain because of the consequences of their not being adequately followed up medically, it is likely that there are also many cases of psychosomatic conditions arising more from the donors' being misguided or misinformed.

Livelihood assistance and/or job placement are also important components of the compensation package. Without a job or means of livelihood, a person cannot be expected to have reasonable access to things that are necessary for promoting a reasonable health status. Many organ donors are jobless and have a very undependable means, if any, of livelihood.

Educational assistance is another appropriate component, considering that many organ sellers have a very low educational attainment. Like all the other components mentioned above, educational assistance ought to be seen as part of the proposal's response to the organ donor's vulnerability to exploitation.

What emerges from this compensation package is a framework where the organ donor is regarded as a highly valuable contributor to a health and social security system that should be competent to provide certain basic and important goods and services to its members. Being such a contributor, the organ donor is regarded as entitled to a reasonable level of benefits that can be provided by that system. Unfortunately, such a broad and comprehensive system is not yet in place in many countries where organ selling is taking place. This proposal to provide a social amelioration package is also a proposal to set in motion a process toward the establishment of a broad and comprehensive system that is responsive to the needs of the population. That system should be able to provide a reasonable level of medical services and a social security system that effectively caters to employment, educational, and other emergency needs of its members.

Even when that broad and comprehensive system is not yet in place, it is useful (even essential) to view organ donation within that system's framework. This approach to developing a culture of altruism is supported by our continuing experiences with the uncontrolled and unregulated organ market.

The establishment of a broad and comprehensive health-care and social security system requires a financing program that has yet to be developed. In the meantime, a moderately sized program can be initiated on a manageable scale—depending on the amount of available resources—so that an example could be put forward and monitoring and evaluation could be undertaken.

Conclusion

This paper proposes a model for the social amelioration of organ donors that makes it possible for the health-care system to generate more human organs for transplantation and for people to make their organs available for transplant while receiving compensation that takes various forms, to emerge out of the transactions in better health than otherwise, without loss of dignity, and having taken part in a collective undertaking that promotes the interests of organ donors and recipients alike. It recognizes that the implementation of presumed consent or opt-out systems has probably led to an increased supply in organs. However, it would be risky to implement such a system in developing countries where regulatory bodies and health services are not run efficiently and the dissemination of information is not fully reliable. Many developing countries are also plagued by rampant corruption. In those places where we would probably want a presumed consent system to succeed, the above-mentioned barriers to effective governance can be seen to prevail.

The willingness of those who are eager to be reciprocated for their organ donation can be regarded as "soft" altruism. This soft sense of altruism is a "middle ground" alternative to the "strong" altruism assumed in opt-out regimes and to money-only market that insults the poor's capacity to care despite the lack of genuine choices. Accepting this soft sense of altruism is important to this paper's proposal because it explains why the exchange cannot be understood in purely material terms.

Under the proposed system, the role of organ brokers is going to be taken over by the government's primary agency for providing social services, subject to strong account-ability and transparency audits by the public and other stakeholders. The goal is holistic and goes beyond increasing the supply of organs. It is uplifting the conditions of oth-erwise exploitable organ donors. The program seeks to address broader needs not only of those desperately needing organs but also those of potential providers of organs and their families. Neither a superficial ban on organ markets nor an equally exploitable opt-out system could obviate the need for a broader institutional support mechanism in organ donation (cadaveric or otherwise) with material and financial benefits to the donors and their families who, in developing countries, are usually poor. Organ dona-tion and social amelioration are inseparable solutions. Preventing such material support mechanism for the desired health outcomes is unjust, if not downright cruel.

Trust in the medical profession and the transplant community is not necessarily enhanced by the ban on organ markets. Coming from the ranks of the same profession and group are those who continue to exercise willful ignorance towards black markets for organs (Caplan 2014) that will persist so long as the there is a much greater need than the altruism of organ donors could meet. What undermines trust in the context of organ transplantation is not the money that changes hands but the reduction of the whole process into a purely monetary matter. On the other hand, structures can be put in place to simultaneously value the donation and improve the well-being of donors and their families. Organ donation without an accompanying social amelioration package for donors is ethically "business as usual" for the transplant world maintained by either opt-out or opt-in regimes.

References

Awaya, T. et al. (2009). "Failure of Informed Consent in Compensated Non-Related Kidney Donation in the Philippines," *Asian Bioethics Review*, 1(2): 138–43.

Caplan, A. (2014). "Trafficking and Markets in Kidneys: Two Poor Solutions to a Pressing Problem?" in A. Akabayashi (ed.), *The Future of Bioethics: International Dialogues*. Oxford: Oxford University Press, 407–16.

Dizon, D. (2010). "Conditional Cash Transfer Helps Pinoys Beat Poverty Trap," July 31, ABS-CBNnews.com, http://www.abs-cbnnews.com/nation/07/30/10/conditional-cash-transfer-helps-pinoys-beat-poverty-trap (accessed January 19, 2013).

Gertler, P. (2004). "Do Conditional Cash Transfers Improve Child Health? Evidence from PROGRESA's Control Randomized Experiment," *American Economic Review*, 94 (2): 336–41.

Gil-Diaz, C. (2009). "Spain's Record Organ Donations: Mining Moral Conviction," *Cambridge Quarterly of Healthcare Ethics*, 18:256–61.

Mendoza, R. L. (2010). "Kidney Black Markets and Legal Transplants: Are They Opposite Sides of the Same Coin?" *Health Policy*, 94:255–65.

Mossialos, E. (2008). "Does Organ Donation Legislation Affect Individuals' Willingness to Donate Their Own or Their Relative's Organs? Evidence from European Union Survey Data," *BMC Health Services Research*, 8:48.

Philippine Information Agency. (2011). "Pantawid Pamilya Shows Positive Effects on Filipino Families," January 10, http://pantawid.dswd.gov.ph/index.php/news/181-4ps-shows-positive-effects-on-filipino-families (accessed August 19, 2013).

Son, H. H. (2008). "Conditional Cash Transfer Programs: An Effective Tool for Poverty Alleviation?" Manila, Philippines: Asian Development Bank.

Zargooshi, J. (2001). "Quality of Life of Iranian Kidney Donors," *Journal of Urology*, 166:1790–9.

12.6

Response to Commentaries

Arthur L. Caplan

The four thoughtful commentaries on my arguments against organ markets and in favor of presumed consent for lessening the demand for organs for transplant raise many important issues. Each commentator has usefully engaged my arguments and offered many points worthy of consideration.

Daniel Fu-Chang Tsai (Tsai 2013) supports my argument against trafficking and markets. He notes that his country, Taiwan, has a huge need for kidneys for transplantation and that the shortage in kidneys has fostered trafficking in kidneys for transplantation. This has led to strenuous and, in my view, commendable efforts by government and private groups to identify, discourage, and penalize trafficking (Tsai 2013).

Tsai is skeptical, however, that a presumed consent strategy can work in Taiwan or in other nations. He points to alleged abuse in Singapore and worries on the part of physicians in Taiwan about the trustworthiness of a presumed consent policy. He wonders if it is right to,

take advantage of people's indifference or lack of interest in social/medical policy. If so, is it ethical to harm a few in order to benefit many? (Tsai in this chapter)

I would agree that a shift from an opt-in strategy to an opt-out policy of presumed consent must only be undertaken with full-throated public debate and then a consensus to do so. Presumed consent, like any other change in donor policy, ought not be imposed by authority. To work well it must be a response to the public's desire to try and improve the supply of organs with a change in policy that respects autonomy and choice while affording every protection to those who wish to opt out.

It is important to keep in mind that claims of abuse are not limited, as Tsai might be read as suggesting, to opt-out systems. Opt-in systems generate plenty of complaints, lawsuits, and charges of coercion and inequity as well (Lisberg 2005). Moreover, in those nations operating with presumed consent systems the number of persons complaining that every effort has not been made to insure that any objections on the part of the deceased to donation were not zealously pursued and heeded is negligible. Given the growing need for kidneys in Taiwan, an aging population and a growing transplantation capacity for all organs and tissues, it would seem useful to engage in a publicity campaign and political dialogue about a presumed consent policy.

Professor Nakajima in his commentary (Nakajima 2013) notes concerns about presumed consent. He wonders how a family could make a decision to donate the organs of an infant,

without the infant's intentional expression of the will to donate organs (Lisberg 2005).

This issue troubles Professor Arima as well (Arima 2013).

In countries that have *opt-in* systems, parents are allowed to make decisions in favor of organ donation for infants and young children in the absence of any possible wish or expression of choice on the part of the child. The issue then is not presumed consent, as Nakajima and Arima both suggest, but, rather, the extent to which parents and guardians are allowed to make any decisions at all about organ donation for newborns, infants, young children, and those with severe mental disabilities who never attained competency during their lifetimes. This is a difficult problem but one that is not a strong counterargument against presumed consent. Rather it is a general concern about using anyone as a cadaver donor who, lacking any capacity for having autonomy, never was able to express a wish about donation and permitting third parties do so.

Nakajima also wonders whether in trying to preserve the rights of those who do not wish to donate, any cost savings can be achieved relative to educating the public about opt-in versus opt-out systems. I suspect he is right—a shift in policy will require a large-scale educational effort that would be costly. The issue, however, is not whether it would be cheaper than the current costs of trying to encourage the citizens of Japan to opt in, but whether spending money on a national campaign favoring presumed consent might deliver more organs to those in need while still respecting voluntary choice. Such a campaign must include making clear to families that they may opt out of donating without fear of penalty or stigma of any sort.

I do agree with Professor Nakajima that scarcity is a function not only of supply but also of priority. Not all organs are of equal quality, some in need have rare blood and tissue types, and some live far from transplant centers and services. In truth, cadaver organs cannot meet the true demand for transplants—what we might see if persons of all ages were added to wait lists along with those with various co-morbidities. As I note in my paper, demand is far greater worldwide than any policy regarding cadaver organ procurement is capable of meeting whether opt-in, opt-out, or markets. The only long-term solutions to organ and tissue shortage involve stem cells, xenografts, or artificial organs. But we can and should do better then we are now doing in getting organs, and presumed consent, adopted with public support and strict protections for voluntary choice, is worth exploring as one ethical way to do so.

Professor Arima does not take issue with my critique of trafficking or markets but believes that the road to presumed consent policies may be rockier than I concede. Obviously it is an empirical question whether a presumed consent approach will produce more organs for transplant. The data on this question shows no negative results and trends that are positive. If that is so, then the case for trying to persuade the public in Japan and elsewhere of the merits of helping those in need is surely strong.

But this shift is only worth attempting if presumed consent is consistent with the core moral values—respect for persons, individual autonomy, informed consent, and altruism—that, as I maintain, have long grounded cadaver transplant policies since the inception of organ transplantation in the 1950s.

In the United States the majority of people answer polls by indicating that they wish to be organ donors upon their death. So it is not a long leap to the view that the proper default for public policy is to presume consent rather than the opposite. In Japan, China, and other nations where public willingness to donate may not be as strong, a sustained campaign to persuade the public that donation is the right thing to do, prudent—should a family member or friend need an organ—and a sign of social solidarity may need to precede a policy shift defaulting to the presumption of donation.

Professor Arima's main concern with presumed consent, however, is that the family may not really know what the deceased's wishes were regarding cadaver donation. In the absence of a stated objection, families may tilt toward allowing donation due to the possible pressure they may feel from a presumed consent policy.

It is interesting to note that in the United States and other nations, families are given no ability to override a stated wish about donation one way or another. They are used as surrogates only in the face of complete uncertainty about what the deceased may have wished.

Surely a shift toward presumed consent will engender more discussion among families about their wishes. Decisions that now must often be made in ignorance by families, whether under an opt-in policy or a presumed consent policy, may well be better informed.

The core question raised by Arima is whether families have a role to play in donation when the deceased has stated no wish. Even if it is not true that a presumed consent policy is harder to resist than an opt-in policy as Arima argues, I think families must have the final say but not for the reason given by Professor Arima.

Families should try as best they can to honor what they believe the deceased would have wanted. But, sadly, in many instances, the deceased was not sure about, never thought about, did not wish to think about or, due to a lifelong lack of capacity, could not have thought about donation. In such circumstances families are allowed to decide not just as surrogates for the deceased but also as the persons responsible for the disposition of bodily remains. In other words, there is a default to family when autonomy is not present.

Autonomy is important, and I would say is of primary importance regarding organ donation. That said, when it cannot be accessed in matters of organ donation, or for that matter, autopsy, funeral arrangements, burial, or distribution of the resources of a deceased person who dies intestate, all such decisions are left, default, to the family. This is not because they can always be amplifiers of autonomy but because they are the most likely to make prudent and respectful decisions about their loved ones. Who better than the family to decide when we know not what the deceased might have wanted? This is a presumption that makes the best of a flawed situation. If organ donation is a social good and if we believe it is the right thing to do in lieu of any known objection then allowing the family discretion to choose in the context of a presumed consent policy seems consistent with the ethical values that have been and should remain the foundation for cadaver organ procurement.

Professors de Castro and Sy (2013) argue that presumed consent may be more exploitative of the poor than regulated markets. They note that it is difficult to implement a shift in policy toward presumed consent in developing nations that may be beset with limited infrastructure, corruption, and communication inefficiencies. These are, certainly, huge challenges to shifting policy regarding cadaver donation, but without making some effort many nations that lack any cadaver donation system will invoke these reasons and thereby have no effort to move away from trafficking.

China is a prime example of a nation with significant transplant capacity, significant need, some trafficking (Anonymous 2011), and a near-complete reliance on executed prisoners for most of its organ supply. Without pressure to change, even in the face of limits and severe challenges, the reliance on prisoners and trafficking seems likely to endure (Caplan 2011; Caplan et al. 2011).

Moreover, the limitations de Castro and Sy note also work against their own suggestion of a social amelioration approach that is a form of a regulated market strategy. Will corrupt, inefficient, underdeveloped nations really offer those who sell kidneys medical insurance, life insurance, psychological counseling, livelihood assistance, and educational assistance? This strains credulity far more than my argument that poor and developing nations ought debate and consider presumed consent.

More to the point, should the citizens of every nation not expect some of these forms of social aid whether they agree or not to have an organ removed from their bodies? And should physicians agree to remove a kidney from the poorest of the poor knowing that there is no medical reason to do so and that the only reason the seller would choose to undergo such a surgical procedure is to gain access to basic benefits that otherwise will not be offered. Add to this the fact that social amelioration schemes involving regulated markets using offers of access to core benefits will do nothing to solve the shortage of hearts, lungs, livers, intestine, pancreas, cornea, bone, ligaments, and other organs and tissues that the creation of some sort of cadaver donor system—opt in or opt out—seeks to address. What de Castro and Sy propose is a regulated kidney market offering access to the poorest of the poor to crucial social benefits if they will have their kidneys cut out to use for the rich. That may help a few in the short run but does nothing to solve the more basic long-term challenge of getting more organs and tissues of all types or providing basic social benefits to all.

References

Anonymous. (2011). "Oz Kidney Buyers Giving China's 'Transplant Tourism' a Boost," *Sify News*, February 6, http://www.sify.com/news/oz-kidney-buyers-giving-china-s-transplant-tourism-a-boost-news-international-lcgpOcbgcgj.html (accessed August 17, 2011).

Arima, H. (2014). "Presuming Minor Consent and Allowing Family Veto: Two Moral Concerns about Organ Procurement Policy," in A. Akabayashi (ed.), *The Future of Bioethics: International Dialogues*. Oxford: Oxford University Press, 426–34.

Caplan, A. L. (2011). "The Use of Prisoners as Sources of Organs: An Ethically Dubious Practice," *American Journal of Bioethics*, 11(10): 1–5.

Morton College Library Cicero, ILL

Caplan A. L. et al. (2011.) "Time for a Boycott of Chinese Medicine and Science Pertaining to Organ Transplantation," *Lancet*, 378:1218.

de Castro, L. D., and Sy, P. A. (2014). "Organ Donation and Social Amelioration," in A. Akabayashi (ed.), *The Future of Bioethics: International Dialogues*. Oxford: Oxford University Press, 435–43.

Lisberg, A. (2005). "Critically Ill Woman Gets Liver: Donor System Successful after Search Controversy," *Daily News*, August 9, http://www.nydailynews.com/archives/news/critically-ill-woman-liver-donor-system-successful-search-controversy-article-1.616497 (accessed January 19, 2013).

Nakajima, T. (2014). "Can a Presumed Consent System Stop Organ Trafficking?" in A. Akabayashi (ed.), *The Future of Bioethics: International Dialogues*. Oxford: Oxford University Press, 421–5.

Tsai, D. F.-C. (2014). "Against Organ Markets but Be Cautious in Adopting Presumed Consent," in A. Akabayashi (ed.), *The Future of Bioethics: International Dialogues*. Oxford: Oxford University Press, 417–20.

13.1

Primary Topic Article

Ethics Without Borders? Why the United States Needs an International Dialogue on Living Organ Donation

Mark P. Aulisio, Nicole M. Deming, Donna L. Luebke, Miriam Weiss, Rachel Phetteplace, and Stuart J. Youngner

Introduction

The number of individuals that could benefit from organ transplantation is far greater than the number of organs available for transplantation. This has led to a variety of efforts to increase organ supply worldwide. Some strategies include adopting an opt-out or presumed consent model (Spain) and providing individuals with donor cards priority should they require an organ transplant (Israel). In the US such efforts have included public awareness campaigns, driver's license and donor registry initiatives, "required request" and mandatory Organ Procurement Organization (OPO) notification of impending patient deaths, use of expanded criteria for deceased donors, and "donation after cardiac death" (Institute of Medicine 1998; Siminoff and Lawrence 2002: 754–60; Siminoff, Burant, and Youngner 2004: 217–34; Bernat et al. 2006: 281–91).

Globally, efforts to increase organ supply have also extended to increasing the numbers of living organ donors, arguably the greatest growth area in transplant over the last decade. A recent study of living kidney donation, for example, indicated a growth rate of 50 percent or more over the last decade in 62 percent of the 69 countries studied, with almost 40 percent of all kidney transplants worldwide coming from live donors by 2006 (Horvat, Shariff, and Garg 2009: 1088–98). In the US, the numbers of living organ donors actually surpassed those of deceased donors over a three-year period from 2001 to 2003 and growth in living donation outpaced that of deceased donation by more than 3:2 from 1996 to 2005 (http://optn.transplant.hrsa.gov/latestData/step2.asp). This growth, which encompasses not only the traditional category of living related donation but also degrees of non-related living donation (i.e. close friendship to anonymous donors), raises a number of ethical questions that have yet to be fully confronted in the US. Here we highlight some of these ethical challenges for living organ donation in the

US, offer suggestions as to how such challenges might be met, and invite international dialogue on what are, ultimately, ethical issues without (national) borders.

Rise of living organ donation in the United States

Before turning to the ethical questions raised by living organ donation, we will look briefly at its emergence as a leading source of organs for transplant in the US. Initially, living donors were the primary sources of organs for transplant in the US. Shortly thereafter successes with cadaveric organs led many in the transplant community to question the ethics of using organs from live donors (Starzl 1987: 174–5; Starzl 1992). The primary concern involved the potential harm of removing an organ from healthy people who themselves had no medical need for surgery. The organ procurement itself entails injury, pain, risk of a variety of complications, and even death. To this day, the long-term outcomes for living organ donors remain uncertain. The development of immunosuppressant drugs and advances in surgical intervention led to great success in deceased donor transplant. This success, coupled with ethical concerns, led to the removal of prisoners as potential sources of organs and the near-complete absence of living organ donation outside a familial context for many years. Gaining true consent, free from coercion or undue influence, is the main problem in retrieving organs from individuals with limited or no options. For example, one physician from Virginia proposed to increase organ donation by acting as a broker between indigent foreigners brought to the US as donors and the recipients' payers—Medicare or Medicaid (Joralemon 2001: 30–5). This proposal was met with near-universal horror and condemnation in our country, prompting Congress to prohibit the sale of organs.

The numbers of living organ donors began to increase both in absolute terms and as a percentage of total donors starting in the early 1990s. For example, OPTN/UNOS data shows that there were 2,571 living donors, 36.3 percent of all donors, in 1992. By 2001, living organ donors as a *percentage* of all donors in the US reached 52.1 percent, and by 2004 the number of living organ donors topped 7,000 (7,004). Since peaking in 2004, living organ donation in the US has decreased slightly, but the number of living organ donors has remained above 6,000—almost 350 percent higher than its 1988 level (http://optn.transplant.hrsa.gov/latestData/rptData.asp, accessed December 8, 2011). Interestingly, living unrelated donation (neither blood nor marriage relationship) was by far the biggest growth area, rising from single or low double digits in the early 1990s to over 1,500 by 2004, a level it has since maintained even as overall numbers of living organ donors trended down slightly from 2005 to 2009 (http://optn.transplant.hrsa. gov/latestData/rptData.asp, accessed January 18, 2011).

What might account for the rapid increase in living organ donation, in general, and living unrelated donation, in particular? There are, of course, many factors but several are worth underscoring. As the wait list grew and potential sources for deceased donor organs remained stable, living organ donors became one of the few potential growth areas for increasing organ supply. Growing public awareness of the wait list and education of the public regarding living organ donation no doubt played an important role, as did direct appeal by desperate wait-listed patients through news or media outlets, particularly with respect to living unrelated donation. In addition, the rise of the Internet has made direct appeal much easier and probably more effective, whether facilitated through pay commercial websites like http://www.matchingdonors.com, Craigslist, or other noncommercial sites and chat rooms that allow desperate patients to advertise their need in the hopes that a sympathetic person will make a directed donation of a kidney, or a liver or lung lobe (Zink et al. 2005: 581–5; Delmonico and Graham 2006: 37–40).[1]

Ethical questions in the United States

The growth in living organ donation has been welcomed by many as an answer to the shortage of deceased donor organs for transplant. This growth, however, raises a number of very serious ethical challenges that must be addressed by the transplant community if living organ donation is to be performed responsibly (Biller-Andorno 2002: 199–204; DuBois 2002: E1–E4; Caplan 2004: 1933–4; Zink et al. 2005: 581–5). This is particularly true where non-related, or "acquaintance," directed donation and anonymous donation are concerned. Here, we will highlight just a few of the many ethical questions raised by living organ donation.

Autonomy, harm, and health professional participation?

Some might argue that, given the centrality of the value of autonomy in US society, living organ donation should be viewed as ethically unproblematic. There are two problems with this line of argument.

First, even in the US, it is one thing to harm oneself; it is quite another to participate in the harming of another—and the procurement of organs from the living requires the participation of others (i.e. health professionals) in what is at least a prima facie harming of the donor. Importantly, the *consent* of an individual to being harmed does not in itself count as either justification or excuse for another's doing the harming. A charge of murder cannot be escaped, for example, by arguing that the (now dead) person consented to being shot to death even if they did in fact so consent. This is true even if one argues that the harming is done with the consent of the harmed person *to promote a good that the harmed person him- or herself wanted to see promoted*. No surgeon would be legally justified or excused in amputating the right arm of a healthy person merely because that person ardently desired to have his or her arm amputated and donated to science, even if the consent were genuine and the benefit cohered with the deeply held values of the patient or his or her interpretation of the will of God (Aulisio, Devita, and Luebke 2007: S95–101).

Second, within health care, patient autonomy itself is not without limits. Patient autonomy is and should be a core value, but it is normally so only for selecting among a range of medically acceptable options or refusing medical intervention altogether. For example, if a perfectly healthy person announces that he or she wants a new liver,

---

[1] See, for example, http://www.matchingdonors.com (accessed January 15, 2013).

health professionals obviously are not obliged to honor the request. This is true even if the "patient" is well informed and the request coheres with his or her most deeply held values. The reason, of course, is that there is no medical indication for a liver transplant. This is not because of the scarcity of livers for transplant. Even if livers grew on trees and were plentiful, the fact that there is no medical indication for transplant would take precedence. "Best treatment" must be identified in light of the values of a competent adult patient but only within the range of medically acceptable options—and these are not set merely by reference to patient values.

Both of these points are directly relevant for living organ donation. Prospective living donors plainly do not have a medical condition that warrants the removal of an organ as among the range of medically acceptable options. The removal or resection of an organ from a healthy patient constitutes a prima facie harm, even if done with the consent of the patient and for a greater good such as saving another's life. The point of calling this a prima facie harm is to distinguish it from being called a "harm" relative to donor values, which it clearly is not. Furthermore, the removal of an organ from a healthy patient which is not medically indicated for that patient and which therefore constitutes a prima facie harm to that patient, *requires the participation of others,* i.e. health professionals (Aulisio, Devita, and Luebke 2007: S95–101).

Living organ donation, therefore, constitutes a unique exception to basic limitations on autonomy and participation of others in bringing about a prima facie harm. Because of its unique place in this regard, it is imperative that the transplant community ensure that the highest ethical standards are met.

The historical paradigm: living related donation?

As mentioned above, living organ donation early on paradigmatically involved living related donation, where the relationship was either biological or familial. What is an otherwise unusual choice—the choice to have a healthy organ removed—is contextualized and rationalized by the fact of the biological or familial. This is the primary reason that living related donation was the only type of living donation that was traditionally accepted by the transplant community. The biologic or familial relational context is so important that in some cases the courts have permitted minors to donate organs to siblings on the grounds that it is in the *best interest of the minor donor* to be allowed to do so (Aulisio, May, and Block 2001: 408–19).

Living related donation itself is not unproblematic despite being the traditionally most accepted form of living organ donation. The powerful bonds of a biological or familial relationship help to contextualize and rationalize the wish to donate but they also raise the risk of coercion. To address this, physicians have historically been willing to give prospective living related donors who do not wish to be donors a way out by claiming (even falsely) that they are not compatible with the needy relative. The risk of coercion is very real and must be taken seriously if living related organ donation is to be conducted in a responsible manner. This risk, combined with the fact that the removal of a kidney, liver lobe, or lung lobe constitutes a prima facie harm to the prospective living donor and the fact that health professionals must participate in organ procurement *ethically requires that high standards for living organ donation be developed and maintained.* To guard against the dangers of coercion, rigorous standards of care for psychological evaluation of prospective donors and a robust consent process should be developed, maintained, and monitored by the transplant community. The fact that no such standards currently exist is a serious ethical issue that cannot continue unaddressed (Caplan 2004: 1933–4; Zink et al. 2005: 581–5; Aulisio, Devita, and Luebke 2007: S95–101). As we have argued elsewhere, organ category-specific standards of care should be developed for (1) rigorous assessment of the decision capacity and psychological state of the prospective donor and (2) a robust informed consent process that unfolds gradually over time and includes significant educational components (Aulisio, Devita, and Luebke 2007: S95–101).

In addition, the published academic literature on living organ donor outcomes in the US consists primarily of self-reports from transplant centers with little or no long-term tracking of living donor health and well-being. This serious gap in the academic literature is more concerning given the growing number of disturbing anecdotes of botched procurements and poor short- and long-term aftercare for living donors (Ommen, Winston, and Murphy 2006: 885–95). For example, the *St. Louis Post-Dispatch* did a special series in May 2005 which, among other things, chronicled the stories of at least 11 living organ donors who have experienced serious short- and long-term health problems following donation, one of whom (Rita Kocian) apparently had a known history of depression, drug abuse, and a recent suicide attempt.[2] Similarly, the emergence of various living donor advocacy groups in the US such as the Living Organ Donor Advocate Program founded by live kidney donor and nurse, Kimberly Tracy, and the Live Organ Donor Education and Protection Project founded by Rhonda Boone and Vicki Hurewitz, widows of live liver donors Danny Boone and Michael Hurewitz, suggests that there may be much deeper problems for living organ donors than the published academic literature indicates.[3] These problems range over a host of issues from short- and long-term aftercare to emotional and psychological well-being, to health and life insurance.

Robust and comprehensive short- and long-term donor outcome data must be gathered if living organ donation is to be responsibly practiced in the US. The most comprehensive and effective way to gather such data would be through a living organ donor registry that longitudinally tracks donor health and well-being. Unlike much of Western Europe and Japan, the US has no such registry.[4] In addition, it is hard to see how a robust informed consent process can be done in the absence of the data a comprehensive registry would provide.

Living unrelated donation in a relational context?

There are at least two types of living unrelated donation that occur in a relational context: paired donation, where incompatible donor–recipient pairs are matched, and living

---

[2] See Shelton 2005a. For Rita Kocian's story see Shelton 2005c.

[3] Living Donors Matter https://www.facebook.com/LivingDonorsMatter, Living Organ Donor Advocate Program at http://www.lodap.com, and Live Organ Donor Education and Protection Project at http://www.lodepp.org (this site is now defunct).

[4] This is true despite repeated calls for the development of a registry. See, for example, the recent call for a living kidney donor registry in the US in Ross, Siegler, and Thistlethewaite (2007: 48). Also, Davis and Cooper (2010: 1873–80).

donation by a friend. The latter, friendship donation, is only a modest stretch of the original biological or familial paradigm for living organ donation and poses no special problems. The former, paired donation, occurs when a sibling, spouse, parent, or child is willing to donate to another, D1–R1, but is not compatible. A second incompatible pair, D2–R2, is then matched with the first incompatible pair so that D1 gives to R2 and D2 gives to R1. In the US, groups such as the North American Paired Donation Network have facilitated paired donation for a number of years (http://www.facebook.com/pages/Paired-Donation-Network/116174520328). Though all of the concerns articulated above concerning living organ donation apply here, as with friendship donation, it could be argued that there is nothing uniquely ethically problematic about paired donation, at least when the procurements and transplants occur simultaneously as is normally the case. If paired donation and transplant are not carried out simultaneously, however, the prospect of a potential donor backing out after the first donor's procurement and transplant exists.

This concern is more pressing for a more recent form of paired donation–paired donor chains. This occurs when multiple pairs are grouped to form an organ exchange chain. Johns Hopkins, for example, performed a quintuple transplant in 2006 and six-way transplant in 2008 (Dominguez 2008). Donor chains raise the risk that a donor further down the chain might back out after the up-the-chain procurement has been made, breaking the chain and leaving some prospective recipients without organs because donors must be permitted to change their minds even at the 11th hour. Similarly, prospective donors who might want to change their minds might feel undue pressure if an entire donor chain were to collapse should they change their minds. To our knowledge neither of these potential problems has occurred, but they remain real concerns for donor chains and become more exigent as the chain lengthens.

Straining the paradigm: acquaintance-directed donation or anonymous non-directed donation?

Acquaintance-directed donation and anonymous non-directed donation push even further from the living related donation paradigm, arguably straining it to the breaking point. The desire of a living person to donate an organ to an acquaintance or a possibly never-to-be-known stranger is more difficult to rationalize. The reasons for donation outside a relational context vary. Some may have a loved one who was successfully given the "gift of life" by another and wish to give in kind. Others may be motivated by religious belief such as, for example, members of the Jesus Christians, a group founded by David McKay, who donated a kidney at the Mayo Clinic in 2003 to an acquaintance he met online (http://jesuschristians.com/). Whatever any particular individual's motivations might be, given the fact that the living unrelated donor candidate is (1) considering consenting to a prima facie harm, (2) considering a prima facie odd choice (no existing relationship with the prospective recipient that contextualizes or rationalizes the choice), and (3) requires the participation of health professionals to effectuate that choice, it would be appropriate for the transplant community to raise the bar for the psychological evaluation and consenting of these prospective donors even higher in order to avoid unwittingly taking advantage of persons with psychological or psychiatric illness. *This is not to say that all or even the majority of prospective living donors in this category are driven by mental illness. The important consideration, rather, is that safeguards be put in place to avoid exploitation of those who do have such an illness.*

In the case of living directed acquaintance donation, there is the ever-present fear of quid pro quo or financial compensation. Unlike anonymous living donation, this type of donation also raises the ethical issue of recipients unfairly jumping the queue through direct appeal and public solicitation. The medium of the Internet seems particularly susceptible to these problems. Commercial efforts like that of MatchingDonors.com (at http://www.matchingdonors.com, accessed January 15, 2013) raise very serious ethical concerns. MatchingDonors.com helps potential recipients find potential donors via the Internet, essentially enabling the prospective recipient to "jump" the waiting list by finding their own donor. Patients in need of transplant can list on the site for life for a flat fee of $595.00, 90 days for $441.00, 30 days for $295.00, and seven days for $49.00. The incentive for prospective recipients is, obviously, huge and it would not be surprising if some patients offered significant financial compensation for being chosen to receive the "donor's" organs, effectively buying an organ. Matchingdonors.com and other similar commercial organizations risk enabling a commodities market for human organs, a very serious infringement upon the Uniform Anatomical Gift Act. In one controversial case, Robert Smitty of Chattanooga, Tennessee repeatedly posted to http://www.livingdonorsonline.org (accessed January 15, 2013) looking for a buyer of one of his kidneys. In one post, he reportedly sought $175,000. Robert Smitty eventually donated to Bob Hickey of Edwards, Colorado, whom he found on MatchingDonors.com. Though Smitty reportedly failed four lie detector tests for the TV show *Lie Detector,* he claimed that he just wanted to do a good deed so his young son would look up to him (Shelton 2005b: A7).

Even if there is no clandestine financial quid pro quo, sites like Matchingdonors.com, despite their best intent, enable prospective donors to select possible recipients on the basis of race, ethnicity, social status, or any number of possible criteria that the Organ Procurement and Transplantation Network (OPTN) wait list explicitly precludes. As such, these sites raise questions about the ideal that all should have equal access to donor organs based on the complex broadly agreed-upon scoring system that is supposed to prioritize recipients in a socially neutral way.

Conclusion

In conclusion, we have argued that the growth of living organ donation in the US, from living related donation to all forms of living unrelated donation, has raised a number of serious ethical questions that need to be answered if living organ donation is to be performed responsibly. Living organ donation straightforwardly involves a healthy person, with no medical condition for which the removal of an organ would be among the range of medically acceptable options, consenting to a prima facie harm—for the greater good of saving or improving the quality of another's life. This prima facie harm requires the participation of health professionals—the transplant community. Interestingly, the US societal context does not normally construe the consent of an individual to being harmed as either justification or excuse for other parties' participation in the harming. The fact that living organ donation has this unique feature is a powerful reason for the transplant community setting high ethical standards for this practice. Against this backdrop, we considered ethical issues across and within three categories of living organ donation: living related, living unrelated in a relational context, and acquaintance-directed or anonymous non-directed donation.

All forms of living donation require the development of standards of care for (1) assessment of the psychological state and decisional capacity of prospective living donors and (2) a rich and detailed informed consent process. Standards of care for assessment of psychological state and decisional capacity of prospective donors will guard against risks of coercion, especially in living related donation, and exploitation of those with mental illness, particularly in forms of living unrelated donation such as acquaintance and anonymous donation. A robust informed consent process itself requires the maintenance of a living donor registry in the US so that short- and long-term living donor outcomes can be rigorously tracked. This alone would fill a serious gap in current data in the US, a gap which is all the more concerning in light of the number of disturbing anecdotes of poor donor short- and long-term aftercare and even botched procurements.

As the paradigm of living related donation is stretched to include living unrelated donation in a relational context, additional ethical questions emerge. While friendship donation and traditional paired donation involve essentially the same ethical issues as living related donation, the emergence of paired donor chains raises new concerns (see Appendix for examples of different types of paired donor chains). Chief among these, we suggested, are the related risks of (1) the timing of paired donor chains procurement and transplant, which raise the risk that a donor further down the chain might back out, leaving some prospective recipients without organs, and (2) that prospective donors may feel undue pressure as paired donor chains lengthen and the ramifications of changing one's mind grow.

Finally, straining of the living related paradigm for living organ donation to include acquaintance-directed donation and anonymous non-directed donation raises still more ethical issues. The absence of a relational context requires an alternative rationalization that will contextualize the choice. In order to avoid unwittingly taking advantage of persons with mental illness, we suggested that it would be appropriate to raise the bar for psychological and decisional capacity assessment for this category of live donation. In addition, the emergence of the Internet as a medium for direct appeal itself risks facilitating bias and prejudice in organ allocation, unfair jumping of the wait-list queue, and even illicit organ sales.

As we conclude, we want to emphasize that despite the very real concerns articulated herein, we strongly support organ donation and transplantation. The ethical value of donated organs means it is imperative that living organ donation be performed according to the highest standards—not just technical but also ethical—for the sake of donors and recipients alike.

Appendix: Examples of Swaps and Chains

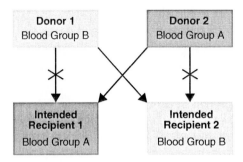

Figure 13.1 A balanced living paired exchange between two donor–recipient pairs. The pairs are incompatible because of ABO blood group mismatch.

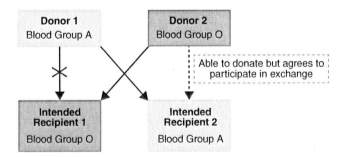

Figure 13.2 An altruistically unbalanced living paired exchange between two donor–recipient pairs. Recipient 2 is able to receive Donor 2's blood group O kidney. They agree to participate in an unbalanced exchange.

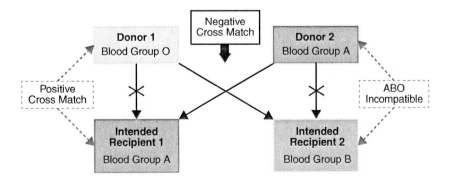

Figure 13.3 A balanced living paired exchange between two donor–recipient pairs. In this exchange the cause of incompatibility is different for each pair.

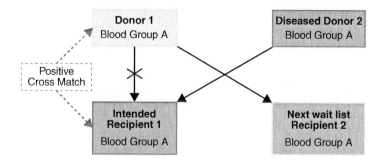

Figure 13.4 Live donor/list exchange or indirect exchange. This exchange combines living and deceased donor kidney transplantation.

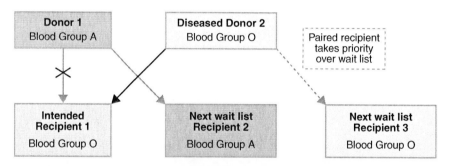

Figure 13.5 Live donor/list exchange or indirect exchanges may disproportionately harm waiting-list blood group O recipients, by increasing their time on the list.

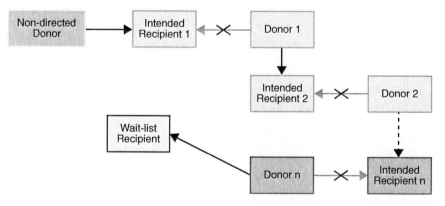

Figure 13.6 A non-directed donor initiates a chain exchange. The diagram shows a "closed chain" model where the last transplant goes to a recipient on the deceased donor waiting list. This pattern has also been termed a "domino transplant."

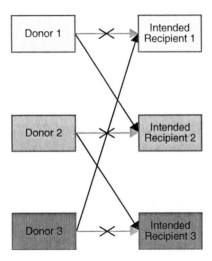

Figure 13.7 Diagram of a simultaneous three-way exchange. Three-way exchanges increase the logistic complexity of matched exchanges.

References

Aulisio, M. P., DeVita, M., and Luebke, D. (2007). "Taking Values Seriously: Ethical Challenges in Organ Donation and Transplant for Critical Care Professionals," *Critical Care Medicine*, 35(2): S95–101.

Aulisio, M. P., May, T., and Block, G. D. (2001). "Procreation for Donation: The Moral and Political Permissability of 'Having a Child to Save a Child,'" *Cambridge Quarterly of Healthcare Ethics*, 10(4): 408–19.

Bernat, J. L. et al. (2006). "Report of a National Conference on Donation after Cardiac Death," *American Journal of Transplantation*, 6(2): 281–91.

Biller-Andorno, N. (2002). "Gender Imbalance in Living Organ Donation," *Medicine, Health Care, and Philosophy*, 5(2): 199–204.

Caplan, A. L. (2004). "Transplantation at Any Price?" *American Journal of Transplantation*, 4(12): 1933–4.

Davis, C. L., and Cooper, M. (2010). "The State of US Living Kidney Donors," *Clinical Journal of the American Society of Nephrology*, 5: 1873–80.

Delmonico, F. L., and Graham, W. K. (2006). "Direction of the Organ Procurement and Transplantation Network and United Network for Organ Sharing Regarding the Oversight of Live Donor Transplantation and Solicitation for Organs," *American Journal of Transplantation*, 6(1): 37–40.

DuBois, J. M. (2002). "Is Living Organ Donation Ethically Acceptable?" *Health Care Ethics USA: A Publication of the Center for Health Care Ethics*, 10(2): E1–E4.

Dominguez, A. (2008). "Six-Way Kidney Transplant Carried out in US," *Associated Press*, April 10 [online], http://www.guardian.co.uk/world/2008/apr/10/usa.sciencenews (accessed January 15, 2013).

Horvat, L. D., Shariff, S. Z., and Garg, A. X. (2009). "Global Trends in the Rates of Living Kidney Donation," *Kidney International*, 75(10): 1088–98.

Institute of Medicine. (1998). *Non-Heart-Beating Organ Transplantation: Medical and Ethical Issues in Procurement.*

Joralemon, D. (2001), "Shifting Ethics: Debating the Incentive Question in Organ Transplantation," *Journal of Medical Ethics*, 27:30–5.

Ommen, E. S., Winston, J. A., and Murphy, B. (2006). "Medical Risks in Living Kidney Donors: Absence of Proof is not Proof of Absence," *Clinical Journal of the American Society of Nephrology*, 1:885–95.

Ross, L. F., Siegler, M., and Thistlethewaite, J. R. (2007). "We Need a Registry of Living Kidney Donors," *The Hastings Center Report*, 37(6): 48.

Shelton, D. (2005a). "A Post-Dispatch Investigations: Lives on the Line," *St. Louis Post-Dispatch*, May 8–12: May 8: A1 and A5-8; May 9: A1 and A6; May 10: A1 and A6-7; May 11: A1 and A10-11; May 12: A1 and A14-15.

Shelton, D. (2005b). "Total Strangers," *St. Louis Post-Dispatch,* May 10: A7.

Shelton, D. (2005c). "What Happened to Rita Shouldn't Have Happened," *St. Louis Post-Dispatch,* May 8: A8.

Siminoff, L. A., Burant, C., and Youngner, S. J. (2004). "Death and Organ Procurement: Public Beliefs and Attitudes," *Kennedy Institute of Ethics Journal*, 14(3): 217–34.

Siminoff, L. A., and Lawrence, R. H. (2002). "Knowing Patients' Preferences about Organ Donation: Does It Make a Difference?" *The Journal of Trauma*, 53(4): 754–60.

Starzl, T. E. (1987). "Living Donors: Con," *Transplant Proceedings*, 19(1): 174–5.

Starzl, T. E. (1992). *The Puzzle People: Memoirs of a Transplant Surgeon.* Pittsburgh: University of Pittsburgh Press.

Zink, S. et al. (2005). "Living Donation: Focus on Public Concerns," *Clinical Transplantation*, 19(5): 581–5.

13.2

Commentary
Can Living Donation Be Justified?

Yohei Akaida and Kohji Ishihara

In their paper, Aulisio and others discuss the ethical challenges posed by living organ donation with reference to recent trends in the US. In the first section of this commentary, we compare living donor organ transplantation trends in the US and Japan. In the second section, we examine the authors' discussion on ethical concerns specific to each kind of living organ donation with reference to the situation and cases in Japan. In the last section, we address the ethical challenges posed by living donor organ transplantation itself.

1 Living donor organ transplantation in the US and Japan

Aulisio and others point out that the number of living donor organ transplants began to increase from the early 1990s. Living organ donors as a percentage of all donors in the US peaked at 52.1 percent in 2001, and the annual number of living organ donors peaked at 7,004 in 2004. In particular, the annual number of living unrelated donations has increased substantially, from the single or low double digits in the early 1990s to over 1,500 in 2004 (Aulisio et al. in this chapter). As possible reasons for this rapid increase in living donations, particularly living unrelated donations, Aulisio and others suggest the following factors: 1) increase in waiting-list figures and the drain of potential sources of cadaveric organs, 2) growing public awareness of the waiting list coupled with direct appeals by wait-listed patients through news or media outlets, and 3) the rise of the Internet, which has made direct appeal much easier through paid commercial or noncommercial sites.

In Japan, the first living donor kidney transplant was performed in 1964 (Maruyama 2009: 85). Since then, the number of living donor kidney transplants has increased to about 1,000 cases annually in recent years (JST 2009: 19). The total number of living donor kidney transplants reached 16,817 by the end of 2008, while the total number of cadaveric kidney transplants (the number of transplanted kidneys) was only 5,172 (JST 2009: 19). Living donor liver transplants, which were first performed in 1989 at Shimane Medical University (now Shimane University), peaked at 566 in 2005 (JST

2009: 11; Maruyama 2009: 85). The total number of liver transplants reached 5,188, while the number of brain–death liver transplants reached only 58 by the end of 2008 (JST 2009: 11). Instances of other organ transplants in Japan are low: only 76 living donor lung transplants, 15 living donor pancreas transplants (JST 2009: 31, 35), and 12 living donor small intestine transplants (Keio Hospital Information and Patient Assistance Service 2010) were performed by the end of 2008.

Two major differences between living organ transplantation in the US and Japan stand out. First, the proportion of living transplants to cadaveric transplants has been very high in Japan from early on. For example, 137 living donor kidney transplants had been performed by the end of 1970, whereas the number of cadaveric kidney transplants was only 37 (JST 2009: 19). This situation is in contrast to that of the US, where living organ transplants increased rapidly in the 1990s. Second, among living organ donations, unrelated donations are rare in Japan, while they increased rapidly in the US in the 1990s and 2000s.

The high proportion of living donations in Japan may be due to close family relationships, considering that most living donations fall under the "related" category. However, we can also argue that the high proportion of living donations in Japan can be attributed to the small number of cadaveric donations. In 2008, for example, among kidney transplants, the number of living donor transplants was 991 and that of cadaveric transplants was 210 in Japan, while in the US the number of living transplants was 5,966 and that of cadaveric transplants was 10,101 (see Table 1).

With respect to the difference in number of unrelated donations, the regulation governing living organ donations is obviously a factor. In Japan, although there is no law prohibiting living unrelated organ donations, the ethical guidelines of the Japan Society for Transplantation (JST) declares that "cadaveric transplantation is the desirable type of donation," and also stipulates that living donations should be related donations (within

Table 1   Number of kidney transplants in the US and Japan in 2008 (based on OPTN/SRTR 2009: Chap. 3, Table 5.4d and JST 2009: 19–20)

	Patients on the waiting list for kidney transplantation	Kidney Transplants	Living donor kidney transplants		Deceased donor kidney transplants	
US	76,089	16,067*	5,966*	Related**: 4213 Unrelated: 1556 Unknown: 197	10,101*	
Japan	11,814***	1,201	991		210	Cardiac death: 184 Brain death: 26

*Kidney alone transplants.
**Including "parent," "offspring," "sibling," "other relatives," and "spouse" (OPTN/SRTR 2009: Table 5.4d).
***As of November 2, 2009.

blood relationships of the sixth degree or in-law relationships of the third degree). The guideline allows unrelated donations, provided that the ethics committee of the facility individually approves them after considering the JST ethics panel discussion (JST 2007). Given that the number of living unrelated donors was very small even in the US in the early 1990s, and increased rapidly perhaps due to effective appeal through news or media outlets and the Internet as Aulisio and others suggest, there seems to be no reason to deny the possibility that the number of unrelated donations will increase if JST changes its ethical guidelines, and desperate patients and their families begin to advertise their needs through various media outlets. However, we cannot deny that family relationship differences between the US and Japan may be a potential factor. It is reasonable to think that the ethical guidelines that impose a strong limitation on living unrelated donations reflect the Japanese perception of family relationships and attitudes toward organ donation. By scrutinizing this problem, we can find some cue for developing transplantation ethics based on cultural and societal diversity. However, this is beyond the scope of this commentary.

2 Ethical issues specific to the kind of living organ donation

Aulisio and others distinguished three kinds of living organ donation: living related donation, living unrelated donation in a relational context, and acquaintance-directed donation or anonymous non-directed donation. Here, we examine their discussions on the ethical concerns specific to these kinds in the context of Japanese cases.

2.1 Living related donation

Aulisio and others point out that the living biological or familial donation "was the only type of living donation that was traditionally accepted by the transplant community" because "[w]hat is an otherwise unusual choice—the choice to have a healthy organ removed—is contextualized and rationalized by the fact of the biological or familial" (Aulisio et al. in this chapter). They also point to the ethical issue associated with living related donation: it raises the risk of coercion precisely because of the powerful bond of familial relationships. To guard against the danger of coercion, they argue that "rigorous standards of care for psychological evaluation of prospective donors and a robust consent process should be developed, maintained, and monitored by the transplant community" (Aulisio et al. in this chapter). To develop a robust informed consent process, information on living organ donor outcomes is mandatory. However, according to them, "the published academic literature on living organ donor outcomes in the US" is very thin. Drawing on news stories and reports of various living donor advocacy groups, they suggest that "there may be much deeper problems for living organ donors than the published academic literature indicates," and insist that "[r]obust and comprehensive short- and long-term donor outcome data must be gathered" (Aulisio et al. in this chapter).

The lack of rigorous standards of care for the psychological evaluation of prospective donors and donor outcomes data is also true for Japan. There are no detailed guidelines concerning donor selection or detailed surveys on donor outcomes. The JST Ethical Guidelines contain stipulations on donor selection, but they are not sufficiently detailed.[5] As for donor outcomes data, although many books on living donation have been written by recipients or physicians (Nakamura 1990; Korenaga 2003; Kanisyoku Taikensha Iryosha Yushi 2004; Uetake 2004), few surveys on the health conditions of donors exist. An exception is a survey published by the Japanese Liver Transplantation Society (2005).[6] A total of 1,480 donors who were operated on between 1990 and 2003 participated in the survey, which covered physical and mental conditions, and aftercare. About 2.9 percent of respondents answered "approximately half recovered" or "hardly recovered" or "not recovered at all," while 97.1 percent of respondents answered "perfectly recovered" or "almost recovered." Such surveys should be conducted continuously and in greater detail not only for living liver donors, but for all living organ donors.

Given that living related organ donations are allowed (although not self-evident as argued below), avoidance of coercion, development of a robust informed consent process, and provision of sufficient aftercare are the most important ethical issues. However, rigorous standards for donor selection, detailed surveys of donor outcomes, and an aftercare system are lacking in both Japan and the US, and these shortcomings must be addressed.

2.2 Living unrelated donation in a relational context

Aulisio and others describe three types of "living unrelated donation in a relational context": friendship donation, paired donation, and paired donor chain. According to them, there is nothing uniquely or ethically problematic about friendship donation and (simultaneous) paired donation (although all concerns raised regarding living organ donations apply here), while the paired donor chain poses ethical challenges. Paired donor chains, they argue, carry the risk of a prospective donor breaking the chain due to a change of mind, thereby imposing undue pressure on her/him.

However, is it true that friendship donation and paired donation raise no special ethical issues? In the organ purchase case that occurred in Japan in 2006 (*Asahi Shimbun* 2006: 1, 14), the donor was a longtime friend. Usually, friendship as a relationship is not as strong as familial relationships, and may provide an incentive for monetary compensation.

Paired donation may be associated with the risk of coercion. Aulisio and others point out that "physicians have historically been willing to give prospective living related donors who do not wish to be donors a way out by claiming (even falsely) that they are not compatible with the needy relative" (Aulisio et al. in this chapter). Conversely, presenting the possibility of paired donation (and paired donor chain) may block the "way out."

---

[5] For studies on Japanese donors' consent process and professionals' attitudes, see Fujita, Slingsby, and Akabayashi (2004), Fujita et al. (2006), and Fujita et al. (2010). Fujita et al. (2010) carried out a survey on living donor liver transplants in Japan, and pointed out that many Japanese facilities have more conservative regulations and that "[t]he JST guidelines may play a role in guaranteeing the maximum scope of eligibility for each facility" (Fujita et al. 2010: 1457).

[6] Yokota (2007) and Fukunishi et al. (2001) are other exceptions.

It is true that these potential issues concerning friendship donation and paired donation are not different from those arising from living related organ donation, but compared to the latter, friendship donation and paired donation appear to raise the risk of realizing ethical concerns about living donation.

2.3 Acquaintance-directed donation or anonymous non-directed donation

Aulisio and others point out that acquaintance-directed donation or anonymous non-directed donation strains the living related paradigm "to the breaking point" (Aulisio et al. in this chapter). The desire for such types of donations "is more difficult to rationalize." In such donations, they insist, the transplant community should "raise the bar for the psychological evaluation and consenting of these prospective donors even higher in order to avoid unwittingly taking advantage of persons with psychological or psychiatric illness." Furthermore, in the case of living acquaintance-directed donation, "there is the ever-present fear of quid pro quo or financial compensation," particularly via the Internet.

In Japan, there is no system in place to support anonymous non-directed donation or acquaintance-directed donation. Japanese law does not prohibit such types of donations, but as mentioned above, JST ethical guidelines impose rigid conditions on unrelated donations in general, and as a result, there have been few cases of living unrelated transplants in Japan.

The rationale behind raising the bar in cases of directed-acquaintance donation and anonymous non-directed donation, suggested by Aulisio and others, appears to be the high risk of clandestine financial compensation or the exploitation of persons with psychological or psychiatric illness. However, these problems are also shared by living related donation or friendship donation, even if to a lesser degree. Living organ donation is in itself ethically problematic in constituting "prima facie harm." Historically in the US and in Japan, this is why living organ donations have been usually limited to related donations. Although living donor organ transplants as such should be avoided, they have been allowed between related persons as an exception. Acquaintance-directed donations and anonymous non-directed donations may reveal ethical concerns of living donor organ transplants more clearly than living related transplants.

3 Ethics of living organ donation

We conclude by addressing the ethical challenges posed by living organ donation itself. In their paper, Aulisio and others discuss ethical problems on the premise that living organ donation could be allowed against the backdrop of organ shortage. We agree with them in that living organ donation should be carried out according to the highest standards to prevent coercion and to realize a robust informed consent process with detailed information of donor outcomes, which is currently lacking in Japan and the US. However, the question of ethical justification of living organ transplantation remains open.

Aulisio and others (in this chapter) argue that the value of autonomy cannot justify living organ donation, because patient autonomy should be limited within health care for at least two reasons. First, patient autonomy can be allowed only within the range of medically acceptable options. Although not mentioned, this limitation appears to address the beneficence principle. Second, "the consent of an individual to being harmed" is neither justification nor excuse for another's participation in the harming. This limitation appears to address the non-maleficence principle. Considering these limitations on autonomy, it may be rational to argue that living organ donation cannot be justified. However, they insist that

Living organ donation...constitutes a unique exception to basic limitations on autonomy and participation of others in bringing about a prima facie harm. Because of its unique place in this regard, it is imperative that the transplant community ensure that the highest ethical standards are met. (Aulisio et al. in this chapter).

Aulisio and others further argue that living organ donation should be carried out according to the highest ethical standards because, as an exception, it is permitted to exceed the limitation on autonomy. However, the rationale behind this exception was not presented. Should we think that the principle of autonomy takes priority over the principle of beneficence and the principle of non-maleficence in living organ donation? Or can living organ donation be justified on the grounds of a utilitarian argument? Or is it unnecessary to justify living organ donation? As long as living organ transplantation continues to be performed, efforts must be undertaken to improve the organ transplantation system. However, the justification of living organ donation remains an ethical challenge as long as living organ donation constitutes "prima facie harm" to donors, even if the donation system is improved in an ideal way.

References

Asahi Shimbun. (2006). 26 December, Evening Edition, retrieved from *KIKUZO II visual* (accessed July 18, 2013).

Aulisio, M. et al. (2014). "Ethics Without Borders? Why *The United States* Needs an International Dialogue on Living Organ Donation," in A. Akabayashi (ed.), *The Future of Bioethics: International Dialogues.* Oxford: Oxford University Press, 449–60.

Fujita, M., Slingsby, B.T., Akabayashi, A. (2004). "Three Patterns of Voluntary Consent in the Case of Adult-to-Adult Living Related Liver Transplantation in Japan," *Transplantation Proceedings*, 36(5): 1425–8.

Fujita, M. et al. (2006). "A Model of Donors' Decision-Making in Adult-to-Adult Living Donor Liver Transplantation in Japan: Having No Choice," *Liver Transplantation*, 12:768–74.

Fujita, M. et al. (2010). "Attitudes of Medical Professionals and Transplantation Facilities: Toward Living-Donor Liver Transplantation in Japan," *Transplantation Proceedings*, 42(5): 1453–9.

Fukunishi, I. et al. (2001). "Psychiatric Disorders before and after Living-Related Transplantation," *Psychosomatics*, 42(4): 337–43.

Japanese Liver Transplantation Society. (2005). "Report of Survey on Living Liver Donors," (in Japanese). http://jlts.umin.ac.jp/donor_survey_full.pdf (accessed January 15, 2013).

Kanisyoku Taikensha Iryosha Yushi (Volunteers of Donors, Recipients and Health Professionals). (2004). *Shinjiru Kizuna Ikituzukeru Omoi Seitai Kanishoku: Shinjitsu no Koe* (Bond of Trust, Living Feelings, and True Voices of Living Liver Transplantation), Tokyo: Shounsha.

Keio Hospital Information and Patient Assistance Service. (2010). (in Japanese). http://kompas. hosp.keio.ac.jp/contents/000113.html (accessed January 15, 2013).

Korenaga, M. (2003). *Seitai Ishoku wo Ukete: Gan kokuchi kara Happyaku Yonjunichi no Tatakai* (Experiencing Living Liver Transplantation: 840 Days of Fighting Cancer), Tokyo: Kohbunsha Shinsho.

Maruyama, E. (2009). "Seitai Ishoku ni okeru Donor no Yoken: Shinto Seigen (Japanese) (Kinship Relationship Requirement for Living Donor Organ Donation for Transplantation)," in Y. Shirosita (ed), *Seitai Ishoku to Hou* (Living Organ Transplantation and the Law). Tokyo: Nihon Hyoronsha, 125–37.

Nakamura, T. (ed.). (1990). *Ketsudan: Seitai Kanishoku no Kiseki* (Decision: History of Living Liver Transplantation), Tokyo: Jijitushinsha.

OPTN/SRTR. (2009). "Annual Report 2009," http://optn.transplant.hrsa.gov/ar2009/ (accessed January 15, 2013).

The Japan Society for Transplantation (JST). (2007). "Ethical Guidelines, 2003, 2007," (in Japanese). http://www.asas.or.jp/jst/pdf/kaisei20071122.pdf (accessed January 15, 2013).

The Japan Society for Transplantation (JST). (2009). "Transplantation Fact Book 2009," (in Japanese). http://www.asas.or.jp/jst/pdf/fct2009.pdf (accessed January 15, 2013).

Uetake, S. (2004). *Tsuma ni Kanzou wo Morau: Zouki Ishoku no Kakaeru Mondai* (Receiving Liver from My Wife: Problems of Organ Transplantation), Tokyo: Aki Shobo.

Yokota, K. (2007). "Seijin Kan Seitai Kanishoku Donor no Jutuzengo QOL Henka oyobi Fuan Yoin ni kansuru Jyudanteki Kenkyu (Longitudinal Study on Quality of Life and on Anxiety Factors in Living Donors Before and After Adult-to-Adult Liver Transplantation)." *Hiroshima Daigaku Hokengaku Journal*, 7(1): 30–9.

13.3

Commentary
Living Organ Donation and Organ Shortages: Another Perspective

Farhat Moazam

Mark Aulisio and others raise important points in their article. They highlight the lack of attention to the long-term health and well-being of living organ donors, and the absence of national registries to track such data in many countries, including the US. It is only recently that these issues are finally beginning to come under discussion by health-care professionals associated with the field of organ transplantation. The authors also offer lucid arguments about potential perils, a kind of slippery slope, inherent in "stretching" and then "straining" the ethically justifiable paradigm of living related donation, to cover instances that involve acquaintance-directed and anonymous non-directed living donation. In the background of a steady increase in the numbers of non-related living organ donations in America, the authors emphasize the need for ensuring the "highest standards," technical and ethical, in such cases. There is little to disagree with them on these points.

However, in an article that mentions a global community and multicultural ethical perspectives, one would have liked to see a broader take on issues of informed consent and organ shortages that cut across nations and societies, than one restricted to the situation in the US. But perhaps this is understandable. The *weltanschauung* and experiences of those positioned within economically "developed" countries remain the most prominent in international conferences and publications when it comes to addressing various aspects of organ transplantation. However, this ignores the fact that organ transplantation, particularly when involving living kidney donations, is now among the most common surgical interventions undertaken in many "developing" countries. Generally speaking, medical attention tends to focus on finding scientific, technologically driven ways to increase the "supply" of organs, and bioethics revolves around discussions of donor consent that stay within the framework of an individual's right to make autonomous decisions regarding his or her body. The reality is that the act of organ donation, by the living or following death, has complex, multifaceted dimensions which can be neither captured effectively through scientific and technological debates alone, nor comprehended completely through philosophically grounded, rational arguments that reduce the act to a transaction between two individuals, a donor and a recipient, to the exclusion of community and societal values in which the giving and receiving take place.

Having had an opportunity to practice medicine for an equal number of years in America and in Pakistan, I will comment on two broad areas, informed consent for living organ donation and shortages of transplantable organs, which are discussed in this article. My commentary will employ a "non-Western," non-technological gaze in an attempt to move the discussion to a more inclusive level.

Informed consent and the living related kidney donor

The authors note that by perceiving autonomy as the controlling societal value, living related donation is often considered to be ethically unproblematic. However, they argue, correctly, that removing an organ from a "healthy patient" involves inflicting potential harm on the donor (by the physician undertaking donor nephrectomy), and therefore donor autonomy in such cases cannot be considered "unbridled."[7] It is the obligation of the physician to ensure, through a "robust consent process," and psychological assessment when needed, that there is no element of coercion behind the decision to donate a kidney. While the authors do qualify the absoluteness of autonomy by noting its tension with the professional code of do no harm, in the final analysis it is the donor who must make the decision. It can therefore be argued that in this view too the autonomy of the individual, the freedom to make choices free from external influences, which is the cornerstone of contemporary bioethics, *does* remain the controlling societal value.

Juxtaposing this familiar bioethical world against one less well known—the triad of patient–family–physician interactions in Pakistan in the matter of living related kidney donations—may help to deepen our perspectives on both. Clearly, organ transplantation is unique in being the only medical specialty which relies on the generosity of others for its very existence—healthy persons willing to undergo a surgical procedure with potential risks and no direct benefit to them, and others who permit the use of parts of their bodies following death. In both instances, the decision to donate an organ or not, and how this is arrived at, is deeply influenced by the social construct of the self and relationships with others, historical and cultural understanding of kinships and family bonds, indigenous values and belief systems employed to make sense of suffering and death, and, last but not least, prevailing socio-economic realities. Without taking these contextual features into account, which may differ from one society to another, it is difficult to fully comprehend this truly extraordinary human act. To elaborate, I will use some of my findings from an in-depth, ethnographic study I conducted in a

---

[7] The authors' use of the term "patient" in referring to the living organ donor is curious. This is not a value-neutral word. As commonly understood and used, it pertains to someone with an ailment/illness for which he/she seeks treatment from a relevant health-care professional. In contrast, organ donors are healthy individuals who undergo surgery they do not need, to help others. The ethical responsibility of societies to provide postoperative and long-term follow-up does not convert donors into patients.

transplantation institution in Pakistan (Moazam 2006). Readers from other developing countries may find some of these to be not too dissimilar to their own experiences.

Pakistan, a country of 170 million people, most of whom are Muslims, is a low-income, traditional, hierarchical society in which the family and not the individual constitutes the social unit, and moral values are imbibed through religious teachings. As a "collectivistic" society the emphasis is on interdependencies and obligations to the family, particularly to those related by blood, rather than the rights of individual members (Markus, Rose, and Kitayama 1991; Kagitcibasi 1996). Extended families in Pakistan often consist of two or more interdependent generations living together and pooling their resources.

The country has a high prevalence of ESRD, no national health insurance schemes, and insufficient dialysis and transplantation facilities, many of which are in the private sector and thus further inaccessible to the majority. Within this background, the Sindh Institute of Urology and Transplantation in Karachi, a public sector hospital with state-of-the-art facilities and which provides free treatment, shoulders a major burden for dialyzing patients and undertaking the largest number of related living kidney transplants in the country (Rizvi et al. 2010). Unusual to Pakistan, physicians work on a fixed salary and are not allowed private practice. Kidney transplantations are conducted six days a week but at any given time there are many more waiting to be accommodated on the hospital's operating list.

My study reveals that the ethical ethos of, and the language used by, those who work in this institute and the patients and families who seek their care, centralize interdependencies and duties to others rather than rights and autonomy. Among the most common reasons given by family members who donate a kidney is their cultural and religious sense of obligation to save the life of blood kin, an act that is also considered pleasing to God and rewarded in the hereafter. The decision about who in the family should be the donor is often taken collectively and includes pragmatic considerations balancing benefits and repercussions to profoundly interdependent lives, and it is a decision in which physicians play an active, even directive, role. Encounters between physicians and patients do not take place alone but involve family members who usually accompany anyone seeking health care in Pakistan. These interactions are driven by an ethos in which physicians perceive their first and primary moral duty to their patients who require transplantation, and family members perceive it an obligation to provide a kidney to save the life of kin. Within this framework, physicians assume a benevolent parental role as an "elder" of the family and use their socially and religiously legitimized authority to coax, cajole, and occasionally scold members who seem reluctant to donate. The staff is also driven by practical concerns: successfully transplanting one patient means that another among the waiting hundreds can be moved up the list (Moazam 2006: 93–107, 122–45).

This moral world is vastly different from the one that dominates ethical discourse on organ transplantation in which the act of donating a kidney to a family member is considered supererogatory but never obligatory, "praiseworthy but optional," and in which the role of physicians is to ensure that donors face no external pressures while arriving at their decisions (Beauchamp and Childress 2001: 49–51). The findings of my study are not meant to imply that collective decisions and extended systems of kinships are always absolute ideals of unity and selflessness, or that they offer no ethical challenges (Moazam 2006: 145–53). It is my intention merely to illustrate that the ethical framework of the institute's staff and patients, if viewed through a narrow prism of individual autonomy and a right to make choices, would appear distorted. A wider lens is required which takes into account the existing kinship systems, shared religious beliefs and values, and prevailing socio-economic realities; without this, the complexity of ethical realities within which humans live would elude the viewer.

Shortages of transplantable organs

Surgeons who pioneered living organ transplantation in the 1950s did so with a sense of hope while also aware that, in placing an otherwise healthy individual under the knife, they were transgressing the central professional code which stipulates that above all physicians must do no harm. In fact, Renee Fox reports that Tom Starzl called "a permanent moratorium" on using kidneys from living donors due to his concerns that there was neither surety against donor harm nor "complete assurance" that the consent was free from coercion (Fox 2003: 145–60). However, over time, transplantation became routinized as a surgical procedure like any other. With this has also come a preoccupation with finding ways to increase the number of organs, from living and deceased sources, to meet the steadily expanding pool of patients waiting to be transplanted (Fox and Swazey 1992: 43–8). Today, the scarcity of organs is often chosen to be labeled as a "crisis" and supported by publicizing the large numbers of patients on transplant waiting lists. The authors note that it is tragic that since 1995 almost 100,000 individuals in the US have died while waiting to be transplanted. But perhaps we need to place this "crisis" within wider perspectives. As an example, American National Highway Traffic Safety Administration data reveals that, since 1995, more than 30,000 people die each year in the US from vehicular accidents (NHTSA Data Resource Website).

Reference to organ shortages is presented using market-influenced terminologies, such as "demand and supply" ratios in which the focus is almost exclusively on how to increase the supply side of the equation. Little if any attention is directed to underlying factors that may be contributing to the increase in the demand. In reality almost all countries including the US have had a gradual increase in the total number of kidneys transplanted every year, but as the number of patients entering the pool of those requiring transplantation is growing more rapidly, the gap continues to widen. With improving techniques and better immunosuppression, many patients with ESRD who would not have been considered suitable candidates a couple of decades ago are now being considered for transplantation. The ability and willingness of transplant professionals in this regard are matched by growing public expectations, especially in highly industrialized countries, that modern medicine can provide unlimited longevity with surgical interventions as and when necessary (Callahan and Nuland 2011).

But the most significant reason for the rapid increase in the number of those requiring kidney transplantation is a progressive rise in the prevalence of ESRD populations in economically advanced countries. In the US alone these numbers have doubled between 1991 and 2000 (Gilbertson et al. 2005). The increase in the incidence of ESRD, being termed a global epidemic by some, is multifactorial—longevity of life, a shift to chronic diseases in an increasingly aging population, and rise in obesity and diabetes leading to hypertension and other events that are harbingers of kidney disease. As lifespans increase worldwide, and improved material circumstances spread to economically disadvantaged countries, this global burden of ESRD is predicted to become even more severe (McClellan 2006). Clearly then, the problem of organ shortages cannot be resolved through an exclusive focus on increasing the supply of kidneys without simultaneously addressing public health measures and developing strategies for prevention, and early detection and treatment of renal disease. The importance of preventing kidney disease has been highlighted recently, but public health measures have never garnered the same levels of interest among medical and bioethics communities as have "sexier" issues pertaining to tertiary medicine (Nwankwo, Bello, and El Nahas 2005).

To conclude, many ESRD patients are provided a new lease on life through a kidney transplant, a miracle of modern medicine that requires support from all quarters. But it is also important to be clear about the use of the "do no harm" principle as it applies to organ donors. The only donor who cannot be "harmed" in any sense of the word is the deceased donor. In the case of living donors harm can at best be minimized but never eliminated with any surety, and the quantum for potential harm increases as one moves on the scale from the related to the unrelated donor, and from the altruistic donor to the kidney vendor (Moazam, Zaman, and Jafarey 2009). This concern has been voiced recently by international organizations during discussions about measures to increase the number of transplantable organs. The potential for harming living donors was mostly reflected in the Madrid Resolution on Organ Donation and Transplantation which followed the Third Global Consultation in March 2010 organized by the World Health Organization (WHO) in collaboration with the Spanish National Transplant Organization (ONT) and The Transplantation Society (TTS) (The Transplantation Society 2010).

The Madrid Resolution, which sought ways to promote ethical national self-sufficiency in meeting the need for organs, recommends that deceased donations should be considered "the priority source" and must be maximized, while living donations should be encouraged as a "complementary" source. This echoes the position of the WHO Guiding Principles, endorsed by the 63rd World Health Assembly in May 2010, that donations should be maximized from deceased donors while protecting the health and welfare of living donors (World Health Organization 2010). An international subcommittee of participants involved in formulating the Madrid Resolution, and which I co-chaired with Nikola Biller-Andorno from the University of Zurich, was given the task of elaborating on ethical issues related to organ donation and transplantation. In our recommendations to the Congress we prioritized deceased over living donation, while also making the point that this may help to produce a normative shift in perceptions of organ donation as a matter of rights of donors and recipients to one of shared responsibility and solidarity across all levels of society.

References

Beauchamp, T. L., and Childress, J. C. (2001). *Principles of Biomedical Ethics*. 5th ed. New York: Oxford University Press.

Callahan, D., and Nuland, S. B. (2011). "The Quagmire: How American Medicine is Destroying Itself," *New Republic*, June 9: 16–8.

Fox, R. C. (2003). "The Transplant Surgeon, the Sociologist, and the Historian: A Conversation with Thomas E. Starzl," in C. M. Messikomer, J. P. Swazey, and A. Glicksman (eds), *Society and Medicine: Essays in Honor of Renée C. Fox*. New Brunswick: Transaction Publishers, 145–59.

Fox, R. C., and Swazey, J. P. (1992). *Spare Parts: Organ Replacement in American Society*. New York: Oxford University Press.

Gilbertson, D. T. et al. (2005). "Projecting the Number of Patients with End-Stage Renal Disease in the United States to the Year 2015," *Journal of the American Society of Nephrology*, 16:3736–41.

Kagitcibasi, C. (1996). "The Autonomous-Relational Self: A New Synthesis," *European Psychologist*, 1(3): 180–6.

Markus, H., Rose, H., and Kitayama, S. (1991). "Culture and the Self: Implications for Cognition, Emotion and Motivation," *Psychological Review*, 98(2): 224–53.

McClellan, M. W. (2006). "The Epidemic of Renal Disease: What Drives It and What Can Be Done?" *Nephrology Dialysis Transplantation*, 21(6): 1461–4.

Moazam, F. (2006). *Bioethics and Transplantation in a Muslim Society: A Study in Culture, Ethnography, and Religion*. Bloomington, IN: Indiana University Press.

Moazam, F., Zaman, R. M., and Jafarey, A. M. (2009). "Conversations with Kidney Vendors in Pakistan: An Ethnographic Study," *Hastings Center Report*, 39(3): 29–44.

NHTSA Data Resource. http://www-fars.nhtsa.dot.gov/Main/index.aspx (accessed January 15, 2013).

Nwankwo, E., Bello, A. K., and El Nahas, A. M. (2005). "Chronic Kidney Disease: Stemming the Global Tide," *American Journal of Kidney Diseases*, 45(1): 201–8.

Rizvi, S. A. H. et al. (2010). "Living Related Renal Transplants with Lifelong Follow-up: A Model for the Developing World," *Clinical Nephrology*, 74(Supplement 1): S142–9.

The Transplantation Society. (2010). "The Madrid Resolution on Organ Donation and Transplantation: Third Global Consultation Organized by the WHO," http://www.tts.org/index.php?option=com_content&view=article&id=746:the-madrid-resolution-on-organ-donation-and-transplantation&catid=67:august-2010-newsletter&Itemid=565 (accessed January 15, 2013).

World Health Organization. (2010). "Sixty-Third World Health Assembly, Resolution WHA63.22, Agenda Item 11.21, Human Organ and Tissue Transplantation," May 21, http://apps.who.int/gb/ebwha/pdf_files/WHA63/A63_R22-en.pdf (accessed January 15, 2013).

13.4

Commentary
The Paradigm of Living Related
Donation: Stretched, Strained, and Abused?

Leonardo D. de Castro

The high value we give to living related organ donation has its roots in the medical and scientific context that made living organ transplantation possible in the first place. In the early days, the recipient and the donor had to be genetically related (as closely as possible) in order to minimize the risk of rejection and thereby improve the likelihood of success. Additionally, there was a related consideration in that the procedure carried risks for the donor. Thus, it helped to have a donor who was willing to take risks for the sake of the organ recipient. As relatives (especially the closest ones) were the most likely to be willing to undertake such risks, it was useful for living organ transplants to be carried out with related donors.

Since those early beginnings of living organ donation, a lot of things have changed. Factors affecting the characteristics of qualified donors have evolved and many new doors for possible organ donors have been opened that were clearly shut previously. As a result, the context of living related donation is said to be stretched and strained (Aulisio et al. 2013). Is it also being abused? Are non-traditional organ donors being unduly exploited? This paper seeks to clarify possible answers to these questions by examining developments and scenarios involving living organ donation focusing on the transplant of kidneys. The aim is to identify the ethical implications of some policy and legislative options.

The authors observe that living related donation is being stretched in cases of living donation by friend and paired donation. They also refer to the living related paradigm being strained to breaking point by acquaintance-directed donation or anonymous non-directed donation. One can see that the paradigm is truly being stretched and perhaps strained to breaking point in the ways mentioned. One may even cite additional ways in which the stretching and the straining are taking place.

At the same time, the concepts of friendship and kinship are quickly evolving. Specific friendships, families, and other relationships are being stretched and strained to breaking point. These are even abused in a way that leads to questions about their continuing significance in the context of living organ donation. It is important to see these developments as providing an occasion to reexamine the pertinent concepts in relation to the core foundations of the ethics that govern the dominant paradigm for organ donation.

Kinship and friendship: stretched and strained

The stretching and the straining of the concepts of friendship and kinship can be a bad thing in that the situations in which these are invoked represent examples of unjustified exposure of individual human beings to risks. They could also indicate abuse of trust and confidence. On the other hand, one may accept that the forces of globalization in the field of medicine have ushered in changes in our understanding of friendship and kinship and we have to be open to a reinterpretation of the impact of these on the living related paradigm for organ donation and transplantation.

The following case examples illustrate some of the considerations that have acquired importance in regard to our appreciation of living organ donation:

1. A member of the cabinet in a developing country was the recipient of a kidney transplanted from a donor who was employed as his chauffeur. Some members of the recipient's family said the donor was "virtually" one of them. He was also from the same town and was treated well by the employer's immediate family. When he was absent from family gatherings, people often asked where he was. One family member claimed that the donor was so close to the recipient that the latter considered him one of his children. Another relative said it did not seem difficult for the donor, a father to four daughters, to give up his kidney in order to give it to his boss. According to someone else, the chauffeur would have donated voluntarily as "you can't scare him into giving up his kidney."

   The donor said he "did not ask for payment in return but he was happy about the [recipient's] statement that his family would be taken care of." Moreover, "when there is someone in need, don't deny them your help. It feels good to help your fellowman." (Salaverria 2007)

2. This donor used to serve as a helper for the family of the recipient. As a young boy he lived with the recipient's family after his father died. His mother realized that she was in no position to provide a good future for her son so she left him in the care of the family where she herself was employed as a maid before getting married. The donor grew up providing house help while also being a playmate of the future recipient's children. He was not paid wages but he was provided food, clothing, and bed space. He was also sent to primary school and the first of four years of high school. He was occasionally referred to as having been informally "adopted" by the family although he was understood to have work obligations and he never truly achieved status as a child of the recipient. When the oldest of the future recipient's children went to the big city to work as manager of a factory, he recruited the future donor to work as a utility man. In the big city, he found his own bed space but still visited the "adoptive" family once a year. During one of those visits, the factory manager asked him if he would be willing to donate an organ to transplant to the manager's father. He felt compelled to say "yes."

3. Kate belonged to a poor family that was going through a very challenging period economically. Kate's father had died when she was still very young and her mother was left to fend for five children. Kate had a second-degree cousin, Lita, who needed a kidney for transplant and had offered her a sum of money if she agreed to be a donor. The anticipation of material reward enabled Kate to overcome her fears of undergoing a nephrectomy. She agreed to be tested and to subsequently make the donation. After the successful transplant, the two families were drawn closer together. Lita and her family felt compelled to reciprocate the help provided by Kate and to come to the aid of Kate's family in their times of need.

4. Jerry sold his kidney through an underground broker. When he was asked why he did it he said: "Of course, life being so difficult for us, why wouldn't we be encouraged [to sell]? Where can we get money if we do not do such a thing?" His kidney was priced at US $2,500 but he received only US $1,500—the rest went to the broker.

    Jerry used a huge chunk of the money to buy a television set and a DVD player so his five very young children could have a source of entertainment at home. According to the local village head, organ vendors like Jerry live a "good life" for about a month before going back to their usual level of subsistence. Very few of them manage to transcend poverty through the sale of a kidney. As a construction worker he was paid about US $4 per day when he had a job. Jerry said he was jobless at the time of the interview. While he did not regret having sold his kidney, he felt bad that he did not know where to get money to buy medicines that he needed.

5. William lived in the same village as Jerry, where there are about 15 organ donors a year, according to the elected leader. He said the recipient went to their place with a small monetary gift. "I pitied him because of his condition so I received the gift and went on to donate my kidney." He received a little more than US $1,000. Although he acknowledged that he was paid, when the interviewer referred to William as an organ vendor, he got mad and said, "Not a vendor, I was an organ donor!"

The discussions below refer to these case examples to illustrate the flexibility of kinship boundaries and the impact that this flexibility has had on human interdependence, reciprocity, and moral responsibility.

Globalization and its impact on organ transplantation

Globalization has had a profound and extensive impact on human relationships in various fields of human activity. Efficient travel and migration have provided opportunities for human contact and interaction beyond those that were previously limited to people sharing geographic location. Globalization has also had a significant impact on the nature of human relationships that provide the context for the practice of organ transplantation. While some aspects of globalization have resulted in more benefits to transplant recipients and organ donors alike, the facilitation of movement has also resulted in ethical challenges, some of which have been mired in controversy.

One of the challenges arising from easy movement across boundaries has to do with transplantation between total strangers sharing no genetic or ethnic ties. This has proven to be a challenge because the prevailing bioethical milieu puts a high value on organ donation carried out within a context of kinship or altruism. Now this context is being eroded because of scientific and medical developments.

Pressures to expand the pool of organ donors to non-relatives and to the living

The current state of biomedical science and technology has made it possible for non-relatives to become viable donors. Among other things, the use of advanced immunosuppressant drugs has enlarged the donor pool for organ transplantation to include those who are not so closely related or even those who are not genetically related at all. Rejection issues are being overcome and incompatibilities between donor and recipient have become less of an obstacle to safe transplantation. Studies such as those undertaken in more than 200 American transplant centers in 2000 established that "kidney grafts from living unrelated donors continue to have excellent long-term survival rates despite a high degree of HLA incompatibility...[and] living unrelated donors exhibited short- and long-term graft outcomes similar to values of sibling donor transplants" (Gjertson and Cecka 2000: 496).

Another study found that "although LURD recipients have poorer HLA matching and older donors, their patient and graft survival rates are equivalent to those of non-HLA-identical LRD recipients" (Humar et al. 2000: 1942). There was even a lower incidence of biopsy-proven chronic rejection in LURD transplants. Similar findings have been reported in Germany.

Subsequently, a long-term follow-up with 2,155 cases in Iran (Sinforoosh et al. 2006) showed that the results of living unrelated kidney transplantation are as good as those in living related kidney transplantation. On this basis, the authors confirmed that transplants from living unrelated donors may be proposed as a good therapeutic alternative for management of patients with ESRD.

Research findings such as these have put tremendous pressure on societies to support and encourage non-related living organ donation. After all, more living donor organs for transplant from any source means longer or higher-quality lives for more people in general. Kidney transplant beneficiaries have experienced a higher quality of life than people who have been provided other forms of therapy (Keown 2001). Moreover, studies have indicated lower expenses for organ transplantation because of more appealing cost–benefit ratio (Miranda et al. 2003).

There has been increased pressure also for living donation in general because transplants from living donors have led to better results than those from cadavers. Figures from the OPTN in the United States indicate that patients receiving kidneys from living donors have higher survival rates than patients receiving kidneys from cadavers. The five-year survival rate for transplants performed between 1995 and 2002 was 90.5 percent for living donors compared to 82.5 percent for cadaveric donors. For liver transplants, the five-year survival rate was at 80.0 percent for living donors compared to 72.1 percent for cadaveric donors.[8]

Additionally, it has been established that graft survival rates are significantly better overall for living donor than for cadaver organs. For transplants performed between 1995 through 2002, the five-year survival rate for kidney transplants was 78.6 percent for living donors compared to 65.5 percent for cadaveric donors. For liver transplants, the five-year survival rate was 70.8 percent for living donors compared to 64.4 percent for cadaveric donors.[9] These comparative survival rates encourage doctors and patients to pursue living rather than cadaveric donors. The phenomenon could also explain why the annual number of living donors of kidneys steadily rose in the United States at the turn of the century and even exceeded the number of cadaver donors at some point.[10] In the Philippines, kidney transplants have been hugely sourced from living donors (Manauis et al. 2008; Mendoza 2010).

The ever-growing number of patients throughout the world who are in need of transplantable organs is obviously a source of growing pressure that extends to possible organ donors, related or unrelated. As the number of people throughout the world with ESRD has continued to rise, the number of kidneys that become available for transplantation has not proportionately risen, leaving a widening gap between need and availability. People are dying while waiting to receive organs. The mortality rate for people on waiting lists ranges from 5 to 30 percent depending on country and type of organ (Miranda and Matesanz 1998). This gap cannot even come close to being filled by the ability and willingness of genetically related donors. Instead, advances in biomedical science and technology have provided ways of addressing the gap (but not necessarily narrowing it) without remaining dependent on the genetic family as the comparable success of transplants from living unrelated renal donors has indicated.

---

[8] All Kaplan-Meier Patient Survival Rates For Transplants Performed: 1995–2002. Based on Organ Procurement and Transplantation Network data as of March 11, 2005 (OPTN 2005a). This work was supported in part by Health Resources and Services Administration contract 231-00-0115. The content is the responsibility of the authors alone and does not necessarily reflect the views or policies of the Department of Health and Human Services, nor does mention of trade names, commercial products, or organizations imply endorsement by the US government.

[9] All Kaplan-Meier Patient Survival Rates For Transplants Performed: 1995–2002. Based on Organ Procurement and Transplantation Network data as of March 11, 2005 (OPTN 2005a). This work was supported in part by Health Resources and Services Administration contract 231-00-0115. The content is the responsibility of the authors alone and does not necessarily reflect the views or policies of the Department of Health and Human Services, nor does mention of trade names, commercial products, or organizations imply endorsement by the US government.

[10] Donors Recovered in the US by Donor Type. Based on Organ Procurement and Transplantation Network data, accessed on February 17, 2005 (OPTN 2005b). This work was supported in part by Health Resources and Services Administration contract 231-00-0115. The content is the responsibility of the authors alone and does not necessarily reflect the views or policies of the Department of Health and Human Services, nor does mention of trade names, commercial products, or organizations imply endorsement by the US government.

Growing human interdependence

These developments foreshadow an expanding sphere of interdependence among human beings in matters of health in general and, in particular, in medical matters that can be addressed by organ transplantation. Rightly or wrongly, patients have been travelling to find organ donors, organ donors have been travelling to places outside their own countries in response to others' needs, transplantable organs have been flown across national boundaries in order to be made available to patients in need, and doctors have done their own travelling in order to provide services. Indeed, some of the travelling has taken place—and continues to take place—under suspicious (if not clearly reprehensible) circumstances. Good or bad, these developments indicate a perception of an enlarging sphere of interdependence—of people looking beyond their immediate families or community boundaries to seek help or to respond to the needs of others.

There was a time when the willingness to make a direct contribution with transplant organs was expected only among close relatives. With widespread public awareness of the options for organ donation being made possible by advanced technology the call for contributions is now extending way beyond the confines of the recipient's genetic family.

For a while, kidney patients thought their chances of getting a lease on life or a better quality of life rested exclusively on the availability of cadaver donors or living related donors. Now they have a reason to seek contributions from non-relatives. On the other hand, there are people whose lives would not ordinarily have been relevant to others. Somehow, those lives have become relevant. Modern technology has made it possible for them to provide much-needed assistance. In the context of globalization and modern technology, people who were previously distant and uninvolved have been afforded an opportunity to be close and involved. People who would not have been regarded as having a role in the treatment of particular patients in the past are now seeing the burden of helping to save or extend lives by organ transplantation offered to them.

In effect, the genetic distance between pairs of non-related patients and donors is being bridged. Parties that may have been previously distant and genetically unrelated are being drawn closer together by the essential health need of one party and the capacity of the other to fill that need. The genetic distance is being bridged by advances in science and technology, resulting in increased interdependence among unrelated persons in this area of critical care.

Extended family: extended moral responsibility?

Where there is a prevailing culture of extended families, one could expect society to be more accepting of living non-related organ transplantation. People from such societies have been willing to extend the boundaries of family care and interdependence beyond the genetic family. Helpers, maids, drivers, unemployed distant relatives and in-laws, friends, and associates could all be part of an extended family. When they are, they could be drawn even closer to one another by the need for an organ on the part of one and the ability and willingness to meet that need on the part of another. This combination of factors creates the natural context for relationships of interdependence and reciproc-ity. Some of these relationships could be founded on a sense of gratitude for past favors received or for long-standing dependencies. In some societies, the recognition of a debt of gratitude could be equated with a recognition of responsibility for a lifetime. It means a lifetime of being beholden. This is the reason why the bonds can be sealed even more tightly than genetic ties. Neither the chauffeur in case example 1 nor the helper and her family in case example 2 could be held back by a rule limiting organ donation to rela-tives. Within their culture, they consider themselves and the recipients of their donated organs part of the same family. Thus, the search for an organ donor is not taking place in an unfamiliar territory. In the kind of setting described, it occurs as a normal event often beyond the radar of moral criticism. This could explain the observation that in a number of societies, the implementation of laws limiting organ donation to close rela-tives appears to have stalled. These laws have been widely breached, misunderstood, and unappreciated.

This is not to say that extended families are taking the place of genetically rooted core relationships. Genetic relationships are at the center of varying levels of attach-ment defining the interdependence and responsibilities of specific members. Many of us are familiar with the coercion that immediate family members could be subjected to when one of them is discovered to be in need of an organ transplant. Often, there is strong pressure on parents, children, or siblings to have themselves tested for compat-ibility and, if appropriate, to donate an organ. In some cases, we have seen a need to mitigate the effects of such pressures in order to enable an individual's expression of self-determination. Yet, while it is useful to avoid the coercive impact of external factors, it would also be necessary to acknowledge that many family members have to deal with internal pressures that they impose on themselves as they acknowledge a responsibility to come to the aid of a loved one.

What is especially significant about internal pressures imposed by individuals on themselves is that these constitute an acknowledgement of responsibility transcending genetic boundaries. The example of the chauffeur who donated a kidney to his employ-er in the first case described above illustrates this acknowledgement of responsibility. It shows a closeness that transcends genetic kinship. The same can probably be said of the former helper in the second case example, in that the motivation to donate an organ could, at least in part, be attributed to an emotional bond. Such acknowledgement of responsibility beyond the immediate family—or even beyond an extended family—confirms the expanding sphere of interdependence and reciprocity. The first two case examples illustrate a degree of relationship that could easily be higher compared to a genetically based relationship such as that described in case example 3.

This does not mean that the emotional bond between the individuals concerned can always be presumed to give rise to equitable and just undertakings. The balance of power among the parties involved can be so uneven that the weaker one is taken advantage of. An exploitative relationship may arise because of the presence of such fac-tors as inadequate or misleading information, the one-sided nature of benefits, or the use of coercive force. As a result, the strain on the living donor paradigm could become unbearable and an organ donation could thus be exploitative. Obviously, the nature of the emotional bond when there is an offer of a donation has to be closely examined. The newspapers are not lacking in accounts of exploitation being perpetrated on organ donors under such circumstances. Case example 4 and case example 5 are representative of many experiences that have been anecdotally reported and statistically accounted for in various publications. Warnings such as those made by Aulisio et al. have to be heeded if unrelated transplants are not to be exploitative.

However, when the interdependence and reciprocity are founded on equality and justice, one should also wonder why public policy or the law should step in and prohibit a life-saving or quality-enhancing organ donation. Prohibiting organ donation from non-relatives under such circumstances fails to recognize the fact that contemporary society has transcended the genetic paradigm for the family. This kind of policy would effectively penalize possible recipients of transplantable organs and would thus be unethical. Genetic ties aside, emotional bonds among non-relatives could be just as strong, if not even stronger than, those that prevail among family members. The implications of these for contemporary society have to be recognized and appreciated.

The main point is that the sense of responsibility that relates to organ donation cannot be confined only to the genetic family. Arising from the realization (1) that there is another person requiring help, (2) that the person requiring help is someone with whom the prospective donor is related in a special way, and (3) that the prospective donor is in a unique position to provide the help needed, this sense of responsibility is capable of flourishing outside as well as inside a genetically based kinship. This conclusion arises more strongly as we are now told that blood relatives are not necessarily more medically suitable donors if only because of the great advances in anti-rejection drugs.

The fact that blood relationship has been rendered minimally significant for the medical success of organ transplants puts into question genetically rooted conceptions of the family. Genetic relationships continue to play a special role in the way that human beings relate to one another. However, there are specific concerns that have begun to transcend genetically centered interpretations. As social beings, human beings have learned to engage in emotive relationships that transcend blood ties. It would be wrong to continue to predicate organ transplant policies primarily on genetic relationships. While there is a need to be wary of commercially motivated "kinships," this wariness must be tempered by openness to emerging types of human bonds and to flexible conceptions of the family.

Moreover, it is about time that human beings looked at the emerging pressures in terms of the challenge to extend the frontiers of human responsibility beyond the boundaries set by genetics and limited reciprocities.

To some extent, the family is a social unit for reproduction. In the face of assisted means of reproduction, the family paradigm is already facing challenges. Other challenges haunt that paradigm in other areas of biotechnology and health care. It appears that those challenges require flexibility in defining the boundaries that define membership of a family. Among other things, the frontiers of interdependence, reciprocity, and responsibility are having to be adjusted. Responsibility for health concerns is extending way beyond genetic family borders. This is an empirical fact that will continue to exist whether we recognize it or not.

References

Aulisio, M. et al. (2014). "Ethics Without Borders? Why *The Unites States* Needs an International Dialogue on Living Organ Donation," in A. Akabayashi (ed.), *The Future of Bioethics: International Dialogues.* Oxford: Oxford University Press, 449–60.

Gjertson, D. W., and Cecka, J. M. (2000). "Living Unrelated Donor Kidney Transplantation," *Kidney International*, 58:496–7.

Humar, A. et al. (2000). "Living Unrelated Donors in Kidney Transplants: Better Long-Term Results than with Non-HLA-Identical Living Related Donors?" *Transplantation*, 69(9): 1942–5.

Keown, P. (2001). "Improving the Quality of Life: The New Target for Transplantation," *Transplantation*, 72:567–74.

Manauis, M. N. et al. (2008). "A National Program for Nondirected Kidney Donation from Living Unrelated Donors: The Philippine Experience," *Transplantation Proceedings*, 40:2100–3.

Mendoza, R. L. (2010). "Kidney Black Markets and Legal Transplants: Are They Opposite Sides of the Same Coin?" *Health Policy*, 94:255–65.

Miranda, B. et al. (2003). "Organ Shortage and the Organization of Organ Allocation," *European Respiratory Monograph*, 26:62–77.

Miranda, B., and Matesanz, R. (1998). "International Issues in Transplantation: Setting the Scene and Flagging the Most Urgent and Controversial Issues," *Annals of the New York Academy of Sciences*, 862:129–43.

Organ Procurement and Transplantation Network (OPTN). (2005a). "All Kaplan-Meier Patient Survival Rates for Transplants Performed: 1995–2002 Based on OPTN data as of March 11, 2005," http://optn.transplant.hrsa.gov/latestData/step2.asp (accessed March 15, 2005).

Organ Procurement and Transplantation Network (OPTN). (2005b). "Donors Recovered in the US by Donor Type," http://optn.transplant.hrsa.gov/latestData/step2.asp (accessed February 17, 2005).

Salaverria, L. (2007). "It Feels Good to Help: Gonzalez's Kidney Donor," *Philippine Daily Inquirer*, September 18, http://newsinfo.inquirer.net/breakingnews/metro/view/20070918-89345/percent91It_feels_good_to_help percent92--Gonzalez percent92s_kidney_donor (accessed January 19, 2013).

Sinforoosh et al. (2006). "Living Unrelated versus Living Related Kidney Transplantation: 20 Years' Experience with 2155 Cases," *Transplantation Proceedings*, 38(2): 422–5.

13.5

Response to Commentaries

Donna L. Luebke, Nicole M. Deming, Rachel Phetteplace, and Mark P. Aulisio

We thank Drs. Farhat Moazam, Yohei Akaida, Kohji Ishihara, and Leonardo D. de Castro for their commentaries on "Ethics Without Borders? Why the United States Needs an International Dialogue on Living Organ Donation." Our goal was to generate a conversation on the many issues surrounding organ donation by highlighting the ethical challenges in living organ donation in the US; recognizing that there will be both differences and similarities among countries. Our paper outlines our concerns regarding the current transplant situation in our country and offers a perspective on the stretching and straining occurring within our borders so as to open international dialogue within an ethics framework. Due to pressure to increase the donor pool in both developed and developing countries, we must continue to challenge the suggested practices to increase donation and never assume that living donation is a "resolved" issue.

Although we have had an organized system of organ donation and transplantation since the National Organ Transplant Act (NOTA) of 1984 created the Organ Procurement and Transplantation Network (OPTN), the promise of NOTA was never realized. The promise was that an unlimited pool of deceased donor organs existed and would be readily available once we organized our system of procurement and allocation. This same promise is being used today regarding kidney and liver transplants—only the unlimited supply is now the living. In 2006, the US Department of Health and Human Services Health Resources Services Administration added to the OPTN's responsibility calling for the development of living donor policies with emphasis on donor safety. To date there are no living donor policies, especially with regard to medical evaluation (suitability) and informed consent (http://optn.transplant.hrsa.gov).

In 2007, two key initiatives were put forth here in the US. The Centers for Medicare and Medicaid Services (CMS) Rules and Regulations for Transplant Programs, Final Rule mandated an independent donor advocate to assure proper donor evaluation and consent. In addition, transplant programs were required per mandatory policy (OPTN Final Rule) to submit donor follow-up data for 24 months post donation (previously 12 months). Assessment of risks and complications has been hampered by incomplete submissions of follow-up data. The obligation to submit follow-up data was previously met by designating the donor as "lost to follow-up" or even returning an empty form. Of the 6,732 living donors who donated an organ in 2006, more than 30 percent were lost to follow-up with some centers declaring no available follow-up for 100 percent of their donors (Klein et al. 2010: 973–86).

Historically, the supply of organs suitable for transplantation from deceased donors has not kept pace with the demand (especially for kidneys). In the US, efforts to "promote" living organ donation include getting organs from non-familial or non-related donors, anonymous donors, and publicly solicited donors—from public appeals via the media to bulletin boards and the Internet. Davis and Cooper (2010: 1873–80) note a dramatic change in the relationship between live donors and their recipients (1988–2008) as we have moved beyond blood and genetics. Axelrod et al. present the "changing face of living donation" (Axelrod et al. 2010: 987–1002) and suggest the transplant community focus on increasing living donors and "consider greater economic support" for donors. Additional efforts to expand living organ donation include desensitization protocols, a movement toward a national paired kidney donation program, donor chains, and acceptance of expanded criteria or marginal live donors which includes those who are older, obese, or even with hypertension. These trends and suggestions raise concerns that the transplant community is desensitized to the dangers of live donation to the donor and instead focus primarily on the benefit to the recipient. As the demographics of live donors change and the motivation for donation is less explicable by the nature of familiar relationships, we must be sensitive to how these changes impact the ethical issues of transplantation both on an individual patient level and on a larger scale. As Drs. Akaida and Ishihara stated, "the justification of living organ donation remains an ethical challenge" and we must be vigilant in responding to changes in practice. We want to help the recipient without undue threat to the donor.

Creating high standards regarding the proper consent and evaluation of donors is a necessary step to promote ethical live donation, but it is not sufficient. As Dr. de Castro made clear in his case examples, a wide range of relationship exists between donors and recipients. The dynamics in these donor–recipient relationships are an important piece when trying to understand the motivations for live donation and often play a key role in determining whether a donation is ethical or an abuse of power. If the transplant community does not seek answers to the question of why a donor volunteers to donate, then we are being responsible for the harm that results from our willful ignorance.

While we highlighted the lack of attention to the long-term health and well-being of living organ donors and the absence of national registries, we are not alone in this regard (Emara et al. 2008: 525–31). As shared by Moazam, it is only recently that the transplant community is discussing donor issues at international meetings such as those that took place in Amsterdam (2004), Vancouver (2005), Istanbul (2008), and Madrid (2010). The primary objective of the forums in Amsterdam and Vancouver was to develop an international standard of care for the living organ donor. Despite a clear recognition of need, these robust standards for evaluation and consent still do not exist. Attention to the health and well-being of live organ donors (most specifically, the live kidney donor) is not new, as noted by the Council of the Transplantation Society in 1985 (Council of the Transplantation Society 1985: 715–16) and the Live Organ Donor Consensus Group in 2000 (The Live Organ Donor Consensus Group 2000: 1–11). We offer that another reason for "recent" discussion is increased public awareness that: living donation is "not always heartwarming" when donors suffer adverse events like ESRD or death (Shelton

2009; Cherikh et al. 2009; Segev et al. 2010: 959–66; Zoler 2011); there is little data on which to base consent in the absence of donor registries which track both short- and long-term outcome (Ommen, Winston, and Murphy 2006: 1873–80); and there is increased concern for those donor populations at risk by racial variations (Lentine et al. 2010: 724–32).

In Pakistan and Japan the emphasis is on the family and implied moral obligations; where duty to others prevails over autonomy. However, generalizations only help identify what is common, not what is occurring in a specific situation. We acknowledge the diversity among patients' values but remain convinced that these values must be discovered rather than presumed. The benefit of using the principle of autonomy to justify this position is that the authority and knowledge reside in the patient (donor or recipient), not the health-care professional.

The Live Organ Donor Consensus Group (Abecassis et al. 2000: 2919–26) concluded that the live organ donor be competent, willing to donate, free of coercion…yet in Pakistan the physician plays an active role along with the family as to who should be the donor. According to Moazam, the physician is a coaxer or cajoler. Moazam later recommends the use of a wider lens beyond autonomy and individual rights—one with focus on kinship, religious beliefs and values, and prevailing socio-economic system. We would argue that the donor should remain as the focal point in the picture even when viewed with a wider lens that incorporates the larger social context. Allowing the recipient or religious norms greater consideration over another individual's right violates the duty and care owed to the donor. The idea of physicians using their knowledge and positions of power to coax or cajole donors is an extremely uncomfortable description of the doctor–patient relationship.

Our use of the word "patient" when describing a healthy donor is intentional. Moazam says that a patient is someone who needs care or treatment and concludes that live donors do not fit this definition. We disagree. Healthy individuals that see physicians for annual checkups are and should be considered patients. Physicians are obligated to use their knowledge for the benefit of the patient whether healthy or unwell. A physician's fiduciary duty and duty to care do not diminish as a patient gets healthier; these duties are constant. The term "patient" arises as a result of the relationship between the doctor and the patient, not the amount of services provided by the doctor to the patient. Potential donors are patients when they enter a health-care system (transplant hospital) for evaluation. They continue to be patients when they undergo surgery (nephrectomy) and when they are recovering from the surgery. Some may even argue that living organ donors are patients for the rest of their lives. The failure to afford live donors the rights and protections granted to patients seems to be a major hurdle in establishing long-term follow-up programs or donor registries. Donors have not been viewed as in need of care, and as a result, have been classified as unworthy of care.

Where do we go from here?

Moazam comments that the emphasis is on increasing the supply of organs with little attention to demand. The Madrid Resolution has changed the tone. Each nation is encouraged to meet the health-care needs of its people in a comprehensive manner and to address those conditions that lead to end-stage organ disease, from prevention to treatment. Every country should proceed through regulated and ethical regional and international cooperation. Deceased donation should be maximized where possible and living donation seen as complementary (WHO Principles 2011: S29–31).

Moazam also shares that in the case of living donation harm can at best be minimized but never eliminated...and the potential for harm increases as one moves on the scale from related to unrelated donors, and from the altruistic donor to the kidney vendor. In conclusion, we echo and support the recommendation to shift from the perception of organ donation as a matter of rights of donors and recipients to one of shared responsibility and solidarity across all levels of society and across all borders.

de Castro states that preventing non-relatives from donating fails to recognize that contemporary society transcends the genetic paradigm for the family. We need to be open to emerging types of human bonds and to a flexible conception of family/friendship. There is growing human interdependence—people looking beyond immediate family for help or to respond to the needs of others. The flexible conception of family and friendship establishes a greater need to examine the donor–recipient relationship rather than rely upon traditional definitions and our presumption regarding the motivations for donation.

We end with a response to Akaida and Ishihara. They say we argue that living donation should be carried out according to the highest standards and permitted to exceed the limitations of autonomy but offer no rationale. We did not argue for living donation based on autonomy but presented the US model that often uses autonomy to justify a patient's choice or action on the basis that the individual most affected should have the power to decide. However, this traditional use of autonomy fails in the context of live donation because of the high degree of involvement of other parties (health-care professionals) in causing the harm to the individual.

We look forward to continuing these discussions and learning from our colleagues in the future.

References

Abecassis, M. et al. (2000). "Consensus Statement on the Live Organ Donor," *Journal of the American Medical Association*, 284(22): 2919–26.

Axelrod, D. A., et al. (2010). "Kidney and Pancreas Transplantation in the United States, 1999–2008: The Changing Face of Living Donation," *American Journal of Transplantation*, 10(Part 2): 987–1002.

Cherikh, W. S. et al. (2009). "Prior Living Kidney Donors Subsequently Placed on Waiting List: An Organ Procurement and Transplantation Network (OPTN) Analysis," *ASMHTP Annual Meeting*. Las Vegas, NV, September 25, 2009.

Davis, C. L., and Cooper, M. (2010). "The State of U. S. Living Kidney Donors," *Clinical Journal of the American Society of Nephrology*, 5(10): 1873–80.

Emara, M. et al. (2008). "Evidence for a Need to Mandate Kidney Transplant Living Donor Registries," *Clinical Transplantation*, 22: 525–31.

Klein, A. S. et al. (2010). "Organ Donation and Utilization in the United States, 1999–2008," *Americal Journal of Transplantation*, 10(2): 973–86.

Lentine, K. L. et al. (2010). "Racial Variation in Medical Outcomes among Living Kidney Donors," *New England Journal of Medicine*, 363(8): 724–32.

Ommen, E. S., Winston, J. A., and Murphy, B. (2006). "Medical Risks in Living Kidney Donors: Absence of Proof Is Not Proof of Absence," *Clinical Journal of the American Society of Nephrology*, 5:1873–80.

Segev, D. L. et al. (2010). "Following Live Kidney Donation Perioperative Mortality and Long-term Survival," *JAMA*, 303(10): 959–66.

Shelton, D. L. (2009). "Living Organ Donations: Not Always Heartwarming Human Interest Stories," *University of California Annenburg School of Communication*. http://www.reportingonhealth.org/resources/lessons/live-organ-donations (accessed December 11, 2012).

The Council of the Transplantation Society. (1985). "Commercialisation in Transplantation: The Problem and Some Guidelines for Practice," *Lancet*, 2(8457): 715–6.

The Live Organ Donor Consensus Group. (2000). "Consensus Statement on the Live Organ Donor," *JAMA*, 284:1–11.

The WHO Principles. (2011). "The Madrid Resolution on Organ Donation and Transplantation: National Responsibility in Meeting the Needs of Patients," *Transplantation*, June 15, 91(Supplement 11): S29–31.

Zoler, M. (2011). Kidney Donor Death Highlights Lingering Clip Ligation Problem, International Medicine News Digital Network.

14.1

Primary Topic Article
The Future of Altruistic Medicine

Jacqueline J. L. Chin

Contemporary medicine and the value of altruism

Altruism, as a fundamental value of medicine, has become an idea of substantial complexity in our time. For over 50 years, altruism has been studied and debated in a wide range of medical contexts, including voluntary participation of healthy persons in clinical trials; donation of blood, organs, stem cells, gametes, and genetic materials; and in addressing challenges to medical professionalism in doctors' dealings with patients (Steinberg 2010: 249).

Altruistic behaviour has reported psychological benefits for actors such as healthy research volunteers or body donors, in enhancing their self-respect through free and beneficent actions (Westlie et al. 1993: 1146; Schover et al. 1997: 1596; Johnson et al. 1999: 717; Vlaovic et al. 1999: 859; Corley et al. 2000: 43; Jansen 2009: 26). Some argue that nudging families, communities, and whole populations to act altruistically for the sake of common interests, while guaranteeing substantial forms of freedom to act, is indispensable for the long-term survival of affective ties, a collective conscience, and pro-social behaviour extending beyond kinship and particularistic community ties (Titmuss 1971; Murray 1987: 30; Voo 2011). In addition, the value of altruism has been viewed as central to understanding medicine as a profession and social service for the universal benefit of the vulnerable sick (Relman 2007: 2668).

Conversely, many altruistic acts may be misdirected (Steinbrook 2006: 324), unduly pressurizing for individuals (Kaplan and Williams 2007: 497; Scheper-Hughes 2007: 507), compulsively or otherwise unreasonably heroic (Knibbe and Verkerk 2010: 149). Certainly, altruism has served as a euphemism for exploitative acts (Raymond 1990: 7) and legal fictions (Epstein and Danovitch 2009: 357). There is also much current debate over which acts, be they forms of donation or medical services, should be 'purely altruistic' (uncompensated by material considerations), 'predominantly altruistic' (mixed with some compensation), or commercialized for public benefit (Steinberg 2010: 249), and how altruistic behaviour would be affected by being mixed together with commercial elements (Arrow 1975: 13; Etzioni 1998; Archard 2002: 87; Schweda and Schicktanz 2009: 1129).

Thus, altruism in medicine is not an unmitigated good and warrants ethical scrutiny within the agenda of bioethics (Steinberg 2010: 249). A contemporary ethics of altruism will be defined by many issues, which may be summarized here as follows:

1. How medicine as an altruistic profession might justify the imposition of serious risk on healthy individuals through imperatives to participate in research or in body donations for saving the health of others; what the nature and extent of acceptable risk are for consenting altruists, and what methodologies may be used for making such determinations. Over and above physical harms, the nature of risk in body donations, given the body's significance beyond an individual's disposition towards it, differs in offers made by universal altruists and by family members. The acts of altruistic strangers create forms of relationship with attendant normative implications that should be studied and better understood. Family donations create distinctive risks whose impact on decision-making, family ties, and family ethics point to new and critical areas of research. Methodologies for determining acceptable risk in these domains are also emerging.

2. Whether altruism is for everybody: who may be found suitable for accepting altruistic risks, whether solicitation of altruists is appropriate, and how the nature of informed consent for altruists is to be characterized. For instance, presumed consent regimes for organ donation have been confronted with diverse cultural understandings of the meaning of the body, including solid organs, tissues, and regenerative parts of bodies. This has drawn attention to the need for procurement and/or legislative systems to consult with indigenous groups in order to frame appropriate parameters and boundaries for solicitation of altruists in accordance with their cultural and religious beliefs and world views.

3. What provisions should be made for preventing harm to altruists; the methodologies to determine harms and benefits to such individuals; and means and standards of monitoring, regulation, and oversight that should be in place to protect them. This concerns inquiry into what forms of reciprocal obligation fall upon systems that are placing demands on individuals to act altruistically. In mitigating harms to altruists, professional standards of care and risk assessment must be guaranteed before donation, and access to follow-up care should take a high priority within these systems. Interestingly, it has been an unexpected consequence of organ donation that the health of donors in some developed countries has been found to improve post donation (Westlie et al. 1993: 1146; Corley et al. 2000: 43). But the question of rewards and benefits (which has stirred animated debate in psychology, biology, sociology, and philosophy on how far the term altruism is a coherent description of actions taken by individual agents for the benefit of others) has no generalizable answer at this juncture, but seems to require contemporary and sociologically informed accounts of non-exploitation that operate in actual and relevant social settings across different societies.

4. How best to procure, allocate, and reciprocate the benefits of altruism; whether altruism and commercialism should mix, and what that might do to motivation and agency in the public domain. Some benefits of altruism, as earlier mentioned, include benefits to the needy, and psychological and reputational (and from this,

often material) benefits for altruistic individuals; other potential benefits include social cohesiveness, social trust, and freedom (for individuals, and collectives such as a family or religious order) to pursue higher-than-ordinary moral attainments. Should benefits for the needy be directed or non-directed, and who should have the power of allocation? What forms of reciprocation, and by whom, would best enable the sustained circulation of altruism's benefits?

Against this overview of emerging concerns regarding the value of altruism, this essay explores the possibilities for altruistic medicine in one sphere by presenting a case study within the challenging arena of transplant tourism. Our reason for selecting transplant tourism for discussion in this volume on the future of bioethics is that it combines the problems of globalization, commercialization, and the increasing bodily invasion that is entailed by modern medicine (key areas would include reproductive tourism, biological enhancement, clinical trials, biobanking, and large-scale genetic research); these problems, along with the enduring question of altruism in medicine, can be expected to remain live issues in the next 50 years.

Medical tourism: benefits, hazards, and the case for better practices

Travel for organ transplantation is a special category of the increasingly significant practice of cross-border medical treatment dubbed 'medical tourism' that has burgeoned in the past decade. The term 'medical tourism' denotes travel by persons from one country to another for medical care or treatment. In the past, this commonly referred to visits abroad to health spas and resorts for convalescence or to seek rare medical expertise that was unavailable in one's own country, and would often include rest and recreation. Medical tourism ballooned in the last decade, and was estimated in 2010 to be a US $100 billion industry worldwide, including all procedures ranging from cosmetic enhancements to transplants. This development has been attributed to greater freedom of movement of goods and services globally, ease of international travel for affluent patients, and availability of information on the Internet with regard to health care in countries that have made the export of lucrative health services a focus of their economies. Patients are seeking health services abroad due to the unavailability of domestic expertise, lack of coverage by health insurance and long waiting times at home, and lower costs for health services and expertise in emerging economies. From the receiving country's point of view, export of health services generates revenue for investments in national public health-care infrastructures and technologies, providing advanced training for local health-care professionals, and introducing new management techniques including quality management regimes and professional regulatory requirements. Many countries, including Canada, India, Singapore, Thailand, the United Kingdom, and the United States, have spawned 'medical brokerage' businesses advertising affordable procedures, health care, and recreation to international patients. These entities include private companies, individual hospitals, private hospital chains, and in some cases, well coordinated private–public initiatives coordinated by governments.

The ethical risks of medical tourism have been well documented (Pennings 2007). The Global Agreement on Trade in Services (GATS) has tried to liberalize four modes of trade in health services: overseas consumption, movements of skilled personnel and service providers, direct cross-border trade in professional services (telemedicine), and foreign direct investment in health care and health insurance. These developments have disrupted local health-care provision for citizens in a variety of ways.

1. They have spurred an outmigration of skilled professionals and trained health-care providers from exporting countries to receiving countries that are establishing themselves as health-care 'hubs', thereby compromising health-care capabilities at home in some countries, and non-reciprocation of a duty on the part of professionals to the communities that have invested in their training.

2. Within 'hub' countries, a migration of health-care professionals from public to private health-care facilities to service a growing foreign pool of fee-for-service patients can create an imbalance between private and public health-care provisioning. This threatens to compromise the principles of:

    a. universal health provision on the basis of need rather than ability to pay;[1]
    b. non-discrimination in relation to the quality of health-care provision for financially subsidized domestic populations versus foreign paying populations;[2]
    c. prioritizing public health, preventive medicine, primary health care, and other essential community health services over investments in non-essential but lucrative high-tech treatment procedures that are revenue-generating means to improving overall health-care provision, but threaten overconsumption and waste of critical national resources.

3. Medical tourism, if relied on as a quick solution to serious flaws in the domestic health-care provisioning of certain countries, may impede needed reform within those jurisdictions. For example, unreasonable waiting times, or weak government controls over private investor-owned businesses that sell health insurance and deliver medical care with a view to maximizing income are already fuelling runaway health costs, and putting pressure on some national health budgets. Sending patients overseas for cheaper health care of uncertain quality would spell an abdication of the duty of states to provide safe and reliable health care for their citizens.

4. Within professional practice, quality of health care may be compromised by both physical and cultural distance between doctors and patients.

---

[1] Some countries have successful two-tier health systems that strive to capture a range of benchmarks of fairness based on WHO criteria of equity of access to care, quality of care, and efficient use of resources. Extended criteria have been developed by Norman Daniels and colleagues: 1. Reducing exposure to health and other risk factors; 2. Limiting financial barriers to equitable access to health care; 3. Limiting non-financial barriers to access the comprehensiveness of benefits and tiering; 4. Equitable financing; 5. Efficacy; 6. Efficiency; 7. Quality of care; 8. Democratic accountability; 9. Patient and provider autonomy (Daniels et al. 2000: 74).

[2] Limiting the size of the tourism sector and selecting the range of health services and medical procedures available are approaches in response to b. and c.

5. Some categories of medical tourism pose special problems of law evasion. In addition to the common reasons of unavailability, higher cost, and longer waiting time, some patients travel for treatment because certain types of medical procedures are domestically outlawed or legally cumbersome; have yet to be certified safe; or are denied to certain categories of persons on account of socially and administratively sanctioned norms. The availability of cross-border treatment increases autonomy, but may also mean law evasion, and increase in exploitative or criminal activities.

Travel for transplantation might, or might not, fall within the special category of medical tourism described at 5 (Budiani-Saberi and Delmonico 2008: 925). Some international transplant practices are legal and appropriate such as when, under vigilant regulation and oversight by recognized authorities, donor and recipient pairs travel from countries without transplant services to those with the required expertise, or when individuals travel to donate or receive a transplant made possible by a relative, universal donor, or under a paired-exchange agreement or reciprocal organ-sharing programme. However, *transplant tourism* has been associated with increased exploitation, syndicated crime, and the use of law to mask illegal activities. Indeed, there has been a tendency in the literature to *define* the term transplant tourism by its *risks and hazards* rather than its essential activities. For example, the United Network for Organ Sharing (UNOS) has defined transplant tourism as 'the purchase of a transplant organ abroad that includes access to an organ while bypassing laws, rules or processes of any or all countries involved' (Barr et al. 2006: 1373). Likewise, the Declaration of Istanbul (DOI) states that *travel for transplantation,* which it defines as 'the movement of organs, donors, recipients, or transplant professionals across jurisdictional borders for transplantation purposes', 'becomes *transplant tourism* if it involves organ trafficking and/or transplant commercialism or if the resources (organs, professionals, and transplant centers) devoted to providing transplants to patients from outside a country undermine the country's ability to provide transplant services for its own population' (Participants in the Istanbul Summit 2008: 1227).

The confused positions represented here have not been helpful, for they have been ineffective for stemming transplant tourism which is, arguably, an integral part of the policies for economic and scientific development in many countries. Instead, a regulated practice of international transplant medicine might be defined by the following activities:

1. The movement of organs, donors, recipients, or transplant professionals across jurisdictional borders for transplantation purposes ('travel for transplantation', as defined by DOI).
2. Brokerage activities (transplant commercialism), though not necessarily organ sales (commodification of the body, the main idea defining 'transplant commercialism' in DOI) or organ trafficking ('the recruitment, transport, transfer, harboring or receipt of living or deceased persons or their organs by means of the threat or use of force or other forms of coercion, of abduction, of fraud, of deception, of the abuse of power or of a position of vulnerability, or of the giving to, or the receiving by, a third party of payments or benefits to achieve the transfer of control over the potential donor, for the purpose of exploitation by the removal of organs for transplantation', as defined in DOI).

3. Transplant surgery and medical treatment in a foreign jurisdiction for at least one of the parties, which *could well be* lawful in that jurisdiction and subject to regulation and professional scrutiny.

Those who oppose transplant tourism recommend a global ban on transplant tourism (Participants in the Istanbul Summit 2008: 1227; Turner 2008: 101; Epstein 2009: 134). They rightly point out that, among the many forms of medical tourism, it poses special dangers and risks which include the following:

1. Transplant tourism creates a strong demand for transplantable organs and magnifies the risk of organ trafficking and exploitation of the poor in the receiving countries and their hinterland.
2. It has been noted that in spite of enacting legislation to curb organ trading in countries such as India, Pakistan, and Colombia, trafficking persists because of the marketing of 'all-inclusive' transplant packages which procure organs for transplantation on behalf of the receiving patient.
3. Research on donor welfare shows that they receive substandard medical care following nephrectomy, suffer a decline in self-assessed health status, and those who receive payments in compensation for their 'donation' experience no long-term benefits.
4. Governments and professional institutions such as hospitals are ethically compromised by their causal role in the problems of trafficking, related crimes, and failure to guarantee donor welfare, which can be arguably eliminated by ceasing to practise transplant tourism.
5. States may be faulted for inequities in treatment of citizens and foreign patients if attention is directed towards transplant tourism activities rather than achieving national self-sufficiency.

Transplant tourism does indeed pose significant risks. Like some aspects of reproductive tourism (such as discrimination against girls and exploitation of women), it carries special risks to bodily integrity and increases exploitation of the economically disadvantaged. However, this fact alone may be insufficient reason to impose a ban on transplant tourism on a global scale. Greater proliferation of such medical options internationally is a likely future prospect (Pennings 2002: 337). Can a systematic examination of the kinds of risks involved pave the way for transforming the present landscape of transplant tourism into ethically robust practices of international transplant medicine? Might reflecting on altruistic medicine serve to deepen scholarly and practical understanding of what is at stake?

In a personal viewpoint published in the *American Journal of Transplantation,* I described aspects of Singapore's fledgling attempt at a coordinated strategy for addressing the ethical issues posed in receiving foreign patients for live transplants, and set about an examination of the risks of its being exploited by some international patients and/or operatives of illegal organ markets. In this essay, I revisit Singapore's hybrid ethical position, which attempts to combine national development needs with an ethics of altruistic donation (a reimbursement-only model proposed by DOI), and consider how some recent thinking might provide directions for addressing important gaps (and indeed, describing what these are) within a purported practice of altruistic medicine.

Transplant medicine in Singapore: priorities and ethical responsibilities

Economic and social progress, and ethical responsibilities

After an initial miscalculation of its role in the emerging global 'value chain' of contemporary medicine, transplant medicine is now considered by policy, economic, and health-care elites in Singapore to be an indispensable part of Singapore's bid to become a global biomedical hub. Performing living donor transplants for foreign patients is not ostensibly aimed at increasing supply of organs for local and international patients, but rather to generate a large enough patient load in excess of local streams for cultivating expertise and retaining medical talent. In addition, procedures like transplant surgery are on the high end of the value chain, generating profits that could be used for building public health infrastructures and improving the quality of medical care for all. Authorities reckon that failure to achieve these goals in professional medicine would turn Singapore into a 'backwater', undermining the quality and ultimately the integrity of its health-care system (Lee 2006: 11; Turner 2007: 303).

To increase the supply of organs, two separate pieces of legislation have been designed to address the organ shortages and to govern their procurement within a multicultural and multi-religious society: the Medical (Therapy, Research and Education) Act 1972 (MTERA) and the Human Organ Transplant Act 1987 (HOTA).

Under the provisions of s7 of the MTERA, persons have the legal right to donate parts of their body to approved hospitals, medical or dental schools, colleges, or universities for 'medical or dental education, research, advancement of medical or dental science, therapy or transplantation' or to 'any specified individual for therapy or transplantation needed by him'.

The HOTA instituted in 1987 provided an opt-out system where individuals were presumed to have consented to organ donation upon death. Family members have no legal right of objection, although in practice, organ retrieval is carried out with due regard to families. This system applied to all Singaporean citizens and permanent residents other than Muslims, who were automatically considered objectors because under the Muslim Council's interpretation, removal of organs at death constitutes desecration of the deceased, and the consent of *waris* (paternal next-of-kin) was necessary for organ donation. Muslims in Singapore could opt in to organ donation under HOTA, or pledge their organs under MTERA. Muslim exemption from presumed consent was removed in 2007 following a religious ruling by the Islamic Religious Council of Singapore permitting Muslims to come under the HOTA.

In 2004, to increase the pool of donors, the Act was amended to permit retrieval of other types of organs besides kidneys (livers, hearts, and corneas), and all causes of death rather than only death by accidental causes. At the same time, living donor transplants were legalized, but written authorization by a hospital ethics committee was required and applicants had to be screened for eligibility. In 2009, amendments to the HOTA removed the upper age limit of 60 years for deceased donations to allow transplantable organs to be assessed for medical suitability (in line with practice in Norway, Spain, the United Kingdom, and the United States) so as to help increase supply. In addition, paired exchanges and reimbursement of donors for documentable or reasonable costs[3] were allowed. Furthermore, regulatory oversight of all living organ donations was established under Section 15A (3) through appointment of doctors and laypersons to a National Panel of Transplant Ethics Committees (TECs). Over the years, these legislative changes were undertaken with serious intent *both* to expand the supply of transplantable organs, *and* to ensure that organ donors are not exploited, unlawfully induced, or forced into organ retrieval by others.

While increasing the supply of organs is an important priority for developing transplant medicine, Singapore has in place legislation and oversight mechanisms through working TECs to help stem organ trafficking and transplant commercialism. In attempting to dissociate its practice of transplant tourism from organ trafficking and commercialism, it has aimed to achieve a reputation for ethical self-regulation and strengthen its status as an advanced nation. The 'all-in transplant packages' advertised in other regional transplant hubs are avoided or, at least, have not yet come to light. Live organ transplants are legally performed for donor–recipient pairs who usually have an existing emotional relationship, being either family members or close friends (although donations from strangers are not strictly excluded). They may be both residing in Singapore, both from another country, or from different countries. Organ commercialism is outlawed, and heavy penalties including hefty fines (up to SG $100,000) or a jail term (up to ten years), or both were introduced in an amendment to the HOTA in 2009.

On the equitable distribution of transplant provisions, there is overcapacity of transplant expertise and services in Singapore for patients suffering from organ failure, but demand for transplantable organs has continually outstripped supply (Ministry of Health Figures, http://www.liveon.sg/content/dam/moh_liveon/docs/info_booklets/LiveOnStats2011a.pdf, accessed 16 January 2013). The supply of kidneys from the deceased donor pool managed are allocated by the National Organ Transplant Unit (NOTU) first to citizens and permanent residents on a centralized wait list who have not opted out of donation under the Human Organ Transplant Act, then to those who have opted out, and finally to foreigners. Almost all *living* kidney and liver donations are *directed donations* by relatives or friends. Thus, the question of competition with foreigners for access to organ transplants does not arise for the local population, and distribution of organs in the common pool is based on a principle of communal participation. However, the possibility of being reimbursed for the cost of transplant procedures and other documented expenses means that recipients who have no means of paying for such costs would be unfairly disadvantaged in their search for a donor. In response, the National Kidney Foundation currently offers up to SG $5,000 for reimbursement of lost income to citizens and permanent residents who make a live organ donation. Available aids for payment of transplant and other medical costs of recipient and donor (even if the donor is non-Singaporean) include government subsidies available through means testing, national insurance schemes for catastrophic illnesses, or permitted use of compulsory health-care savings. Those who are unable to afford even subsidized charges may receive help through Medifund, an endowment fund set up by the government as a social safety net for needy patients.

---

[3] Under Section 14 (3)(c) of the HOTA, costs that may be reimbursed include expenses incurred for medical procedures, childcare, loss of earnings, short- or long-term medical care as a consequence of organ donation.

While legislation and policy measures have had some real effect in controlling organ trafficking and transplant commercialism in Singapore, there remain some clear risks. In the first case of organ trafficking prosecuted in Singapore in which a potential recipient (*Public Prosecutor* v *Tang Wee Sung* [2008] SGDC 262), potential Indonesian donor (*Public Prosecutor* v *Sulaiman Damanik and Another* [2008] SGDC 175) and the middleman who brought them together (*Public Prosecutor* v *Wang Chin Sing* [2008] SGDC 268) all received sentences, though of varying severity. However, the activities of brokerages remain unmonitored and there is little information about their operations, and whether Singapore's organ trafficking laws have been violated by these agencies. In particular, any commercial exchanges that may have occurred outside Singapore are nearly impossible to detect, much less investigate and prosecute. The economic relationship between doctors and these 'middlemen' remains a murky area, and no information about the involvement of doctors and other health-care professionals emerged in the case, which was concluded just months before the 2009 HOTA revision of penalties for organ trafficking. There remains a need for more information, regulation, and transparent, accountable practice in these areas.

In addition, the accountability of TECs has been an unexamined question. This is made difficult by the guidelines on altruistic organ donation, including roles and responsibilities for transplant centres, TECs, transplant physicians, and donors and recipients seeking transplantation surgery being confidential information under statutory law. The guidelines and recommendations for TEC process are positioned as work-in-progress. The government acknowledges that many lacunae remain and conducts closed-door discussions with TECs to debate problems and perspectives arising from their experiences so far.

But apart from identifying regulatory gaps, there are issues at hand for what I have referred to as 'a contemporary ethics of altruism'.

How can the ethics of altruism apply to international transplant medicine?

From the outset, the very practice of transplant medicine raises ethical questions because it imposes serious risk on healthy individuals through created demands on them to participate in organ donation to save the health of others. According to a contemporary ethics of altruism that has taken shape since Titmuss produced his groundbreaking work, *The Gift Relationship,* moral justification for doing so rests in the idea that, in liberal societies, opportunities to freely choose acts of high moral achievement must be made available to the individual (Titmuss 1971). But under certain economic, social, and cultural conditions, the argument that freedom to make organ donations is a hallmark of the good society will be hard to accept wholeheartedly. The practice has created new psychological pressures on persons which, under certain conditions, for example poverty and marginalization, shade into near-irresistible inducement (Zargooshi 2001: 1790; de Castro 2003a: 142). For certain individuals, perhaps family members or devotees of a religious order, the choice of saving the health of an intimate could present to these individuals unexamined ideas of moral necessity that call into question how free some of their decisions to donate actually are (Crouch and Elliott 1999: 275; Scheper-Hughes

2007: 507). The right of prisoners to participate in organ donation has also been contentious in recent years (de Castro 2003b: 171). That said, the importance of preserving equal rights to freedom for all persons is clear, and it would be wrong to deny disadvantaged and incarcerated persons equal opportunities for high moral attainments. It would fall on those who argue against permitting altruistic organ donation by the poor, educationally disadvantaged, and prisoners to prove their vulnerability. Argument is also necessary to show that exploitation by some is incompatible with the exercise of freedom; indeed, it seems quite plausible that providing non-exploitative opportunities for the exercise of freedom can serve to empower the disadvantaged to escape other conditions of exploitation.

Even when individuals are guaranteed real (or at least unquestioned) freedom to take serious risks in their own health-care decisions, medical ethics requires an account of acceptable risk that guides medicine in its professional duty of care. Acceptable risk, in its bare bones, is the measure of harm that will be tolerated by individuals in exchange for perceived benefits or advantages that may accrue from taking the risk in question. In organ donation, this notion is quite a complex one. Since risks are taken by two patients rather than one, there is already a baseline amplification of psychosocial risks. Such risks have been set out in terms of the relationship created between the donor–recipient pair in the course of the altruistic or gift transaction, and current guidelines on informed consent have sought to capture these risks (The Ethics Committee of the Transplantation Society 2004: 491; Barr et al. 2006: 1373). However, extant reports of organ donor experiences reveal a far more complex range of psychosocial risks which have to do with (a) desecration of the body and losses to self-esteem and social standing (Zargooshi 2001: 1970); (b) communal claims on bodies which engender competing interests in keeping the individual's organs in reserve for 'more important' familial or other relationships; (c) unique family dynamics that could mean unproblematic identification with the act of donation, or less happily, resentment on account of past or existing conflicts, rivalries, or perceptions of abuse.

There is also the question of what donors perceive as advantages that would motivate their risk taking. The conventional answer to this is that body donors receive psychological benefit such as enhanced self-respect, and perceive the benefits of contributing to the common interest. But increasingly, academic discussion (particularly on tissue donation) has drawn attention also to the importance of keeping faith with donors who give altruistically without expectation of external (particularly commercial) rewards to forge sustainable systems of procurement and distribution (Dickenson 2008). Notably, some have argued that the one-way altruism in some tissue economies is unstable; if the commodification happening somewhere down the line is acceptable in global tissue economies, to insist on non-compensated altruistic donation is morally schizophrenic (Mahoney 2000: 163). The parallel argument in organ transplantation would be that there is an inherent moral instability in the idea that international transplant medicine, which thrives through large and lucrative commercial concerns, should insist on altruistic organ donation. While all large concerns must deal in money, it is profit taking without returning something back to the society which supports these enterprises that is morally odious. In addition, the prevailing moral ideal within medicine is that of service to humanity and the exercise of fiduciary responsibility for the benefit of societies. Thus, to stabilize an altruistic system of transplant medicine, some form of third-party reciprocation that offers fitting responses to donors' conceptions of benefit may be called for. For example, third parties, which could be governments or commercial concerns, might respond appropriately by giving as much priority to improving the health of organ donors as to saving the health of organ recipients. Additionally, they might explore creative and practical means of enhancing donor reputation and increasing social cohesiveness.

In the case of Singapore, the decision to implement an altruistic system of organ donation within its practice of international transplant medicine followed in the wake of public disquiet over the Tang Wee Sung organ trafficking case. The government's apparent compromise for pursuing a globally controversial policy of international transplant medicine was to accept the terms of DOI and the World Health Organization for living organ donation; while paying compensation to donors was initially discussed, a reimbursement model was eventually adopted to signal commitment to prevailing international ethical guidelines. But a hybrid model of transplant medicine, which combines commercial and altruistic elements, is inherently unstable, as was observed. It will be a matter of time before current academic debates on reciprocity gain traction and take the system into its next phase of development.

At present, novel demands on professional and stakeholder responsibility are already being felt and recognized. Transplant teams are falling into line with the prohibition on organ trafficking, after the sentencing of Mr Tang Wee Sung. TECs, which represent the government, have the responsibility of determining the adequacy of the informed consent process for patients. The complexity of this task is not lost on these committees, which are regularly confronted with an array of exotic cultural rules that operate within combinations of modern and traditional family structures and religious communities, and circumstances of life that are near-unimaginable to (or very likely incorrectly imagined by) those of us who are used to social conditions within a modern metropolis. Determinations of voluntariness, and understanding of risks and benefits, cannot be disentangled from an informed appreciation of what risks and benefits are pertinent to donors from different societies, and how they measure risk against perceived benefit. Research into methodologies of risk determination in organ donation is much needed in medical ethics, without which incorrect decisions on informed consent would be the unfortunate (indeed tragic) outcome for patients.

Beyond informed consent, there is the challenge of implementing practices that safeguard donors' well-being. Follow-up care for foreign donors is hardly possible. Medical insurance is undeveloped in some of these countries, and there is no guaranteed provision for paid follow-up health care through the voluntary reimbursements by recipients. Currently, the standard of donor care is limited to rigorous patient education pre and post transplant, availability of well trained translators to overcome language barriers, strict rules against premature discharge and travel, adequate supply of immunosuppressive medication and good records on the donor, the surgery, and post-surgical treatment that might be preferably transferred to a central transplant organization in the donor's country. But the prospect that private commercial entities could be incentivized to establish access to cross-border follow-up facilities is not too remote given current expansion trends.

Concern about inappropriate solicitation of body donors is expressed in the 'flagging' of certain types of cases for special scrutiny by TECs, for instance with impoverished, educationally disadvantaged, or socially marginalized persons who *may* be vulnerable to targeting, harassment, and coercion by powerful group members or commercial brokers. A somewhat different dimension of this issue became better appreciated in Singapore through the experience of its Muslim community's decisions to first opt out of, and then seek inclusion under, the HOTA's provision of presumed consent to organ donation upon death. This has been instructive in bringing about greater social awareness of cultural attitudes to the body and body donation. On the other hand, the practice of organ donation is welcomed and held in high esteem within certain communities. For instance, our experience has been that Buddhist donors are apt to look upon organ donation as a means of creating merit in preparation for the next life; and Buddhist monastic orders have systematic rules within their communities for taking responsibility for any future reciprocal needs of donor monks or devotees.

The future of altruistic medicine

In tracing an agenda for altruistic medicine in the contemporary landscape of globalized biomedicine, we have suggested that adequate weight should be given to current realities faced by nation-states and policymakers. We have considered some current issues facing transplant medicine in Singapore as a case at hand. Emerging nations have prioritized the modernization of their health-care systems as a means to conserve medical talent and expertise at home. Competing for high-value clients in the emerging global system of medical tourism is seen as an inevitable course of action by governments seeking to stem decline in the quality of their domestic health-care systems. Under these imperatives, what meaning and value can be given to altruism in medicine? Developing nations may seek international standing by normalizing new regimes of medical practice through internal self-regulation and adherence to ethical standards prescribed by international bodies such as the World Health Organization, the World Medical Association, and various taskforces and patient lobby groups. Hence, progress in understanding and implementing stakeholder responsibilities is occurring in some of these countries, a project that can be developed and advanced by a serious engagement with some of the pertinent questions for altruistic medicine raised near the beginning of this chapter. By discussing a live example in this essay, I have explored what could be at stake in sustaining an altruistic system of organ donation.

Note: the truth about ethical boundaries

A field of applied ethics, including medical ethics, is a form of ethics directed towards practical attainments—a form of ethics that is a *praxis,* in the sense that:

1. it needs good information about the way that people in a particular cultural context actually think;

2. it makes observations about the practical consequences of their ways of thinking and acting; and
3. it attempts to discern, through their thought-life, the goals and values that people living within a cultural context believe to be important.

But to move beyond steps 1–3 to arrive at its goal, that is, *ethical knowledge,* a field of applied ethics (e.g. medical ethics) needs knowledge of a method of doing so. It must then describe the applications of this method, which yields ethical knowledge within that culture. Then it has to translate the meaning of this gain *as ethical knowledge,* which consists in such attainments as: knowledge of the environment, and of better ways of attaining goals expressive of values that people believe to be important in the (or sometimes only *their*) world. To be a successful translator of this sort, a person working in the field of applied ethics need not be a member of the culture he or she studies, but such a person has to understand (a wide range of methods is available for this) the goals and values of that culture and people, in the light of which any ethical knowledge is to be had at all.

Ethical knowledge, as described, is thus practical knowledge. *Qua* practical knowledge, it is attained through *praxis* (action which yields experiential knowledge), and using such knowledge to succeed in carrying out planned actions. Where actions do not succeed, experiential knowledge thereby gained may lead to the revision of beliefs about the valuable, or the attainable, or a cultural world and environment or, if one looks beyond that, *the* world and the wider environment. To attain ethical knowledge requires constant experimentation in action to gain new experiential knowledge as a basis for trying to further act successfully to achieve some set of desired goals. Again, that which is experienced as successful or failed action forms the basis for future action. In the light of this, an essay which considers the prospects for medicine to contribute to the formation of altruistic societies should pay special attention to policy experiments, their known implications, and suggestions for further experimentation and consolidation of experience.

In the contemporary globalized world, there is real danger of believing in, and submitting to, a 'flat world' thesis, which may spell deep losses in ethical knowledge. We need to recover cultural knowledge that has been 'lost'. Except in the rarest of cases, human communities and cultures have never have been sealed off from one another, but instead share complex intertwining histories. This means that there is no quick way of gaining understanding of the tapestry of beliefs and values of a particular society. Now more than ever before (in part due to the spread and democratization of information, and consequently the spread of egalitarian ideals in academia) we better appreciate the need for more 'data' from well conceived empirical studies of complex cultures of health care in 'particularistic' societies. A society such as Singapore which has inherited its constitution, based on the ideals of political liberalism, is sometimes described as a 'highly Westernized Asian culture' in extreme shorthand terms that are anything but informative today, being the language of a hopefully bygone age of naive globalized medical ethics. What is needed is detailed information gathering and careful interpretation of cultural values, histories, social goals, and configurations of needs and interests within societies seeking to survive and flourish in their environment. To gain—indeed to recover—ethical knowledge against a flattening world, we must have *confidence* to act in the world in the light of our values and beliefs. As cultures meet with increasing frequency and intensity, we may well clash at first, then converge, or converge too quickly, then clash. The former situation holds out the only real prospect of shared, culture-respecting universalistic ethics; the latter will only produce, variously, familiar patterns of domination and dissent.

References

Archard, D. (2002). 'Selling Yourself: Titmuss's Argument against a Market in Blood,' *Journal of Ethics*, 6(1):87–102.

Arrow, K. J. (1975). 'Gifts and Exchanges,' in E. S. Phelps (ed), *Altruism, Morality, and Economic Theory*. New York: Russell Sage Foundation, 13–28.

Barr, M. L. et al. (2006). 'A Report of the Vancouver Forum on the Care of the Live Organ Donor: Lung, Liver, Pancreas, and Intestine Data and Medical Guidelines,' *Transplantation*, 81(10):1373–85.

Budiani-Saberi, D. A., and Delmonico, F. L. (2008). 'Organ Trafficking and Transplant Tourism: A Commentary on the Global Realities,' *American Journal of Transplantation*, 8(5):925–9.

Corley, M. C. et al. (2000). 'Attitude, Self-image, and Quality of Life of Living Kidney Donors,' *Nephrology Nursing Journal*, 27(1): 43–50.

Crouch, R. A., and Elliott, C. (1999). 'Moral Agency and the Family: the Case of Living Related Organ Transplantation,' *Cambridge Quarterly of Healthcare Ethics*, 8(3): 275–87.

Daniels, N. et al. (2000). 'Benchmarks of Fairness for Health Care Reform: A Policy Tool for Developing Countries,' *Bulletin of the World Health Organization*, 78(6): 740–50.

de Castro, L. D. (2003a). 'Commodification and Exploitation: Arguments in Favour of Compensated Organ Donation,' *Journal of Medical Ethics*, 29(3):142–6.

de Castro, L. D. (2003b). 'Human Organs from Prisoners: Kidneys for Life,' *Journal of Medical Ethics*, 29(3):171–5.

Dickenson, D. (2008). *Body-Shopping: The Economy Fuelled by Flesh and Blood*. Oxford: Oneworld.

Epstein, M. (2009). 'Sociological and Ethical Issues in Transplant Commercialism,' *Current Opinion in Organ Transplantation*, 14(2): 134–9.

Epstein, M., and Danovitch, G. (2009). 'Is Altruistic-directed Living Unrelated Organ Donation a Legal Fiction?' *Nephrology Dialysis Transplantation*, 24(2): 357–60.

Etzioni, A. (1998). *The Moral Dimension: Towards a New Economics*. New York: Free Press.

Jansen, L. A. (2009). 'The Ethics of Altruism in Clinical Research,' *Hastings Center Report*, 39(4): 26–36.

Johnson, E. M. et al. (1999). 'Long-Term Follow-Up of Living Kidney Donors: Quality of Life after Donation,' *Transplantation*, 67(5): 717–21.

Kaplan, B., and Williams, R. (2007). 'Organ Donation: The Gift, the Weight, and the Tyranny of Good Acts,' *American Journal of Transplantation*, 7(3): 497–8.

Knibbe, M., and Verkerk, M. (2010). 'Making Sense of Risk: Donor Risk Communication in Families Considering Living Liver Donation to a Child,' *Medicine Health Care, and Philosophy*, 13(2):149–56.

Lee, K.Y. (2006). 'Globalisation of Medicine: Excerpts of Speech by Minister Mentor Mr Lee Kuan Yew at the SGH's 185th Anniversary Dinner on 16 April 2006 at Ritz-Carlton Millenia,' *SMA News*, 38(5): 11–12, 15.

Mahoney, J. D. (2000). 'The Market for Human Tissue,' *Virginia Law Review*, 86(2): 163–223.

Murray, T. H. (1987). 'Gifts of the Body and the Needs of Strangers,' *Hastings Center Report*, 17(2): 30–8.

Participants in the International Summit on Transplant Tourism and Organ Trafficking Convened by the Transplantation Society and International Society of Nephrology in Istanbul, Turkey, 30 April through 2 May 2008 (Participants in the Istanbul Summit). (2008). 'The Declaration of Istanbul on Organ Trafficking and Transplant Tourism,' *Clinical Journal of the American Society of Nephrology*, 3(5): 1227–31.

Pennings, G. (2002). 'Reproductive Tourism as Moral Pluralism in Motion,' *Journal of Medical Ethics*, 28(6): 337–41.

Pennings, G. (2007). 'Ethics without Boundaries: Medical Tourism,' in R. Ashcroft et al. (eds), *Principles of Health Care Ethics*. Chichester, West Sussex: John Wiley and Sons, 505–10.

Raymond, J. G. (1990). 'Reproductive Gifts and Gift Giving: The Altruistic Woman,' *Hastings Center Report*, 20(6): 7–11.

Relman, A. S. (2007). 'Medical Professionalism in a Commercialized Health Care Market,' *JAMA*, 298(22): 2668–70.

Scheper-Hughes, N. (2007). 'The Tyranny of the Gift: Sacrificial Violence in Living Donor Transplants,' *American Journal of Transplantation*, 7(3): 507–11.

Schover, L. R. et al. (1997). 'The Psychosocial Impact of Donating a Kidney: Long-Term Follow-Up from a Urology Based Center,' *Journal of Urology*, 157(5): 1596–601.

Schweda, M., and Schicktanz, S. (2009). 'Public Ideas and Values concerning the Commercialization of Organ Donation in Four European Countries,' *Social Science and Medicine*, 68(6): 1129–36.

Steinberg, D. (2010). 'Altruism in Medicine: Its Definition, Nature, and Dilemmas,' *Cambridge Quarterly of Healthcare Ethics*, 19(2): 249–57.

Steinbrook, R. (2006). 'Egg Donation and Human Embryonic Stem-cell Research,' *New England Journal of Medicine*, 354(4): 324–6.

The Ethics Committee of the Transplanation Society. (2004). 'The Consensus Statement of the Amsterdam Forum on the Care of the Live Kidney Donor,' *Transplantation*, 78(4): 491–2.

Titmuss, R. (1971). *The Gift Relationship: From Human Blood to Social Policy*. London: George Allen and Unwin.

Turner, L. (2007). '"First World Health Care at Third World Prices": Globalization, Bioethics and Medical Tourism,' *BioSocieties*, 2: 303–25.

Turner L. (2008). '"Medical Tourism" Initiatives Should Exclude Commercial Organ Transplantation,' *Journal of the Royal Society of Medicine*, 101(8): 391–4.

Vlaovic, P. D. et al. (1999). 'Psychosocial Impact of Renal Donation,' *Canadian Journal of Urology*, 6(5): 859–64.

Voo, T. C. (2011). 'The Social Rationale of the Gift Relationship,' *Journal of Medical Ethics*, 37:663–7.

Westlie, L. et al. (1993). 'Quality of Life in Norwegian Kidney Donors,' *Nephrology Dialysis Transplantation*, 8(10): 1146–50.

Zargooshi, J. (2001). 'Quality of Life of Iranian Kidney "Donors,"' *Journal of Urology*, 166(5): 1790–9.

14.2

Commentary
Local and Global Contexts of Praxis of Bioethics: 'Transplant Tourism' and 'Altruistic' Medicine

Yosuke Shimazono

In 'The Future of Altruistic Medicine', Chin questions the value of altruism in medicine in a globalizing world. In endorsing the 'praxis' of medical ethics grounded in particular social, economic, technological, and cultural circumstances, Chin states that altruism is a significant value for medical practice, but not an 'unmitigated good'. Chin asks if we should categorically oppose altruism and commercialism, and focuses on transplant medicine in Singapore, especially the issue of 'transplant tourism'. In what follows, I would like to make a few critical comments based on my experience studying organ transplantation from an anthropological perspective.

Let me begin with the major topic of Chin's article, 'transplant tourism'. Goods and services in transplant medicine are highly profitable commodities in the globalizing market of health-care services. According to Chin, they are seen by policymakers in Singapore as 'an indispensable part of Singapore's bid to become a global biomedical hub'. In spite of the DOI, which includes a call for an internationally concerted effort to curtail 'transplant tourism', Chin argues that 'adequate weight should be given to current realities faced by nation-states and policymakers'. She describes a scenario in which promotion of 'transplant tourism' to meet the economic demands of a health-care system can be reconciled with transplant medicine based on altruism.

A possible source of confusion is that 'transplant tourism' is used differently by various authors.[4] Those who oppose transplant tourism define the term by its *risks* and *hazards,* rather than its essential activities. Chin uses it in the broader sense of medical tourism in the field of organ transplantation. Chin has trouble with the former definition, but the reason is not presented clearly. She states: 'the confused positions represented here have

---

[4] Let me note that in when I was trying to publish the results of my study on 'transplant tourism' commissioned by the WHO, a reviewer asked me to retract this term, at least from the title, given its pejorative connotation (e.g. 'sex tourism'). The term 'reproductive tourism' has been out of use now and replaced by 'cross-border reproductive care' for the same reason.

not been helpful, for they have been ineffective for stemming transplant tourism which is, arguably, an integral part of the policies for economic and scientific development in many countries' (Chin in this chapter). However, my experience as a (very) peripheral participant in the consultative process leading up to the DOI suggests that this statement overlooks the fact that the process and the DOI were instrumental in encouraging health authorities in some countries to combat organ trade within their borders and discouraging others from promoting 'transplant tourism' involving transplant commercialism (e.g. Pakistan and Philippines).

In principle, cross-border provision and consumption of transplant medical services may not be inherently immoral, unethical, dangerous, or risky. However, I call attention to the fact that an increase in medical tourism in the area of transplant medicine during the last decade has usually involved problematic activities, such as organ trafficking, transplant commercialism that involves excessive commodification of the human body, or inequitable allocation of deceased donor organs. This suggests that there are reasons to be very cautious about considering transplant medicine as a lucrative source of revenue. In fact, Chin astutely points out that economic interests to promote 'transplant tourism' and attempts to curtail organ trafficking or transplant commercialism are not easily reconciled. The danger of 'compromised judgement' abounds. Chin also admits that 'any commercial exchanges that may have occurred outside Singapore are nearly impossible to detect, much less investigate and prosecute' (Chin in this chapter).

I suggest, in dealing with transplant tourism, that not only the commercial interest of the nation-state, but also the *praxis* of bioethics in a global context, should be taken into account. Globalization of transplant medicine led to diversification of transplant medicine practices. Obtaining a global consensus on the wide array of ethical, social, and legal issues among divergent stakeholders has become an enormously complicated task. In this context, achieving a certain degree of 'harmonization' between jurisdictions has emerged as an important pragmatic goal. Therefore, policymakers in Singapore are held accountable for ensuring transparency of their practices to the international community, and are responsible for ensuring, rather than undermining, the moral integrity of transplant medicine in other countries by promoting the provision of transplantation-related medical care to foreign patients.

I shall now comment on 'altruism'. The social role of gift giving in various societies is an old topic in anthropology. In describing various kinds of gifts, anthropologists have carefully distanced themselves from the Western tendency to characterize gift giving as an altruistic behaviour. The motivation that drives people to give, receive, and give in return in various societies is much more complex than the 'egoistic' and 'altruistic' dichotomy. In studying transplantation, I have been perplexed with the casual use of 'altruism' in bioethical discourse. The term is too insensitive to differentiate between donation of bodily substances to close kin and donation to an anonymous stranger or the nation as an imagined community. Different body parts may also have different values. We bleed as part of life, sometimes intentionally (bloodletting, for instance). In contrast, internal organs lie deep within our bodies. Different body parts have different symbolic meanings as well. The word 'altruism' was coined by Auguste Comte, and the cultural history of this term is intertwined with a reaction to popularization of the view of a human being as a rational decision-maker and utility maximizer. However, this term is too 'flat' a term, and cannot capture the complexity of social lives. Therefore, it may not be enough to question the value of altruism as the author does; the value of the *concept* of altruism itself needs scrutiny.

Reference

Chin, J. J. L. (2014). 'The Future of Altruistic Medicine,' in A. Akabayashi (ed.), *The Future of Bioethics: International Dialogues*. Oxford: Oxford University Press, 488–502.

14.3

Commentary
Altruism in the Service of the Market and the State, and the Ethics of Regulation

Amar Jesani

In a world increasingly dominated by a market which promotes self-interest and egoistic behavior on a large scale, Dr. Jacqueline Chin has correctly identified altruism as an important moral challenge of the future in her paper titled, "The Future of Altruistic Medicine." Evolutionary biologists and psychologists have studied the nature of altruism in detail and, as yet, there is no consensus on it. There is substantial agreement on defining an altruistic action as one that is intentional and voluntary, done for the welfare of others without expectation of any external rewards. At the same time, there is wide variation in the interpretation of altruistic behavior. Something that was thought of as "pure altruism" could be easily reinterpreted as investment for immediate or future reward (expectation of reciprocity). Besides, the context that motivates individuals to resort to such action could, when there exists an imbalance of power, render the altruism harmful and exploitative. Motives for an action are difficult to separate from the pressures of situation that could indirectly force individuals and groups to act in a cooperative manner.

Dr. Chin's paper also explores the use and potential abuse of altruism in the context of the health-care service system. Such altruism may take the form of cooperation, solidarity, or acting to secure future rewards associated with state policies and the market. Human societies are not organized primarily on the basis of self-interest, but also on the basis of the human social needs of cooperation, family and community ties, cultural and religious values, and above all, a broad empathy even for those with whom we are not involved in close personal relationships. People have a high stake in the health system and so our altruism to help each other is quite understandable; but at the same time, the altruism of other stakeholders—health professionals, the corporations running health-care institutions in the market setting, managers and policy makers—is equally pertinent to understanding how the altruism actually plays out in the broader system.

These issues are, as Dr. Chin has asserted, complex and difficult to resolve. They constitute a major moral challenge for the future. My comments therefore will address four connected issues: (a) altruism of, and in, the medical profession; (b) institutional arrangements by the state to scale up altruism through solidarity and reciprocal rewards; (c) institutional arrangements to scale up altruism in the domestic and international markets; and (d) the role of regulation to protect altruists in the form of transplant ethics committees. In the process of explaining these issues, I will suggest a few questions, in addition to those identified by Dr. Chin, for future research and policy initiatives.

Altruism in, and of, the medical profession

The ideal public image of the medical profession is still that of an occupation of healing, with its practitioners committed to following a calling to care for others. That is the reason why, despite all efforts by the market, and despite market-friendly policies of governments around the world, the idea of health care as a public good keeps pressuring societies to either reorganize or regulate the system to fulfill the historical mission of medicine. Medical altruism involves not only the altruism of people—the users of services—helping each other in times of medical needs, but also the altruism of the providers, the other stakeholders of the system. The providers are also part of society and, as human beings, they are under equal obligation to participate in the system of cooperation and not get swayed by self-interest.

Therefore, an obvious question to ask is: To what extent do medical practice and the medical profession currently exhibit altruistic characteristics or virtue?

In the Singapore case described in the paper, a lack of fulfillment of professional ambition in high-end practice led to an exodus of doctors both out of the country and from the public to the private sector. We cannot argue with doctors' expectation that the system in which they work should enable them to fulfill their professional ambitions in serving those who need organ transplants. However, their individualistic and self-interested decisions to abandon the system rather than use their corporate power to persuade policy makers to change it does not show any altruistic intention or support for the users of their services. Unfortunately this behavior of medical professionals is not new. In fact, it is rare to find the medical profession using its corporate power to change the system to one that provides universal access to all, from primary to super specialty tertiary care, through a democratically derived structure and governance. Historically, there are more examples of doctors, individually or corporately, opposing the state's/ society's attempts to institute universal access to care by public financing and/or provisioning. This happened even in some developed countries where associations of doctors now favor universal access, since many actively opposed it when the health-care system was first established. For example, the Beveridge Report, which was instrumental in establishing universal access in the UK, was not supported by the premier medical association of the country; something similar occurred in Canada. The same is happening in India today as the state is under increasing pressure to make the transition to universal access, and its efforts to put in place even basic market regulations are being opposed. Such an attitude of the profession has massive implications for developing countries where the inequities in health and access to health care are unacceptably high. In addition, the international medical bodies of the professions have not done enough to ensure that members from developing countries sit at the negotiation table with policy makers to ensure a change to universal access.

Therefore, we need more research to generate evidence of altruism *of* the medical profession—including how it fares in comparison with laypeople, particularly those who are poor and vulnerable, who are making some altruistic commitment by participating in the system of cooperation by providing organs, blood, and other biological material, and accepting risks by participating in clinical trials of products that could improve the welfare of millions. Unless health-care providers become role models by themselves exhibiting altruism, the altruism in medicine exhibited by others will not be sustainable in the long run. If the moral value of altruism is to be nurtured, we need to consider whether the current state of medical practice and the medical profession, along with their internal ethical governance mechanisms and commitment, are appropriate. And, of course, as medical professionals we need to reflect on the changes needed to strengthen altruism of and in medicine. The issue of contemporary ethics of altruism in medicine is one that warrants further exploration.

State intervention for scaling up altruism

While attempts to understand "pure" altruistic behavior by individuals have merit, in present-day complex societies "pure" altruistic actions that conform to all definitions are relatively rare. However, what we observe are altruistic impulses and/or behaviors of individuals, groups, and communities, leading to reciprocity, cooperation, empathy, or solidarity. Irrespective of the methodology used, none of them is attainable on a large scale in the unregulated market environment. All of them demand an appropriate state intervention. Singapore's legislation to provide the right to donate organs and its provision for an opt-out system to allow harvesting of organs after death, combined with the allocation of those organs for transplantation, show the state's progressive commitment to channel altruistic behavior for a more equitable system.

Developing countries may learn something from Singapore's approach. It shows that a progressive state can play a positive role in evolving political consensus and in creating institutional arrangements. There is, of course, a need to document the sort of democratic political process that leads to a consensus among all stakeholders, and that convinces laypeople to participate in the state's attempt to make institutional arrangements to nurture and scale up people's altruistic behavior. Research on the evolution of such good practices would help other countries to achieve the same ends within their own socio-economic and political systems. For instance, India has adopted, through law, a regulatory regime to minimize exploitation in the market governing organ transplantation. It has done so without establishing the sort of political consensus that could persuade people to become organ donors, and persuade the health system to reciprocate by allowing those in need of organ transplantation the right to receive one regardless of their capacity to pay. Learning from examples such as that of Singapore would be very useful in cases like this.

Domestic market and medical tourism: two-systems approach

All nations have their priorities, and Singapore's ambition is to become "a global bio-medical hub." On the one hand, it has established a public system for harvesting organs and providing transplantation to those in need, regardless of their capacity to pay. On the other hand, it has created an international private, market-based economy of medical tourism to cater to the rich domestic and international clients needing organs.

This dual system is created ostensibly for two reasons. One, to conserve medical talent and expertise. The paper shows that it has not only succeeded in doing this, but it has also attracted medical expertise from abroad in order to maintain its annual 20 percent growth of the medical tourism market. Two, the medical tourism market generates revenue for financing the domestic system of universal access to health care and transplantation. Even so, evidently, attempts are also made to regulate this fully commercialized market system in order to nurture some aspects of altruism, by restricting the sale and purchase of organs and the international trafficking of organs.

This is an interesting case study involving two systems with diametrically opposite objectives and value systems, in which the public system is to some extent dependent on the business of the private system. While the going is good—20 percent annual increase in the market—the system looks robust. But how will such an arrangement be affected by fluctuations in the international market? How are these two systems insulated from each other within the country? What happens when the supply of medical talent from abroad can no longer sustain the growing international market, resulting in the migration of doctors from the public to the private system? How ethical would it be to poach medical talent from other countries to keep such a system going? Would it in the long run jeopardize the institutionalized altruism of the public system? At the same time, is the international market system a poor role model when adopted in a partial manner? That is, although the ethical and political justifications for Singapore's system emanate from its attempts to retain doctors who have no altruistic commitment, and from its generation of revenue for universal access to the public system, what happens when the international competition becomes unhealthy, prompting other nations to create market-based medical tourism hubs without attempting to provide universal access to the public system, as India seems to be doing at present? These are some broad questions that bioethics must grapple with in the future.

Transplant ethics committee as regulator

Regulation by ethics committees is, in general, fraught with many complex problems, as we in India are discovering with our system of ethics committees at institutional and private levels regulating clinical trials. Their role in clinical trials is very precise, and must follow legal regulations. Ethical reflection by such committees is rare, if it happens at all. Such committees are overburdened with ticking a checklist and clearing trials or procedures, given the demand for timely review and the lives or money at stake.

While issues related to conflicts of interests are very important, we must also address the problem of assessing the genuine independence—structural and financial—of such ethics committees. There has been very little work on this problem, and therefore the question of whether the decision-making process of such committees is vitiated by a lack of independence has also remained largely unaddressed.

To what extent are merely reviewing and approving a proposal adequate for ensuring that what has been approved will be procedurally implemented in an ethical manner? Some research has been done on what measures should be introduced to the process of reviewing and assessing proposals in order to ensure the protection of participants and patients; but there is scant material on whether and how such work actually provides protection to the participants. Investigating this latter issue requires data about the capacity and feasibility of ethics committees to investigate and assess, including to investigate when donors are brought from other countries. More challenging yet would be the availability of resources, competence, and power to follow up long-term care of the donors.

In India, the ethics committees for clinical trials disclose very little data on their work; thus they lack transparency and accountability. In the case of Singapore, it should worry us that despite all efforts made by Dr. Chin, there was no disclosure of crucial information by the TECs. Interestingly, while the process of fostering altruism in organ donation has many democratic aspects—including allowing religious communities to take their time in joining the opt-out system—the governance of the system remains shrouded in secrecy. When the business of regulatory bodies involves experts reviewing the work of experts, without any transparency and accountability, it should become a real cause for concern. Could such a situation lead to transplant ethics committees becoming facilitators of business rather than protectors of ethics and patients? While at present it would be prudent to reserve judgment on such an issue, there is no doubt that more investigation of the work of ethics committees is needed. More so because reducing the rate of approvals could slow down commerce, consequently having a negative impact on domestic public health-care finances and provisioning.

Regulations are means to control or prevent abuse of altruists by the market or the state. In order to prevent people losing trust in medical altruism, the ethics of regulation and its processes, including governance, must constitute one of the research and policy challenges of the future.

14.4

Commentary

Altruism in Organ Donation: Would Reciprocity Offer an Alternative Explanation?

Mala Ramanathan

Altruism in organ donation and the legal framework in Singapore for organ donation

Altruism in medicine warrants ethical scrutiny, as has been pointed out by Dr. Chin (Chin in this chapter). In this case study, she examines the situation with regard to altruistic organ donors in Singapore and the regulations that have evolved to encourage organ donation, encompassing both cadaver and live donor options. It is indeed remarkable that the state would consider policy review on an ongoing basis and make relevant corrections to address lacunae that have been identified. It is also important to note that this is part of an effort to generate ethical knowledge that includes plural voices. This effort is one of several that aim to include the voices of the vendors (Moazam, Zaman, and Jafarey 2009) and that of the physician surgeons (Danavitch and Leichtman 2006). The ethical understanding that emerges from such an empirical exercise makes the ethical knowledge inclusive of the multiple stakeholders' perspectives.

In viewing altruistic organ donations under the legal regime in Singapore, I would like to take a sceptic's perspective. This is not to deny the potential for altruism in organ donations, but to look for additional factors that might also explain citizens' acquiescence with the state's rulings as being morally acceptable. My commentary is limited to an examination of whether the framework of altruism alone is sufficient to explain organ donation in Singapore, or if there are other equally competing and empirically tenable explanations that can be considered.

The two legal instruments that facilitate it are the MTERA and the HOTA. The MTERA legalizes the donation of human organs and the HOTA facilitates an opt-out arrangement for individuals who were presumed to have consented to organ donation upon death. There were exceptions to this law that assumed that members of the Muslim communities would not be able to consent to organ donations, as removal of organs would be seen as desecration of the deceased. After a 20-year period, the Islamic Religious Council of Singapore also permitted the Muslims in Singapore to join the mainstream with regard to the pledging of organs for transplantation. Therefore, those groups which were exempted under Singapore law could also now consider the option of HOTA. The extension of this legal mandate in 2004 made it possible to increase the list of organs that could potentially be harvested; it also extended the age limit for organ donation by including all causes of death, and legitimized living donor transplants. In 2009, the upper age limit was relaxed from 60 to include all medically suitable donations.

The allocation of kidneys from the diseased donor pool prioritizes donations to citizens and permanent residents on a centralized waiting list who have not opted out of donations under HOTA, then to those who have opted out. Last on this waiting list are foreigners who have opted to use Singapore's excellent health-care facilities for their own transplantation needs. Thus, within the community, access to organ transplantation is based on the principle of communal participation. It has also been pointed out that all living donations are directed donations by relatives or friends. Some ethical problems associated with this aspect of transplantation therapy have been identified, but they are nearly universal across the developing countries.

I cannot but agree that ethical knowledge gleaned from the various participants in the process of organ donation has to be viewed as work-in-progress, and corrections applied as the need arises. The government of Singapore should be congratulated for its quick policy corrections, and also for putting in place evidence-based policy processes. All of these measures have contributed to enhancing the supply of organs. Yet the demand for transplantable organs has outstripped the supply.

I propose to comment on the attribution of altruism to the pledging of organs after death for future use by others, within a system that provides an opt-out option. While accepting the possibility that people would indeed pledge organs (in this case refrain from declining to pledging them) with no expectation of any returns, I would like to look at other equally compelling explanations for doing this.

A sceptical perspective: an alternative explanation

It is possible to obtain a social contract in a society like Singapore where literacy is nearly universal (Department of Statistics Singapore 2011).[5] The state can reach out to all its residents with key information and disseminate it, encourage debate, draw inferences, and make policy decisions. Decisions about organ donation can be made with greater assurance by citizens where pledging of organs is rendered feasible through state intervention to minimize information asymmetry. Moreover, its implementation by law is indicative of the state's commitment to safeguard against potential injustices characteristic of information asymmetry, which results in organ trade.

This social contract is enforced through sanctions against those who opt out. While this is not visible, those citizens who opt out and subsequently need an organ transplant will be placed further down the waiting list than those who have not opted out. Such regulation helps achieve the desired policy goal by providing an incentive for people to

---

[5] The literacy level in Singapore among residents aged 15 and above for men is 96.1 and for women is 94.1.

refrain from opting out; and that the Muslim Religious Council eventually withdrew its objections and enabled Muslims to pledge organs are evidence of its effectiveness.

The issue of enforceability is moot, and is particularly interesting viewed from the context of India, where it would seem almost impossible to obtain this form of social contract. This is because the diversity of the community in question would make it difficult even to formulate a universal social contract that is likely to be accepted by the required number of individuals. A possible explanation for this is the size of Singapore's population (Department of Statistics Singapore 2011),[6] which is just short of 4 million;[7] but I would also like to look beyond these simplistic explanations.

In addition to the social contract, there is the ubiquitous acceptance of the idea of being part of a 'highly Westernized Asian culture' within Singapore (Chin in this chapter). Such a society is expected to profess liberal values and to respect all religions and rights of individuals. Therefore while sanctions against nonconformism are possible, complete exclusion is not. This also serves to bring recalcitrant groups within the fold of the social contract.

Why, then, would people who are generally unwilling to be generous with organs for which they have a current need and long-term utility be willing to donate an organ? Here I am not talking of people who are extraordinarily motivated either by religious or personal benevolent proclivities (Gohh et al. 2001) that border on heroism. Would people acquiesce to such a proposal if they did not stand to receive any direct benefits? The potential for direct benefits is limited in this case, since donors provide their organs after death. Therefore those who do not opt out of donations in Singapore do not stand to gain either in terms of organs or in terms of financial benefits. However, it can result in a sense of solidarity with fellow citizens, a sense of having contributed to society even after death. In Hinduism the ability to be charitable during one's life brings salvific religious merit to the one practising it, and in Buddhism it is a form of communal insurance which is efficient in a society with a lot of uncertainty (McCleary 2007).

In the case of organ donations after death, clearly there is no scope for direct benefits for donors, if we view such benefits as those that can be enjoyed only after a donation has taken place. If voluntary donations are the norm, as is the case in Singapore, who or what would represent the target of these benevolent acts by individuals?

The value of reciprocity as a possible explanation

Rather than looking at altruism in its various versions, pure or commercialized or a combination of both, I wish also to look at another relevant value in these societies: that of reciprocity across kinship ties and across generations. It is difficult to view organ

---

[6] The size of the population of Singapore considering only Singapore citizens is 3,257,200. Including all Singapore residents, the population is 3,789,300.

[7] A population of 3.25 or 3.78 million is not large compared to larger metros in India, which have populations of over 10 million. The population of Mumbai is 12.5 million, and of Delhi is 11.01 million. Census of India 2011. City Census, 2011, accessed from http://www.census2011.co.in/city.php, (accessed 5 July 2012). (Census of India 2011).

donation as indicative of reciprocity with a society when the donor is not in a position to benefit.

Under MTERA, it will not be possible to direct donations except in the case of live organ donations; a dead donor will not be in a position to indicate the preferred recipient of their generosity. How, then, is a plea for recognizing reciprocity tenable? In societies where kinship ties and familial ties are strong (as in Singapore) and valued, and where this is recognized by the state (Government of Singapore 2012), most donors would recognize that the benefits would accrue indirectly. Any donation of organs is likely to benefit all members of one's family—and others—uniformly, since anyone could potentially come to need an organ transplant. There is no certainty that such a need would not arise within one's own family or extended kinship ties. In that sense, organ donation can be seen as a risk-avoidance strategy. The benefit of pledging to donate is direct since the individual in their own lifetime would stand to gain by being in the priority group for receiving donations, and their being prioritized in this way is due to their participating in the practice of reciprocity. In return for this prioritization, pledging to donate organs is reasonable compensation to make to those who exist now and those who might exist in future, as the individual who dies has no further use for their organs. This trade-off is particularly attractive when there is no assurance that those near and dear would not be in need of similar donations made by others. In this context, sanctions against those who do not conform is a form of punishment that those who expect reciprocity in organ donations would condone (Fehr and Gächter 2000).

Another question to examine here in the context of altruistic donors is whether all people are situated in equal positions, both in life and in society, and therefore whether they are equally able to practise altruism or reject demands to practise it for the benefit of others. When not all participants in a society are equal, how can individuals enhance their value to others? Such value enhancements could take the form of the moral merit that accrues through sacrifice, and the possible claims to which those who make such sacrifices are entitled. Making sacrifices, as a result, could seem an attractive proposition for vulnerable individuals in unequal societies. Distributive justice requires that one recognize this inequality within societies and therefore look beyond altruism for possible explanations for generosity involving organ donation.

It is important to note that the moral merit that accrues to those who make a sacrifice could also extend to the direct descendants of donors, and to their extended kinship ties, as it would not accrue to those who have already died. This would thus help to extend the possibility of reciprocity within altruistic organ donations—even after death.

Possible caveats

The perspective that assumes rationality and risk minimization as a value is also shared by economists working in the area of game theory.

References

Census of India (2011). 'City Census, 2011', http://www.census2011.co.in/city.php (accessed 5 July 2012).

Danavitch, G. M., and Leichtman, A. B (2006). 'Kidney Vending: The "Trojan Horse" of Organ Transplantation', *Clinical Journal of the American Society of Nephrology*, 1:1133–5.

Department of Statistics Singapore (2011). 'Key Annual Indicators 2011. Literacy and Education', http://www.singstat.gov.sg/stats/keyind.html#litedu (accessed 15 January 2013).

Fehr, E., and Gächter, S. (2000). 'Fairness and Retaliation: The Economics of Reciprocity', *Journal of Economic Perspectives*, 14(3): 159–81.

Gohh, R. Y. et al. (2001). 'Controversies in Organ Donation: the Altruistic Living Donor', *Nephrology Dialysis Transplantation*, 16:619–21.

Government of Singapore (2012). 'Family Values Remain the Cornerstone of Our Society', http://www.youtube.com/watch?v=YVcCPrrzwHs&list=PL87B679CA66E6B722&index=11&feature=plpp_video (accessed 15 January 2013).

McCleary, R. M. (2007). 'Salvation, Damnation and Economic Incentives', *Journal of Contemporary Religion*, 22(1): 49–74.

Moazam, F., Zaman, F. M., and Jafarey, A. M. (2009). 'Conversations with Kidney Vendors in Pakistan: An Ethnographic Study', *Hasting Centre Report*, 39(3): 29–44.

14.5

Commentary

A New Twist on Altruism: Survivors of Japan's 3/11

Michael C. Brannigan

Professor Jacqueline Chin's splendid essay is instructive on many levels such as her especially noteworthy considerations regarding ownership in relation to our embodied selves. This, in turn, unearths inescapable questions of bodily ontology for which cultural worldviews are profoundly influential. Spurred on by her marvelous account, I will here address the issue of altruism through a less conventional lens. This involves more closely examining the relational dynamic that acts as the undercurrent of her view of 'ethical boundaries,' namely the synergy between a culture's worldviews (beliefs, goals, values, desires, etc.) and ways of behaving or living within that worldview. And I will do so within the distressing context of disaster.

There is perhaps no more compelling framework to examine the relationship between culture, worldviews, behavior, and possibilities for altruism, particularly altruism's implications for health care (clinical, epidemiological, and public health) than within the context of severe social trauma, or what we ordinarily label 'disaster.' In my estimation, crisis, personal and/or collective, local and/or widespread, is the litmus test of deeply held values. Consequently, expressions of altruism, demonstrated through actions not just immediate but sustained over time, reflect measures of altruistic disposition which in turn disclose a culture's worldviews, just as it does on the micro level of individual belief systems and priorities.

Professor Chin's final section is particularly relevant. She rightfully warns us against acquiescing to a "flat world" vision in which cultural, philosophical, and moral boundaries are no longer considered significant. This flattening process is evident, for example, within the overused rubric of "multiculturalism," which, via a teleology of tolerance, can in effect meld down and blur noteworthy distinctions among cultural boundaries and their worldviews. Ethically, the principal challenge here lies in constructing fair and reasonable limits to tolerance, which, while not our focus here, remains crucial in intercultural research. As Chin wisely puts it, cultures "share complex intertwining histories." No culture is an island. Therefore, applying monolithic nets violates each culture's complex and rich character (Brannigan 2008: 346).

The first major step in ethical understanding is ultimately the most challenging. It requires that we attempt, in the most reasonable way we can, to wear the lens of the Other, the Other being Other because he/she/they are other than I. Can we somehow see the world through the Other's perspective? Because we are all inherently linked, sharing "complex intertwining histories," such effort enhances self-understanding precisely *through* other-understanding. Again, one particularly poignant framework in illustrating this lies in circumstances of disaster.

In January 2012, I traveled northward to stricken areas in the prefectures of Miyagi and Iwate, regions that remain severely debilitated from the 3 March 2011 Tohoku earthquake and tsunami, now officially dubbed the Great East Japan Earthquake, and widely known as "3/11." The area closer to the nuclear power plant in Fukushima Prefecture was off bounds to visitors. My aim was simple. I wanted to meet with and listen to those who experienced deep, personal loss, to learn from them what helped them to endure the catastrophe, how they viewed their futures, and what hopes and fears they carry. In essence, I was hoping to learn from them what really matters.[8]

Post-disaster narratives tend to acquire their own sort of mythologies of altruism. For instance, there is the heroic account of Wallace Hartley, the bandleader on the *Titanic* who urged his musicians to play to the bitter end, with "Nearer My God to Thee." Post-disaster tales, particularly media fed, also convey the seedier, self-centered side of humanity, like the Hollywood version of *Titanic* passengers' pure panic overriding decorum and fair play. Likewise, following Japan's 3/11 tragedy, news accounts describe elderly patients abandoned by their physicians and swept away by deadly waves. In my personal encounters, however, I heard other stories, ones that will most likely not reach headlines. We will probably not read of the physicians in the coastal town of Otsuchi who, after bracing the powerful 9.0 magnitude earthquake, immediately left their homes to be with their patients at Otsuchi Hospital, only to be crushed along with their patients by a massive wall of seawater carrying mud and debris.

My encounters with the many people I spoke with taught me precious lessons regarding altruism in its bare bones. We can more commonly define altruism as an inner disposition that generates actions whereby regard for others trumps self-regard. As Chin insightfully reveals in her essay, altruism thereby rests upon deep-rooted values and beliefs. These values and beliefs represent the core of who and what really matters.

My steadfast companions Aoki Kunio, Naito Mizuki, and Suzuki Hiroko accompanied me throughout these conversations with survivors (Brannigan 2012a).[9] Kunio is a top-level manager in Tokyo for the East Japan Railway Culture Foundation, which aims to enhance international links with the country's marvelous railway system. Mizuki is his skilled chief assistant. She offered invaluable support through her keen translation and interpretation of these conversations throughout our visit, particularly when it came to capturing our conversations' more subtle and all-important nuances. I hesitate

---

[8] Some of the following anecdotes (Kanayama, Imai, and Iwasaki) I refer to in more condensed version in my newspaper piece (Brannigan 2012b).

[9] First references to Japanese names follow the traditional order of family name first, followed by personal name.

to refer to these as "interviews," at least in any formal sense. I had no preset written questionnaire. Rather, though I carried certain questions internally, when meeting with survivors, I let them share at their own pace. I simply listened with full attention, occasionally responding and raising questions.[10] Hiroko manages the town of Tono's Furusato Village, a precious colony of houses and scenic mountain land in the *Nanbu Magariya* tradition of the Edo period (1600–1867).[11] Hiroko works diligently with her staff to preserve the memory of and respect for this tradition and its communal spirit. She moved to Tono prior to 3/11 after working as a travel agent in nearby Sendai, where she lost family and friends to the tsunami. Indeed, it was through her contacts that we were able to meet the many kind people we encountered. In her gracious, gentle, and selfless disposition, Hiroko embodies altruism in pure form.

Throughout my encounters with survivors, what struck me first and foremost was how each one with whom we spoke graciously welcomed us into his and her personal world of misery, loss, and endurance. Each person shared openly with us their profound sadness, fears, and hopes. Even more remarkable, each person expressed their deep gratitude *to us* for offering them this opportunity to share. They were truly my teachers, embodying lessons of resilience and deep, genuine selflessness. They all personified altruism, even in the face of looming helplessness.

Some narratives of altruism particularly stand out, like Kanayama Bunzo's total dedication to plant mustard seed flowers throughout the devastated areas of Otsuchi where nearly 2,000 people have perished. His daughter was swept away by the monster waves. He also lost many friends as he witnessed raging fires set off from toppled ships' fuel colliding with cars strewn everywhere. Yet, by planting seeds for these yellow flowers, yellow being the color for happiness and a color used at memorial services, he intends to express hope to surviving residents. The retired truck driver exudes charm and charisma. At first, he no doubt cut a lonely figure with his picks and shovels, planting his flowers along the dry riverbed of Otsuchigawa. In short time, however, his example grew contagious, and he now leads a large band of committed volunteers, mostly young, who work alongside him every day.[12]

And there is the youthful Imai Jin, who, after spending days searching fearfully for his wife and son, finally found them alive. He now speaks often to groups throughout the district and regularly insists that what really matters in life is that survivors work to strengthen family and rebuild community. In our conversations he repeatedly insisted that true community will not come about from digital communication devices like cell phones. Rather, real community can only come from interpersonal, human-to-human engagement with each other. Imai now leads a growing group of volunteers to help

---

[10] This listening is a double-edged sword. While it allows a survivor to recount her experiences and may help to be somewhat cathartic, it can also bring about a deepening of her grief.

[11] In this tradition, people and horses lived in the same dwelling. For the website of Furusato Village, see http://www.tono-furusato.jp/ (accessed 15 January 2013). Furusato Village has recently sponsored the 'Beacon of Rebirth' project, at http://fukkou-noroshi.jp/en/ (accessed 15 January 2013).

[12] The news story of Bunzo Kanayama is at 'Happy Yellow Flower Strategy, the Town Spread Circle of Support Sledgehammer' (trans. from Japanese), *Yomiuri Online*, 14 June 2011. http://www.yomiuri.co.jp/feature/20110316-866918/news/20110614-OYT1T00099.htm (accessed 15 January 2013).

reconstruct parts of Otsuchi, and he also acts as a guide for visitors who come to Otsuchi and surrounding villages.[13] He offers them the same lesson he offers us.

These personal accounts are magnified through numerous reported instances of altruistic behavior during and after the triple impact of earthquake–tsunami–radiation meltdown. Miki Endo stayed on the second floor of the three-story Disaster Readiness Center in coastal Minamisanriku when the earthquake and tsunami struck. She continued to broadcast nonstop over the emergency loudspeaker system, imploring residents to climb to higher ground. The thousands who heeded her pleas survived. Endo and her supervisor stayed at their posts as she issued warnings until massive waves swept over the building. Her body has not been recovered.

There are many Miki Endos. Countless firemen died while staying on ground level directing people to evacuate and climb to higher ground. Kunio Aoki described to me how workers from Japan Railways West immediately came to the aid of the crippled Japan Railways East transport system and offered openhanded assistance. Hiroko Suzuki told me of the numerous physicians who immediately left their homes to be with their patients in coastal hospitals, and how many of them died staying with their bedridden patients who could not be brought up to the roofs.

Here are more stories we will not read in the headlines. The good citizens of Tono, Hiroko's mountain village well known for its tradition and emphasis on Japanese folklore and community, were the immediate hub of aid for nearby ravaged coastal towns. Bear in mind that the powerful earthquake seriously damaged mountain areas and villages so that many roads were impassable. Tono residents therefore climbed down difficult mountain paths to deliver blankets, food, and water. They also organized the delivery of 10,000 *kasa* (umbrellas) to villagers, vital during the rainy season ahead. Moreover, trucks delivering water from Japan's southern island Kyushu (where I was born in Fukuoka) arrived in Tono after four days of nonstop driving, often having to avert roads damaged by the earthquake. Tono citizens then carried the water by themselves down to the coastal towns.

Especially noteworthy is the response of survivors when Tono townspeople reached them. The survivors went out of their way to reassure the Tono helpers that "All was alright" and urged them to take care of themselves first. Kunio pointed out to me that understanding this response is crucial. This response illustrates how many Japanese victims generally responded to aid. The victims wanted to empower the helpers, who themselves suffered hardships in the process of helping, to feel permitted to support each other as well. In this way, the victims of disaster demonstrate altruism just as do those who come to their aid.

Another memorable encounter was our meeting with Iwasaki Akiko on the ten-month anniversary of 3/11. With her vibrant yet soft personality Akiko radiates reassurance. She runs a ryokan, or traditional inn, called Houraikan on the edge of the small port town of Kamaishi with a stunning ocean view.[14] Kamaishi, like other towns, was nearly wiped out by the tsunami. There, like all towns along the coast, volunteers

[13] For more on Jin Imai, see http://www.kenpokukanko.co.jp/knp (accessed 15 January 2013).

[14] For the website of Houraikan, see http://houraikan.jp/ (accessed 15 January 2013). This depicts the beautiful setting of Akiko's inn overlooking the sandy beach eastward towards the rising sun.

and crew work daily clearing away massive mountains of debris. The Great Hanshin Earthquake at Kobe in January 1995 compelled Akiko to build a more disaster-resistant structure, so that Houraikan was one of the few buildings left standing after 3/11. Yet even though her ryokan is not on beach level but sits on a small hill protected by trees, it was severely damaged by waves which reached the top of the third floor.

Akiko reopened Houraikan in early January 2012, less than a week before we arrived. Many of her regular guests wanted her to reopen in December. Yet because December is a special month for families to be together in anticipation of the New Year, she set that month aside as a time for her employees. She herself lost family as well as three employees to the tsunami, and remaining employees also lost relatives and friends. For all whose lives were turned upside down and for whom the sea still appears dark and ominous, Houraikan's official reopening represented light and promise, a new beginning.

Akiko herself played a key role in saving many from the onslaught of seawater, debris, and mud. When she spotted the receding water soon after seemingly interminable tremors from the 9.0-magnitude earthquake 130 km northeast and seaward off Kamaishi, she ordered her guests to climb up the path she had built some years ago behind her inn, and ran to neighbors pleading that they do the same. While she was doing this, onrushing waves swept her under. She described how it felt like an eternity before a neighbor's hand clutched her and pulled her up. She had just enough time to make it to her fourth floor with others who gathered there and watched as the waves reached as high as the floor beneath them. Those who bounded up the hill were saved.

In recounting her experience, Akiko stressed repeatedly that as difficult it is to survive this impact, what is more difficult is to face life afterwards, to pick up the pieces, "to go on living." Throughout the devastated Tohoku region, particularly along the coastline, there continue to be reports of suicide among survivors who find it impossible to live on without their spouse, children, and livelihood, as is especially the case with farmers whose crops will be completely ruined for years. Some of these survivors find little in the way of security living in the numerous clusters of temporary shelters scattered throughout the region. Akiko's daughter, who now stays at the inn with her child, recently celebrated "Coming of Age" day in Japan, a time for all 20-year-olds to celebrate their entry into adulthood with its obligations and rights, now contributing and belonging to the community as an adult. Her close friend and classmate, however, did not celebrate "Coming of Age." She had lost her entire family to the tsunami and had been missing since December. There is no trace of her body, and many fear she most likely took her life.

Akiko shared with us the lesson she had learned through all of this, one to always "keep in mind." Namely: "We need human connection in order to survive the days ahead" and "to go on living." Akiko reminded us, and this is the lesson that Hiroko, Bunzo, Jin, and all others embody, that we can never claim that "I'm recovered" so long as any one other person is not. For her, this way of thinking of "human connection" lies "in our DNA." Ultimately, this sense of human connectedness, this emphasis upon "we" rather than "I" is what drives altruistic behavior. I still wonder whether Akiko was speaking for all us humans regarding this inherent component "in our DNA," or her villagers, or Japanese in general. Are there cultural dispositions that more easily enable the resuscitation and sustenance of genuine community in Akiko's sense?

Akiko went on to describe how she and other survivors now resist town officials' move to set up 14.5-meter-high levees to protect against future tsunamis. They argue that levees would further destroy the surrounding environment, trees, and sandy beaches. For Akiko and many Japanese, we can never overcome Nature's force and power. Therefore, as she insists, the key to future survival lies not in artificial measures of protection and concrete. The key to survival and future posterity lies in educating and supporting each other so that all know what to do in the face of threatening disaster. All this requires community collaboration and effort. Akiko's dream is to build a broad path up the small mountain behind her inn, one that is visible throughout the neighborhood and beach, a path with wide steps and even a small arena for theater and concerts. With many in the village dead or missing, this dream will only come alive if outsiders come to live in Kamaishi, outsiders who are willing to live together in genuine community.

Professor Chin's keen insights remind us that altruism expresses itself within a rich texture of contexts. These voices above embody altruism in deep ways. They not only articulate their owners' extraordinary kindness. They also convey their singular trust in us by sharing with us their personal stories. These survivors are also victims, and they inspire those of us who are "safe." The victims become the altruists. Indeed, they revitalize us, and I feel especially privileged to share their stories with others. Just as each survivor expressed deep indebtedness to us for this opportunity to share, I, in turn, can never sufficiently express to them my heartfelt gratitude for being my memorable and lifelong teachers.

References

Brannigan, M. (2008). '*Ikiru* and Net-Casting in Intercultural Bioethics,' in S. Shapshay (ed), *Bioethics at the Movies*. Baltimore, MD: Johns Hopkins University Press. 345–65.

Brannigan, M. (2012a). Interviews above Recorded with Akiko Iwasaki, Bunzo Kanayama, and Jin Imai, at Kamaishi and Otsuchi, Iwate Prefecture, Japan, from 10–14 January 2012.

Brannigan, M. (2012b). 'First Person Plural: Japan One Year Later,' *Times Union*, 4 March.

14.6

Response to Commentaries

Jacqueline J. L. Chin

I am grateful for the very insightful and helpful comments offered by Yosuke Shimazono, Amar Jesani, Mala Ramanathan, and Michael Brannigan, and provide replies to them in turn.

Transplant tourism

Dr Shimazono's commentary raises a number of very important issues which occasion further thinking and clarification of my claims in this paper. First, he defends the Declaration of Istanbul's stipulative definition of transplant tourism for its effective influence on encouraging health authorities in some countries to combat organ trafficking within their borders, and to discourage others from promoting transplant tourism involving commercialism. While the influence of the DOI in the global fight against organ trafficking is enormous and unquestionable, and has led to concerted legal and policy action in many countries, including Singapore, the focus of my point about its 'confused positions' relates to its unclear statements and omissions in connection with forms of cross-border transplant medicine. Not all of these should be dismissed; and transplant tourism as DOI defines it is but one facet (albeit a very important one) of the larger picture of globalized transplant practices. My position is stated in a paper I published with Alastair Campbell entitled, 'Transplant Tourism or International Transplant Medicine: A Case for Making the Distinction' (Chin and Campbell 2012: 1700–7), in which we argue that routine denunciation of the practices of transplant tourism by the WHO, DOI, and other international bodies has failed to consider what governments should do to ensure that their citizens have access to all forms of transplantation. In advocating that national deceased donor schemes and multinational organ-sharing programmes are the only acceptable avenues for addressing the organ shortage crisis, these agencies ignore the fact that, for some small states and developing countries, meeting the obligation to provide transplant services to their citizens may well depend on navigating global trading systems. Nimbleness is needed to address complex risks, both to the integrity of these health-care systems, and to citizens and all international patients who use increasingly accessible global transplantation services. These same guidelines ignore the impact of current international trade agreements, which strongly influence the policy priorities of developing countries and small states. Among developing countries, the pursuit of complex and myriad forms of modernization, including globalization of their health-care systems, forms an overarching ideal of 'progress' that frames and animates a range of ethical concerns in medicine. Admittedly the present demand for self-sufficiency in organ supply responds to risks such as poor clinical outcomes, and exploitation of the poor through the various commercial practices of transplant tourism. However, countries like Singapore, which accept the principle of self-sufficiency in organ supply (patients seeking transplant services in Singapore must find their own donor) demonstrates that providing international transplant services is quite compatible with the logic of self-sufficiency. In that paper, we set out a systematic account of risks that indicate areas in which gaps between ethics and practice should be closed, and a preliminary set of practical suggestions for doing so.

Global bioethics

A second important point in Shimazono's critique of the paper is that 'not only the commercial interest of the nation-state, but also the *praxis* of bioethics in a global context, should be taken into account'. He urges as well that 'policy makers in Singapore are held accountable for ensuring transparency of their practices to the international community, and are responsible for ensuring, rather than undermining, the moral integrity of transplant medicine in other countries by promoting the provision of transplantation-related medical care to foreign patients' (Shimazono in this chapter). Our case study on an altruistic system of international transplant medicine that is being attempted in Singapore indicates some early commitments to patients and the international community. The hugely difficult task of achieving global consensus on the wide array of social, ethical, and legal issues among divergent stakeholders (and we might add, competitor countries) is the very reason that the Singapore experiment as described can offer a tactical means of drawing competitor nations in the region and around the world into practices that better secure their reputations and commitment to the safety and welfare of patients; it will not be lost on medical professionals and commercial entities that ethics can also promote good business (in more than one sense of 'good').

Altruism and conceptual clarification

On Shimazono's warning against casual uses of the term 'altruism' that do not take due account of anthropological and other literatures, I fully agree that it is a term of art that requires careful conceptual analysis. In the contemporary globalized and commercialized practice of transplant medicine, altruistic organ donation is neither a kind of almsgiving nor gift exchange, but a new animal as it were.

On this note, Dr Jesani's commentary provides an illuminating account of some of the core features of contemporary altruism in medicine, and an inspiring contribution from a medical professional to understanding the role of good faith among medical professionals and other stakeholders in sustaining citizens' commitment to altruistic action including body donations for medical therapy or research. Respecting the freedom to donate (and to *not* donate) for all citizens and citizen groups should certainly be secured by states that participate in globalized transplantation practices; and these practices, as he argues, must not be allowed to supplant the foundations of human societies, which are 'not organized primarily on the basis of self-interest, but also on the basis of the human social needs of cooperation, family and community ties, cultural and religious values and above all, a broad empathy even for those with whom we are not involved in close personal relationships' (Jesani in this chapter).

Mixed systems of health care

Jesani considers helpful ethical questions that arise for a country's reliance on international markets, including the market in medical talent, to preserve the integrity of its public health-care system. He quite rightly asks how public and private systems can be 'insulated from each other within the country'. This is an issue that has not been lost to Singapore's leaders. The former prime minister Lee Kuan Yew declared in 2006 that the government needed to be vigilant in ensuring that the public health-care system would always maintain superior standards to those of private health-care institutions, through the backing of state resources. Only then, he argued, would the public sector be able to retain the country's best medical talent and attract foreign medical talent. Indeed, the latter engenders questions of global justice and the ethical imperative of not damaging the capacities and integrity of health-care systems in other countries. Thus, the language that is used by Singapore leaders is that of creating networks of medical expertise with neighbouring countries; ostensibly, the expansion of Singapore's private hospital chains in the region is one such method of networking professional expertise and capacity internationally.

Transplant ethics committees

Valid arguments have been offered by Dr Jesani on the need for public accountability of transplant and other kinds of ethics committees. It is understandably alarming that a democratic nation should resist information sharing to the extent that its regulatory guidelines for transplant ethics committees are confidential. But one consideration is worth noting: the work of Singapore's transplant ethics committees would be as closely watched by organ traffickers as it is by international organ-trading watchdog organizations. It is well known that much coaching of interviewees through the application process for living organ donation takes place by middlemen prior to the TEC sessions. The twin demands of public transparency and regulatory efficacy are not easy to reconcile, and one might surmise that prudential considerations are preventing disclosure of the workings of TECs at the moment.

Altruistic motivation and reciprocity

Professor Mala Ramanathan focuses on the altruistic basis of procurement of deceased donor organs, politely casting aside the concept of altruism in favour of reciprocity as a motivational basis for organ donation within state-organized systems. Her analysis relies on empirical studies in moral psychology that have informed game theoretic explanations of the motivation to act in the interest of others. As mentioned above, the term 'altruism' is a term of art, and could encompass notions of indirect reciprocity of the kind that she describes. If I read her proposal correctly, the idea of reciprocal benefits in organ donation extending across kinship ties and generations is a hybrid form of directed donation that privileges family members on the priority list. One problem with this is that persons who are unmarried, orphaned, estranged from their families, or who belong to small families would be marginalized under such a system. As for reciprocity across generations, the same objection applies. However, it is interesting that if such a system motivates those with heritable disease it is not stated how many generations are to enjoy the benefit, which may have implications for its practicability.

Altruism and solidarity in wider society

Professor Brannigan's fascinating piece deals with the important question of the impact of altruism on social solidarity and draws materials from other contexts, in particular disaster emergency settings. The 'twist' on altruism that he provides is well taken; it is a reminder that the study and critique of altruism in organ donation settings must be viewed against the broad spectrum of other realms of social action that contribute to the web of social understandings which determine public attitudes to altruistic organ donation in its particular forms in particular societies.

It would be a fascinating study to examine public attitudes to altruistic organ donation in Japan after '3/11', when the discipline and social cohesion of ordinary Japanese citizens became a subject that drew worldwide admiration and praise. The provenance of this approach can be traced to Richard Titmuss, who often referred to the wartime experiences of British citizens of his generation as an important factor in public support for unpaid blood donation in the United Kingdom.

References

Chin, J. J., and Campbell, A.V. (2012). 'Transplant Tourism or International Transplant Medicine? A Case for Making the Distinction,' *American Journal of Transplantation*, 12(7): 1700–7.

Jesani, A. (2014). 'Altruism in the Service of the Market and the State, and the Ethics of Regulation,' in A. Akabayashi (ed.), *The Future of Bioethics: International Dialogues*. Oxford: Oxford University Press, 506–10.

Shimazono, Y. (2014). 'Local and Global Contexts of Praxis of Bioethics: "Transplant Tourism" and "Altruistic" Medicine,' in A. Akabayashi (ed.), *The Future of Bioethics: International Dialogues*. Oxford: Oxford University Press, 503–5.

SECTION B

Public Health Ethics

15.1

Primary Topic Article
What is 'Public Health Ethics'?

Angus Dawson

1 Introduction

We might think of public health ethics as consisting of a list of topics or issues reflecting the day-to-day practice of public health practitioners. The list would be a long one and include different kinds of programmes (e.g. vaccination, screening, restaurant inspection, health promotion, etc.) or different methods (e.g. epidemiology, monitoring air and water quality, surveillance, etc.) or particular ethical issues (e.g. how do we weigh the interests of individuals against those of populations, should we always get informed consent before conducting routine surveillance, how important is the pursuit of equity within medical practice? etc.). If nothing else, this provides a quick sense of how the area of public health differs from many of the issues that have been at the forefront of discussions in bioethics for the last 40 years. It should also be immediately apparent to anyone who knows the field of bioethics that such topics and issues have been relatively neglected.

However, this has begun to change over the last ten years, and there is an increasing interest in public health ethics, with numerous articles, edited collections, and a dedicated journal. These developments have had a number of causes. One important inspiration has been the sudden reappearance of mass infectious disease as a threat in the richer parts of the world. (The continuing infectious disease burden in low- and middle-income countries could, of course, be largely ignored.) The belief that such threats were a thing of the past has proven to be overoptimistic with the rise of SARS, H5N1 (avian) flu, H1N1 (swine) flu and drug-resistant forms of tuberculosis. Infectious disease is the area of public health activity that has received the greatest coverage in the ethics literature in recent years. However, it is important to make clear that when we think of public health ethics we ought to notice that it is about more than just issues relating to infectious disease. Public health ethics will include ethical issues relating to health promotion, mental health issues such as suicide, chronic disease, environmental factors, threats to health from radiation, air particulates or contaminated water, health priority setting, health equity, methodological issues relating to population health and epidemiology, etc.

I suggest that thinking of public health ethics as a list of topics is a useful first step in gaining a sense of the field. However, such an approach sees public health ethics as merely *additional* to topics to be covered in the bioethics literature. I want to suggest that this is inadequate and that we ought to think of public health ethics as requiring something more radical, what I will call a *substantive* public health ethics. This view takes as its starting point not a list of topics but the very concept of 'public health' and sees it as foundational to how we ought to think of public health ethics. So what do we mean when we talk of 'public health'? The concept is highly contested. This is hardly surprising as the concept of 'health' itself is notoriously hard to define (Nordenfelt 2007). For example, health can be thought of in narrow, biological terms (perhaps normal functioning) or in broader, more social terms. If we then add the word 'public' to that of 'health', we further complicate the story as there are (at least) two senses of public that can be seen at work here, and both are important (Verweij and Dawson 2007). The first is 'public' as a noun (a public) in the sense of a group or a population. We can talk of this as population health. A population's health can change over time (it can improve or decline, or the distribution of health states of individuals within that population can grow narrower or wider, etc.). It is also easy (perhaps too easy) to see how such a notion of population health lends itself to the idea of population health as the aggregate health of the constituent individuals.

The second sense of 'public' is different and tells us something about the nature of the required response. It is 'public' in a different way, in that much public health activity requires the coordinated actions of many individuals through group or collective interventions. It is because of this feature that the paradigm cases of public health activity are carried out by or on behalf of the state. Such state action is often seen to be the guarantor that the required action occurs, perhaps through the provision of universal programmes or, ultimately, in at least some cases, legal enforcement. This is an important reason why much public health activity can be seen as controversial.

A substantive view of public health ethics sees public health activity as a certain kind of practice, with a particular set of aims and methods. It aims to articulate the relevant values, and defend them and subject them to critique. If accounts of public health ethics do not fit in some way with the practice, then they risk changing the subject. Such an outcome would not count as answering how we ought to think about issues in public health ethics. This does not mean that a substantive account need be uncritical of public health activity as it is envisaged or practised. On a substantive view, public health activity can be unethical, but we should not start with another perspective about how to think about ethics, developed in a different area of health care, and then be surprised if we discover that it clashes with routine public health work performed by sincere and well-meaning public health officials. It makes no sense, I suggest, to start from a position that just presumes that large parts of public health are an illegitimate practice (Dawson 2011).

2 A quick history of public health ethics

Of course, public health threats to human health are as old as humankind. Virtually all cultures contain historical and literary discussion of threats from infectious disease and catastrophic environmental change. The impact of infectious disease can be seen in human bones found through archaeological investigation, and the need for better hygiene and sanitation drove much early government action in the nineteenth century, in relation to work on clean water and better sewage systems for the growing, and increasingly crowded, urban population (Rosen 1993). Concerns about the poor quality of life of many citizens drove legislation to improve workplace conditions and prevent food adulteration, despite the opposition from those with financial interests in the existing state of affairs. Many of these changes used ethical and political arguments, but there was no public health ethics (as such).

It was the 1970s before writers were consciously exploring concepts and arguments that are recognizable today as public health ethics. A leader in the field was Dan Beauchamp (1976; 1985), proposing the importance of the concepts of 'community' and 'social justice' for thinking in this area. A new wave of interest in thinking about infectious disease began with discussion of the often blatantly discriminatory policy response to HIV and AIDS in the early 1980s. This work was led by key, influential figures in public health ethics such as Ron Bayer and Larry Gostin. Another influence on thinking about public health ethics can be seen in the development by bodies such as the American Public Health Association of professional codes of ethical conduct for public health practitioners, as well as the attempt to draw up curricula for courses in public health ethics, to try and establish and encourage the idea of ethical conduct as central to the professional practice of public health (ASPH 2002).

Over time, there has been a consolidation of the field, and an attempt to provide a more systematic approach to thinking about public health ethics, through the development of various frameworks for decision-making. Many of these adopt an approach focused on trying to establish the relevant principles or values for thinking about public health ethics. I will briefly outline three influential accounts here.

Ross Upshur (2002) proposes using four principles to deliberate about public health ethics as follows:

- Harm principle;
- Least restrictive or coercive means;
- Reciprocity principle;
- Transparency principle.

Larry Gostin (2005) proposed a set of public health values as follows:

- Transparency;
- Protection of vulnerable populations;
- Fair treatment and social justice;
- The least restrictive alternative.

James Childress et al. (2002) offered a more complex two-tier approach to decision-making with a distinction between goals and constraints. They suggested three relevant considerations as goals for public health:

- Producing benefits;
- Avoiding, preventing, removing harms;
- Maximizing utility.

And five 'justificatory conditions' for interventions, that act as constraints upon the pursuit of the proposed goals:

- Effectiveness;
- Proportionality;
- Necessity;
- Least infringement;
- Public justification.

How to construct and use frameworks raises many complex issues that cannot be explored here (Dawson 2009). However, we should note not only the different values and principles that are listed in each approach, but also the strong influence of traditional liberal ideas (see below). Even if we agree with a set of proposed principles or values, there are still many questions to ask about the relationships between the different elements, whether we are to rank them or see them as equal, and how they are to be used in actual decision-making. One alternative approach, that does offer clear assistance with deliberation about how we ought to make decisions, is the kind of framework proposed by Nancy Kass (2001). This approach has the advantage that it is focused on a particular issue rather than being over-general. Unusually for a framework, it also provides guidance on how it is to be used and how the different elements are related to each other. Kass offers an ordered series of questions as a means to explore the justifiability of any proposed public health intervention. However, despite this, a careful reading of the descriptive and justificatory paragraphs in the article make clear that individual liberty ends up being the dominant value in this approach after all. This can, however, be questioned, as it is not clear that this is appropriate for a framework about how to make ethical decisions in relation to public health (even assuming it is elsewhere).

An alternative to a principles approach would be to focus on developing a more theoretical perspective towards public health, that is then able to provide some robust policy implications. Key examples would be discussions of health-related justice such as the work of Norman Daniels (2008) and that on social justice by Madison Powers and Ruth Faden (2008), or where there is appeal to a particular theoretical view such as the capabilities approach (Ruger 2009; Venkatapuram 2011). Another option would be to appeal to some overarching theoretical view such as the recent defence of the idea of 'stewardship' by the UK's Nuffield Council (2007) as a means of providing a modified form of liberalism. The central metaphor of 'steward' is used to describe the role and attitude of the state towards individual citizens. The approach is an attempt to avoid both paternalism (which is defined as being a bad thing) and a straightforward libertarianism. However, despite the rhetoric about it being a new approach, it tends to produce the same answers on policy issues because of the central role given to liberty in the use of such things as the intervention ladder (Dawson and Verweij 2008).

3 The dominant approach to public health ethics

Despite all the activity in the area of public health ethics, I suggest that, on the whole, the dominant approach to thinking about these issues has been rather narrow. It has tended to be influenced by models developed over the last 40 years in the context of medical ethics and medical law. They in turn have been dominated by a particular idea about which values ought to be seen as important. Of course it is a vast simplification but the dominant tradition in bioethics has been to invoke a rather simplistic form of liberalism or even libertarianism, held to be derived from John Stuart Mill's famous essay, *On Liberty* (1859). I think we have reason to reject this as being Mill's settled view, and think we have good evidence for seeing him as holding a richer view of ethics than this suggests (Dawson and Verweij 2009; Jennings 2009). Hence, I prefer to see this approach as 'Millian' rather than Millian. The distinction between a libertarian and a liberal is hard to draw. As I use it here, a libertarian holds that liberty (defined as freedom from constraint) is either the only value that matters or the value that must always take priority over other considerations. A liberal, on the other hand, holds liberty to be important to the extent that there ought to be a presumption in its favour, but that it can sometimes be overruled by more important considerations. On this view, being a libertarian is an all-or-nothing affair, whilst liberals come in many varieties. Liberal views in public health ethics are perhaps best represented by Stephen Holland (2007). He provides a thorough and consistent defence and application of this position to a number of different areas of public health. A more sophisticated, but still liberal, view has also recently been developed by John Coggon (2012).

This dominant model sees liberty as captured by the idea of non-interference (Radoilska 2009). That is, there is a *presumption* in favour of liberty unless there is 'good reason' not to allow it to occur. Good reasons are centralized upon the idea of preventing harm to other people. Whatever we might think of this as an approach for other areas of activity, it seems, intuitively, to be a very odd approach to public health. If we have to focus on just one value in public health, why should it be liberty, rather than, say, harm? Indeed, why focus on only one value at all? Surely it makes more sense to argue for a form of value pluralism? On the latter view we accept a range of different values with no prior commitments as to which value takes priority over any others. The danger of focusing on liberty as non-interference is that it is then too easy to frame our discussions of public health ethics merely in terms of an eternal struggle: the individual *versus* the population (or society or state, etc.).

Indeed, this approach is problematic for a number of reasons. First, it fails to account for the fact that the individual is also a member of the population. This means that we ought to be cautious in holding that issues in public health ethics ought to be seen as framed in these either/or terms. What an individual wants might well be in conflict with what is in the interests of a community or population. But merely stating things in these terms is not enough to settle the ethical issue about which ought to take precedence. It will surely depend upon the context. Sometimes we need to ensure that individuals are not merely sacrificed for the public good, but there will be plenty of situations where it is appropriate to hold that individual interests do not take priority. Second, the kinds of issues and values that can be appealed to in this dichotomous approach are limited. It might work, at least to some extent, when we are thinking about whether or not to detain someone refusing to take their tuberculosis medication. But how can it help when it comes to thinking about measures to address poor air or water quality, or issues related to climate change? In these kinds of cases, our thinking ought to turn to ideas about public and common goods, common interests, and values such as solidarity and justice.

So, medical ethics, medical law (Dawson 2010), as well as, arguably, the dominant 'Millian' voice in public health ethics, all seem to point in the same direction: towards a focus on individuals and their liberty as the paramount value. We could, of course, approach public health ethics in this way, but the result will be that much routine public health work ends up being considered unethical. This conclusion seems, at least to me, to be bought at too great a cost.

4   In defence of substantive public health ethics

An alternative view of public health ethics seeks to discover and articulate the values that are (and ought to be) part of public health as a practice. The starting point has to be with what public health is, what it aims to achieve, and what methods it uses to pursue those ends. What might count as the aims of public health is subject to dispute (Munthe 2008), but if we look at public health as a practice, the aims can be seen to be to prevent or reduce harm, to promote health, and to identify and reduce health inequities. It will be instantly apparent that seeking to attain such ends will require both individual and collective action. This links with the suggestion made earlier that we can think about using our account of public health as the basis for a different, more substantive, public health ethics.

In developing such a substantive public health ethics we can look to more social values, values that are visible and emerge from the fact that as human creatures we are social beings. Such values will not only include the kinds of values that have dominated discussions in medical ethics such as respect for autonomy, beneficence, and non-maleficence, but will also include such things as solidarity, reciprocity, common goods, trust, and social justice. Many of these can be linked to the necessary conditions for a flourishing life. Decision-making will involve articulating these values, and accepting that sometimes we will have to sacrifice some values, for the sake of others, when they are considered to be more important at a particular time. However, this does not mean that the 'defeated' values are to be discarded. All such values can be seen to be equal, in the sense that no value has priority or a presumption in its favour. Decision-making involves the use of discussion and experience to find the best solution to the problems we face together. Health is not always the critical factor, but it is often vitally important, because of the foundational role that it plays in our lives, whatever we wish to pursue. Seeing the value of health, including the aspects of our health that can only be pursed through the activities of public health, is not a merely prudential matter, nor does it require any individual declaration or endorsement by the individual themselves. In addition, at least some public health practice is concerned with protecting the weak and the vulnerable, in the sense of those unable to protect themselves. This substantive approach will be one focused on ideas about human interests, goods, and the harms that can damage these considerations. We have no good reason to think that all goods are individual goods or that they are merely linked to that which is desired (Dawson 2011). It is by living within families, social groups, and communities that we become who we are.

Such a substantive view of public health ethics will be aligned with other areas of applied ethics such as global and environmental ethics. The links to global ethics come about, as there is no good reason to delimit what counts as public health as being circumscribed by the boundaries of a state. Public health is about all health, even if pragmatically we tend to see it as primarily the responsibility of the state. It can also be linked to global ethics, because of a common concern to act to bring about greater social justice. The link can be made to environmental ethics as many public health problems link with issues relating to animal health (e.g. zoonotic diseases), food production, water, air and land management, climate change, etc.

The substantive approach is not, of course, beyond criticism. It remains vague, and needs to be filled out. However, at this stage all I seek to do is to provide the opportunity to move away from the dominant set of assumptions shaping much of the current discussion in public health ethics. Critique of this alternative should not just consist of repeating the idea that individual liberty ought to be the supreme value. A substantive account provides no reason to see individuals as necessarily being 'sacrificed' for the greater good. Liberty is an important value, but it can be weighed against others, and those others can tip the scales. It may also be objected that this approach gives too much power to public health professionals and/or governments. However, there is no reason to think that it is incompatible with democratic structures that can provide legitimacy to action, after consultation and debate. If such social structures are in place and liberty is curtailed for the sake of the public's health, why should we think this is necessarily wrong?

5 An example: smoking policy

We can see how such different approaches work out by exploring an example. Smoking policy over the last 30 years can be used to illustrate how a 'Millian' approach has come to define the limits of state intervention for many. On this view the key occasions when the state can intervene legitimately in individual choices is when it is seeking to inform about the risk of harm, protect those unable to protect themselves, or to protect third parties from harm. Different elements of smoking policy over the last 30 years can be used to illustrate this approach. Warning labels on cigarette packets provide information about the possible cumulative effects of smoking. Policy to protect those not able to make a fully informed decision about whether to smoke is illustrated by restricting access to cigarette vending machines by removing them from open public places such as station platforms, to make it harder for young people to get access to cigarettes. Banning smoking in cars when children are present or in public places such as workplaces, bars, and restaurants, protects third parties from the harm resulting from so-called 'passive' smoking.

However, this is about as far as the 'Millian' arguments will get us. Other policies that have been implemented may be condemned as illiberal. For example, high taxation on cigarettes where the intention is to prevent or reduce consumption by smokers can be seen as aimed at reducing the harm to an individual, even if that individual may wish to smoke. (Of course, politicians might just cynically use this as an excuse, when they are really seeking to raise revenue.) Policies such as placing cigarettes in plain packaging (as in Australia) or removing cigarettes from public display at the point of sale (as in Ontario, Canada), or controlling when or where cigarette advertising occurs may be more difficult to justify on the liberal approach. Does this mean they are unjustifiable? Not necessarily.

We might look to other possible arguments to justify such restrictive smoking policies. They might not be ones that the libertarian is happy to accept, but of course that is not itself a rebuttal. The first argument focuses on smoking as a social practice. This argument appeals to the idea that individuals do not simply make their choices in a social vacuum. Our choices are influenced or shaped by the choices that others make. If I grow up in a society where all around me are smoking, there is a higher probability that I am likely to accept this norm and smoke myself. However, if I grow up in a place where few people smoke, particularly where few of my family or friends smoke, then the norm is set against smoking, and it is more likely that I will not smoke. Of course, individual willpower might mean that I choose to go against any such norms, but this point can be used to illustrate the power of culture, tradition, and social norms upon the choices that we all make. This provides an argument for more restrictive smoking policies where the aim is to try and shape smoking norms in relation to smokers by making it harder to smoke and easier to give up, and in relation to non-smokers (particularly children) by making it less likely that they are exposed to smoking behaviour as a normal part of life.

The second argument appeals to the idea of social justice and builds upon the first. We know that there is a social gradient in relation to smoking, in that you are more likely to smoke if you belong to a lower-income group. As a result, all other things being equal, if you are a child brought up in a lower-income group it is more likely that you will smoke than if you are raised in a higher-income group. Is this an inequity that we wish to tolerate? It is not clear that we should do so, and the argument for using this as a justification for further restriction on smoking and cigarette sales can appeal to the idea of social justice as a justification. We have no reason a priori to think that the freedom to smoke must take precedence over greater equity in health outcomes. We might choose to prioritize an individual's freedom to smoke, but if we do so, we must accept the true costs of that action; in this case, the likely result is more smokers, with more harm as a result, and greater inequity in the distribution of that known harm. The libertarian can again assert the priority that ought to be given to liberty, but this looks less plausible as we explore these other arguments. Indeed, as time goes by, and despite the practical objections related to smuggling, etc., given our knowledge about the harms, it becomes harder and harder not to think that an eventual total ban on tobacco makes sense (Proctor 2011).

6 Conclusion

Public health ethics is a flourishing area of activity within bioethics. There is a growing body of work, expanding to take in more and more topics and approaches. However, I have argued here that it must take care not to lean too heavily upon the resources from elsewhere as this may result in an inappropriate framing of public health issues with the resultant presumption that much routine activity is morally wrong (Dawson 2011). Of course, it could be that such actions are unethical; but such a claim requires argument, not just an inference from a contestable assumption. I have argued, instead, for what I have called substantive public health ethics, a perspective building upon a critical but sympathetic evaluation of the aims and methods of public health as a practice.

References

Association of Schools of Public Health (ASPH). (2003). *Ethics and Public Health: Model Curriculum*. Washington DC: ASPH. http://www.asph.org/document.cfm?page=782 (accessed 15 January 2013).

Beauchamp, D. E. (1976). 'Public Health as Social Justice', *Enquiry*, 13(1): 363–70.

Beauchamp, D. E. (1985). 'Community: The Neglected Tradition of Public Health', *Hastings Center Report*, 15(6): 28–36.

Childress, J. F. et al. (2002). 'Public Health Ethics: Mapping the Terrain', *Journal of Law, Medicine, and Ethics*, 30(2): 170–8.

Coggon, J. (2012). *What Makes Health Public?* Cambridge: Cambridge University Press.

Daniels, N. (2008). *Just Health: Meeting Health Needs Fairly*. Cambridge: Cambridge University Press.

Dawson, A. (2009). 'Theory and Practice in Public Health Ethics: A Complex Relationship', in S. Peckham, and A. Hann (eds), *Public Health Ethics and Practice*. London: Policy Press, 191–209.

Dawson, A. (2010). 'The Future of Bioethics: Three Dogmas and a Cup of Hemlock', *Bioethics*, 24 (5): 218–25.

Dawson, A. (2011). 'Resetting the Parameters: Public Health as the Foundation for Public Health Ethics', in A. Dawson (ed), *Public Health Ethics: Key Concepts and Issues in Policy and Practice*. Cambridge: Cambridge University Press, 143–53.

Dawson, A., and Verweij, M. (2008). 'The Steward of the Millian State', *Public Health Ethics*, 1(3): 1–3.

Gostin, L. O. (2005). 'Public Health Preparedness and Ethical Values in Pandemic Influenza', in S. L. Knobler et al. (eds), *The Threat of Pandemic Influenza: Are We Ready?* Washington, DC: National Academies Press, 357–72.

Holland, S. (2007). *Public Health Ethics*. Cambridge: Polity Press.

Jennings, B. (2009). 'Public Health and Liberty: Beyond the Liberty Paradigm', *Public Health Ethics*, 2(2): 123–34.

Kass, N. E. (2001). 'An Ethics Framework for Public Health', *American Journal of Public Health*, 91(11): 1776–82.

Munthe, C. (2008). 'The Goals of Public Health: An Integrated, Multidimensional Model', *Public Health Ethics*, 1(1): 39–52.

Nordenfelt, L. (2007). 'The Concepts of Health and Disease', in R. Ashcroft et al. (eds), *Principles of Health Care Ethics*. 2nd ed. Chichester: Wiley, 537–42.

Nuffield Council on Bioethics. (2007). *Public Health: Ethical Issues*. London: NCB.

Powers, M., and Faden, R. (2008). *Social Justice: The Moral Foundations of Public Health and Health Policy*. Oxford: Oxford University Press.

Proctor, R. N. (2011). *Golden Holocaust: Origins of the Cigarette Catastrophe and the Case for Abolition*. Berkeley, CA: University of California Press.

Radoilska, L. (2009). 'Public Health Ethics and Liberalism', *Public Health Ethics*, 2(2): 135–45.

Rosen, G. (1993). *A History of Public Health*. Expanded ed. Baltimore, MD: Johns Hopkins University Press.

Ruger, J. P. (2009). *Health and Social Justice*. Oxford: Oxford University Press.

Upshur, R. E. G. (2002). 'Principles for the Justification of Public Health Interventions', *Canadian Journal of Public Health*, 93(2): 101–3.

Venkatapuram, S. (2011). *Health Justice: An Argument for the Capabilities Approach*. Cambridge: Polity Press.

Verweij, M., and Dawson, A. (2007). 'The Meaning of 'Public' in Public Health', in A. Dawson, and M. Verweij (eds), *Ethics, Prevention, and Public Health*. Oxford: Oxford University Press, 13–29.

15.2

Commentary
What is 'Substantive Public Health Ethics'?[1]

Keiichiro Yamamoto

The question 'What is "public health ethics"?' is indeed perplexing, just as most philosophical problems are. In his splendid paper, Professor Dawson takes a courageous step to address this issue and argues that we need a more radical approach toward public health and should part company with the dominant model in traditional bioethics. He then attempts to develop his own approach, namely what he calls 'a substantive public health ethics'. Although this attempt is certainly noteworthy, several important questions remain unanswered, given the radial basis of his public health ethics. In order to understand it, I raise a few questions in the following sections and demonstrate that his substantive public health ethics is, overall, inscrutable.

One of the main reasons why Dawson regards his own public health ethics as 'radical' and 'substantive' is that it differs from the dominant tradition in bioethics: a form of libertarianism and/or liberalism. What is it that distinguishes his approach from this dominant model? In my view, there are at least two important differences. First, his substantive public health ethics presupposes a form of value pluralism, which demands that we compare a range of different values without any prior commitment as to which value takes priority over others. Second, he proposes a different methodology to develop public health ethics, starting with the very concept of 'public health' and focusing on public health as a practice. Here, my attention centres on these two differences.

On the first difference

According to Dawson's definitions, unlike libertarianism, liberalism accepts a form of value pluralism and thus allows commensurability or trade-offs among certain values (see also Griffin 1986: 77–92). It is clear that Dawson also argues for a kind of value pluralism in this chapter. Given this, there appears to be no distinction between his public health ethics and this sort of liberalism. A significant difference, however, lies in

[1] I am grateful to Drs. Satoshi Kodama, Akifumi Shimanouchi, Eisuke Nakazawa, and Atsushi Tsuchiya for helpful comments and discussions on the topic of this chapter.

the requirement of having no prior commitments when deciding which value takes precedence over others.

This requirement raises both philosophical and practical issues. First, despite Dawson's intention, it seems to imply that we should assume a neutral position or a tolerant attitude when comparing different values. If so, does this not mean that we have a prior commitment to some liberal value, namely neutrality or tolerance? (see Dawson 2011: 7; also Gray 1996; Berlin 2002). It seems that the harder we try to comply with this requirement, the more we commit to such a liberal value.[2] Second, because the liberalism Dawson has in his mind allows comparability between certain values, is it not possible for the liberal to alter his or her commitment as to which value should take priority *after* a debate on public health ethics, even if s/he was committed to a liberal value such as autonomy *before* the debate? If this change is possible in practice, I do not see any problems with having a prior commitment to a certain value.

Furthermore, as a matter of practice, I think it may be acceptable for an individual to have a prior commitment to not all but *a certain* liberal value when discussing *certain* types of public health activities, if their history is given serious consideration. As Dawson describes in this chapter, public health activities are diverse, ranging from prevention of infectious diseases to health promotion, which also means that there are different kinds of public health interventions. For instance, the Japanese government passed a law on the segregation of leprosy patients in 1907. Segregation was maintained under the revised law, the Leprosy Prevention Law, even after a new government was established at the end of World War II and Promin was shown to be effective in those patients. The law was finally abolished in 1996. Hajime Sato and Minoru Narita, who studied this segregation, explain why the Japanese government upheld the law for almost 90 years as follows:

> This study demonstrates that the segregation of leprosy patients was introduced in Japan soon after the disease was found to be contagious, but maintained long after it became known that patient isolation is not necessary in the majority of cases. Segregation or isolation of leprosy patients was advocated and justified in the language of science and *public health*. (Sato and Narita 2003: 2535; italics added)

If we take a closer look at the history of public health, we may well discover other similar interventions implemented in the name of public health, for example the Tuskegee Syphilis Study. In light of these historical facts, it does not appear too irrelevant to the discussion of certain public health activities that we are committed to a certain kind of liberty, such as the idea of non-interference, prior to its comparison with other important values.

---

[2] If we seriously consider this requirement of no prior commitment, it may lead to a Rawlsian veil of ignorance and detract from communitarianism, such as that proposed by Michael Sandel. This could be one reason why Dawson hesitates to consider communitarianism as a political philosophy for his public health ethics (see Dawson 2011: 12–13).

On the second difference

Another important distinction that we can find in Dawson's approach to public health relates to his method of developing public health ethics—likely another important reason why he considers his public health ethics as 'substantive'. It is one thing to advocate value pluralism and another to explain how a certain value can take precedence over others. In other words, no matter how vehemently we defend his value pluralism, we need another argument to demonstrate how certain values given great importance in public health practice can take priority over others, including certain liberties. Dawson's substantive public health ethics is expected to provide this argument. He then proposes a new approach to develop such a public health ethics, which begins with the very concept of 'public health' and captures the nature of public health as a practice. Indeed, he all too often highlights the gravity of framing public health ethics on the basis of public health as a practice. This substantive public health ethics can in turn refer to the social values he mentions in this chapter, which may justify a certain public health practice, such as smoking regulations.

This approach may have several advantages, but I will venture to pose a series of questions. It is true that Dawson's approach can be 'radical' and quite different from that of traditional bioethics. For unlike his substantive public health ethics, traditional bioethics, I believe, did not simply set out with the very concept of medicine or the nature of medicine as a practice. Aside from the difficulties associated with capturing the nature of medical practice, if we accept his methodology and inquire into medical practice per se, is it possible for us to discover, other than its professional ethics, bioethics as we have now? The answer may be negative. It can be said that traditional bioethics must have been introduced to provide a critical scrutiny of medical practice: something external to such practice. By contrast, his substantive public health ethics appears to have developed from public health practice itself: something internal to that practice. If so, how can it provide a critical perspective on such practice?

Of course, the form of value pluralism Dawson presents can offer a critical perspective to a certain extent, because it requires that we accord equal consideration to a set of values, including certain liberal values. On the other hand, his substantive public health ethics goes a step further to show how certain social values can take priority over others. I wonder what his justification for those values in a political situation would be at this stage. Put another way, as Dawson states in his other paper that 'it makes sense to see [political philosophy] as being at the core of public health ethics' (Dawson 2009: 121), what is his political philosophy?[3] In my view, he offers no details on grounds of those social values in this chapter, except for the implication that they 'can be linked to the necessary conditions for a flourishing life'. Moreover, he appears to think that institutions of democracy can provide another critical perspective. It can, however, be argued that they do not always work as expected. For instance, all we need is to remember the history of public health, such as the segregation of leprosy patients in Japan mentioned above. Yutaka Fujino, an authority on segregation policy issues, opines that it was

---

[3] Arguments for the need of some kind of political philosophy to think about public health can also be found in O'Neil (2002), and Powers, Faden, and Saghai (2012).

Japanese democracy after World War II that needed it and justified it on account of public welfare (Fujino 2006: 19–20). Undoubtedly, one can point out the idiosyncrasies of Japanese democracy, but cases like this can also be found in other democratic societies.

Conclusion

A closer perusal reveals that Dawson may not fully answer the question he himself raised in this chapter: 'What is "public health ethics"?' This may reflect the fact that at this moment what his 'substantive public health ethics' really is remains elusive. On the other hand, as Dawson points out, it is indeed problematic that we make it a rule to ensure that liberties of all sorts always trump other values. Should we maintain that kind of extreme libertarianism, it would become difficult to have a meaningful discussion on public health or even to develop public health ethics. If we pay sufficient attention to his arguments in this chapter, we will likely avoid that pitfall.

References

Berlin, I. (2002). *Liberty*, edited by H. Hardy. Oxford: Oxford University Press.

Dawson, A. (2009). 'Editorial: Political Philosophy and Public Health Ethics', *Public Health Ethics*, 2(2): 121–2.

Dawson, A. (2011), 'Resetting the Parameters: Public Health as the Foundation for Public Health Ethics', in A. Dawson (ed), *Public Health Ethics*, Cambridge: Cambridge University Press, 143–53.

Fujino, Y. (2006). *Hansenbyo to Sengo Minshushugi* (Hansen's Disease and Postwar Democracy). Tokyo: Iwanami.

Gray, J. (1996). *Isaiah Berlin*. Princeton, NJ: Princeton University Press.

Griffin, J. (1986). *Well-Being*. Oxford: Clarendon Press.

O'Neil, O. (2002). 'Public Health or Clinical Ethics: Thinking beyond Borders', *Ethics and International Affairs*, 16(2): 35–45.

Powers, M., Faden, R., and Saghai, Y. (2012), 'Liberty, Mill and the Framework of Public Health', *Public Health Ethics*, 5(1): 6–15.

Sato, H., and Narita, M. (2003). 'Politics of Leprosy Segregation in Japan: The Emergence, Transformation and Abolition of the Patient Segregation Policy', *Social Science and Medicine*, 56:2529–39.

15.3

Commentary
What are Collective Values?

Ryoji Sato

In his paper, Dawson criticizes what he calls 'the dominant approach' in public health ethics and argues for 'substantive health ethics'. He claims that the dominant approach to public health ethics focuses too much on individual liberty. According to the dominant approach, individual liberty should be maximally preserved unless there is a reason to do otherwise, such as others being harmed. In doing so, Dawson claims, the dominant approach fails to capture the legitimacy of many practices in public health ethics. Dawson admits that even from the liberalist point of view, some practices such as vaccination against infectious diseases are justifiable, as avoidance of vaccination may cause harm to others and thereby violate the harm principle. However, he suggests that it is mysterious how the approach can justify our current actions toward environmental issues that involve air and water pollution, and climate change. On the other hand, Dawson writes that substantive public health ethics 'seeks to discover and articulate the values that are (and ought to be) part of public health as a practice' (Dawson in this chapter), and hence incorporates values other than individual liberty. He names public and common goods, common interests, and social values (hereafter, 'collective values') as candidates of values without which 'much routine public health work ends up being considered unethical' (Dawson in this chapter).

In this commentary, I hope to concentrate on the notions of collective values, since it seems that there are two entirely different ways of unpacking the notions. This, in turn, might produce two entirely different ways of coping with public health-related issues. To illustrate this, I will first invoke Dawson's example of substantive public ethics, because I think one interpretation is implicitly adopted there.

Dawson considers the policies on and legal restriction of smoking as examples of substantive public health ethics. He argues that while many policies such as those aimed to prevent passive smoking and to protect minors are justifiable in the liberalist framework, policies such as high taxation on cigarettes or hiding them from display in stores (see section 5 in this chapter for more detail) are not easy to defend. This is primarily because those policies violate the liberty to smoke at will. He does contend, however, that these may be justifiable from the perspective of substantive public health ethics.

Dawson lays out two arguments to justify these policies and restriction. The first deals with the fact that smoking is a social practice. If the norm encourages smoking in society, more people tend to smoke, and if the norm discourages smoking, more people tend to not smoke. While this sounds plausible, it is unclear why this fact supports political intervention against smoking. One possibility is that the norm relegates one's decision with regard to smoking; the decision seems to be regulated exclusively by an individual, but society actually plays a large role to influence this as well. Another possibility is that changing the social norm relevant to smoking involves minimal (and thus permissible) infringement of liberty and brings in a greater benefit to society. If the social norm is successfully changed to discourage smoking, fewer people would want to smoke, leading to less infringement of liberty. The exception to this would be during the transition period, when a substantial amount of infringement would occur. Either way, Dawson tries to argue that liberty is not the supreme value, and under certain circumstances, it is comparable to the benefit of not smoking.

The second argument is much more straightforward. Dawson mentions that people raised in a lower-income group are more likely to smoke. Policies that try to put cigarettes out of reach of these people are justifiable from the viewpoint of social justice. In this case, he explicitly refers to the value of social justice as a value which might be able to trump liberty.

As revealed by these arguments, when Dawson writes of 'public and common goods, common interests, and values such as solidarity and justice', they are conceived as something that can diverge from what people *actually value*. In a pro-smoking society, smoking is associated with positive stereotypes, and people value that. Dawson recommends abandoning the habit, simply because it is *objectively* bad. This point is clearer in his previous work. He says: 'The goods I am interested in here are those things that are good for humans (or allow human flourishing or the good life). They will include some of the same things that are often appealed to during the formulation of arguments over the objective list forms of consequentialism (for example, autonomy, pleasure, health, etc.)' (Dawson 2011: 14). However, a more subjectivistic (or what might be called communitarian) interpretation of 'collective values' is also possible, and would state that collective goods are conceived as what the majority of the population actually regards as important. In this interpretation, the policies discussed above might not be recommended in highly pro-smoking societies. Indeed, while global enthusiasm exists toward reducing smoking, perspectives on alcohol consumption or drugs vary widely across countries. As such, it might be best to defend the status quo according to cultural trends. In this way, these two interpretations of 'collective values' can produce two different sorts of public health policies.

Of course, it would be absurd to count only subjective values or to count only objective values. If only subjective values are considered, no 'progressive' policies that the majority of population does not support could be implemented. We could not even say we make progress if we succeed in reducing smoking. Moreover, there is the danger of sacrificing minorities; policies must be in accordance with current values of the group. On the other hand, paternalism and chauvinism could result from being wholly objective. As such, inclusion of both subjective and objective values is the most intuitive, and is likely to be most in line with Dawson's intention. I would contend, however, that just incorporating both values is not sufficient to justify certain policies because the balance between them is critical for determining what types of public health policies are justifiable. For example, if you place more importance on subjective values, the policies on and restriction of smoking would not be justifiable.

One reason the dominant approach has been dominant may be the fear of the latter, more subjectivistic interpretation of 'collective values.' Oppression of minorities for the sake of the majority has occurred historically in the fields such as eugenics policies, and concerns certainly exist for the future. For example, genetic screening would benefit the majority of people, but the benefits for those with the genetic 'risks' might be impaired in terms of health insurance or family relationships. A similar concern is anticipated for the recent enterprise to prevent mental illness, which involves identification of people with the risk of psychosis.[4]

Faced with these possibilities, some may wish to remain in the liberalist account, and try to respond to Dawson's criticism that the liberalist position cannot justify everyday practice in the domain of public health ethics. It might be carried out by applying principles they can also adopt. For example, a liberalist could justify policies relevant to smoking (discussed above) by making use of the harm principle. More people smoking would lead to more people with lung cancer. This would produce an unnecessary economic burden on the public insurance system, which would create economic harm to others. From this point of view, one might conclude that every effort should be made to reduce the amount of smoking.

It is not clear how many of the daily practices in public health are actually covered by these arguments, but it seems that most types of activities would apply. While some explanations may sound unnatural or ad hoc, lacking elegance may be preferable to the most unwanted consequences such as oppression of minorities.

References

Dawson, A. (2011). 'Resetting the Parameters: Public Health as the Foundation for Public Health Ethics,' in A. Dawson (ed), *Public Health Ethics*. New York: Cambridge University Press, 143–53.

Dawson, A. (2014). 'What is 'Public Health Ethics'?' in A. Akabayashi (ed.), *The Future of Bioethics: International Dialogues*. Oxford: Oxford University Press, 529–38.

Schaffner, K. F., and McGorry, P. D. (2001). 'Preventing Severe Mental Illnesses: New Prospects and Ethical Challenges,' *Schizophrenia Research*, 51 (1): 3–15.

---

[4] See Schaffner and McGorry (2001) for details of prevention research of psychosis and ethical problems related to it.

15.4

Commentary
What is Expected of Public Health Ethics?

Taketoshi Okita

As Dawson points out, public health includes many activities. Although one must consider the issues common to these activities, there are also issues specific to particular activities. Ethical discussion of these issues cannot be advanced without considering how these individual activities are practiced. In that sense, public health ethics should not be simply regarded as an extension of medical ethics and bioethics which treat medical institutions as the primary setting. Instead, it is necessary to carry out discussions by confronting the activities that constitute public health.

The present discussion divides the activities of public health into two broad categories. One involves formulating countermeasures against acute infectious diseases such as H1N1 influenza virus infection that emerged as a worldwide epidemic in 2009. The other includes health promotion measures, such as the smoking policies discussed by Dawson. This is, of course, not to say that all public health activities fall into one of these categories. Even in the case of acute infection countermeasures for infectious diseases like H1N1 infection, there are other issues such as the stockpiling and distribution of vaccines and antiviral drugs that do not fall under the category of non-pharmaceutical interventions. Moreover, there are issues that overlap with health promotion within routine influenza countermeasures that individuals are expected to take (in particular, wearing of masks in Japan). Thus, in commenting on Dawson's arguments, I will make two overall points using the above distinctions mainly for convenience.

First, with respect to countermeasures against acute infectious diseases such as H1N1 infection, I will consider non-pharmaceutical interventions, in particular quarantines. After infections with the new H1N1 influenza virus were first reported in Mexico and elsewhere overseas in 2009, there was growing alarm about travelers and returnees from North America in Japan and its mass media. Day after day there was talk about whether or not travelers with symptoms such as high fever were infected with H1N1 influenza virus. For a time, the minister of health, welfare and labor personally came out to make statements in front of the media. In cases in which H1N1 virus infection was suspected, the concerned person's freedom of movement was restricted, and if an infection was confirmed by test results, the person was confined to lodgings or medical institutions near airports for a set period of time. Those who had come into contact with the infected and thus were suspected of infection were similarly confined to a specified place. The measure known as 'restriction of activities' or 'quarantine' was adopted.

This could be regarded as a representative example of an ethical problem related to public health. The problem fits neatly into the typical schema of argument in that it involves the protection of society's interest in preventing the spread of infection and the restriction of individual freedom. As Dawson points out, the thinking that regards only individual freedom as a dominant value or takes a position of noninterference with individual liberty is unable to implement necessary countermeasures. There is no time to spare when establishing countermeasures for highly contagious diseases or infections accompanied by extremely severe symptoms, and even brief hesitation can lead to irreversible harm. From the perspective of preventing the spread of infection, and in order to implement ethically appropriate countermeasures, there is an unquestionable need to establish arguments that are tailored to the public health-specific event of preventing infection, but are not based on zero-sum thinking.

At the same time, however, this does not eliminate the fact that the freedom of quarantined individuals has been restricted. Even if this is an unavoidable act taken to prevent the spread of infection, consideration must still be given to the individual whose liberty is restricted. In the context of Japanese H1N1 countermeasures, there was a leak of personal information, such as the location of residence and institutional affiliation, of quarantined individuals found to be infected, which led to panicked, hyper-inflated reporting and even bashing of the infected. Furthermore, in some cases, the infection was apparently reported on television before the infected individual was personally informed, and thus some people learned of their infection from the news. Although the infected were directed to dispose of their clothing, it is said that no compensation was offered. This treatment of individuals subject to quarantine was never confirmed even at official settings that reviewed H1N1 influenza countermeasures, and was only corroborated by medical practitioners who privately felt there was a problem.[5]

When discussing the ethical implications of measures that result in violation of individual freedom of movement or privacy, there appear to be dangers in the way that arguments are formulated based on justification. Is there not a danger that in discussing the issue in either/or terms of whether or not the measures are justified, the detailed circumstances faced by those subject to measures such as quarantine might be taken lightly? Certainly no time can be wasted in implementing influenza countermeasures, as they require swift decision-making. Discussions that simply obstruct timely action would seem meaningless. Yet, regardless of the degree to which public health activities are justified as appropriate and based on ethical considerations, this does not cancel out the violation of individual rights. In public health activities, there always remains something that cannot be justified, and I think there is a need for a framework for debate

---

[5] http://apital.asahi.com/article/takayama/2012111500024.html (accessed 16 January 2013). It has been reported that although in official discussions the government was aware that the scientific grounds were weak for the series of measures, including quarantines, these measures were nevertheless implemented.

premised on unflagging verification of activities, even after the fact.[6] In that sense, the "Millian" approach described by Dawson could represent an important approach to public health ethics, given the constant pursuit of individual freedom. It may not be appropriate to discuss public health ethics solely based on the "Millian" approach, but that does not mean that it should be completely replaced with another approach.

Next, I would like to briefly touch on health promotion activities, such as cigarette smoking policies. As Dawson accurately points out, these activities go beyond disease prevention and health promotion, and have a character that can lead to the construction of social norms.

Dawson points out that public health, in aiming to realize the values it aspires to, is moving more and more beyond the framework of the state. This applies not only to infectious diseases such as influenza infection, but to health-promotion issues related to smoking and alcohol consumption. This is clear from a look at recent trends at the World Health Organization. Yet it must not be forgotten that the primary actor in making changes to the legal system and similar activities is the state. As Dawson points out with respect to the work of Rosen, public health came into being together with the establishment of the modern state. When it comes down to issues primarily concerned with the health of individuals, why does the state become involved in constructing social norms? This cannot be discussed without considering economic dimensions such as health-care costs.

Similarly, Foucault is one figure who, while citing Rosen, analyzed how public health was related to the establishment of the modern state and the ways it contributes to the maintenance of the current state and society (Foucault 1994a: 40–58; Foucault 1994b: 207–28). Foucault's analysis, while somewhat unrefined, offers extremely rich insight of particular use in investigating the aims of new public health including health promotion, and in critically verifying its functions. For some reason, however, it seems that Foucault's ideas are rarely brought up in discussions of public health ethics.[7]

As Dawson argues, it is necessary to discuss the value of public health sympathetically, as nothing will come of merely pointing out its problems. Public health, however, is an activity implicated in social norms—which is to say that, if we are forced to build a society using the means of public health, then it is necessary to have a perspective that questions what the goals of public health are and considers what kind of society public health helps construct. Such a perspective is necessary if public health ethics is truly to be substantive. Foucault is just one example that provides such a perspective. I think it is necessary in public health ethics to strive for a cross-discipline discussion that brings in perspectives from political thought, sociology, and so on.

---

[6] In discussions by Gostin et al. (2003), for example, individuals subject to quarantine are treated as people who contributed to preventing the spread of infection, and it is argued that their opinions must be heard by a third-party organization and any damages incurred must be compensated.

[7] A search for the name Foucault within *Public Health Ethics* edited by Dawson yielded very few hits (as of 19 July 2012).

References

Foucault, M. (1994a). 'Cris de la Médecine ou Crise de l'Antimédecine?' *Dits et Écrits III*, Paris: Gallimard, 40–58.

Foucault, M. (1994b). 'La naissance de la médecine sociale,' *Dits et Écrits III*, Paris: Gallimard, 207–28.

Gostin, L. O. et al. (2003). 'Ethical and Legal Challenges Posed by Severe Acute Respiratory Syndrome: Implications for the Control of Severe Infectious Disease Threats', in R. Bayer et al. (ed), *Public Health Ethics: Theory, Policy, and Practice*, Oxford: Oxford University Press, 261–78.

15.5

Commentary
Public Health as Civic Practice

Bruce Jennings

The fields of ethics and political theory have undergone a veritable renaissance in the past two generations. This is due in part to the emergence of many outstanding individual thinkers whose innovative and influential work has elevated the level of philosophical and theoretical creativity in these fields. However, in large part this revitalization is also due to the practical or applied turn of normative inquiry, which has taken moral and political philosophy out of the academy and into the wider polity and society. The discourses of professional ethics, including physician and nursing ethics, government ethics, environmental ethics, bioethics, and now public health ethics have all developed apace, bringing large numbers of scholars, educators, policy advisors, and consultants into this domain.

What are the place and contribution of public health ethics in this complex intellectual and cultural formation, this 'practical turn' in ethics? Angus Dawson offers a persuasive answer to this question and takes an important step forward in mapping and clarifying the distinctive identity for this rapidly developing field. His essay is more than merely a snapshot of the discipline or a review of work in the field so far; I read it as an exercise in what might be called the meta-theory of public health ethics. In my view, Dawson makes an important contribution to this meta-theoretical discussion.

The field of public health ethics needs philosophical and methodological self-consciousness and self-scrutiny at this time for several reasons. For one thing, public health ethics is emerging out of the larger background field of bioethics. Bioethics has certainly established itself both intellectually and institutionally, but it also has meta-theoretical and conceptual blind spots of its own, and past work in bioethics is not in every way a model that public health ethics should imitate. Even more fundamentally, public health ethics requires self-scrutiny because public health itself poses unique challenges to ethics inquiry and normative discourse. Public health policy and practice are a complex domain with a rich, but chequered, political and ideological history. Contemporary global health problems, and consequently the profession of public health itself, are also embedded in a dynamic system of political economic and governance that is at a particularly crucial historical moment. The present forces of global capitalism and neoliberalism are transforming the post-World War II system of national welfare states, and thereby altering the foundations of contemporary public health. This leads to normative confusion and ethical challenge for the authority and public legitimacy of public health functions within most countries today. Public health ethics must be conceptually well equipped to address this dynamic of legitimization and to preserve the progressive, humanitarian values of the public health tradition and profession at its best. I shall return to this point later.

Dawson avoids two shortcomings that have marked many similar discussions in recent years. First, he does not simplistically pit an individual health perspective against a population health perspective, as some have done via the contrast between bioethics and public health ethics. And second, he does not define public health ethics in terms of some particular agenda of topics.

Bioethics and public health ethics are often opposed to one another as if the former were the champion of individualism and the latter the defender of collectivism. This dichotomy is too crude to shed any light on ethical questions of health at either the clinical or the population level, and Dawson is careful not to ground his conception of the distinctiveness of public health ethics upon it. To be sure, Dawson does make note of the relative neglect by mainstream bioethics of many social and health problems (including but not limited to infectious disease) that are significant at the population level. But he does not conclude from this that the role of public health ethics is to be merely a kibitzer or a special advocate for neglected problems. He argues instead that public health ethics should be grounded on what he calls a 'substantive conception' of public health itself.

What does that substantive conception amount to? In answering this question Dawson appeals to the notion of a practice, which has become a familiar term of art in ethics. 'A substantive view of public health ethics,' he writes, 'sees public health activity as a certain kind of practice, with a particular set of aims and methods. It aims to articulate the relevant values, and defend them and subject them to critique' (Dawson 2014: 530).

In other words, the ethical assessment of public health policies and programmes grows out of an interpretive understanding of the kind of thing public health is—the study, promotion, and maintenance of it—and a thick description of the human meaning and significance of health and flourishing and of the form of life involved in achieving public health. Ethical assessment should not be based on abstract principles applied from an extrinsic standpoint alone. Rather, ethical judgement and evaluation must engage human conduct from within its active, ongoing conditions and circumstances. In this fashion Dawson distances public health ethics from the engineering model of 'applied ethics,' and the notion that specific action-guiding conclusions can be derived from very general covering principles—two meta-theoretical orientations that have been exceedingly influential in the cognate field of bioethics.

The type of public health ethics that Dawson calls for does not lend itself to armchair philosophy and hypothetical cases. It requires a thick description of circumstance (ethics should be informed by history and social science), and it involves the facilitation of human well-being, capability, and development on the level of both individual agency and social institutions.

This approach to ethics is possible and cogent because human conduct does not consist of isolated acts by discrete individuals, but is structured into social 'practices' embedded within cultural orders of meaning. Practices are patterns of conduct that a given cultural tradition identifies with the meeting of human needs and with the pursuit of human excellences. They are the normative, rule-governed forms of conduct that can be learned and can be done well or badly. The so-called application of ethical principles inevitably occurs within practices, not outside them. It is a contextually situated interpretation that is never merely a logical operation but is itself a value-laden and selective evaluation or 'specification' in its own right.

Dawson insightfully reviews many of the advantages and strengths that accompany a notion of substantive public health ethics developed in this way. It breaks free of libertarian ideology and its underlying atomistic and individualistic understanding of the human person. It provides a solid rationale for interdisciplinary research and dialogue between empirical research and normative analysis. Most important of all, perhaps, it provides an opening for the crucial task, within the setting of public health policy and elsewhere, of re-conceptualizing older dichotomies inherited from the liberal tradition between the individual and society and between liberty and equality.

It is important not to read into Dawson's emphasis on the concrete normative identity of public health as a practice an implicit kind of special pleading for the interests and agendas of public health professionals or agencies. It is often thought that without general universal principles of human rights or social justice, the key agents and power centres of society, including institutionalized public health, will function in a relativistic fashion prone to ethical corruption and self-serving conduct. Dawson clearly intends that his approach have no such implication.

But the philosophical question he raises is fundamental and not easily resolved, touching as it does on understandings of ethics present in the ancient debate between Plato and Aristotle and the modern debate between Kant and Hegel. Working, as I see it, in the Aristotelian and Hegelian line, Dawson locates viable and critical ethical constraints in conditions immanent rather than transcendent, that is, close to home for public health professionals and others whose practices and forms of life are said to have inherent values that provide the requisite ethical ideals and restraints. I wonder, however, how stark our philosophical choice needs to be here. Public health practitioners clearly have general moral obligations as citizens and as human beings. But they have a more concrete set of commitments and obligations as well. The task of public health ethics is not to legitimate the authority and interests of public health professionals, but to give those who answer the call of public health something of inherent value to profess.

In closing I would like to underscore what I see as one of the most important facets and implications of Dawson's analysis: namely the significance that public health ethics can have, not only for public health, but also for ethics. Consider the following analogy with the development (within bioethics and more broadly) of feminist ethics. There is much more to feminist ethics than only serving to remind us of the interests and rights of women, as important as that is. Fundamentally, feminist ethics is significant because it has transformed ethical concepts and our understanding of the human condition in a general way. In a similar vein, public health ethics has done much more than merely tend to overlooked issues or 'inconvenient truths'. Public health ethics has a conceptually transformative potential both for the applied domain of health issues and also for ethics and political theory as a whole. The reason is that public health stands at a central ideological fault line of advanced capitalist society and governance. It is a core health and welfare function of the modern state, and it is at the pivot point of contemporary struggle over the meaning and social embodiment of the two key values of our political and ethical tradition: liberty and equality. The function of the welfare state and the historical compromise of liberal capitalism blending liberty and equality together as human rights and justice are all presently in play and the stakes are very high.

Normatively, public health ethics stands at the epicentre of these upheavals of thought and politics. Its task is not only to ethically guide the pursuit of health but also to conceptually reclaim the notion of things that are 'public'. It is within the discourse of public health ethics that crucial work will be done to determine what individuals in contemporary society share and owe to one another and to determine how the civic or political imagination, civic motivation, and civic sense of responsibility necessary to the functioning of democracy can be maintained, if indeed they can be at all.

Reference

Dawson, A. (2014). 'What is 'Public Health Ethics'?' in A. Akabayashi (ed.), *The Future of Bioethics: International Dialogues*. Oxford: Oxford University Press, 529–38.

15.6

Response to Commentaries
In Defence of Substantive Public Health Ethics

Angus Dawson

It is always flattering when scholars take the time to read your work carefully, critically engage with your arguments, and point out issues requiring clarification. I am grateful to all four of the individuals who have written commentaries and I am conscious that I cannot do justice to all the points that they raise. What I would like to do is to briefly restate to some extent the views outlined in my original paper as a means of responding to some of the issues discussed in the commentaries.

One of the central aims in my recent work has been to argue that when we think of public health ethics we ought to begin with trying to understand the aims and methods of public health (Dawson 2011); indeed, that we ought think of public health as a practice, and begin our critical discussions of ethics from that internal perspective. This does not mean that we have to accept uncritically everything that occurs in the name of that practice either today or when errors have been made in the past. Neither does it mean that public health ethics is a mere systematization of current conventional thinking. It does mean that we should not judge that particular practice by inappropriate and externally created rules. To see what I mean, imagine the practice of a particular game: tennis, hockey, or soccer. Each game can be thought to be a practice, governed by a particular set of formal rules, but also norms of conduct. Such rules and norms are subject to development and change over time. Sometimes this change can be imperceptibly slow (e.g. goal line reviews in soccer) and on other occasions it can be revolutionary (e.g. the fabled creation of rugby football allegedly in an instant). Each change is subject to discussion and debate; past practice can be critiqued or be returned to in the future. However, it makes no sense to judge one game by the rules of another (e.g. chess is very different from volleyball). In an analogous way, we can think of public health as an activity with a particular set of aims (e.g. prevention rather than mere cure, reducing health inequities, a focus on population health, not just individual health, etc.) and particular kinds of methods (e.g. surveillance, epidemiology, screening, etc.). Such aims and methods are open to review and change over time (e.g. a growing concern about minority populations, an increasing focus on non-communicable disease, etc.) and there is plenty of room for disagreement within the practice itself. (Indeed, in relation to public health as a practice there is more of a contribution from norms rather than formal rules than in the case of games.) However, it makes no sense, I suggest, to use a view of ethics developed elsewhere, for a different set of purposes, and think that it will automatically be useful in a very different context. Just as chess is not volleyball, public health is not reproductive medicine. It therefore makes no sense to assume that the ethical values, theories, or frameworks developed for a different context are the appropriate ones to use.

Once you have identified a practice, you can then begin to discuss and articulate the values that are present in that practice. Such a procedure ought to be a critical process, in that it is one of deliberation and debate. In this way progress may be made; elements of the practice might change precisely as a result of this reflective method. This process is not one of neutrality in the sense that we start from nowhere, with no prior commitments: exactly the reverse. Our commitments, as part of the practice, drive the debate. I believe that neutrality in the sense assumed by many liberals and libertarians is a myth (cf. Yamamoto). I do not think that we can specify in advance of a requirement to make a judgement exactly what will be relevant to that judgement. This is why I claim to be both a value pluralist (i.e. there are a number of relevant values) and what we might call a value egalitarian, in that there should be no prior weighting given to particular values (e.g. such as liberty, autonomy). The exact division between liberals and libertarians is unclear. However, what they have in common is a presumption (prior to judgement about a particular case) to hold that, say, non-interference should always take priority; or that it will take priority unless there is some strong, justified reason why not; or there is a presumption in its favour; or that in our choices we should maximize liberty; or ensure the least restriction of liberty possible, etc., etc. Such positions are neither neutral (and this is one reason why it is a myth) nor egalitarian in terms of value weightings. In such positions, liberty is given special or additional weighting *prior to* any particular judgement. Of course, liberty is vitally important, and will in many cases triumph over all other values. But my point is that sometimes it should not, and so it makes no sense to just assume it will (as libertarians, many liberals, and many traditional bioethicists tend to do). What normative ethical or political theory do I want to defend? Jennings points out in his elegant and subtle commentary that this is to ask the wrong question. My central claim is to seek to rebut the unthinking presumption in favour of liberty in our debates about bioethics. As it happens, I think you can support my plural, egalitarian view of values from the perspective of pretty much any theory you like (e.g. most forms of consequentialism, pluralist 'Rossian' deontology, virtue ethics, Scanlonian contractualism, capabilities, etc). I take this to be a strength, not a weakness.

As a result of all this, it is hopefully now clear why I am not committed to accepting the necessity of past (or present) acts of public health authorities as always being legitimate. Some of the criticism of my position (cf. Yamamoto, Sato) appeals to cases (e.g. Japanese leprosy prevention, Tuskegee, etc.) as objections to my general view. Such an approach is, however, missing the point. Counterexamples will not work in this way, because I have not specified any necessary and sufficient conditions for the practice of public health. A practice is not the right kind of thing to be specified in that way. Nowhere do I say or imply that everything that public health officials do is correct. There is no guarantee that inappropriate or out-of-date policies will not continue, often because there is insufficient critical reflection on both relevant evidence and ethical considerations. It is not because something is the act of a public health official that makes it right (or wrong), rather the evaluation of rightness will turn on the facts of each case judged in an appropriate way using the relevant values. Neither is there is anything in my view that entails oppressing minorities (cf. Sato); quite the contrary. My appeal for a more mature, discursive polity is motivated by the importance of seeing and debating the complexity of policy options, critically engaging with policy, and constantly monitoring for the unforeseen consequences of actions. The existence of a democratic form of government does not, of course, guarantee that any resultant policy will be ethically appropriate. But it does, I think, make it more likely, as the government is required to give reasons and evidence for its actions and these can then be openly contested.

I will end with some comments on the main example I discuss in my chapter, that of restrictions on smoking. I chose this because I am interested in how our choices might be thought to be (at least partly) expressions of the norms that govern us. Smoking is an excellent example, at least in most richer parts of the world, of how quickly norms can change. In this case, we have moved from a norm of general acceptance of smoking to viewing it as unacceptable in a 30-year period. This is remarkable. It is not that the change in norm itself justified political action (cf. Sato), but rather that the change in norm is partly the result of, but also itself drives, the change in legal restrictions on smoking. These changes in turn are motivated by evidence of harm, importantly both to others (through passive smoking) but also to smokers themselves. At least one of the possible reasons for this policy is a concern about equity, and if that is the motivation, discussions about paternalism are irrelevant. This also illustrates why we ought not to automatically frame our discussions solely in terms of liberty, but discuss all relevant values. Surely any sensible ethical theory will allow us to sometimes promote justice over liberty? I certainly want to do so, and the more plausible versions of liberalism will do so too.

Many writers are too quick to dismiss the possibility of more objective elements within how we ought to conceptualize the good life. We do, importantly, allow people to make their own health-affecting choices in many cases. We allow them to base their actions upon what *they* value. However, in some cases we do not. These cases are based on various reasons and some will be acceptable to liberals and some not. I am keen to expand the space for discourse about what counts as a valid reason for sometimes restricting liberty. Part of my justification for this would be to appeal to what we share as human creatures, as biological and social beings. The outline for what counts as a good life can be drawn using an appeal to the interests that we have as such beings, and much of this outline is supported by routine public health activity (Dawson 2011). Seeking to protect such interests still allows plenty of room for personal choice. At least some of these interests can only be protected by collective action, and this is often most efficiently conducted by the state on our behalf. Some libertarians and postmodernists (cf. Okita) might not like this, but the important thing is that there is nothing intrinsically wrong with state action, as long as it is open to discussion and debate. One of the (many) problems with Foucault's position is that he sees the state as necessarily being oppressive of individuals, as though individuals have no responsibility for the state taking the form that it does. Any state is only as good as the citizens that constitute that state. The actions of the state can be both negative and positive. The state can act for our good, and also damage it. There is no good reason to necessarily see actions of the state as being a bad thing. Indeed, sometimes the state is the best means of attaining some aspects of our collective good life. Like Jennings, I allow for the possibility of a richer political discourse in relation to policy options, with the result that we find it easier to articulate, defend, and enjoy all aspects of *public* activity, including public health.

Reference

Dawson, A. (2011). 'Resetting the Parameters: Public Health as the Foundation for Public Health Ethics', in A. Dawson (ed), *Public Health Ethics: Key Concepts and Issues in Policy and Practice.* Cambridge: Cambridge University Press, 143–53.

16.1

Primary Topic Article
Accountability for Reasonable Priority Setting

Norman Daniels and James Sabin

1 The problem: ethical disagreement about priorities in health

Many health policy decisions involve setting priorities for the use of resources in meeting health needs. Such decisions often rest on ethical considerations, and reasonable people may disagree about them. These ethical disagreements about priorities raise questions about the legitimacy and fairness of the decisions that are made.

Such decisions are pervasive in health policy. In the context of individual medical care, questions that often attract attention include coverage decisions for a new technology or limits in public or private insurance schemes. These might take place at a national level, as in the case of the National Institute for Health and Clinical Excellence (NICE) recommendations to the NHS in the UK about a specific intervention or as in Israel's decisions about which new interventions to include among a list of candidates for addition to its "basket" of benefits, or when the FDA in the US approves a drug and it is then available within Medicare and Medicaid by legal requirements, or in private insurance schemes by contractual arrangement. They might also take place within a specific local health authority or purchasing agent, as in the UK or Sweden or in a particular private insurance scheme in the US.

But priority setting about medical care is not just about new health technology assessments. It includes decisions about how a hospital or local health authority uses its budget to meet competing health needs in the population it serves. And, in the context of public health, as in health and safety regulation, priority-setting decisions may involve investing in risk reduction for one group versus another at varying cost and intrusiveness.

Where such decisions are made, they create winners and losers. Some people are benefited by them and others are not. These conflicting interests and claims contribute to the disagreement about specific priorities.

One form that ethical controversy takes when priorities are set is whether to maximize aggregate health in a population or to address concerns about health disparities. Both are key goals of health policy, and sometimes they conflict. We have strong ethical reasons to pursue both goals, and much controversy surrounds what trade-offs in those goals are ethically acceptable in specific contexts. Some theories may emphasize one goal over the other—as utilitarianism arguably does by favoring maximizing aggregate population health, but other theories may support a complex blend of both, as in some liberal egalitarian approaches (Daniels 2008).

Other disagreements involve tension between the compassionate use of unproven technologies and careful stewardship of resources (Daniels and Sabin 2008), controversy about the use of a treatment/enhancement distinction as a rough guide to priorities in health policy, or tension between identified and statistical victims (Daniels 2011). Sometimes one side of these disagreements reflects a health-maximizing strategy (e.g. stewardship may be aimed at more cost-effective care), but sometimes not (e.g. if there are the same numbers of identified and statistical victims, but there is a preference for the former).

The shared feature of all these disagreements is that we lack consensus on ethical principles that can resolve these disputes (Daniels and Sabin 1997). If we had such consensus, our disagreements would take the form of controversy about how they should be applied, including controversy about the facts of the context. Unfortunately, the controversy is deeper. As a result, the controversies about priority setting raise hard questions about both legitimacy (who has the moral authority to make these decisions, and how they should be made) and fairness (whether the decisions are fair to the different parties with conflicting health needs and the claims they can base on them).

To illustrate the pervasiveness and depth of the ethical disagreements, we shall argue in section 2 that existing economic tools aimed at helping with priority setting fall short of addressing important distributive issues and that people hold defendable attitudes toward distribution that differ from the maximizing assumptions in these tools. In section 3, we suggest we need a fair deliberative process that holds decision-makers accountable for the reasonableness of their decisions. The main idea is an appeal to a notion of pure procedural justice: in the absence of prior agreement on principles to resolve disputes, the outcomes of a fair process count as fair outcomes (Daniels and Sabin 1997). Though the proposed process faces some important objections, described in section 4, we conclude that it not only enhances the legitimacy of contested decisions, but also yields fair decisions, even if convincing arguments later compel us to modify our views about their fairness. (The fairness of the outcomes is thus defeasible.) This approach has varied applications, and there has been varied uptake of them in different places, less in the US than elsewhere. Some of these applications are briefly described in section 5. Further research is needed to establish the merits of the approach.

2 The limitations of key economic tools

Comparative effectiveness research (CER) and cost-effectiveness analysis (CEA) have important applications for guiding priority-setting decisions. Nevertheless, both kinds of tools fall short of being able to address important questions about distribution and value that many priority-setting decisions must address. Both tools provide important inputs into a broader deliberative process, but they do not substitute for it.

In the US, the Patient Protection and Affordable Care Act (PPACA 2010)[1] promotes CER for the information it gives about alternative interventions, but the legislation bars CER from playing a role in coverage decisions, an unfortunate concession to the politics surrounding limit setting in the US. (Public officials in the US resist acknowledging the need for limits, and candidates for public office score points by accusing their opponents of "rationing." Arguably, the effect is to distract attention from limit setting by insurers.) A typical use of CER compares the effectiveness of two interventions (drugs, procedures, or even two methods of delivery), but in the US context, it largely avoids considerations of cost. Obviously, if there is only one effective treatment for a condition, CER tells us nothing useful. Similarly, it tells us nothing about whether a more effective intervention is worth its extra cost. And, CER cannot help us compare the outcomes of interventions across different disease conditions, since it uses no measure of health that permits such a comparison of effectiveness. Accordingly, there are many questions facing decision-makers about resource allocation in health care that cannot be answered by this approach, even if it can help us avoid investments in things that do not work or that offer no improvement over other interventions.

In Germany, however, CER is combined with an economic analysis that takes cost into consideration and that allows the calculation of "efficiency frontiers" for different classes of drugs (Caro et al. 2010). To calculate an efficiency frontier, the effect of each drug in a class in producing some health outcome is plotted against its cost, and the curve is the efficiency frontier for that class of drugs. It is then possible to project from the performance of drugs in a specific class to see if a new intervention in that class yields an improvement in effectiveness at a price that makes it more or less efficient than that which is projected from the existing efficiency frontier. This use of CER allows German decision-makers to negotiate about the price of treatments, rejecting payments that yield inefficient improvements. The assumption in Germany is that every intervention that has greater effectiveness can be covered, but only at the appropriate price. Still, the German use of CER cannot make comparisons across diseases, and so it allows great differences in efficiency across conditions.

CEA aims for greater scope. It deploys a common unit for measuring health outcomes, either a disability-adjusted life year (DALY) or a quality-adjusted life year (QALY). This unit purports to combine duration with quality, permitting us to compare health states across a broad range of disease conditions. In doing a CEA, we construct a ratio (the incremental cost-effectiveness ratio or ICER) of the change in costs that results from the new intervention with the change in health effects (as measured by QALYs or DALYs). This allows us to calculate the cost per QALY (or DALY) and arrive at a general efficiency measure for a broad range of interventions for different conditions.

[1] Pub.L. 111–48 (http://www.gpo.gov/fdsys/pkg/PLAW-111publ48/content-detail.html), 124 Stat. 119, to be codified as amended at scattered sections of the Internal Revenue Code and in 42 U.S.C.

Critics have noted problematic ethical assumptions in both the construction of the health-adjusted life-year measures and the use of CEA (Nord 1999; Brock 2003; Brock 2004). To see some of these problems, consider the following table:

Rationing problem	CEA	Fairness
Priorities	No priority to worst off	Some priority to worst off
Aggregation	Any aggregation is OK	Some aggregations OK
Best outcomes/fair chances	Best outcomes	Fair chances

CEA systematically departs from judgments many people will make about what is fair. The priorities problem asks how much priority we should give to people who are worse off. By constructing a unit of health effectiveness, such as the QALY, CEA assumes this unit has the same value whoever gets it or wherever it goes in a life ("A QALY is a QALY" is the slogan). But intuitively many people think that a unit of health is worth more if someone who is relatively worse off (sicker) gets it rather than some-one who is better off (less sick) (Brock 2002). At the same time, people generally do not think we should give complete priority to those who are worse off. We may be able to do very little for them, so giving them complete priority means we would have to forgo doing a lot more good for others. Few would defend creating a bottomless pit out of those unfortunate enough to be the worst off.

Similarly, CEA assumes that we should aggregate even very small benefits so that if enough people get small benefits it outweighs giving significant benefits to a few. But intuitively, most people think some benefits are trivial goods that should not be aggre-gated to outweigh significant benefits to a few (Kamm 1993). Curing a lot of colds, for example, does not outweigh saving a life.

Finally, CEA favors putting resources where we get a best outcome, whereas people intuitively favor giving people a fair (if not equal) chance at a benefit. Locating an HIV/AIDS treatment clinic in an urban area may save more lives than reaching out to a rural area, but in doing so we may deny many people a fair chance at a significant benefit (Daniels 2004).

In all three of these cases, CEA favors a maximizing strategy, whereas people making judgments about fairness are generally willing to sacrifice some aggregate population health in order to treat people fairly. In each case, whether it is giving some priority to those who are worse off, viewing some benefits as not worth aggregating, or giving people fair chances at some benefit, fairness deviates from the health maximization that CEA favors. Yet we lack agreement on principles that tells us how to trade off goals of maximization and fairness in these cases.

Determining priorities primarily by seeing whether an intervention achieves some cost/QALY standard is adopting a health-maximization approach. Such an approach will depart from widely held judgments about fairness. Thus, NICE in the UK has had to modify its initially more rigid practice of approving new interventions only if they met a cost/QALY standard in the face of recommendations from its Citizens Council. This Council, intended to reflect representative social and ethical judgments of people in the UK, has proposed relaxing NICE's threshold in a variety of cases where judgments about fairness differed from concerns about health maximization. The judgments of the Citizens Council in this regard are consistent with what the social science literature suggests are widely held views in a range of cultures and contexts (Menzel et al. 1999; Nord 1999; Ubel, Richardson, and Pinto Prades 1999; Ubel, Baron, and Asch 2001; Dolan et al. 2005).

3 Accountability for reasonableness: a proposal

The problem, as we have described it, is that priority-setting decisions are often ethically controversial, and this raises questions about their legitimacy and fairness. In addition, the main analytic tools we have to aid decision-making, CER and CEA, either address only limited questions or adopt controversial approaches that ignore important distributive issues. These tools conflict with widely held views about what is equitable or fair. At the same time, we lack agreement on principles fine-grained enough to tell us what is fair in these cases. Because of this lack of agreement on principles, we shall argue that we need to rely on a form of procedural justice to arrive at decisions we can regard as legitimate and fair. Before making that argument, however, it is worth briefly considering some alternative views.

Despite our characterization of the problem, some may think issues of legitimacy and possibly of fairness are at least already addressed in either of two ways. The first approach is a market argument: at least where decisions are made by private insurance schemes, as in much of the health care delivered in the US, it might be claimed that people who buy such insurance express implicit consent to the limits involved in priority-setting decisions these insurers make. The claim is that consent to these limits means issues of legitimacy are clearly settled and, arguably, fairness is not at issue since we freely gave informed consent to them and they are therefore not unfair to us.

This argument fails both in theory and in practice (Daniels and Sabin 1997). Even if enrollment in an insurance scheme constituted freely given consent, half of all Americans getting employer-based insurance have no choice of plans and so are not freely consenting to one among alternative mechanisms for setting priorities. Basically, the only health insurance they can afford is the plan their employer provides to them, and their employer is in general not their fiduciary agent, bound to pursue the workers' best interests. In practice, then, the argument does not work for many people. But even in theory it is problematic: people lack real information about such priority setting when they enroll in a health-insurance scheme, and they cannot exit from plans and seek alternatives easily when they realize a plan may not meet their needs, as they can when their family's needs outgrow what a given car can meet (too many children) and they sell it to buy another. Even if they could exit a plan and enter another, the market offers them few real options and so may fail to meet their needs or market preferences.

A more promising argument may be that the authority democratically delegated to agencies that manage our health systems mean decisions have at least the legitimacy of other democratically authorized decisions. Since we rely on a representative, democratic political process to make decisions in the face of many ethical disagreements about policy, it is arguably fair, and at least no more problematic than similar decisions that devolve to appropriately delegated authorities. One problem, however, for standard democratic decision-making is that it often rests on the simple aggregation of preferences (Cohen 1996), and few people want to accept that process as determining what counts as ethically right. A racist policy that has popular support from a majority is not thereby the right policy to pursue. In moral deliberation, in contrast, we aim to evaluate the weight that reasons should receive; we do not simply aggregate the preferences people have. This suggests that we need a process that is more deliberative than a simple aggregative democratic vote; such a process can supplement and improve, even if not replace, broader democratic processes that we hope may become more deliberative. The deliberation that the process encourages is intended to emphasize ethical reasoning about what we should count as fair. (Maybe if some existing public procedures that were intended to be deliberative worked better, they would suffice; in any case, what we propose draws on features of process that are widely believed to be necessary to assure proper deliberations.)

Key elements of fair deliberative process will involve at least four conditions: 1) publicity, specifically transparency about the grounds for decisions; 2) relevance, rationales that rely on reasons that all can accept as relevant to meeting health needs fairly (by "all" we mean people who are affected by a decision and who seek mutually justifiable grounds for such decisions); 3) revisability, including procedures for revising decisions in light of new evidence and arguments and other challenges to them; 4) enforcement, meaning assurance that the conditions 1–3 are met. Together these elements assure "accountability for reasonableness" (Daniels and Sabin 1997; Daniels and Sabin 2008).

A fair process requires publicity about the reasons and rationales that play a part in decisions. There must be no secrets where justice is involved, for people should not be expected to accept decisions that affect their well-being unless they are aware of the grounds for those decisions. This broader transparency about rationales is a hallmark of fair process. Fair process also involves constraints on reasons. Fair-minded people—those who seek mutually justifiable grounds for cooperation—must agree that the reasons, evidence, and rationales are relevant to meeting population health needs fairly, the shared goal of deliberation. One important way to make sure that there is a real deliberation about relevant reasons is to include a range of stakeholders in the deliberative process. Such stakeholders should not be token "lay" people who may be intimidated by others; they should be supported so they can clearly express their views about relevant reasons. Including an appropriate range of stakeholders does not make a process more democratic (for they are not elected representatives of the public), but it can improve the quality of the deliberation, provided the process is managed so that it is not simply a lobbying exercise by people who are not really seeking relevant reasons. Fair process also requires opportunities to challenge and revise decisions in light of the kinds of considerations all stakeholders may raise. There should be a mechanism for appeals of decisions by those affected by them.

Accountability for reasonableness makes it possible to educate all stakeholders about deliberation about fair decisions under resource constraints. It facilitates social learning about limits. It connects decision-making in health-care institutions to broader, more fundamental democratic deliberative processes.

Accountability for reasonableness also occupies a middle ground in the debate between those calling for "explicit" and those calling for "implicit" rationing. Like implicit approaches, it does not require that principles for rationing be made explicit ahead of time. But, like explicit approaches, it does call for transparency about reasoning that fair-minded people can eventually agree is relevant. Since we may not be able to construct principles that yield fair decisions ahead of time, we need a process that allows us to develop those reasons over time as we face real cases. The social learning that this approach facilitates provides our best prospect of achieving agreement over sharing medical and other health resources fairly.

Since there are various levels at which priority-setting decisions are made—national, state, health authority, hospital, health plan—it will be necessary to adapt a fair, deliberative process to the institutional level and type of decision being made. One size will not fit all. Even the four general conditions described are not intended to be exhaustive, and some flexibility in applying them may be needed. For example, including a range of stakeholders in the process in general increases the quality of decisions and may increase the "buy-in" that results, enhancing legitimacy and acceptability. But such inclusion may not fit all contexts—indeed, it may be so far from what is legally required in, say, US law regarding private insurance schemes that demanding it would make the approach unrealizable given the obstacles to such inclusion by many organizations. Better to rely on transparency to accomplish some of what stakeholder involvement might achieve than make it a requirement regardless of the legal context.

4 Problems with accountability for reasonableness

In this brief essay, we cannot do justice to many of the objections that have been made to this approach, but we shall briefly consider four.

First, does the approach actually yield decisions we should view as fair and not simply as legitimate?[2] Following Rawls's discussion, we can distinguish two main forms of procedural justice. In pure procedural justice, we lack prior agreement on a relevant principle for determining just outcomes, and we accept the outcome of a fair process as fair. Rawls offers gambling as an example: we accept the outcome of an unfettered spin of the roulette wheel as fair. In contrast, criminal trials constitute an example of impure procedural justice, since we have prior agreement on a relevant principle: convict all and only the guilty. We determine who the guilty are through trials that pit adversaries against each other but are judged by neutral parties. If we later find conclusive evidence that someone we found guilty in a trial is innocent (say, through DNA evidence), then we should overturn the trial result.

Since we lack prior agreement on distributive principles specific enough to yield outcomes to decisions about allocating health-care resources, the proposed process has some resemblance to pure procedural justice. On this view we have no basis for denying fairness to the outcome of a fair process. But the situation differs in two important ways from Rawls's example of gambling. Unlike gambling we should reject outcomes that

---

[2] Dan Brock has urged this objection in conversations with one of us (ND).

violate requirements of justice—say, about non-discrimination. Further, again unlike the case of gambling, we can imagine arriving at a philosophically persuasive view about how to solve the priorities problem or any of the other unsolved rationing problems. Such a view might "defeat" decisions about fairness arrived at through the process. The "defeasible" fairness that results is the most we can claim for the outcome of our fair process—it is as fair as we can determine, given everything we know and believe.

Second, why think we can arrive with more confidence at an account of fair process than we can arrive at an account of fair outcomes?[3] It may well turn out to be the case that we cannot arrive at a widely acceptable account of a fair deliberative process and that we are in the same fix as we are with regard to contested substantive decisions. Indeed, skepticism is often warranted about the many ways a process can be captured by parties who subvert its intended role as a form of procedural justice. On the other hand, many societies succeed in finding agreement about fair procedures in the face of ongoing substantive disagreements. In short, the worry is real, but there are many instances where the search for a fair process that is widely acceptable succeeds. There is to be sure no guarantee it always will.

Third, accountability for reasonableness may yield different answers for cases that seem similar, violating a principle of formal justice that like cases be treated alike. We discuss this issue elsewhere (Daniels and Sabin 2008): a fair process can yield different conclusions when considerations that all see as relevant are given different weight in two applications of a process that meets the conditions of accountability for reasonableness. It does not follow that such a result violates any formal principle of justice, for two cases, however similar they seem, are not being judged the same way if the reasons that play a relevant role in deciding them are given different weights by different groups involved in the two procedures. The rationales explain why the groups treat the cases differently, and so the different outcome is not arbitrary.

Still, how tolerable such differences are, for example between different districts or health authorities in a health system, may depend on differences in their political culture. If the belief is that a national health system, such as the NHS in the UK, cannot accept such "post-code variations" in decisions, then a uniform decision may have to be made for the whole system. Achieving uniform decisions was one of the central rationales for setting up NICE in the UK. If, however, the system has a more federalist structure, intended to reflect locally distinct beliefs, including those about fair treatment when using scarce resources, then variation might be an acceptable result. Whether the variation in outcomes is a problem, then, depends on judgments about how uniform treatment must be in a health system, and those judgments may vary without one view being right and the other clearly wrong.

Finally, is there any evidence that accountability for reasonableness achieves better outcomes? Most of the studies done to date on this approach to priority setting simply accept the theoretical rationale for the framework, ask if the decision-making in that context complies with the conditions, and sometimes propose how to secure better compliance. But a different kind of empirical evidence is needed if the goal is to show

---

[3] Marc Roberts and Michael Reich have urged this objection in conversations with one of us (ND).

that accountability for reasonableness improves outcomes in some way. Producing such evidence is difficult for quite distinct reasons. First, we would need proper comparison cases—cases where there is good compliance with the conditions and cases where the approach is not implemented. If other factors can be controlled for, we may find an appropriate comparison in a before-and-after study of the use of the fair process (but then baseline measures are needed). Getting such cases is difficult. Second, we would need good measures of the ways in which outcomes are better. Given that one of the reasons for the approach is that we lack consensus on principles for what counts as a fair outcome, how can we tell that the decisions are more fair? We lack an independent measure of fairness against which to measure change. We might argue that some accounts of greater equity in health outcomes should be used to measure fairness, but that assumes we can determine what counts as equitable in these cases. We might think that legitimacy is easier to find a measure for: we might be able to find out the attitudes of people affected by the decisions, or even those making them, to see if they judge it to be more legitimate. But finding indicators of legitimacy is itself complex. For example, we might think that greater acceptability would mean fewer appeals of decisions. But how active the appeals process is may depend on how legitimate it is believed to be—people may appeal only if they trust the process to yield reasonable outcomes.

This empirical challenge to accountability for reasonableness is a serious problem: it is hard to persuade people who might, for largely theoretical reasons, be interested in using it to actually adapt it to their needs, which requires a resource investment in it, if we cannot point to evidence that it improves the situation. Practical people are going to ask whether "it works," and answering that question requires evidence we do not have.

5 Applications of accountability for reasonableness

Despite this lack of empirical evidence, accountability for reasonableness has had enough theoretical appeal to motivate significant use of it. We shall begin by describing briefly some of these uses, and then we shall try to explain why these uses primarily occur outside the US, where the approach was developed. We conclude by noting some further contexts where this approach to priority setting may be of use.

Until very recently, NICE in the UK had the assignment of making recommendations to the NHS in England and Wales about coverage for new interventions (exactly what its role will be under the new Conservative–Liberal government coalition is less clear). Its main tool was, as noted earlier, to invoke a cost-effectiveness threshold: interventions whose cost per QALY is below £20,000 per QALY are routinely covered, and those above £30,000 per QALY are rarely covered, but those in the £20,000–£30,000 pound per QALY range are deliberated about more carefully. Because this threshold seemed an unacceptably inflexible standard to some, the Citizens Council, a group of representative laypeople who deliberate about issues a few times a year for two to three days at a time, proposed some forms of flexibility in the standard, such as allowing life-extending treatments to meet a less demanding standard. The Citizens Council has deliberated about a variety of social and ethical issues, and some of its recommendations regarding them have been adopted by NICE as features of its policy toward recommendations. The director of NICE, Sir Michael Rawlins, cites accountability for reasonableness as the inspiration for this kind of stakeholder input into ethical issues (Rawlins 2005). In addition, NICE's recommendations are fully transparent, with all evidence and rationales available on its website. Further, there is provision for reconsidering decisions in light of new evidence and arguments. In short, NICE arguably meets or comes close to meeting the conditions that are central to accountability for reasonableness.

Other examples of the influence of this approach can be found elsewhere in Europe. For example, the Swedes are engaged in a process of identifying and possibly replacing the least valuable 10 percent of services offered in its health systems (Waldau, Lindholm, and Wiechel 2010). The exercise is carried out in local districts, which engage in a highly transparent process that involves a broad range of stakeholders. The Norwegians began to emphasize the importance of fair, deliberative process as opposed to "principles" nearly a decade ago (Holm 2000). And the World Health Organization gave some recognition to the approach in its ethical guidelines for antiretroviral treatment (WHO 2004).

There have also been some experiments using the approach in middle- and low-income developing countries. In Mexico, toward the end of Julio Frenk's administration as secretary of health, a manual was developed for a fair process for incrementally adding coverage to the catastrophic insurance plan that was part of Mexico's new Seguro Popular. The manual explicitly embodied accountability for reasonableness. Though implementation of the manual was suspended in the next administration, perhaps because it required more transparency and stakeholder involvement than were comfortable for the leadership in the Mexican system, there is current interest in using it to make decisions about the formulary in IMMS, the Mexican social security health plan.

There has also been some experimentation with accountability for reasonableness in three low-income African countries. An EU-sponsored project (REACT) in Tanzania, Kenya, and Zambia, for example, examined the acceptability of the central ideas in the approach in the context of district health management plans (Byskov et al. 2009). In Tanzania, improvements were noted in the degree to which stakeholders were involved in some deliberations and in the amount of transparency that surrounded district-level plans. But downward constraints from budgets and planning at higher national levels meant there were significant departures from the conditions central to accountability for reasonableness as well (Maluka et al. 2010a; Maluka et al. 2010b).

In contrast to the theoretical appeal that accountability for reasonableness has had in this range of low-, middle-, and high-income countries, it has had little uptake in the land of its birth. The approach was originally developed to improve the legitimacy and fairness of priority-setting decisions in private, managed health-care plans in the US—possibly the hardest case for the approach. Initially there was some interest in having the approach adopted within the accreditation system for such health plans, but health plans were fearful of the exposure to more transparency and possibly to litigation. We (Daniels and Sabin 2008) have argued that the relative lack of interest in this approach derives from several sources in the US: a highly fragmented system in which public and private agencies do not want to be identified as the source of any limits to care; a political culture that has hidden from the need for priority setting (evidence for which comes from the devastating force the mention of "death panels" had in the debate about US health reform); and a strong, vested interest in the private sector that aims to deflect attention away from the many ways it sets limits to care and to hide behind the view that all "medically necessary" care is available to any insured person in need. Unfortunately, even with the recent US health reforms, there remains an explicit policy of avoiding the kind of deliberation about limit setting that is essential to defining an effective and cost-effective benefit package.

We conclude by noting three applications of the approach that have not been implemented. Health policy not only aims at population health improvement in the aggregate but also at the reduction of health inequalities, especially ethically problematic ones such as those that derive from socio-economic status, race, gender, or various policies of social exclusion. But even when a health inequality is clearly one we judge to be unfair or unjust, devoting resources to reducing it encounters the rationing problems we noted earlier. For example, knowing that we could do something to improve the health of those whose health is likely to have been harmed by an unfair distribution of the socially controllable factors that affect health may involve trade-offs against efforts to improve the health of those equally badly off and to whom we have obligations even if their health states are not the result of social injustice. Since reasonable people will disagree about how those trade-offs should be made, accountability for reasonable priority setting is arguably appropriate.

A second application that invites implementation is using accountability for reasonableness to supplement human rights-based approaches to health. Sofia Gruskin and one of us (ND) have argued (Gruskin and Daniels 2008) that a human rights framework does not yield judgments about priorities—right claims are not prioritized across rights or even within them. One consequence of this is that the priorities among programs improving health that human rights advocates negotiate with government officials fail to provide adequate rationales for the priorities that result. This lack of clarity about how priorities are set adds vagueness to the notion that rights to health or health care are to be "progressively realized." Given the commitment of the human rights framework to transparency, to involvement of stakeholders, and to government accountability for goals and targets, there is a natural fit between accountability for reasonableness and the human rights approach to health.

Finally, other pervasive disagreements that affect resource allocation can be addressed by holding decision-makers accountable for the reasonableness of decisions they make. For example, some philosophers, economists, and others have criticized policies that give some priority to rescuing "identified victims" over "statistical" ones, arguing that statistical lives are still lives that deserve equal respect and attention. This prioritization is pervasive in many contexts that protect people against risks to safety and health. Some social science literature suggests that the attitude that people express in these contexts is a concern about the concentration of risk—identified victims have risk fully concentrated in them, whereas statistical victims are parts of larger populations that face smaller individual risks. If, however, concentration of risk can be morally relevant to consider in some contexts (Daniels 2011), then different people may reasonably assign it different weights. This pervasive problem is therefore one that invites an application of accountability for reasonableness.

We conclude by emphasizing an earlier point: the main arguments so far for account-ability for reasonableness are theoretical justifications of why the conditions can enhance legitimacy and improve fairness. But policy makers are practical people and they demand and deserve some empirical evidence that this approach "works," where what counts as "working" is both hard to specify and harder to operationalize and meas-ure. That is the task still facing those who are moved by the theoretical rationale: show the process improves decision-making in relevant ways.

References

Brock, D. (2002). "Priority to the Worst Off in Health Care Resource Prioritization," in M. Battin, R. Rhodes, and A. Silvers (eds), *Medicine and Social Justice*. New York: Oxford University Press, 362–72.

Brock, D. (2003). "Separate Spheres and Indirect Benefits," *Cost Effectiveness and Resource Allocation*, 1:4.

Brock, D. (2004). "Ethical Issues in the Use of Cost Effectiveness Analysis for the Prioritization of Health Care Resources," in G. Khusfh (ed), *Handbook of Bioethics: Taking Stock of the Field from a Philosophical Perspective*. Dordrecht: Kluwer, 353–80.

Byskov, J. et al. (2009). "Accountable Priority Setting for Trust in Health Systems: The Need for Research into a New Approach for Strengthening Sustainable Health Action in Developing Countries," *Health Research Policy and Systems*, 7:23.

Caro, J. J. et al. (2010). "The Efficiency Frontier Approach to Economic Evaluation of Health-care Interventions," *Health Economics*, 19(10): 1117–27.

Cohen, J. (1996). "Procedure and Substance in Deliberative Democracy," in S. Benhabib (ed), *Democracy and Difference: Changing Boundaries of the Political*. Princeton, NJ: Princeton University Press, 95–119.

Daniels, N. (2004). *How to Achieve Fair Distribution of ARTs in "3 by 5": Fair Process and Legitimacy in Patient Selection*. Geneva: World Health Organization/UNAIDS.

Daniels, N. (2008). *Just Health: Meeting Health Needs Fairly*. New York: Cambridge University Press.

Daniels, N. (2011). "Reasonable Disagreement about Identified vs. Statistical Victims," *Hastings Center Report*, 41(1): 35–45.

Daniels, N., and Sabin, J. E. (1997). "Limits to Health Care: Fair Procedures, Democratic Deliberation, and the Legitimacy Problem for Insurers," *Philosophy and Public Affairs*, 26(40): 202–50.

Daniels, N., and Sabin, J. E. (2008). *Setting Limits Fairly: Learning to Share Resources for Health*. 2nd ed. New York: Oxford University Press.

Dolan, P. et al. (2005). "QALY Maximization and People's Preferences: A Methodological Review of the Literature," *Health Economics*, 14: 197–208.

Gruskin, S. and Daniels N. (2008). "Justice and Human Rights: Priority Setting and Fair Deliberative Process," *American Journal of Public Health*, 98(9): 157–7.

Holm, S. (2000). "Developments in the Nordic Countries: Goodbye to the Simple Solutions," in A. Coulter and C. Ham (eds), *The Global Challenge of Health Care Rationing*, Philadelphia, PA: Open University Press, 29–37.

Kamm, F. (1993). "The Choice Between People, Commonsense Morality, and Doctors," *Bioethics*, 1: 255–71.

Maluka, S. et al. (2010a). "Improving District Level Health Planning and Priority Setting in Tanzania through Implementing Accountability for Reasonableness Framework: Perceptions of Stakeholders," *BMC Health Services Research*, 10: 322.

Maluka, S. et al. (2010b). "Decentralized Health Care Priority-Setting in Tanzania: Evaluating against the Accountability for Reasonableness Framework," *Social Science and Medicine*, 71(4): 751–9.

Menzel, P. et al. (1999). "Toward a Broader View of Values in Cost-effectiveness Analysis in Health Care," *Hastings Center Report*, 29(3): 7–15.

Nord, E. (1999). *Cost-Value Analysis in Health Care: Making Sense out of QALY's*. Cambridge: Cambridge University Press.

Rawlins, M. D. (2005). "Pharmacopolitics and Deliberative Democracy," *Clinical Medicine*, 5(5): 471–5.

Ubel, P. A., Richardson, J., and Pinto Prades, J. L. (1999). "Life Saving Treatments and Disabilities: Are all QALYs Created Equal?" *International Journal of Technology Assessment in Health Care*, 15: 738–48.

Ubel, P. A., Baron, J., and Asch, D. A. (2001). "Preference for Equity as a Framing Effect," *Medical Decision Making*, 21: 180–9.

Waldau, S., Lindholm, L., and Wiechel, A. H. (2010). "Priority Setting in Practice: Participants Opinions on Vertical and Horizontal Priority Setting for Reallocation," *Health Policy*, 96(3): 245–54.

World Health Organization (WHO). (2004). *Guidance on Ethics and Equitable Access to HIV Treatment and Care*. Geneva: World Health Organization. http://www.who.int/ethics/Guidance%20on%20Ethics%20and%20HIV.pdf (accessed July 26, 2011.)

16.2

Commentary
Reasonableness and Politics

Daniel Callahan

It is with some discomfort that I write this response. I have been a friend and colleague of Daniels and Sabin for many years and, more than just that, have frequently cited the principle of "accountability for reasonableness" in my own writing. It always seemed to me both wise and full of common sense. Now I have some doubts and questions. They have been stimulated in great part by our recent experience in the United States of a highly polarized and contentious health-care reform debate. If not the most important part of that debate, one striking feature of it, alluded to by Daniels and Sabin, was an attack on the very idea of a government panel of any kind making decisions and setting policy on rationing, comparative or cost-effectiveness research, or priority setting.

Government panels, it was said, would be run by faceless bureaucrats, unelected and distant experts, and would pose a basic threat to a value at the heart of traditional medicine, that of the doctor–patient relationship. One prominent politician coined the inflammatory but politically effective phrase "death panels" to characterize that kind of decision-making. If that was not quite an all-out attack on rationality, it surely tended to subvert the idea of developing a public procedure for decision-making as a sensible way of setting policy. It put in its place the personal values and choices of doctors and patients—a multiplicity of closed two-person systems—indifferent to their collective impact on the quality and cost of health care. In effect, the very idea of a public accountability for reasonableness was killed. As Daniels and Sabin note, "even with the recent US health reforms, there remains an explicit policy of avoiding the kind of deliberation about limit setting that is essential to defining an effective and cost-effective benefit package" (Daniels and Sabin in this chapter).

I am not sure about the phrase "explicit policy." Neither our Congress nor any federal agency has openly formulated such a policy that I am aware of. Instead, I would characterize it as a perception on both the political right and left that the American public has a strong distaste for the very idea of limit setting. Politicians see it as potentially lethal for them to candidly propose any such thing. Yet this perception paradoxically coexists with a consensus on both sides that our health-care costs are excessive, and those that are government run, Medicare and Medicaid, are not economically sustainable without significantly raising taxes or cutting benefits, or some combination of both. The reason for that paradox is not hard to find: we agree on ends, not means.

But even if we could imagine the acceptance of some kind of decision-making agency or committee for limit setting and committed to "accountability for reasonableness," the political polarity now present in the US would likely make it fail. Consider, for instance, the second element of a "fair deliberative process": "relevance, rationales that rely on reasons that all can accept as relevant to meeting health needs fairly (by 'all' we mean people who are affected by a decision ...)" (Daniels and Sabin in this chapter). That means there must be a "range of stakeholders in the deliberative process." But since medical conditions and illness cut across ideological lines, and since there can be and usually are disagreements on what is just and fair, a failure to achieve consensus would seem almost certain. Participants in the discussion would be unlikely to leave their political and ethical values at the door. At the very least one can ask: What kind of consensus is needed? Complete, or partial but still acceptable with dissents?

I have another problem as well. It is not clear at all, or even dealt with, what the stakeholders are supposed to talk about once they have met to deliberate. Daniels and Sabin effectively and persuasively set forth the limitations of key economic tools. CEA and CER, they say, "fall short of being able to address important questions about distribution and value ... Both tools provide important inputs into a broader deliberative process, but they do not substitute for it." They no less point out the difficulties of "authority democratically delegated to agencies ... we need a process that is more deliberative than a simple aggregative democratic vote" (Daniels and Sabin in this chapter). But our Congress is surely a deliberative body, even if a severely divided body. Its members make speeches favoring their individual views, argue with and challenge each other, and then take a vote; and it is a transparent process.

What remains murky in Daniels and Sabin's approach is what counts as "more deliberative"? Somehow it is meant to transcend the use of the available economic tools and do better than legislative bodies would, but what else is needed, what is the "more"? Moreover, "fair process" requires "fair-minded people." How do you screen for and find such people? How can you tell one when you see one? Are they such people who have a wisdom that can see beyond the limits of the available economic tools and be more perceptive about justice than the average legislator?

They say accountability for reasonableness "makes it possible to educate all stakeholders about deliberation about fair decisions under resource restraints. It facilitates social learning about limits" (Daniels and Sabin in this chapter). But who are the educators here, what is the pedagogical method, and how can one know without some agreed-upon substantive criteria that what they decide is really fair? I cannot find in the paper any answers to questions of that kind. Unless, that is, the answer is of a stipulative kind: if you put together a body of stakeholders who agree that they will be "fair-minded," letting them decide just what that means, and they then show they have worked hard to meet the four "key elements" of "fair deliberative process," by definition and prior agreement their decision will be accepted as a fair one. This will be the case even if, as Daniels and Sabin concede, different committees working with the same issue come to different conclusions. Each one will be stipulated "fair." While that may sound odd, it may reasonably be said to reflect legitimate variations in the meaning of fair, none of which counts as definitive and canonical.

Unfortunately, the requirement of transparency opens the door to inspection by the media. And as the British have learned with QALY-influenced decisions, reporters fan out to discover those who will be the losers because of the decisions. More than once the NHS has had to back down on a decision that provoked indignation and outrage. In 2009 the United States Public Health Task Force (USPHT) made a decision, clearly laying out its reasoning, that routine mammographies for breast cancer were no longer necessary for women under the age of 50, and can even have harmful consequences. That decision was attacked by various medical groups, by cancer survivors, and by cancer advocacy groups. The government backed down, with the secretary of the department of health and human services, Kathleen Sibelius, saying that any such decision should be for the doctor and patient to decide. That government task force was made up of cancer and statistical experts, but with no stakeholders, e.g. women who had, or were at risk for, cancer. But if they had tried to get some kind of representative stakeholders, it would have had to have some women under 50 whose lives were saved by the use of mammography and were glad it did so, and some cancer experts who fervently believe in such screening. It is hard to imagine that such a committee could have achieved a consensus. I doubt that any of the dissenters would consider that they were less fair-minded than their fellow task-force members.

Yet, having pointed to many problems, I nonetheless believe that something like what Daniels and Sabin want is necessary: accountability for reasonableness is a reasonable idea. I say "something like" because some further refinements might make it possible for it to operate in a country like ours, suspicious of government, split along public and private lines, and displaying often nasty ideological battles. It is easier for Sweden and Norway, small countries with more homogeneous cultures and a historical willingness to give a strong role to government in managing health care.

I have three suggestions. One of them is that whatever kind of group is put together should have the services of someone who will act much the way a judge does during a trial: stipulate the rules for discussion, lay out alternative possibilities for a practical solution, outline some of the leading modes of thinking about justice, explain the necessity of adhering to the four "key elements," and offer to be on call for information or even to remain with the group all the time. In short, if accountability for reasonableness requires that it make possible the education of all stakeholders, the judge-like person plays that role. They will themselves have to be educated to do so.

A second suggestion is that, since not "all" potential stakeholders can be represented, a decision will have to be made about which kinds are most important and likely to be credible voices. As with the selection of a jury, potential candidates should be interrogated about their understanding of justice, personal biases they might bring to the deliberations, and any direct conflict of interest they might have. A third suggestion is to determine how much consensus is required for a decision to be binding. The reasoning of the dissenters, if unanimity is not required, will have to be exposed. And, as time goes on, and as Daniels and Sabin emphasize, earlier decisions should be open to review.

Reference

Daniels, N., and Sabin, J. (2014). "Accountability for Reasonable Priority Setting," in A. Akabayashi (ed.), *The Future of Bioethics: International Dialogues*. Oxford: Oxford University Press, 558–70.

16.3

Commentary

Deliberation, Fair Outcome, and Empirical Evidence: An Analogy with Archives

Taro Okuda

In 2011, Japan was struck by the earthquake disaster, which led to the Fukushima Daiichi nuclear crisis. In the aftermath of Fukushima, people living in Japan are facing many problems. In particular, in the northeast part of Japan, people are engaged in continuous reconstruction while living under an imminent and long-term radiation threat—though in fact there are radiation risks everywhere in the country. This situation raises positive and negative allocation issues: a positive one is that which people expect and welcome, namely the allocation of resources for emergency restoration; on the other hand, a negative one is that which people want to avoid if possible, namely the allocation of a huge amount of contaminated radioactive waste. How to resolve these allocation issues is a difficult practical problem.

This commentary was written in response to Norman Daniels and James Sabin's "Accountability for Reasonable Priority Setting" (Daniels and Sabin in this chapter). Daniels and Sabin's argument could help Japanese society to address its current crisis. Accordingly, it will be beneficial to consider their proposal carefully.

An analogy between accountability for reasonableness and archives

We might compare Daniels and Sabin's proposal of accountability for reasonableness with archives. The value of archives consists in their enabling us to learn the lessons of history, and to preserve a historical record of our deeds. "History" in this context refers to activities of present or future people. Everyone should be guaranteed equal opportunities to access archives and to use them as a basis for interpreting past events and behavior. Furthermore, every interpretation of historical documents or materials should be treated equally and evaluated through a fair process, such as academic judgment of historical relevance. Moreover, any appropriate critic should be able to revise a presently accepted interpretation. To gain universal application, these rules relating to archives must be enforced. Accordingly, four conditions of fair deliberative process proposed by Daniels and Sabin, i.e. publicity, relevance, revisability, and enforcement, can also be applied to archives. I believe this analogy can help elucidate their approach in their paper.

Using this analogy, we can raise three questions about their arguments.

Question 1: qualification for deliberation

When a deliberative process is adopted, we face some difficult issues regarding how deliberation is to take place.

First, who is in an appropriate position to deliberate and resolve priority-setting decisions? In the case of archives, the answer will be: qualified historians. Likewise, in the case of accountability for reasonableness in population health, participants in deliberation have to be qualified experts. For instance, we may need to rely on such experts in deciding when to start revising existing decisions. In short, the question is who the stakeholders should be. Can stakeholders include anyone who is affected by the decision? Daniels and Sabin propose that stakeholders must satisfy an additional condition: stakeholders are those who seek mutually justifiable grounds for such decisions. This condition enables us to distinguish between good and bad stakeholders. Furthermore, Daniels and Sabin refer to the educational effect of accountability for reasonableness. According to their argument, there are two educational levels of stakeholders: the high class and educated, and the low class, who need to be educated. Is this acceptable?

Second, who should manage and maintain the results of deliberation? In the case of archives, an archivist is responsible for managing and maintaining resources for revision. With accountability for reasonableness in population health, there needs to be some agent who plays a role similar to that of an archivist, who manages and maintains the records of deliberation as resources available for people to look into the fairness of decision-making. The role of this person should be distinguished from those of rationing or safeguarding fairness. If it is an institution that plays this role, then what conditions must this institution meet?

Question 2: relationship between procedure and outcomes

There is a worry about the relationship between procedure and outcomes that may be expressed with Daniels and Sabin's question: "Does the approach actually yield decisions we should view as fair and not simply as legitimate?" This is their objection 1.

Daniels and Sabin mentioned a similar point in an earlier paper:

[J]ustice requires that [health services] be distributed fairly, and there is no way to assure that outcome without requiring that limit-setting decisions and their rationales be public and be challengeable by those affected by them. (Daniels and Sabin 1997: 312)

According to Daniels and Sabin, justice requires fair distribution, or fair outcome, which can be realized only through a fair deliberative process. Objection 1 questions whether a fair procedure necessarily guarantees a fair outcome. In their paper, Daniels and Sabin respond to this objection with reference to Rawls's two main forms of procedural justice (Daniels and Sabin in this chapter). Yet I think the problem is deeper.

In general, it is implied that a specific type of procedure yields certain outcomes; therefore, a fair deliberative process that meets the proposed conditions (transparency, relevance, and revisability) should constrain the scope of outcomes. These conditions cannot always be applied equally and neutrally, especially given that the condition of relevance may have a strong normative force. Accountability for reasonableness can partly work, so to speak, as a safeguard against certain kinds of outcomes. Therefore, accountability for reasonableness may ensure we avoid some unfair outcomes on procedural grounds. However, by contrast, the deliberative process may silence counterclaims or opposition to a proposal. As this type of constraint is based on procedural grounds, it is extremely difficult for us to identify constraints that are potentially unfair.

On the other hand, the archives process does not exclude specific interpretations in advance. Archivists merely manage and maintain historical records. This highlights the need, as I have already stated, for accountability for reasonableness to have an agent equivalent to an archivist.

Finally, I would like to point out an extreme case. Some people may require outcomes for themselves without deliberative reasons. For such people, the deliberative process may look like a mere political power game, which creates winners and losers. To them, the process may seem rather unfair, and they may consider the top-down process a fairer and more appropriate option for resolving problems like those pertaining to population health. Although both aggregative rationing and deliberative decision-making cannot avoid yielding unfair outcomes, the top-down process may be considered fairer in that it at least cannot be held to account for failing to give equal consideration to stakeholders' views, since it makes no provision for such equal consideration. Those holding such a view may give up on the "deliberative process" itself, because they cannot expect "truly fair" outcomes as long as they participate in that process.

Question 3: necessity for empirical evidence

The final point relates to Daniels and Sabin's objection 4: "Is there any evidence that accountability for reasonableness achieves better outcomes?" They view this empirical challenge as a serious problem. However, must they offer empirical evidence that their approach produces better outcomes in order to be persuasive?

It seems to me that the important question is not whether accountability for reasonableness is more effective in practical terms, but whether it can introduce an ethical basis to decision-making. Indeed, how can one obtain empirical evidence for the realization of an ethics-based procedure? As Daniels and Sabin describe it, accountability for reasonableness is a normative requirement. Whether it works as intended when it is put into practice cannot be assessed by reflecting on the concept alone. And even if one can evaluate accountability for reasonableness empirically, this may not be possible without aggregative reasoning. Otherwise, the evaluation of accountability for reasonableness must be based on the deliberative process—and this, of course, would involve making use in the evaluation of what one is aiming to evaluate. I think it is sufficient to say that the appeal of accountability for reasonableness is purely theoretical, and that this provides motivation for decision-makers to implement it. Whether it is actually used or not may lie in the hands of politicians, or ourselves. To use or not to use: that is an existential resolution in our global society.

References

Daniels, N., and Sabin, J. (1997). "Limits to Health Care: Fair Procedures, Democratic Deliberation, and the Legitimacy Problem for Insurers," *Philosophy and Public Affairs*, 26:303–50.

Daniels, N., and Sabin, J. (2014). "Accountability for Reasonable Priority Setting," in A. Akabayashi (ed.), *The Future of Bioethics: International Dialogues*. Oxford: Oxford University Press, 558–70.

16.4

Commentary

Justice, Fairness, and Deliberative Democracy in Health Care[4]

Akira Inoue

1 What is accountability for reasonableness?

As Norman Daniels and James Sabin argue, priorities must be set in health care given the limited resources available for meeting health needs. Consider the following question: What types of medical treatment ought to be covered by public health systems? In answering this question, some people will give more weight to urgency than to treatment efficacy. Others will be more concerned with the level of gains and side effects than with the cost. It is evident that people disagree on what considerations should count and how they should be weighed for priority setting. The disagreement is deeper because we cannot overlook *ethical* considerations, particularly with respect to priority setting. Daniels and Sabin take this seriously and go so far as to say that there is no consensus on ethical principles that can resolve these issues.

A familiar way of dealing with the disagreement in question is to employ economic methods that favor efficient resource allocation. One such method is CEA. CEA is easy to perform and transparent, for it appeals to an established empirical method; health outcomes are assessed in light of meticulous surveys on people's attitudes toward medical treatment of various types, and a ratio of aggregate costs to preferred medical effects is calculated (Powers and Faden 2006: 150–1). Hence, CEA is often used as a guide by policy makers who must come to terms with strict budget constraints in the allocation of scarce health-care resources.

A serious problem with CEA is that the calculation places too much focus on efficiency; to maximize health, CEA may encourage us to disregard certain populations. For example, CEA may give more weight to the sick whose effective treatment comes at a reasonable cost than to severely disabled patients whose effective treatment is relatively expensive. Daniels and Sabin thus state that CEA often goes against our intuitive

[4] Research for this paper was partly supported by a Grant-in-Aid for Young Scientists (B), the Ministry of Education, Culture, Sports, Science, and Technology, Japan.

judgments about fairness.[5] If this is true, can a fairness-based approach exist in the face of deep disagreements on ethical principles? Daniels and Sabin propose "accountability for reasonableness." Accountability for reasonableness is a democratic idea that argues that priority-setting decisions must be publicly justifiable, even if disfavored on ethical grounds. The deliberative conception of democracy is key to public justification, because through deliberation the reasons must be acceptable to those who deeply disagree with a decision as relevant to social venture for fair cooperation. Daniels and Sabin therefore suggest that, when seeking fair terms of social cooperation that can be reasonably endorsed by all, we should forgo ethically controversial principles, including comprehensive principles of justice.

2   Problems with accountability for reasonableness

Obviously, Daniels and Sabin advance the fairness-based argument for deliberative democracy. In doing so, they appeal to our intuitive judgments about fairness. Setting aside the issue of whether such judgments are really widely held, we can immediately call into question their presumption that fairness favors deliberative democracy without reservation. Several procedures can be judged as fair to all parties; a democratic procedure, deliberative or otherwise, is not the only one. Following John Rawls's idea of pure procedural justice to which Daniels and Sabin have recourse, we can consider a lottery as a fair procedure as long as the prize does not change after bets are placed, lottery tickets are purchased voluntarily, no one cheats, and so on (Rawls 1971: 86). In other words, if such background circumstances are acknowledged as fair by all parties, it can reasonably be said that a simple lottery is fair in terms of pure procedural justice. Undoubtedly, adopting it for priority-setting decisions is not democratic, let alone *deliberatively* democratic.[6]

It could be argued that Daniels and Sabin do not consider procedural fairness alone to be sufficient for justifying the deliberative democracy-based idea of accountability for reasonableness. Indeed, they admit two things that make the situation different from a lottery procedure. First, some fair outcomes are rejected on the grounds that they violate requirements of justice. One of the most important requirements is, as Daniels and Sabin emphasize, to give some priority to the worse off. In other words, although it may be fair, or not unfair, to not rescue those who are worse off because of their own reckless actions, justice requires that their lives be saved in most cases. Second, fairness can be seen as defeasible, such that a philosophically persuasive view could ultimately defeat

---

[5] Note that, in Daniels and Sabin's argument, fairness is fundamentally a procedural notion, but sometimes it has a more substantive sense in that not giving priority to the worse off is considered unfair in most cases. Although it might seem sloppy, my account of justice developed in section 3 purports to give fairness a genuine meaning that can capture Daniels and Sabin's way of appreciating fairness.

[6] Expressed differently, as Ben Saunders (2010: 156) argues, because a simple lottery treats people fairly in a way that assigns an equal probability to each possible outcome, *regardless of the parties' inputs,* it is not democratic at all. One might still think of a simple lottery as nothing more than an example of procedural fairness. In that illuminating paper, however, Saunders demonstrates that lottery voting is not only fair, but also *democratic* in that it meets the condition of equal influenceability over collective decisions.

fair priority-setting decisions. Daniels and Sabin thus address that defeasible fairness is the most we can claim, given everything we know.

However, these arguments contravene their presumption about our lack of agreement on the general conception of justice. To give some priority to the worse off even when not helping them may seem fair, justice ought to be comprehensive in ways that outweigh the value of procedural fairness; anchored by justice (or a similar value), some values, such as the value of normal functioning for human beings, may be judged to have more weight than other values. Yet, if justice can adjudicate those values, what type of role does it play? A principle-based role in governing the rules of adjudication seems a most reasonable answer.[7] Furthermore, as Daniels and Sabin (2008: 30) admit, a principle, or principles, of justice may constitute a philosophical persuasive view of fairness in due time. Daniels and Sabin's arguments for justice in health care therefore fit with the idea that we need a comprehensive conception of justice that enjoins certain rules to resolve value conflicts and elucidate a genuine meaning of fairness.

No doubt Daniels and Sabin would object to this proposal, for they appeal to the conception of deliberative democracy given the lack of consensus on particular principles of justice. This possible objection then prompts us to consider whether deliberative democracy can represent not just a fair procedure, but rather an idea covering the requirements of justice, such as the requirement of giving some priority to the worse off. This is what Joshua Cohen proposes. Cohen's proposal treats the idea of deliberative democracy as more fundamental than that of fairness (Cohen 2009: 20–1). Given the absence of convergence on issues involving evaluative judgments, reasonable people engage in mutual reason-giving deliberation over such issues to seek justifiable collective decisions. While disagreement about ethical values constrains reasons that can be advanced in public justification, the reasons would be egalitarian, such that even the worse off can reasonably accept them as relevant when dealing with ethically controversial issues. Cohen thus advocates that public deliberation would encourage us to prioritize the worse off.

However, are the reasons that can be espoused by reasonable people through deliberation such that the reasoned decisions meet the requirements of justice? Empirical evidence says no. According to popular sociopsychological experiments, competent subjects preserve their own beliefs even after the experimenters correct the false evidence on which the beliefs are based (Gaus 2003: 132–3). It is also well established that deliberation in homogeneous circumstances generates a diversity-reducing pressure on people and promotes unreasonable polarization (Sunstein 2003). These studies show that even through deliberation reasonable people often have unreasonable beliefs that may be insensitive to the requirements of justice. It is important to note

[7] It might be claimed that Daniels and Sabin's philosophical position can be understood as moral particularism, in that no moral principle, including principle(s) of justice, can function as a guide to ethical decision-making at least in the ethically contested context. My response is that, aside from the problem of moral particularism, particularist moral reasoning conflicts with the idea of defeasible fairness that a philosophically persuasive view could ultimately provide a firm basis for fair decisions. Moral particularists deny the existence of such a principlist view at the metaphysical level, not at the epistemic one. For this point, see Little (2000).

that this is not merely an empirical threat, but rather a *theoretical* one to the deliberative democracy-based conception of justice. This is because, if the beliefs held by reasonable people must reflect the requirements of justice despite their tendency to have unreasonable beliefs in actual deliberation, then justice must have a normative force that pushes for corrections of such beliefs, independently of the deliberative process. This is not in line with Cohen's and, so interpreted, Daniels and Sabin's proposals.

3   An equal opportunity-based principle of justice: an alternative proposal

It is increasingly clear that a comprehensive conception of justice should be proposed to cope with ethically controversial issues, of which priority setting is representative. But what principle(s) of justice can be seen as plausible? In the following, I suggest that an equal opportunity-based principle of justice (hereafter, EOPJ) provides a basis for just distribution in health.

Equality of opportunity, or, more precisely, substantive equality of opportunity, implies that all individuals should have effectively equivalent arrays of options in terms of prospects for subjective welfare or objective advantage; thus, it is unfair that some people are worse off than others through no choice or fault of their own. Contemporary political philosophers propose this idea as EOPJ (Arneson 1989; Cohen 1989; Arneson 1990; Roemer 1998).[8] This idea is intuitively appealing because, on the one hand, unequal consequences that people cannot reasonably expect to avoid would be alleviated, and, on the other hand, it avoids an egalitarian "moral hazard," a situation in which people care nothing for the consequences of their own choices. These merits, I think, can be fully applied to justice in priority setting for two reasons. First, EOPJ is no doubt procedurally fair, such that it assigns higher priority in health care to the worse off who have few opportunities for healthy lives. EOPJ thus meets the most important requirement of justice: the requirement of giving *some* priority to the worse off. Second, avoidance of the morally hazardous situation promoted by EOPJ is particularly important under conditions of scarce health-care resources. EOPJ therefore has a definite sense of fairness that covers Daniels and Sabin's appeal to our intuitions and fits well with priority-setting conditions.

Recently, however, some egalitarian philosophers have contended that EOPJ is an implausible principle of justice. Among them is Norman Daniels, who nicely addressed two critical points about EOPJ in the context of health care (Daniels 2008: 71–7). On the one hand, EOPJ is *too expansive* in health policy. EOPJ directly protects against any deficit in welfare or advantage so long as it originates from the natural lottery of talents and skills of any kind, given that it represents the unequal sets of opportunities available to people. On the other hand, EOPJ is *too restrictive* to assist certain sick and disabled people, if the deficit in welfare or advantage results from their own choices. To defend

[8] Although they are often called "luck egalitarians," I am reluctant to use this expression because the notion of luck is ambiguous and confusing. However, I admit that my argument is quite similar to Shlomi Segall's defense of the luck egalitarian conception of justice (Segall 2010).

EOPJ, hence, we need to come to terms with these two apparently counterintuitive points.

Let me address the "too restrictive" concern first. To be sure, EOPJ is a responsibility-sensitive principle that allows certain individuals to be disadvantaged in health if they make risky lifestyle choices from opportunities that are effectively equivalent to those available to others. But pay heed to the big-if-type condition, under which fairness is *fully* realized in cases of health inequalities: all individuals have equally exercisable opportunities for welfare or advantage in their lifetime. It goes without saying that this condition hardly occurs in actual circumstances; equality of opportunity for welfare or advantage should be seen as an *ideal* in its literary sense. This does not entail that people should be exempted from responsibility for any bad health consequences. In view of the gap between an individual's actual set of opportunities and her ideal set of opportunities effectively equivalent to those available to others under perfect information, we can roughly determine how (un)fair it may be to assist that individual. Since fairness and responsibility come in degrees, I do not see anything counterintuitive about this.

It should now be evident that the "too restrictive" worry can be defused. Given the gap between actual and ideal circumstances (in which people face an effectively equivalent array of options), it may seem unfair if some individuals are less healthy than others through choices of their own, for example those becoming ill through their intemperance. This is nearly certainly guaranteed by the following facts: first, no one is fully rational to the extent that the most rational option is effectively chosen at every decisional moment; second, our everyday actions go hand in hand with risks and uncertainties that cannot be reasonably foreseen and are hence unavoidable. With this in mind, we can reasonably justify the establishment of a public health insurance system, which *minimally* covers the entire population under budget constraints. Admittedly, this public health system is not too restrictive in that it rescues the worse-off patients in actual circumstances, regardless of their responsibility for being worse off.[9] Nor is it morally hazardous, because the differential degree of (un)fairness represents a value for attributing the corresponding degree of responsibility to people; for example, people should bear the differential cost of medical treatment beyond the minimal coverage. This, I think, matches our intuitive judgments about fairness.

Let me now turn to the "too expansive" concern. As Daniels (2008: 73) argues, EOPJ does not distinguish normal deficit in health from the lack of attractive appearance, such as beauty and handsomeness; any deficit can be a target of rectification in accordance with EOPJ. This may even allow cosmetic surgery to be covered by the public health systems under EOPJ, if it is publicly acknowledged that an individual's physical appearance constrains her effective array of future options through no fault of her own. This might seem counterintuitive.

---

[9] It might be objected that we cannot exclude possibilities of leaving people unhelped, should they be fully rational and presented with opportunities equivalent to those available to others under perfect information. But this brings me to the following question: Would not rescuing them be truly considered merciless? I doubt it, because they have absolutely no trouble avoiding the distressing situation. To say the least, raising mere logical possibilities makes our intuitive judgments untenable.

However, I believe that there is no need to directly associate EOPJ-stipulated judgments of (un)fairness with medical treatments for the deficit. Resource limit—a distinct feature in priority-setting cases—pushes us to seek inexpensive and effective ways of mitigating ill-health conditions, even in cases where elimination of the resulting inequalities is entirely fair. For example, cosmetic surgery is not the only way of caring for those who always worry that their own outward appearance restricts their opportunities for welfare or advantage. There are cheaper and more effective alternatives to align their situation closer to the EOPJ ideal, such as an educational campaign for changing public awareness about appearance. The application of EOPJ to public policies in this way, in my view, would ward off the "too expansive" concern.

Nevertheless, the lack of a fundamental distinction between normal deficits in health and the lack of talents and skills may be considered too counterintuitive to reasonably accept EOPJ as a promising principle of justice in health care. As a matter of fact, Daniels (2008: 74) argues that EOPJ is likely to promote more disagreement among reasonable people about how to meet health needs than the principle of justice that focuses on normal functioning for a healthy life. Admittedly, this argument relies on our intuitions that go against the duty to assist people beyond the level of normal functioning. However, this reliance upon our intuitive judgments is exactly what I have been questioning here, for they are held with reference to the practical implications of the so-called EOPJ viewpoint that Daniels challenges, which differs in significant ways from EOPJ applied in the above-mentioned way. Given the relevant application of EOPJ in practical issues, including ethical controversies such as priority setting, nothing counterintuitive can be found; the practical implications of EOPJ respect both our prioritarian intuition and our responsibility-sensitive one.

I conclude by emphasizing that EOPJ could be a promising conception of justice; while it prioritizes the worse off in actual circumstances, it meets our intuitive judgments that responsibility matters in health policy. Although it is my hope that EOPJ *is* a convincing principle of justice that provides a philosophically persuasive view about fair distribution in health care, there is a need to expand it in order to gain more extensive support. This is my philosophical and thus inevitably endless task that cannot and should not be devolved to fair-minded people who engage in practical deliberation about priority-setting decisions.

References

Arneson, R. J. (1989). "Equality and Equal Opportunity for Welfare," *Philosophical Studies*, 56: 77–93.

Arneson, R. J. (1990). "Liberalism, Distributive Subjectivism, and Equal Opportunity for Welfare," *Philosophy and Public Affairs*, 19: 158–94.

Cohen, G. A. (1989). "On the Currency of Egalitarian Justice," *Ethics*, 99: 906–44.

Cohen, J. (2009). *Philosophy, Politics, Democracy: Selected Essays.* Cambridge, MA: Harvard University Press.

Daniels, N. (2008). *Just Health: Meeting Health Needs Fairly.* New York: Cambridge University Press.

Daniels, N., and Sabin, J. (2008). *Setting Limits Fairly: Learning to Share Resources for Health.* 2nd ed. New York: Oxford University Press.

Gaus, G. F. (2003). *Contemporary Theories of Liberalism: Public Reason as a Post-enlightenment Project*. London: Sage.

Little, M. (2000). "Moral Generalities Revisited," in B. Hooker and M. Little (eds), *Moral Particularlism*. Oxford: Clarendon Press, 296–311.

Powers, M., and Faden, R. (2006). *Social Justice: The Moral Foundations of Public Health and Health Policy*. New York: Oxford University Press.

Rawls, J. (1971). *A Theory of Justice*. Cambridge, MA: Belknap Press of Harvard University Press.

Roemer, J. E. (1998). *Equality of Opportunity*. Cambridge, MA: Harvard University Press.

Saunders, B. (2010). "Democracy, Political Equality, and Majority Rule," *Ethics*, 121:148–77.

Segall, S. (2010). *Health, Luck, and Justice*. Princeton, NJ: Princeton University Press.

Sunstein, C. R. (2003). "The Law of Group Polarization," in J. S. Fishkin and P. Laslett (eds), *Debating Deliberative Democracy*. Oxford: Blackwell, 80–101.

16.5

Commentary

How to Combine Universal and Particular Elements in the Distributive Process

Wilhelm Vossenkuhl

Daniels and Sabin convincingly apply a modified account of Rawlsian pure procedural justice to solving problems of fairness in the distribution of scarce goods in the sphere of public health. They argue for outcomes which do not contravene any general ethical principles, e.g. the outcomes do not result from pure gambling. I take it that Daniels and Sabin see those generally acknowledged ethical principles such as justice, individual freedom, non-discrimination, accountability, etc., as being implicit in procedural justice without being constitutive of the outcomes themselves. So far, they are arguing on Rawlsian ground. The great advantage of the modified version of pure procedural justice as favoured by Daniels and Sabin is that it flexibly applies universal ethical principles to the allocation of particular and changing resources available for distribution. Their regulative idea is that the distributive process should be fair and that nobody should be disadvantaged. I fully subscribe to this idea.

The problem I would like to raise in my short comment is that the combination of universal and particular elements in the distributive process will not leave either side untouched. Scarcity of resources demands that we make changes to our principles of distributive justice and fairness. The fewer the available goods, the harder decisions about their distribution will be. Inevitably, some of the participants in the process of distribution will be disadvantaged. I would like to substantiate this claim using the distribution of post mortem donor organs as an example.

The type of goods I consider is, of course, a special one. Most donor organs such as kidneys, hearts, and lungs are indivisible goods, compared to divisible goods like livers, money, or time. Indivisible goods, when scarce, cannot be distributed equally to those who are in need and deserving. If only one organ is available for two patients, one will be disadvantaged and will eventually die. In practice this problem is partially bypassed by a combination of heterogeneous criteria such as urgency and waiting lists. While urgency is lexicographic, waiting lists are not. Lexicographic orderings oblige clinics and doctors to observe one principle only, in this case the principle of saving lives. The patient who is most in danger of death gets the available organ, while the needs of number one on the waiting list are postponed.

Waiting lists are non-linear and result from a number of sub-criteria, e.g. 'first come, first served', the compatibility of blood groups, the agreeableness of tissues, etc. Patients on waiting lists are often badly in need of transplants. In Germany about 800 patients die per annum due to the scarcity of post mortem donor organs. Now the sub-criteria that determine patients' positions on waiting lists are questionable. Judgements which are not in accordance with the principle of non-discrimination are easily mixed with and camouflaged by medical ones. Age, sex, life conduct, social standing, etc. may be amalgamated with medical criteria like life expectancy, prognosis, and the quality of life. In the end, waiting lists may favour non-smoking, non-drinking, younger, promising, and socially well-to-do patients over elderly smokers with a weakness for drinking and a limited life expectancy.

While the lexicographic principle of saving the lives of those urgently in need of a donor organ seems ethically defensible as long as the number of urgent cases does not exceed the number of available organs, the waiting list—as it stands—is ethically indefensible. The primary reason why it is indefensible is that everyone ranked on a waiting list has an equal ethical claim to being saved. The list as such is directly opposed to the legitimate claim to equal treatment. Every moment a patient waits longer for a donor organ than any other patient is a disadvantage in terms of health and quality of life. The violation of the claim to equal medical treatment is aggravated by the (at least potentially dubious) way the waiting list is formed.

We need not go into further details of the distribution of donor organs in order to understand that pure procedural justice, which tacitly respects the principles of equality and non-discrimination, cannot per se guarantee compliance with either of these principles. The scarcity of indivisible goods creates the problem that equal claims to donor organs cannot be treated equally under conditions of scarcity. The principle of equality is obviously constrained by the scarcity of life-saving goods. This is a severe blow against fairness for patients with ethically equal claims.

There is, of course, a pragmatic way of addressing this problem, which is more or less identical with the current practice of distributing post mortem donor organs. Ethical equality of claims is ignored and substituted by the inequality of medical claims, which is represented by the waiting list. The only argument in favour of this substitution is that it works and is widely accepted.

Theoretically acceptable alternatives to this pragmatic approach to the problem are less obvious. As I indicated above, adapting the principle of justice to the distribution of scarce indivisible goods will not leave this principle untouched. It will be compromised by those conditions. The question is how far this compromise may go. No doubt, there will be a point where the principle will be seriously deflated and endangered altogether. I have, elsewhere, analysed the mutual influence of universally valid ethical principles of distribution and of particular scarce and badly-needed goods (Vossenkuhl 2006: 296–416). The gist of my analysis is that we need three consecutive steps in a process of procedural justice in order to overcome the problems involved and to offer a theoretical and practical solution to the problem described above. Otherwise, any ethical principle we value and subscribe to in the distribution of life-sustaining goods will cease to guide us when those goods become scarce.

The first step follows the maxim that principled claims to life-sustaining goods, like the claim to donor organs, can be constrained if allocating goods according to those claims would lead to an unacceptable distribution of those goods. In the book mentioned I call this the maxim of scarcity (Vossenkuhl 2006: 349). This maxim denies that ethical principles like the principle of equality are overriding and mandatory beyond actual and undeniable confinements. In effect, this maxim supports the lexicographic criterion of urgency. It is certainly acceptable that those patients most in need of a donor organ get the available one while other patients are still waiting for help. Any alternative to this distribution would not be acceptable. But, of course, urgency cannot be the only criterion of distribution, as it would minimize the prognosis and the quality of life of patients who are generally in need of a donor organ and expecting to be transplanted. So it would not be acceptable if imminent death were the only reason for organ transplantations.

A second maxim follows immediately. It obliges an ethically optimal distribution of scarce goods, i.e. that patients' equally legitimate claims to being helped by the transplantation of donor organs should be respected as much as possible. The greatest possible number of patients should be transplanted. This maxim, which I call the maxim of normativity, supports the best possible allocation of organ transplantations. The number of donor organs correlates with the number of patients, who get the therapy they badly need. It is obvious both that this maxim obliges political institutions to encourage people to donate and that it commits us to distributive justice in the allocation of donor organs. As indicated above, the waiting-lists system presently in use seems to be far from achieving this goal, as the formation of these lists does not respect the equality of legitimate claims of patients waiting for donor organs.

Is there any alternative at hand? Yes, indeed. We have to waive pure procedural justice for a moment and take refuge in the Aristotelian notion of justice, which offers a clear account of the normativity of claims. It says that equal claims are to be executed equally, and unequal claims unequally. Now, the equality of claims of patients is defined by the therapy they need in order to survive. But the therapy needs qualification, as different patients need different therapy. Not only do the organs needed differ, but also their size, their match in medical terms, and finally the prognosis, life expectancy, and expected life quality of patients. The latter heavily depends on the age and general health status of patients. An old patient in poor health should not be treated the same way as a young patient with a good prognosis. Age and health status should not be looked upon as opportunities for unfair discrimination, but as criteria which are to be taken seriously and used in a transparent way.

Are we not back at the pragmatic formation of waiting lists? Not at all, as waiting lists deny the equality of claims. Following the maxim of normativity, the alternative is to form groups of patients with equal claims for equal therapies and treat them equally. Age and health status should be considered in the formation of groups of patients with equal claims the same way as any other criterion of equality. Under conditions of scarcity this means that nobody is preferred and ranked on any list but that a lottery decides who gets the available organ out of the group of equals.[10]

Whatever one thinks about lotteries, they simulate disinterested choice best and are therefore closest to the ethical standards to be respected in procedural justice. Now, the example I chose—the distribution of donor organs—is certainly not the only obligation of hospitals and public health. It has to be integrated into the whole spectrum of public health commitments. We therefore need a third maxim—I call it the maxim of integration—which ensures that the value structure of public health does not get out of balance. The structure of these values depends on what society and politics take to be the indispensable tenets of public health. Organ transplantation will be one of these tenets, but by far not the only one. Whatever the competing tenets will be, the value structure to be served will be manifold and changing with the available funds and bio-technical research and development. The balance needed will only be reached by an ongoing process of bargaining in order to allocate the available funds up to the standards set by the publicly agreed value structure of public health.

Granted, the practice of allocating donor organs will not be revolutionized by my maxim-based account of procedural justice. Patients will still be disadvantaged and die due to the scarcity of donor organs. But the role and impact of ethical standards under conditions of scarcity will be more transparent. The constraints on ethical principles and standards relevant to procedural justice, and caused by the scarcity of indivisible goods, will be more perspicuous. It will be easier to overcome the drawbacks in the distribution of donor organs and in the allocation of goods in public health in general.

Reference

Vossenkuhl, W. (2006). *Die Möglichkeit des Guten*. München: C. H. Beck.

---

[10] See my detailed account of the lottery in Vossenkuhl (2006: 134).

16.6

Response to Commentaries
Further Thoughts on Implementing Accountability for Reasonableness

James Sabin and Norman Daniels

We thank Professors Callahan, Inoue, Okuda, and Vossenkuhl for their thoughtful comments on our chapter. Among the many valuable issues they have raised we have focused our response on one that we see as the primary current challenge for the accountability for reasonableness principle—the feasibility of implementation.

Like Callahan, we are based in the United States. With sadness, we share his view that political discourse in the US has become so intensely polarized that it is difficult to see how a deliberative process at the national political level could at present apply the kind of respectful, probing exchange of reasons the accountability for reasonableness principle calls for. As Callahan noted, the US health reform process was almost derailed by duplicitous accusations that the government planned to create "death panels," (when the health reform simply called for clinicians to be reimbursed for discussions of end-of-life care) and a large segment of the population has been led to fear that if the government is allowed to require citizens to obtain health insurance it will ultimately be allowed to require purchase of broccoli as a public health measure (which is how the issue of an individual mandate to buy insurance has been debated in the US Supreme Court)! In this toxic political climate it is not surprising that public trust of the Supreme Court, which has historically been the most respected deliberative body in the country, has fallen to 44 percent.

We have never thought of accountability for reasonableness as a magic bullet that will solve all political ills. We realized from the start that the approach may well not fit at all in political cultures that are very antidemocratic. We had not anticipated that even democratic cultures can become anti-deliberative. We formulated the idea of a fair deliberative process, after many years of observing *collaborative* policy-making processes at health plans, medical groups, and public agencies in the US, Canada, and the UK. The structures and cultures of the sites we visited encouraged participants to conduct themselves in a fair-minded manner and to seek mutually justifiable grounds for cooperation.

When an organization or agency has clear responsibility for a population to be served within a budget and a culture that welcomes open debate, transparency about the grounds for allocation decisions, policies based on relevant reasons, and revision in accord with experience and new evidence, accountability for reasonableness can often be implemented without enormous difficulty. But even at sites that presented favorable environments for applying the principles of accountability for reasonableness, skilled leadership was required for the process to flourish. The two key requirements were solid support from the top leadership and skillful facilitation of the deliberative process itself.

These observations about leadership requirements are consistent with Callahan's suggestion that "someone who will act much the way a judge does during a trial" is needed. And, Okuda appears to be saying something similar when he suggests that in the sphere of government, whether or not accountability for reasonableness is used lies "in the hands of politicians." If authorities opt for a closed, top-down decision process, or if members of a legislature hold to fixed ideological positions and refuse to consider the perspectives advanced by others, the kind of accountable process we have urged cannot be applied.

We were interested to see that Okuda associates our proposal with "archives." We associate his discussion with our conviction that learning from prior decisions is a core component of accountability for reasonableness. One of us (JES) chairs a quarterly ethics advisory group at a regional health plan in the US. In preparing the policy "case" to be considered, relevant precedents are included. In this way, accountability for reasonableness envisions a process analogous to the development of "case law" in the legal system, where, over time, a body of decisions creates principles that can be applied in subsequent cases. In health policy deliberations these precedents do not have the force of law, but deviating from them requires a clearly explicated rationale.

Inoue argues that "we need a comprehensive conception of justice that enjoins certain rules to resolve value conflicts and elucidate a genuine meaning of fairness" and proposes an "equal opportunity-based principle of justice" for that role. An overarching principle of justice may be desirable, but in our view, large, diverse societies do not have shared principles that are specific enough to resolve questions of resource allocation and limits. While most would probably agree with Inoue that we should be held responsible to some degree for the impacts of our lifestyle choices on our health, and some *might* agree that not rescuing us when these choices impair our health and even threaten our lives is not "merciless" (though we disagree), we cannot envision a free society achieving consensus on this perspective. Although Inoue is correct that the degree of responsibility could theoretically be ascertained in each individual case, to the best of our knowledge there are no examples of this having being done in the health sphere. In the US the Emergency Medical Treatment and Active Labor Act explicitly requires hospitals to provide emergency treatment to all regardless of causation of the emergency or ability to pay.

All of the commentators identify the question of who should participate in the deliberative process as an important concern. We can offer these broad responses under the headings of *process, context,* and *content.*

Deliberative *processes* cannot succeed if those who participate are not open to collaborative inquiry and decision making. It is fine for participants to enter with strongly held perspectives as long as they are prepared to listen to others in a respectful manner. In a highly contested area like reproductive ethics we should not expect those who regard abortion as a moral crime and those equally committed to having abortion services available to a population to change their views. But if they are not open to seeking areas of potential agreement and compromise, they should not participate.

The *context* in which the deliberation is conducted influences the answer to the question of who should participate. There should be voices that can speak from the perspectives of the key stakeholders to the decision or policy. Since stakeholders vary with context, so will the optimal composition of the deliberative body. As examples, in the US health system, employers are the main purchaser of insurance for working-age adults and their families and should be included among the participants in setting policy for the insurance funds they contribute to. But in the UK National Health Service, citizens fund the system through their taxes. As a result, the council that advises the NHS about the values that should govern adoption of new treatments and technologies is chosen to reflect the basic demography of the UK, and employers have no distinctive role as they do in the US.

Finally, with regard to *content,* if the task of the deliberative group is to advise about a framework of values to guide allocation policy, specific technical expertise is not required. This explains the decision in the UK to form the Citizens Council, whose task is to give broad guidance about values to NICE on the basis of demography. But if the allocative task is to create policy for a specific clinical area, experts in the relevant areas of treatment and prevention, and patients who have experienced the condition, should be included. Vossenkuhl's "maxim of normativity" appears to be recommending a process like this involving "society and politics" in order to "allocate the available funds...by the publicly agreed value structure of public health."

The work that led to formulating the approach we call accountability for reasonableness required a combination of fieldwork (observing real-world deliberative processes) and conceptual analysis (ensuring that the emerging theory was formulated in a philosophically consistent manner). We believe that at this point the further evolution of the approach requires two different forms of expertise: *organizational development and leadership,* to foster practical implementation at different levels of health systems, and *evaluation science,* to assess the degree to which accountability for reasonableness fosters decisions that are more fair and better accepted by the public. Hopefully, if the approach is more widely adopted, it may be possible to measure its effects on legitimacy and fairness so that the approach can point to evidence about improved outcomes and not rest on theory alone.

SECTION C

Care in the Aging Society

17.1

Primary Topic Article
Taking Seriously Ill People Seriously: Ethics and Policy Dimensions of the Chronic Disease/ End-of-Life Care Continuum

Nancy Berlinger and Michael K. Gusmano

Introduction

Most individuals in the US and other developed nations die of chronic progressive diseases, such as cancer, heart disease, or dementia. These individuals also live with these diseases for some period before a disease process enters its terminal phase and a patient's health-care needs are identified in terms of end-of-life care. The language of "chronicity" is used differently with respect to these major disease trajectories, and even within them. A life-threatening condition may be framed as a "chronic" disease if an incurable disease can be medically managed, even if the underlying disease process is not stable. The experience of living as a seriously ill person may be termed "chronic" illness, often with the expectation that this person should be able to self-manage their disease. The word "chronic" may be broadly applied to different kinds of care received outside the acute-care setting for an ongoing condition; this broad use of "chronic" to mean "sub-acute" may fail to differentiate between the chronic-care needs of an ambulatory patient at a physician's office, and the more extensive medical, nursing, and other caregiving needs of a patient in a nursing home or home-care setting. How we use language to define problems and to describe our professional and societal accountability to patients with respect to these problems, and how we use policy to create, or fail to create, structures and conditions to support persons who are living with chronic progressive diseases that are likely to result in death will be the topic of this paper. The paper will focus on the US context, with particular attention to cancer care, and with comparisons to non-US contexts.

1 What do we mean by "chronicity"?

Stories about curing life-threatening disease are heroic. Stories about managing and living with chronic progressive disease are not. In the United States, where hospitals compete with one another for patients, it is common to see direct-to-consumer advertisements in newspapers and on billboards along highways that tell heroic stories about beating disease and cheating death ("Cancer—you lost, I won"), that urge patients and their loved ones to "come here" (and, by implication, not to go somewhere else) when they get very bad news. These advertisements are reinforced inside acute-care hospitals, where the vignettes about patients that appear in newsletters, fundraising appeals, annual reports, and websites are stories with proper endings (disease defeated, life saved), and with common themes of hope, courage, strength, and gratitude. These are good stories—great stories—if your disease is potentially curable.

Stories about chronicity—about chronic disease, and the experience of living with chronic illness—are unfinished stories. By their nature, they are personal, clinical, and organizational works in progress. We can imagine the hospital advertisement or billboard that says, in effect, "We create survivors," but not the one that says, "We create people who will live with incurable disease, and the side effects of treatment, for some uncertain period of time, and then will die." And even though half of all deaths in the United States occur in hospitals, and an acute-care or specialized hospital, such as a cancer center, may record hundreds of deaths each year, we cannot imagine the advertisement for a non-hospice facility that says, "Come *here* when you're dying—we know how to take care of you."

Most residents of developed nations will, as they age, live for some period of time with at least one chronic disease, broadly understood in the health policy literature as "conditions that last a year or more and require ongoing medical attention and/or limit activities of daily living" (Warshaw 2006: 5–10; see also Hwang et al. 2001: 267–78). In the United States, two out of three residents live with multiple chronic conditions, and certain conditions, such as diabetes, are nearly always accompanied by comorbid chronic conditions (Hwang et al. 2001: 267–78; Warshaw 2006: 5–10). While not all chronic conditions are also progressive conditions, the three major end-of-life trajectories in the United States and other developed nations reflect the end stages of progressive conditions that often have also been chronic conditions: cancer; diseases of major organ systems; Alzheimer's disease.

Defining chronic disease in terms of its ongoing nature is not, however, the only way to understand chronicity. In ethics as in life, language matters. Patients and health-care professionals use the word "chronic" in a variety of ways, while policy analysts, policy makers, and journalists speak of our global "chronic disease future" in ways that are both depressing and somewhat confusing. Progress against infectious disease means that preventable chronic diseases are a growing cause of death in the developing world. In developed and developing nations with aging societies due to declining birth rates and greater longevity, our ability to medically manage some chronic conditions associated with aging means that an ever-increasing percentage of the population of many nations can expect to be diagnosed with Alzheimer's disease, to become a caregiver for a loved one with this disease—or both. A recent report by the Open Society Foundations'

International Palliative Care Institute notes that in the developing world both cancer and AIDS tend to be diagnosed at an advanced stage, and patients' experiences of these diseases are often chronic-illness and terminal-illness experiences (International Palliative Care Initiative Public Health Program 2010). This report also describes the immense disparities in global access to basic pain medications across nations: in 2002, 78 percent of all legally prescribed morphine worldwide reflected data from just six nations, all of which were developed nations, while the remaining 22 percent reflected data from 142 other nations (International Palliative Care Initiative Public Health Program 2010). According to the Open Society report, legal consumption of opioid analgesics is a "good gross indicator" of access to palliative care in a given nation, as drugs such as morphine are highly effective, relatively cheap, and require minimal technology to deliver. Such immense variation in access to one medication long proven to be effective in treating certain symptoms, such as pain and dyspnea, which are associated with both chronic illness and terminal illness, suggests further inequities with respect to the structure of chronic care and end-of-life care across nations.

Practice variation and structural inequities with respect to the chronic disease/end-of-life care continuum are well documented problems *within* developed nations as well. According to a recent report of the Dartmouth Atlas Project, which analyzes data on practice variation in health care in the United States, even within a specialty (cancer care) in which palliative care is relatively well developed and within a population (patients with a life expectancy of six months or less) in which palliative care services are fully covered by Medicare's hospice benefit, rates of enrollment in hospice among patients who were in their last month of life ranged from under 20 percent to higher than 80 percent across different regions of the US, and even within some regions and communities (Goodman et al. 2010: 28). The authors of this report note that these findings should not be interpreted as disease specific, but rather as "often reflective of more general patterns of care received by patients with chronic illness":

[T]he *style* of care provided to cancer patients near the end of life is very similar to the care given to patients *at the same hospital* who die with other types of chronic disease, such as congestive heart failure, diabetes, dementia, or chronic obstructive pulmonary disease…care patterns often cut across many different patient types and care teams within a hospital. (Goodman et al. 2010: 38; italics added)

There are moral implications to how we use language to define problems and how we are accountable, to individual patients and to society, with respect to these problems. A taxonomy of chronicity would include the following definitions:

Chronic disease as ongoing, medically managed, serious disease: In everyday usage, including in media reports, the word "chronic" can suggest "not curable—but treatable," and not merely "of long duration." Certain diseases, such as advanced cancer and chronic obstructive pulmonary disease (COPD), may be chronic, in that they can be medically managed for long periods. They are also progressive, and at some point during progression, the burdens of treatment will exceed the benefits of treatment. There is therefore a tension between the "chronic" and "progressive" aspects of the same serious disease. A failure to clarify that a chronic disease is also a progressive disease with a terminal prognosis, and what can be foreseen as well as what is uncertain about progression, has consequences for informed decision-making. Being able to manage a serious disease is not the same as being able to prevent a patient from dying from this disease. If a patient or surrogate is making decisions without reference to prognosis, the patient loses the opportunity to consider *how* the patient wishes to spend the rest of his or her life and how useful treatment can be in helping the patient to achieve the patient's goals. This use of "chronic" when a disease process is *also* progressive with respect to its expected trajectory is evident even in clinical, ethics, and policy literature that calls into question the value of non-palliative treatment when a patient is near the end of life. For example, in the aforementioned citation from the Dartmouth Atlas report, patients who are dying are described as having "chronic" disease or illness: while these patients have been chronically ill in the sense that they have been ill for months or years, these dying patients are now suffering from rapidly or inexorably progressing disease.

Chronic disease as stable disease: The relationship of "chronic" disease to "stable" disease varies from disease to disease, within different types of the same disease, and from patient to patient. As with the relationship between chronic disease and progressive disease, how patients, loved ones, and clinicians understand and discuss this aspect of chronicity has consequences for informed decision-making. With respect to certain chronic diseases such as diabetes, multiple behavioral factors—adherence to a treatment regimen, diet, exercise, monitoring of comorbid conditions—can determine how stable or potentially stable this disease will be, even when medical treatment is integral to efforts to control disease. With respect to certain other diseases, even perfect adherence to a currently effective treatment regimen cannot guarantee that a chronic disease will be a stable disease process.

Chronicity in cancer offers a case in point. Stabilizing an incurable or recurrent form of cancer tends to involve treatments that interfere with cell development. In the past decade, chronic myelogenous leukemia (CML) has become a stable form of incurable cancer through the introduction of a "biological" drug therapy (imatinib mesylate) that inhibits the development of an enzyme necessary for the growth of this type of cancer cell: in effect, it shuts the cancer down. Other cancer drugs, such as those that target specific hormones implicated in the growth of some breast cancers, have further expanded the modalities for controlling incurable forms of cancer with less toxicity than cytotoxic chemotherapy, which kills rapidly dividing cells. The natural history of some cancer as chronic disease may mean that the emerging paradigm for its management may resemble that for a disease such as HIV/AIDS, in which disease control is more reliant on response to treatment than on behavioral factors under the patient's control; multi-drug treatment regimens can be expected to change as resistance develops; treatment side effects may create their own significant burdens that must also be managed; and the patient's physician must have knowledge of treatment options (Aziz 2007). However, the experience of keeping cancer stable is not like that of keeping HIV/AIDS stable— different diseases, different treatment paradigms, and with respect to cancer, the need for specialist care consistently. If an oncologist treating a patient with metastatic cancer views this patient's disease as "chronic," meaning "stable," as long as the production of cancer cells can be interrupted, and as "progressive" when these modalities are no longer effective, should the physician share this conceptual framework with the patient, or not? This is not only a question of communication style. If the oncologist views chemotherapy, radiation, or another treatment modality in a patient with progressive advanced cancer as a palliative therapy, with the goal of relieving symptoms and helping the patient to feel better, but does not share this view with the patient, then this patient lacks crucial information about the goal of future treatment. This patient may continue to take on treatment burdens in the belief that benefits that are no longer attainable are, in fact, still attainable. At the most basic level, this patient does not know that what matters about treatment is whether or not it is contributing to or detracting from her quality of life as she perceives it: is treatment helping her to spend time as she wishes to spend it, or is treatment now a barrier to doing this? Would hospice care be a more effective way to relieve symptoms and reduce burdens?

Chronic disease as symptomatic illness: Over the past 40 years, bioethicists working from medicine, nursing, sociology, and the humanities have drawn a distinction, in theory and practice, between disease as pathology and illness as the experience of the suffering person. As the result of this theoretical framework and the development of specialties such as palliative medicine, hospice medicine, pain medicine, and reha-bilitative medicine that reflect this theory of illness, the treatment of the symptoms of a disease or injury may be framed as the treatment of chronic "illness" even if an underlying symptom-causing disease process is unstable or is inexorably progress-ing—or, conversely, if a disease or injury has been successfully treated but the patient suffers from post-treatment symptoms. These developments of theory and practice have helped to advance the clinical recognition of the patient's experience of living as an ill person, and of the ethical necessity of integrating the treatment of symptoms into the treatment of disease. The results of a recent randomized controlled trial con-ducted by investigators at Massachusetts General Hospital, added empirical weight to these descriptive and normative accounts. Investigators comparing outcomes among patients diagnosed with metastatic non-small cell lung cancer found that patients who received palliative care integrated into treatment from diagnosis reported better mood and quality of life than patients in the control (treatment only) group; chose less intensive life-sustaining interventions—and also lived an average of three months longer (Temel et al. 2010).

However, the treatment of pain and symptoms continues to be undervalued in cure-oriented medicine. Even when posters in hospitals assure patients that they have a "right" to pain relief, it can be hard to exercise this right, particularly when pain man-agement is conceptualized and organized as an inpatient, "bedside" consultation service that relies on referrals, rather than as a service that is normative—and normal—for all patients. Moreover, some health care professionals tend to steer clear of "pain," whether because they do not like to work with patients who are in pain, or they are unsure of how to treat pain, or they are wary of working with opioids. Some specialists categorize symptom management as "Not [Name of Disease]," therefore, Not *My* Job, even when symptoms of a patient's disease and treatment are foreseeable and treatable. Also, there can even be tension between professionals who would seem to be natural allies in caring for chronically ill patients: is "pain" management a different specialty from "symptom" management, or are they both "palliative care"? Do pain and symptom management require specialist care, or should the same professionals who treat disease also be capable of treating pain and symptoms? The answer to these questions can differ from institution to institution, specialty to specialty, clinician to clinician, and perhaps even nation to nation.

Chronic as "not acute" or "sub-acute": Some clinicians use the word "chronic" to refer to the place in which care is delivered, and also as shorthand for a patient who receives care in a particular setting: outpatient clinics, community health centers, rehabilitative facilities, and home care are associated with "chronic" patients, hospitals are associated with "acute" patients. "Chronic" and "acute" often overlap. A patient who has chronic or worsening symptoms of progressive illness, such as COPD or cancer, may have recurrent bouts of pain or dyspnea that constitute acute episodes of illness. The non-inpatient settings associated with "chronic" care and "chronic" patients encompass a wide range of sickness and relative health. Patients who are chronically ill, with somewhat burdensome, potentially or foreseeably progressive but currently manageable conditions such as diabetes and asthma, should be able to rely on their primary care provider as their "medical home," whether this setting is a physician's office, health center, or outpatient clinic. Chronically ill home-care or nursing-home residents are often seriously ill or disabled, although much of the medical and nursing care they need can be provided outside a hospital setting and their care should be organized to avoid preventable hospitalizations. Organizing ongoing chronic care for patients with Alzheimer's disease, who are likely to need behavioral health services and whose condition may sharply deteriorate during hospitalizations due to delirium, is particularly challenging. Some chronically ill patients, such as cancer patients, require specialist care in the outpatient setting. However, in the United States, patients who live with cancer as a chronic and progressive disease may lack a reliable "medical home" that integrates their primary care and their specialized needs. Even in countries like France, Germany, and the UK, in which general practitioners play a more important role and patients are more likely to have a regular source of care, coordination between primary care and specialists can be a problem (White 1995; Klein 1997: 1267–78; Brown 2003: 52–6; Rodwin and Le Pen 2005: 2259–61).

Within the culture of health care, outpatient settings are less visible than inpatient settings, and settings such as home care are invisible. The medical, legal, and philosophical tools that clinical ethics relies on to address moral dilemmas arising in inpatient care, often concerning end-of-life decision-making, may not offer sufficient tools to professionals and patients collaborating inside a chronic-disease paradigm. A hospital's clinical ethics consultation service, oriented toward "bedside" inpatient consultations, may lack clear authority to consult on dilemmas arising in its own outpatient clinics, and may have no relationship with local primary health-care providers or outpatient specialists.

Professionals who treat patients with chronic and potentially or foreseeable progressive disease may be uncertain as to what constitutes ethically sound practice when discussing treatment options, making treatment recommendations, presenting information about clinical trials, or when disagreements arise. For example, a patient with end-stage renal disease (ESRD) who is undergoing dialysis as an outpatient may, as a consequence of comorbid conditions, lack decision-making capacity or have fluctuating or uncertain capacity. Such a patient may, on occasion, refuse dialysis, leading to episodic hospital admissions to stabilize his condition. On these occasions, the patient may come to the attention of the hospital's clinical ethics consultation service, but there may be no clear way for the consultation team either to resolve this dilemma—namely, how should the changing preferences of a patient with uncertain capacity be understood and honored?—or to collaborate with the patient's other health-care providers concerning this and similar cases. Enlarging the scope of ethics in health care would acknowledge that ethical dilemmas in the treatment and care of seriously ill patients arise in the care of seriously ill but nonhospitalized patients who receive much of their care in a chronic-care setting. The policy and practice challenge would then involve how to create mechanisms for addressing these dilemmas outside the convenient institutional setting of a hospital or nursing home. In more fragmented outpatient delivery systems, such as France and the US, this may be particularly difficult.

Chronic disease as "self-managed" disease: The outcomes-based chronic-disease paradigm described by clinicians and researchers in the United States rests on the understanding that these patients are—and must be—their own principal caregivers (Bodenheimer et al. 2002). This paradigm identifies physicians and nurses as the patient's collaborators in integrating treatment into everyday life, by supporting the patient's ability to consider and make treatment decisions, and by teaching the patient how to identify problems and participate in solving them. This triadic paradigm may not work for every disease that is experienced as both a chronic condition and a progressive disease process. For example, cancer is a challenging disease to self-manage, as treatment regimens change as the disease becomes treatment resistant, and as symptoms and side effects change when treatment changes. Alzheimer's disease and other conditions that cause progressive cognitive impairment, behavioral changes, or deterioration in motor skills will require the continuous involvement of paid or unpaid caregivers to support the patient's self-management capacity. Enlarging the scope of ethics in health care would also acknowledge that the treatment and care of seriously ill patients includes the patient as provider, when a patient, or a family caregiver, is held responsible for self-managing chronic disease and for making treatment decisions in this context.

Narratives of chronicity: How the story of a chronic disease is told, and how this story shapes the clinical and everyday experiences of a person living with this disease, are different for different conditions. Narratives about living with HIV/AIDS are still taking shape 15 years after the introduction of effective antiretroviral therapies. An HIV prevention campaign launched in late 2010 by the New York City Department of Health carried the message "It's never just HIV," in an effort to correct misperceptions about the health consequences of HIV infection even when antiretroviral therapy is available. Narratives of different cancers as chronic diseases are emerging, although stories about living with cancer can be conflated with stories about surviving cancer. In the United States, the National Cancer Institute counts as "cancer survivors" anyone living with a previous diagnosis of cancer: this "survivor" population therefore includes persons with incurable cancers, as well as persons with past diagnoses of early-stage cancer that was treated and has not recurred (Howlader et al. 2012). However, programs designed for cancer "survivors" tend to focus on patients who do not have active disease. Stories about living with cardiac disease, and with various types of cardiac implantable electronic devices, can also be unclear about how living with a device that helps to preserve good health or prevent problems differs from living with a device that sustains life but cannot prevent disease progression, and also from living with a device whose value may be questionable or that adds to a dying patient's burdens.

As much of the action in a patient's chronicity story happens outside the hospital, this is not a story that hospital staff hear on morning rounds. Staff involved in clinical ethics consultations or who take part in clinical ethics education may not hear these stories, either. It is a story that the person living with a serious illness, and the effects of treatment, may have to piece together on her own, uncertain whether her story is a good story—a satisfactory story, a meaningful story, a lucky story—or not, and also uncertain at what point this story becomes a story about dying from a serious illness.

2 Taking seriously ill people seriously: toward ethically sound policy on chronicity

Mindful of these myriad ways in which the experience of chronicity is defined with reference to different disease processes, care settings, and social relationships—including a patient's relationship to herself, in the role of self-manager, and to loved ones in their capacities as caregivers, how can organizational and public policy reflect the nature of living with progressive illness of long duration, and support the ability of individuals to *live with* the diseases they are likely to die from? Direct comparisons between different health-care systems are difficult, particularly when these comparisons involve the United States, in which health care is fragmented into different systems according to payer and in some cases diagnosis. However, in considering how policy can support ethically sound health care for seriously ill patients, some general considerations may apply across different systems. Here are two:

Take seriously ill people seriously by relieving suffering: integrate palliative care into health-care systems

Even when pain and symptoms are foreseeable due to a patient's diagnosis, patients who live with serious illness may have great difficulty learning about and securing ongoing palliative care. In the United States, the typical organization of non-hospice palliative care as an inpatient consultation service does not guarantee that patients in other care settings will have reliable access to this same service, while historical patterns of late enrollment in hospice and of immense variation in referral practices nationally and regionally continue to result in underutilization of hospice services and in inequitable access to these services (Goodman et al. 2010). In Japan as in the US, lack of provider and family experience with palliative care in the context of serious illness outside hospice serves to reinforce these patterns, resulting in late referrals that, following a patient's death, are perceived by survivors to have been too late (Morita et al. 2005; Morita et al. 2006).

Underutilization of palliative care and hospice is a special problem among patients with a terminal diagnosis other than cancer. A 1999 study found that hospital-based physicians in the US had difficulty determining whether "seriously ill hospitalized patients with advanced chronic obstructive pulmonary disease, congestive heart failure, or end-stage liver disease" met the prognostic threshold for the Medicare Hospice Benefit—the so-called "six-month rule," confirming that a patient's life expectancy is six months or less with or without treatment (Fox et al. 1999: 1638–45). Another recent study, also from the US, identified another barrier to hospice referral: physicians' concerns that "patients or their family members would construe hospice referral as a cost-saving technique," and would therefore reject this referral, particularly if a patient was insured through a managed-care plan (Brickner et al. 2004: 411–18). In other words, the actions of physicians were influenced by their beliefs that patients on managed-care plans would perceive a hospice referral not as a sound clinical recommendation based on the patient's prognosis and condition, but as an effort to ration care in the interests of the managed-care organization. In the US, a minority of patients with ESRD receive palliative care and hospice services, even after dialysis is withdrawn, symptoms that can be relieved are foreseeable, and death from renal failure is certain to occur within days or weeks (Murray et al. 2006: 1248–55). In the UK, the use of palliative care by patients with ESRD is also low, with significant practice variation (Gunda et al. 2005: 392–5). While the modern hospice movement was founded in the UK and has long been integrated into the health service, a 1999–2000 survey found that fewer than 5 percent of non-cancer patients in the UK received hospice care (Gunda et al. 2005).

Meeting the palliative care and hospice needs of patients with progressive dementia, with or without common comorbidities such as frailty, presents special ethical and policy challenges. In the US, the "six-month rule" was adopted with a terminal cancer trajectory in mind. However, there is a poor match-up between the needs of the Alzheimer's population and the hospice scope of services. Alzheimer's carries a terminal prognosis, but a patient diagnosed with Alzheimer's may have a life expectancy far exceeding six months, and may need a level of geriatric-psychiatric care difficult to obtain in hospice or deliver in a home setting. Physicians caring for Alzheimer's patients may be unclear about their patients' eligibility for hospice and concerned about recommending hospice services too soon, and as a result, often recommend hospice too late (Mitchell et al. 2007: 7–16). The rate of hospice enrollment among nursing-home residents in the US is also lower than the projected need for hospice services, due in part to the financial disincentive of hospice enrollment for nursing-home operators. Medicare reimburses nursing homes at a lower rate for a "hospice" bed than for a "skilled nursing" bed for the same resident. Long-standing nursing-home practices of repeatedly transferring dying residents to acute-care hospitals as their condition deteriorates, or using feeding tubes in an effort to prevent weight loss in residents with end-stage dementia despite overwhelming evidence that this intervention is harmful in this context, can also be traced to financial and regulatory disincentives to recognizing nursing homes as end-of-life care settings (Meier, Lim, and Carlson 2010; on tube feeding, see Finucane, Christmas, and Travis 1999; Ganzini 2006; Gillick 2006; Gillick and Volandes 2008; Teno et al. 2009; Teno et al. 2011; on proposal on comfort feeding, see Palecek et al. 2010).

Understanding the ethical dimensions of the chronic disease/end-of-life care spectrum requires acknowledging, once again, that the first obligation of health care is to relieve suffering and whenever possible, to prevent. Disease cannot always be defeated, death is not optional for anyone, but research-based knowledge of how to relieve suffering over the course of different serious illnesses is now widely available to health-care professionals. It should be integral to all health-care education and practice; patients' access to this knowledge should not depend on their skill—or luck—in finding a health-care professional who self-identifies with palliative care and is skilled in its delivery.

Taking seriously ill people seriously will require institutions who care for individuals at all stages of chronic and progressive illness to invest in palliative care training for their staff, to self-identify with the goals of palliative care, and to promote ethical reflection aimed at challenging practices, systems, and habits of thought that fail to place the relief of suffering at the center of the health-care enterprise.

Take seriously ill people seriously by acknowledging how care works, what it costs, and how it can fail: Assess and improve existing systems of population-level health-care delivery in terms of the current and projected needs of aging populations and equity for family caregivers. On institutional and societal levels, consider what a society owes to those who live with chronic illness, and to those who are dying.

Due to declining birth rates and increasing human longevity, the world is growing older. By 2020, 20 percent of the population in most developed countries will be over 65 years of age. By the year 2050, every third person on the planet will be over 60 years of age. Persons aged 85 years and over, the fastest-growing segment of the population in most developed countries, tend to be less healthy, and more likely to need medical care for chronic conditions, compared to younger segments of the population. While there is some evidence that disability rates among older people have been declining in recent decades, the absolute number of the elderly is growing, and the number of years that those with disabling conditions may need assistive care may also be increasing (Vita et al. 1998: 1035–41). For example, in the United States, Medicare beneficiaries 85 years and over are more likely to have two or more chronic conditions, at least one functional limitation, and mobility and social activity limitations, than younger Medicare beneficiaries (Centers for Medicare & Medicaid Services). They are also less likely to be engaged in paid employment and more likely to live below the poverty line (Rodwin and Gusmano 2006).

All this translates into a foreseeably greater demand for medical, nursing, and other services needed by the oldest members of aging populations, immense economic and structural challenges for societies, and an urgent need to enlarge the scope of health-care ethics beyond the clinical setting, to include resource allocation and social justice questions that tend to be identified with public health or human rights scholarship and advocacy.

Population aging and the growing prevalence of chronic illness place immense pressure on a particular segment of society: family caregivers, particularly women, who shoulder responsibility for coordinating and providing care for their elderly parents, and who may also serve as the surrogate decision-makers for patients who lack decision-making capacity. Women who are in the labor force are just as likely to serve as family caregivers as women who are not (Pavalko 1997: 170–9). Family caregivers (who may also be friends or neighbors rather than biological or legal family members) are at increased risk of stress and depression, have less time for outside relationships and pastimes, and experience other social consequences of sustained caregiving (Arno, Viola, and Gusmano 2010). Caregivers for elderly people with chronic illnesses are likely to be aging themselves, and so may be experiencing the outset of chronic diseases even as they are required to function as the "well" member of a caregiving relationship.

As growth in household incomes in most developed countries has leveled off, assuming family caregiving responsibilities is likely to add to a caregiver's economic burdens, if the caregiver is also responsible for covering out-of-pocket medical or home-care costs, or for taking on the immense cost of long-term residential care. Among developed nations, Japan, Germany, Austria, and some Scandinavian countries have universal systems of long-term care, but in most countries, long-term care services that support people with chronic illness and their families are limited and means tested. Despite the growing need for reliable, publicly funded home care that would allow a chronically ill person to remain at home and to maintain social relationships, most developed nations have an institutional bias when it comes to funding long-term care. Public funding for in-home nursing services and for long-term residential care is most restricted in the US, where non-hospice patients requiring continuous care must meet the strict income requirements of Medicaid if their care needs exceed the limited periods for which Medicare will reimburse (Rodwin and Gusmano 2006). The health-care reform legislation passed in the US in 2010 (Patient Protection and Affordable Care Act) includes a plan for a federal insurance program that will provide a cash benefit to individuals with functional limitation to help them to pay for home-care services and so maintain greater independence. If fully implemented, this program will not begin providing benefits for five years, so the evaluation of its impact on people with chronic illness and their families is many years in the future (Arno, Viola, and Gusmano 2010). At present, Medicare reimbursement in the US does not encourage the effective management of chronic illness by elderly or disabled beneficiaries, even though about 80 percent of beneficiaries report having at least one chronic condition. For example, routine telephone and email communications between health-care providers and their patients are recognized as "essential to high-quality and efficient care" for patients with chronic illness, who have ongoing medical needs and may have great difficulty traveling to appointments (Berenson and Horvath 2003). However, Medicare does not reimburse health-care providers for these types of communications, due to concerns about moral hazard. From an indemnity insurance perspective, promoting these communications through reimbursements could generate "excessive" phone calls and emails from patients. Medicare's failure to reimburse for routine communications undermines the goal of supporting patient self-management in a patient population for whom face-to-face communications may be particularly burdensome (Berenson and Horvath 2003). From the perspective of chronically ill patients and their caregivers, it makes no sense.

Understanding the ethical dimensions of the chronic disease/end-of-life care spectrum requires acknowledging the extent to which family caregivers are integral to the well-being and choices of individuals who live with chronic disease, including progressive diseases with terminal prognoses, around the world. Taking seriously ill people seriously will require collaboration between formal systems of care and informal caregivers. This is true for nations with fragmented health care systems, such as the US, and for nations with more centralized but increasingly unsustainable health and social welfare systems. Simply put, it is not possible for national government policies and programs to meet the needs of their aging societies without close and sustained partnerships among local governments, nonprofit organizations, community and neighborhood groups, and family caregivers themselves.

Another challenging problem concerns how we talk about economic as well as physiological treatment burdens. Physicians should not bear sole responsibility for addressing economic issues; social workers, for example, may be better able to assist patients with these questions. However, physicians should be prepared to talk about cost when discussing treatment options and making recommendations. Failure to do so may suggest to patients and families that it is wrong to consider cost when assessing treatment options, or that high cost is associated with high value. Physicians, and the institutions in which they work, should recognize their obligation to provide patients and families with information about costs in the context of treatment decision-making, and to prevent economic hardships triggered by poorly informed decision-making or by inattention to the long-term consequences of a treatment decision.

Clinical oncologists who treat patients with advanced cancer are confronting these concerns in different ways in different nations. In the US, oral chemotherapies, which are prescription drugs, present special concerns (Boodman 2010). Depending on the adequacy of their prescription-drug coverage, patients may incur out-of-pocket costs associated with oral treatments (Tangka et al. 2010: 1–8). These patients may also rely on prescription pain medications and supplemental therapies to counteract treatment side effects, adding to their financial burden if insurance does not fully cover these costs. Use of "off-label" medications can also add to a cancer patient's out-of-pocket costs, as insurers are not obligated to cover the cost of drugs not approved for the treatment of a particular condition (National Cancer Institute 1999; Berlinger and Gusmano 2010; Tangka et al. 2010).

Patients in the US, even if they are insured, are responsible for a far greater percentage of their health-care costs than are patients in France. Almost all public and private insurance coverage in the US includes deductibles and co-payments, so total out-of-pocket expenses increase with the use of health-care services. By contrast, French national health insurance (NHI) coverage *increases* when a patient's costs increase. French NHI does not include deductibles, and pharmaceutical benefits are extensive. Moreover, patients with debilitating or chronic illness are exempted from paying co-insurance (Gusmano, Weisz, and Rodwin 2010).

Cost is an ethical issue in health care. The ethical goal of equity requires health-care institutions to grapple with the moral as well as the fiscal dimensions of resource allocation and health-care cost (Berlinger, Jennings, and Wolf 2013). This is much more easily accomplished in centralized health-care systems than in the US, where institutions that provide hands-on care may or may not offer health-care professionals any guidance in how to talk about costs with patients when a treatment option will include economic burdens, or in how ethically sound policy on resource allocation can be developed and supported. The intersection of justice and cost is always a challenging discussion in health care, and clinicians may prefer to avoid these issues. However, these clinicians may also find themselves questioning policies that seem unfair, or that appear to prioritize reimbursable procedures ahead of the welfare of patients, including chronically ill and dying patients.

In its 2010 report, *Easing the Pain: Successes and Challenges in International Palliative Care,* the Open Society Foundations argued that pain relief and palliative care are a "pressing human rights issue." The use of rights language in connection with health care has a long history. Article 25 of the Universal Declaration of Human Rights, adopted by the United Nations in 1948, claims that "everyone has the right to a standard of living adequate for the health and well-being of oneself and one's family, including food, clothing, housing, and medical care" (United Nations 1948). While the claim that patients have a right to palliative or other forms of medical care may be helpful if there are legal or other barriers that prevent patients from receiving it, it does not tell us anything about how this care should be financed. In 2008, for example, the Democratic National Platform in the US claimed that "affordable health care is a basic right," but it did not define "affordable" (Democratic National Convention Committee 2008). In the US, "rights" appeals are also strongly associated with libertarian positions that value personal freedom and limited institutional, including governmental, involvement in the lives of private citizens. This can lead to arguments that suggest—incorrectly—that there is a right to demand whatever medical care one wants, and can, in clinical settings, reduce the ethical goal of supporting patient self-determination to "giving the patient what the patient wants, and can pay for," rather than thinking seriously about what can be of benefit to this patient.

In contrast to "rights" language, whether in terms of an explicit human rights approach or in other philosophical appeals to rights, a bioethics framework may be more useful to health policy makers in thinking about the extent to which patients with chronic, progressive illness should be responsible for the costs of their care.

Understanding the ethical dimensions of the chronic disease/end-of-life care spectrum requires acknowledging the immense role of cost in shaping the options that are available to individuals who are living with, and dying from, chronic and progressive illnesses. Taking seriously ill people seriously will require thinking about what our societies owe these citizens, not merely with respect to investments in high-intervention technologies, but with respect to our willingness to talk about what we want from health care, what we value when we are seriously ill, and what we hope will be in place for us and for our loved ones when we are dying.

References

Arno, P., Viola, D., and Gusmano, M. (2010). "The Caregiving Workforce in the United States," Presented at the London School of Economics, September 9.

Aziz, N. M. (2007). "Cancer Survivorship Research: State of Knowledge, Challenges, and Opportunities." *Acta Oncologica*, 46(4): 417–32.

Berenson, R.A., and Horvath, J. (2003). "Confronting the Barriers to Chronic Care Management in Medicare," *Health Affairs*, Web Exclusive: W3–37.

Berlinger, N., and Gusmano, M. (2010). "Cancer Chronicity: New Research and Policy Challenges," *Journal of Health Services Research and Policy*, 16(2): 121–3.

Berlinger, N., Jennings, B., and Wolf, S. M. (2013). "Institutional Discussion Guide on Resource Allocation and the Cost of Care," in *The Hastings Center Guidelines for Decisions on Life-Sustaining*

Morton College Library Cicero, ILL

Treatment and Care near the End of Life, Revised and Expanded 2nd Edition. Oxford and New York: Oxford University Press, 187–95.

Bodenheimer, T. et al. (2002). "Patient Self-Management of Chronic Disease in Primary Care." *JAMA*, 288(19): 2469–75.

Boodman, S. G. (2010). "Gaps in Insurance Policies Make Oral Drugs Too Pricey for Some Cancer Patients," *Kaiser Health News*, April 27, HE01.

Brickner, L. et al. (2004). "Barriers to Hospice Care and Referrals: Survey of Physicians' Knowledge, Attitudes, and Perceptions in a Health Maintenance Organization," *Journal of Palliative Medicine*, 7(3): 411–18.

Brown, L. (2003). "Comparing Health Systems in Four Countries: Lessons for the United States," *American Journal of Public Health*, 93(1): 52–6.

Democratic National Convention Committee. (2008). "The 2008 Democratic National Platform: Renewing America's Promise. As Approved by the 2008 Democratic National Convention," Monday, August 25, 2008, Denver, CO.

Finucane, T. E., Christmas, C., and Travis, K. (1999). "Tube Feeding in Patients with Advanced Dementia: A Review of the Evidence," *JAMA*, 282(14): 1365–70.

Fox, E. et al. (1999). "Evaluation of Prognostic Criteria for Determining Hospice Eligibility in Patients With Advanced Lung, Heart, or Liver Disease," *JAMA*, 282(17): 1638–45.

Ganzini, L. (2006). "Artificial Nutrition and Hydration at the End of Life: Ethics and Evidence," *Palliative and Supportive Care*, 4: 135–43.

Gillick, M. R. (2006). "The Use of Advance Care Planning to Guide Decisions about Artificial Nutrition and Hydration," *Nutrition in Clinical Practice*, 21(2): 126–33.

Gillick, M. R., and Volandes, A. E. (2008). "The Standard of Caring: Why Do We Still Use Feeding Tubes in Patients with Advanced Dementia?" *Journal of the American Medical Directors Association*, 9(5): 364–7.

Goodman, D. C. et al. (2010). "Quality of End-of-Life Cancer Care for Medicare Beneficiaries: Regional and Hospital-Specific Analyses," A Report of the Dartmouth Atlas Project. Lebanon, NH: Dartmouth Institute for Health Policy and Clinical Practice.

Gunda, S. et al. (2005). "National Survey of Palliative Care in End-Stage Renal Disease in the UK," *Nephrology Dialysis Transplantation*, 20(2): 392–5.

Gusmano, M. K. et al. (2010). *Health Care in World Cities: New York, Paris, and London*. Baltimore, MD: Johns Hopkins University Press.

Howlader, N., Noone, A. M., Krapcho, M. et al. (eds). *SEER Cancer Statistics Review, 1975–2010*, National Cancer Institute. Bethesda, MD, http://seer.cancer.gov/csr/1975_2010/, based on November 2012 SEER data submission, posted to the SEER website, April 2013. Last accessed May 14, 2013.

Hwang, W. et al. (2001), "Out-of-Pocket Medical Spending for Care of Chronic Conditions," *Health Affairs*, 20:267–78.

International Palliative Care Initiative Public Health Program. (2010). *Easing the Pain: Successes and Challenges in International Palliative Care*. New York: Open Society Foundations.

Klein, R. (1997). "Learning from Others: Shall the Last Be the First?" *Journal of Health Politics, Policy, and Law*, 22(5): 1267–78.

Meier, D. E., Lim, B., and Carlson, M. D. (2010). "Raising the Standard: Palliative Care in Nursing Homes," *Health Affairs*, 29(1): 136–40.

Mitchell, S. L. et al. (2007). "Hospice Care for Patients with Dementia," *Journal of Pain and Symptom Management*, 34(1): 7–16.

Morita, T. et al. (2005). "Late Referrals to Specialized Palliative Care Service in Japan," *Journal of Clinical Oncology*, 23(12): 2637–44.

Morita, T. et al. (2006). "Knowledge and Beliefs About End-of-Life Care," *Journal of Pain and Symptom Management*, 31(4): 306–16.

Murray, A. M. et al. (2006). "Use of Hospice in the United States Dialysis Population," *Clinical Journal of the American Society of Nephrology*, 1(6): 1248–55.

National Cancer Institute. (1999). "Learn About Clinical Trial," http://www.cancer.gov/clinicaltrials/learningabout/approval-process-for-cancer-drugs/page5 (accessed January 21, 2013).

Palecek, E. J. et al. (2010). "Comfort Feeding Only: A Proposal to Bring Clarity to Decision-Making Regarding Difficulty with Eating for Persons with Advanced Dementia," *Journal of the American Geriatrics Society*, 58(3): 580–4.

Pavalko, E. K. (1997). "Women's Caregiving and Paid Work: Causal Relationships in Late Midlife," *Journal of Gerontology Series B: Psychological Sciences and Social Sciences*, 52B(4): S170–9.

Rodwin, V. G. and Le Pen, C. (2005). "French Health Care Reform: The Birth of State-Led Managed Care," *New England Journal of Medicine*, 351(22): 2259–61.

Rodwin, V. G., and Gusmano, M. K. (2006). *Growing Older in World Cities: New York, London, Paris, and Tokyo*. Nashville, TN: Vanderbilt University Press.

Tangka, F. K. et al. (2010). "Cancer Treatment Cost in the United States: Has the Burden Shifted over Time?" *Cancer*, 116(14): 3477–84.

Temel, J. S. et al. (2010). "Early palliative care for patients with metastatic non-small-cell lung cancer". *New England Journal of Medicine*, 368(8): 733–42.

Teno, J. M. et al. (2009). "Churning: The Association between Health Care Transitions and Feeding Tube Insertion for Nursing Home Residents with Advanced Cognitive Impairment," *Journal of Palliative Medicine*, 12(4): 359–62.

Teno, J. M. et al. (2011). "Decision-Making and Outcomes of Feeding Tube Insertion: A Five-State Study," *Journal of the American Geriatrics Society*, 59(5): 881–6.

United Nations. (1948). *Universal Declaration of Human Rights*, http://www.un.org/en/documents/udhr/index.shtml (accessed January 3, 2011).

Vita, A. J. et al. (1998). "Aging, Health Risks, and Cumulative Disability," *New England Journal of Medicine*, 338: 1035–41.

Warshaw, G. (2006). "Introduction: Advances and Challenges in Care of Older People with Chronic Illness," *Generation*, 30(3): 5–10.

White, J. (1995). *Competing Solutions: American Health Care Proposals and International Experiences*. Washington, DC: Brookings Institution.

17.2

Commentary

End-of-Life Care in Korea: The Tradition of Filial Loyalty in the Area of High-Tech Medicine

Ilhak Lee

As Nancy Berlinger and Michael Gusmano note, providing treatment for patients suffering from chronic conditions is an important part of population health-care policy. I sympathize with their argument that policy initiatives should focus less on institutionalized health care, and more on home care or patient-friendly care. This would inevitably focus the burden of care on patient family members. As a patient's chronic condition progresses into a terminal one, "quality of death" becomes an important issue, not only for patients and their families, but for policy makers as well. The long and lonely last days of one's life usually lack proper care. This lack of concern for the quality of death arises from many causes, including policy unpreparedness, provider indifference, and public silence on end-of-life issues.

It is time to shift our focus from biomedicine to human aspects of caring. From a policy perspective, this means that health policy limited to health-care reimbursement is no longer an effective means to address the current situation. Instead, the focus should be on more general welfare issues. Specifically, an understanding of the beliefs and attitudes required for fulfilling familial responsibilities is urgently required. I attempt here to demonstrate an ideal policy initiative required to achieve this goal. In some societies, where the responsibility of caring for dying patients rests on family members, the care burden becomes unbearably heavy, especially when combined with policy unpreparedness. Here, I hope to highlight the importance of understanding the cultural and social contexts that surround end-of-life care. In particular, I hope to demonstrate that policy should allow a more diverse delivery of health care and encourage family- and home-based care. Finally, increasing the role of the patient's family must be accompanied by a consideration of the economic aspects of caring for a dying family member, or for others in chronic conditions.

I

Korea is currently experiencing problems with patient care similar to those described by Berlinger and Gusmano. Specifically, health care is provided primarily at acute hospitals, palliative care is difficult to access and does not meet patient needs properly, and there is a lack of consensus regarding the scope and limits for families caring for patients. In addition, multiple issues exist regarding health-care decision-making.

While the cost of end-of-life care, especially expenses for the last three months of life, represents nearly half of all medical expenses required for cancer patient care, care provided in the intensive care unit (ICU) and cutting-edge technologies cannot alone meet the needs of terminal cancer patients. Palliative care requirements are not being fulfilled: dying patients must currently choose between a cure-oriented, high-tech medical approach, the scope of which is limited to biological aspects, and which may involve dying a miserable death on the ICU bed connected to lines and machines; or dying outside the health-care delivery system, being ignored entirely. Neither of these scenarios is acceptable, as patients' needs are not fulfilled and their dignity is overlooked. As more people come to understand that ICU care cannot be the best type of care, a movement has arisen among the older generations, entitled "writing advance directives campaign (from overtaken by death to inviting death)." Adherents to this movement refuse to accept the idea of being tied to a machine until death, and wish to clarify that what they want is not ineffective life-sustaining treatment, but the ability to die in more familiar places such as home. Unfortunately, home-care services are difficult to access and have not been proven effective at this point.

A survey conducted in 2010 showed interesting differences in attitudes towards the death of one's parents versus one's own death. Almost half of respondents (46 percent) listed home as their preferred place of death, yet fewer respondents (36 percent) chose home for the preferred place of death for family members (10 percent chose hospitals) (Park 2011). Let us consider some reasons for this discrepancy.

First, elderly people do not want to be a burden after they are gone, and this may explain why so many die in hospital. It is possible that people value their family interests over their own comfort. For example, in Korea, funeral services are provided by hospital-affiliated facilities. Thus, if a patient dies in a hospital, the funeral service can be provided in a seamless manner by the professional funeral service. The fact that most of the urban population lives in apartments adds to the difficulties of arranging a funeral from home, since it is awkward and unpleasant to move corpses or coffins in and out of the home. On the other hand, economic factors might lead people to choose home as their own preferred place to die. People may prefer that family members remain in the hospital so that they receive the best (albeit expensive) curative treatments; while for themselves, they may prefer to die at home so that they avoid spending money on treatment. In reality, they may be passing up potentially beneficial medical treatment so that they do not become a burden to their children. That they are often not kept informed of their medical condition exacerbates this tendency to succumb to death early by forgoing treatment.

As is the case in other Asian countries, many patients in Korea are not given basic information about their disease. Instead, family members, most often the eldest son of the patient, make medical decisions and are responsible for hospital charges not covered by insurance (50 percent of net expenses). Koreans consider care for older parents as offspring responsibility, which is understood as filial loyalty (ko, hyo, or xiāo). Worldwide, it is seen as quite natural for children to love and care for their aging parents; but in Korea, caring for parents is considered the most fundamental duty of a human being

(Confucius, The Analects, 1:2,6,11; 2:5,7; 4:18.19. 21). In fact, people are evaluated by their attitude towards parents, as filial loyalty is fundamental to all ethics. Ignoring this duty is equal to committing a serious sin and one becomes an object of social blame and scrutiny. There is an old saying, "Serve your parents with everything: it would be of no use to mourn after they passed away." This cultural belief therefore supports the idea that a good child would be willing to cut off their finger so that the dying parent might swallow the blood and be revived by the sacrifice as well as the vitality of blood.

As such, offspring feel that it is their duty to keep a parent alive and provide every possible curative care, regardless of the likelihood of recovery. Even in cases where parents explicitly refuse aggressive medical care, children feel (or are expected to feel) guilty if they give up on providing every possible medical treatment. In modern Korea, offspring will sacrifice their jobs, houses, and savings to pay hospital expenses in order to allow their parents to remain in hospital longer. Understandably, because children seek and accept every measure available, the economic burden is huge.

What becomes of these sacrifices? Many patients spend their last days in the ICU attached to ventilators. However, in the end, there can be no "loyal children after years of caring for a sick parent," and children are forced to terminate treatments for which they are unable to pay (Dae 2008: 524–9). Conservative bioethicists argue that economic concerns should be excluded from the medical decision-making process, and support the notion that giving up aggressive medical treatment is a criminal offense (Kim 2005: 213–29).

As a result, decisions are not made by the patient or for the good of the patient. Instead, they are made according to old and outdated traditions and economic concerns. In other words, in their last days, the patient disappears from the decision-making process.

2

Two features characterize Korean health-care delivery: universal (but not full) health insurance coverage and dominance of Western medicine. When combined, these two features yield neglect for dying patients. Universal health insurance is certainly a great achievement, but the resulting bureaucracy that ends up determining what is included in and excluded from care is not. Moreover, this bureaucracy results in negligence when scientific, cure-oriented biomedicine is offered to chronically ill patients.

Some policy issues exist that prevent health-care providers from seeking alternatives to aggressive care. Currently, Korea's NHI program is facing financial difficulties. As Korean society has become more aged and the government has tried to provide health care to more citizens, the NHI budget has suffered and more loss is expected if the current situation (fewer premium policies and aging of society) continues. Under current circumstances, introduction of more care categories into the NHI is difficult, if not impossible.

It is clear that this problem could arise if hospice/palliative care is introduced for cancer patients. Currently, hospice/palliative care is not recognized as a legitimate care category in the NHI system. The first-phase trial to introduce palliative care was carried out in 2009–10, but the cost was not fully covered by the NHI, so many institutes are doubtful that successful introduction of palliative care could occur in Korea. Home nursing care for cancer patients has been practiced for nearly a decade, but only for reasons of scholarly interest; it is not widespread. This lack of palliative care for cancer patients means that most of them receive cure-oriented medical services until these services can no longer be offered. In some cases, anti-cancer treatments are provided until a few days before the patient dies (Ko 2009). A survey has shown that many cancer patients receive aggressive medical care including invasive life-sustaining treatments. Notably, these are paid for by the patient, as they are not covered by NHI.

This case study of Korean belief and culture shows that caring for dying patients reflects a cultural background that does not easily adapt to changing technology and medical knowledge. While concern for the dying is justifiable within Korean tradition, Koreans adhere unquestioningly to the tradition. As a result, a successful policy must take into account cultural change. In the case of Korea, medical professionals are the group that should be targeted for change, and they in particular must prepare to care for the ill outside hospital walls. A model is required which guarantees quality care and financial sustainability. While not impossible, achieving these changes will likely require a great deal of time.

References

Confucius. The Analects, 1: 2, 6, 11; 2: 5, 7; 4: 18, 19, 21.

Dae, S. H. (2008). "End-of-Life Decision in Korea," *Journal of the Korean Medical Association*, 51(6): 524–9 (in Korean).

Kim, K. (2005). "The Medico-Legal and Ethical Problems of Withholding/Withdrawing of Futile Life-Sustaining Mechanical Respirator Treatment," *Tuberculosis and Respiratory Diseases*, 58(3): 213–29 (in Korean).

Ko, Y. (2009). "Proposal for Social Agreement on Foregoing Useless Life-sustaining-treatment," National Evidence-Based Health Care Collaborating Agency. Proposal for Social Agreement on Foregoing Useless Life-Sustaining-Treatment. Seoul (in Korean).

Park, J. Y. (2011). "Home Health Care Services for Terminally Ill Patients and Dying at Home," Ph.D. thesis (Yonsei University).

17.3

Commentary
Chronic Disease and Mental Care

Yukihiro Nobuhara

Living with a chronic disease such as cancer or heart disease requires enduring some form of pain, and thus patients with chronic diseases require proper pain treatment. Berlinger and Gusmano note various uses of the term "chronicity" and clarify how a chronic disease differs from an acute one. They also suggest that unique treatment is necessary for chronic diseases, and that professionals are required to administer this. The present commentary will review their considerations and argue that chronic diseases require various types of mental care, and that professionals who can provide comprehensive treatment including mental care for patients with chronic diseases are needed.

Cure and care

By examining various uses of "chronicity," Berlinger and Gusmano discern one central feature of chronic diseases: they are not curable but treatable. Here I focus on this perspective in order to consider the uniqueness of chronic diseases.

Disease can be roughly defined as the state of losing health. We can say that the goal of treating a disease is, first of all, to recover the state of health from its state of loss. However, not every disease is treatable in this sense. In some diseases, the healthy state cannot be recovered by means of current medicine. Moreover, some diseases exist for which the healthy state cannot be recovered even by means of advanced medicine in the future. However, this does not mean that such diseases cannot be treated in any sense. Some treatments can decelerate disease progression or palliate pain that accompanies the disease.

In the following commentary, I refer to a treatment that restores the state of health as a "cure" and all other treatments as "care." By these definitions, diseases are not necessarily curable, but care can still be provided. Once this distinction is made, we can establish a category of long-term diseases which are not curable but amenable to care. I define chronic disease as one such disease. If I am not mistaken, it roughly corresponds to the sort of chronic disease which Berlinger and Gusmano think is not sufficiently treated under the current medical system.

Thus defined, chronic disease is not curable. However, the curability of a disease is not always obvious. In some cases, doctors have no clear idea of whether a patient will make a complete recovery from these diseases or not. In these cases, doctors can only guess about the curability. If the disease is considered curable, a cure will be attempted; if not, care will be provided. As such, some diseases for which care is provided may, in fact, be curable, i.e. they may not be truly chronic.

Some treatments seem to cure but in reality do not always do so. For example, patients with diabetes may recover and maintain their health through medication, in which case their bodily state is no different from the healthy state. However, this is achieved through medication, and the patient cannot maintain this healthy state without it. Technically speaking, a healthy state is one that can be maintained without the help of medicine. Thus, maintaining a healthy state through continuous medication does not represent the recovery of health, and therefore is not a cure.

Mental care

Patients with chronic diseases require various types of special care because they are afflicted by long-term incurable diseases. In particular, they require mental care given the uniqueness of chronic disease.

As Berlinger and Gusmano note, it is important to palliate bodily pain if it accompanies chronic disease. Palliating pain may lead to neither a cure of disease nor the delay of its progression. Nevertheless it is critical for one's quality of life. Living with pain is difficult, and pain can deter one from achieving goals. Enduring pain which accompanies a disease contributes no meaning in life, so if at all possible, pain should be palliated. Even if pain palliation reduces one's lifespan, it is still better to choose it, as long as the outcome adds to the total value of life. It is difficult to assess the total value of life, but lifespan is not always the most valuable outcome measure.

It is important to provide appropriate advice and encouragement so that patients can self-manage their chronic disease if necessary. For example, patients with diabetes often maintain their health through regular medication and dieting. However, daily administration of medication is not easy, and dieting even more so, as the temptations to eat and drink are strong. Treatment of diabetes, a lifestyle-related disease, requires a change in patients' lifestyle. It is nearly impossible for patients to go on a complete diet on their own accord without an extraordinarily strong will.

Successful treatment of diabetes, therefore, requires not only strong self-management skills, but also mental support from physicians. Physicians must carefully instill fear into patients who might easily succumb to the temptation to eat sweets by reminding them of the dreadful complications of diabetes, or by reprimanding them for losing self-control. They must also praise patients who are maintaining the necessary diet. This type of mental support does little more than complement self-management, but is indispensable when it comes to empowering patients to self-manage their health.

At some points, patients may lose focus on the meaning of life or lose hope for the future. If this happens, they must be assisted in identifying or establishing a new meaning in life, as their chronic diseases are not curable. Patients with incurable cancer may have to endure painful treatments or live an inactive life, even if their life is extended by treatment. This may lead them to disregard reasons for living which they held when healthy, and they may need to find new reasons for living their life with cancer. However, this is not trivial, and some patients choose to end their lives because they cannot find a new reason. They require mental support through this critical process.

Of course, the risk of losing one's reason to live is not restricted to those with chronic disease. Patients who have little time to live due to a serious disease or who have lost a limb in an accident are at a higher risk for this. Consider the case of a young, healthy person who cannot identify the meaning of his or her life when they are told that they have only a few months to live due to the onset of a sudden heart disease. Excellent athletes would also find it extremely difficult to hold to the same reasons for living if they lost a limb in an accident. Compared to these cases, those with chronic disease are less likely to lose the meaning of life. Still, there remains a risk, and thus we must assist patients with chronic diseases as they reconstruct their meaning of life.

Professionals for chronic disease care

One important question posed by Berlinger and Gusmano is whether professionals who treat chronic disease should also treat pain and symptoms accompanying it or whether there should be specialists who exclusively treat pain and symptoms. According to them, it depends on the circumstances. In my opinion, professionals who treat chronic disease must also treat pain and symptoms. That is, there should be professionals who provide comprehensive care for patients with chronic disease. This care could be divided into bodily care and mental care. Patients with chronic disease could receive better care if the same physicians are providing both bodily and mental care, compared to a scenario in which different physicians provide such care separately.

While bodily care and mental care for patients with chronic disease differ, they are also closely related. The pain and moods experienced by patients with chronic cancer depend on whether their treatment involves radiation or anticancer agents. In addition, the different pains and moods can influence the patient's will to live. Thus, the nature of bodily care can often dictate the necessary mental care. At the same time, the bodily care provided often depends on the mental care. Physicians can administer bodily care which may cause excruciating pain if mental care to help patients endure the pain is available. Thus, a comprehensive consideration of bodily and mental care is necessary to determine the best possible treatment for each patient. Once this has been determined, one and the same physician should be responsible for administering both bodily and mental care.

Physicians who care for patients with chronic disease should provide mental care beyond bodily care, the latter of which is medical care in the narrow sense of the word. Mental care for patients with chronic disease may not currently be considered part of the physician's job description for those who provide bodily care, but it should be. However, for this to be successful, physicians who care for patients with chronic disease must have extensive knowledge and multifaceted abilities. They will require not only medical knowledge and skills, but also a well rounded knowledge of psychology and the human mind and the philosophical ability to consider the meaning of life. They do not need a stereotypical view of psychology and human values, but rather a flexible view of these, enabling them to make comprehensive assessments of patients, depending on their conditions.

As Berlinger and Gusmano point out, care for patients with chronic disease also requires cost consciousness. It is impossible to choose the best bodily care unless the cost for each possible care is considered. Patients themselves may choose a certain course, but it is the physician's duty to provide them with materials for deliberation. Physicians themselves should know the cost of each bodily treatment and be able to weigh these against other factors for deliberation.

In sum, physicians who treat chronic disease must be well-versed in the humanities and have a sense of economy in addition to their medical knowledge and abilities.

17.4

Commentary
Navigating the Twilight Zone

Michael Dunn

Introduction

Issues raised by the care and treatment of chronic diseases currently languish in the backwaters of biomedical ethical discourse. Slow, progressive decline heralds none of the bells and whistles of life-and-death decision-making or radical technological advancement that has proven to be so seductive to contemporary bioethicists. Nevertheless, there is an extensive body of evidence showing how chronic diseases are posing, and will continue to pose, significant political and practical challenges to public service infrastructures within both developed and developing nations that are already straining under economic and demographic pressures. It is to their credit, then, that Berlinger and Gusmano interrogate the ethical question of how health-care organizations—and society more generally—ought to respond to the challenges of chronic disease.

For Berlinger and Gusmano, identifying the obligations that exist in relation to those living with chronic health conditions depends, first, on being clear about what is meant when the concept of "chronicity" is invoked, and, second, on determining how different ways of conceptualizing chronicity establish different normative pathways for ascribing responsibility in the treatment and care of chronic diseases. In this commentary it is argued that, however chronicity is defined, and whatever chronic condition is being described, chronic disease can be distinguished from other health conditions on the differential—and morally significant—kinds of impact that they have on individuals' everyday lives. The claim is made, on the basis of this argument, that Berlinger and Gusmano's directions for reforms in both policy and practice relating to the management of chronic disease point us in the right kinds of directions, but do not go far enough.

Conceptualizing chronic disease

Contemporary arrangements in chronic disease care are complex and multifaceted. The management of long-term progressive health conditions straddles an ever-widening void between acute and end-of-life health care that incorporates multiple institutional arrangements, geographical locations, and professional and nonprofessional actors. This picture is perhaps even less clear in the UK, where, despite the proliferation of primary health care, the historical divide between the provision of "health care" and "social care" functions in practice to exacerbate this dynamic further.

Even more problematically, however, Berlinger and Gusmano show how this gap in service provision is not only difficult to map, but also challenging to navigate. This, they argue, is because different ways of conceiving of chronicity lead to problematic inconsistencies within clinical encounters, and broader difficulties in the development of consistent and defensible policy responses. Determining whether chronic disease ought to be understood as being i) curable, treatable, or manageable, ii) progressive or stable, iii) clinical or sub-acute, and iv) pathological or experiential have important implications for making ethical judgments about clinical responsibility within (and beyond) health-care institutions, and decision-making in the context of the practitioner–patient relationship.

Making judgments, for example, about eligibility for pain medication, or about policies for the development of hospital- and community-based palliative care services, hinges on recognizing that "chronic disease is also a progressive disease with a terminal prognosis" is linked inexorably with the values and priorities of end-of-life care. Judgments about the provision of information required for valid consent in a temporally extended chain of decision-making will depend on whether defining a disease as chronic precludes it being understood as curable.

Whilst Berlinger and Gusmano do not explicitly endorse one or more of the ways of conceptualizing chronicity that they consider, they conclude by giving primacy to patients' narratives of how they experience their illnesses as chronic. Such stories of patients' illnesses are understood in terms of the account of suffering and symptom management contained within them, and their situatedness in a range of institutional and noninstitutional environments. It is from these kinds of accounts that Berlinger and Gusmano ground their claims about the need for a palliative care revolution across health- and personal-care contexts, and patient-centered policies that are responsive to the experiential burden of identified personal, economic, and social difficulties.

Chronicity and disability

One way of making sense of chronicity not entertained by Berlinger and Gusmano is to understand chronicity as disability. Or, to put it another way, that to have a chronic disease is conceptually equivalent to being described as having a disability. Whilst the concept of disability is itself contested, with its descriptive and evaluative meaning open to different interpretations (Dunn 2011), this interpretation would, I believe, require an account of chronic disease to be situated primarily in terms of its effect on the functioning of individuals' everyday lives.

At least for the argument here, it matters little if this effect is fleshed out in terms of the objective statistical deviation from "normal" species functioning, in terms of the negative impact on well-being, or in terms of a phenomenological account of the challenges of a life lived with impairment. What is important, however, is to differenti-ate the disabling impact of chronic diseases from the effects of other non-chronic health conditions.

This difference lies in the ways that chronic diseases *transform* rather than *disrupt* the ways that individuals function in the world. The impact of chronic diseases is not transi-tory; chronic diseases have long-term effects that become inscribed onto individuals' bodies, and into their everyday lives. In contrast to acute conditions, chronic condi-tions centre broader metaphysical questions about, for example, embodiment and per-sonhood, rather than evidence-based pathways for "good" models of treatment or the narrow application of clinicians' ethical principles. This understanding certainly seems to be borne out of the illness narratives brought to our attention by Berlinger and Gusmano. Whilst Berlinger and Gusmano make sense of these narratives of individuals' experiences of living with HIV/AIDS or cancer in terms of a health-orientated empha-sis on pain relief and suffering, I believe that they are more appropriately interpreted as powerful and emotive stories of a broader metamorphosis that accompanies the transi-tion to a life lived with chronic ill health.

What follows normatively from such an account? Again, numerous arguments could be made. It could be concluded that the normative force of the obligation to act in response to such transformations lies in the value of increasing individuals' pleasurable experiences, or in the value of enabling individuals to flourish by having certain mini-mum capabilities to pursue real opportunities in the world based on personal and social circumstances. Reasoning about specific obligations will need to take place in the prac-tical settings in which chronic disease is managed; the task here, in contrast, is to make sense of the meaning of chronic disease itself, and the broad philosophical and ethical implications that follow from this. In relation to the discourses of chronicity discussed by Berlinger and Gusmano, understanding chronicity as disability would require any definition of chronic disease to be anchored in the realities of the transformations that it brings about in a person's everyday life. This definition would need to be sensitive to the multiple webs of support that constitute an individual's interconnectedness with other individuals, rather than clinical disagreements over stability and progressiveness that lie at the heart of current policy debates. Responding to this understanding of chronic-ity as disability will, as is now discussed, require nothing less than a new kind of ethical framework for thinking about values and obligations in the context of the lived realities of long-term chronic conditions.

Taking seriously ill people seriously

Berlinger and Gusmano draw attention to two general considerations for the develop-ment of ethically defensible policy and practice in the management of chronic disease. These considerations are how we can best respond seriously to the health-care chal-lenges facing seriously ill people, and are derived—at least in part—from their claim that chronicity can be best understood in terms of patients' narratives of living with chronic ill health. Their first consideration is to focus on the relief of suffering by advo-cating a palliative care revolution across different care contexts, and the second is to address a range of social, institutional, political, and economic biases against the prior-itization of chronic disease-related concerns. Whilst these considerations are important, I believe that understanding these diseases in terms of their disabling effects on indi-viduals' everyday life experiences requires us to recognize the need for a broader and more ambitious response.

Extending ethical practice and the practice of ethics

The interpretation of suffering and pain management issues in Berlinger and Gusmano's analysis of patients' narratives of chronic ill health leads to them arguing for the exten-sion of palliative care services from hospice settings into acute and community-based health-care services. They wield an abundance of evidence in support of this exten-sion, and their claim is hard to disagree with. Individuals living with chronic condi-tions would clearly benefit from the management of symptoms that often fall outside or between particular medical specialties, and, therefore, involve a failure to meet these individuals' medical needs.

Although this argument is convincing, because patients' narratives about living with chronic diseases are not best interpreted solely in terms of medical need and symptom management, the implications for policy and practice that follow from these narra-tives is greater than meeting medical needs and managing symptoms effectively. Thus, rather than focusing on improving ethical decision-making around pain within clini-cal settings, I contend that the priority must lie in extending our understanding of the ethical dimensions of living with chronic disease, and to approach any ethical issues that arise from a broader nonclinical perspective. As Berlinger and Gusmano themselves recognize, the legal and philosophical tools that clinical ethics relies on to address moral dilemmas in medicine may not be suitable for those working within a chronic-disease paradigm. Crucially, extending ethical practice outside the clinic will require ethical frameworks to be tailored to the multiple realities of the transformations that define everyday life with chronic ill health. It must not simply be about bringing clinical eth-ics to the masses. Herein, therefore, lies the danger of prioritizing the obligation to relieve suffering, rather than seeing this obligation as a component part of a broader ethical framework applicable across institutional and non-institutional care and support environments.

The challenge then is how ethics can be extended out of health-care institutions in ways that do not simply involve, for example, imposing medical ethical principles onto nonmedical considerations that involve different kinds of value judgments about how individuals ought to be supported in pursuing the good life. This challenge will be a considerable one, not least because the conception of the good in personal and social support remains, in contrast to medical care, under-theorized. If we were to understand this value broadly in terms of individuals' long-term well-being, enacting the obligation to assist these individuals to adapt to the transformations in their everyday functioning will be more akin to experiments in living, than identifying optimal treatments. When it is reasonable to conclude that ethical principles do overlap between health care and other contexts in which personal support is provided, extending the practice of ethics into these non-institutional contexts will require this ethical decision-making to be responsive to care philosophies with different kinds of social, political, and philosophical heritages. An example from the UK is contemporary policy and practice in social care where the value of autonomy is interpreted in terms of the goals of facilitating independent living, personalization, and financial control over a support package, rather than in terms of procedural requirements around information provision and the assessment of competence (Department of Health 2010).

A partnership approach endorsed by Berlinger and Gusmano seems to hold the most promise here. Indeed, partnership services are already being rolled out in the UK, where health-care services for complex conditions that give rise to different kinds of needs, such as dementia or intellectual disabilities, are integrated with local authority services responsible for the provision of personal and social support. (Department of Health 1998; 1999) The resulting partnership arrangements involve, for example, psychiatrists working alongside housing officers, and community nurses working alongside occupational therapists. The extension of these services to the care of other chronic diseases ought to be prioritized, as should the further step to develop ethics support that is tailored carefully to these partnership services. New initiatives in this direction, such as the Community Ethics Network (http://www.communityethicsnetwork.ca) are gaining momentum, but are currently limited in scope.

Aligning ethical considerations with sociopolitical considerations

Within Berlinger and Gusmano's second consideration is the compelling claim that responding to the increasing pressures that chronic disease are exerting on public services requires ethicists working in chronic-care settings to focus on questions of resource allocation and social justice. Indeed, the requirement to align ethical questions with political-philosophical questions is brought into even sharper focus when chronic disease is understood in terms of the transformative and disabling effects that it has on individuals' functioning in their everyday lives.

Whilst public debate about the challenges that chronic disease poses to questions of distributive justice, economic productivity, and intergenerational fairness must be encouraged, these challenges will need to become integrated into the questions that arise on a daily basis at the front line of providing care and support to people with chronic diseases. As Berlinger and Gusmano recognize, this will require practice, and models of ethics support and education in practice, to become increasingly orientated towards questions debated at length in political philosophy, public health, and human rights scholarship.

This move will be particularly difficult because making correct judgments about the nature and scope of the obligation to respond to the different ways in which chronic disease disables an individual's daily functioning will require carefully elucidated evaluative judgments to be made. Then, when the nature and scope of the obligation to respond are clarified, decisions about allocating resources will require a robust framework within which this support can be balanced against parallel support arrangements built upon the same values (e.g. the provision of welfare payments to homeless or unemployed individuals, or the long-term care provided to people with profound intellectual impairment). These kinds of support will also need to be balanced against care and treatment built upon different kinds of values (e.g. the value in curing a life-threatening acute condition).

Ultimately, it matters little whether such decisions need to be made within public or private health and personal-care systems. Whilst the challenge might be even greater—and an adequate conclusion will be less likely to be reached—in a marketplace where profit making and efficiency are competing imperatives, the ethical questions will be the same. Established theoretical approaches for resource allocation that focus on, for example, cost effectiveness, need, or the "rule of rescue" will need to be developed around the different ways within which needs, effectiveness, or rescue can be conceptualized and measured correctly given the different support arrangements that are being compared. This is an issue that extends to all personal and social support settings, and is not limited solely to the context of managing chronic disease.

References

Department of Health (1998). *Partnership in Action: New opportunities for Joint Working between Health and Social Services—A discussion document*. London: Stationery Office.

Department of Health (1999). *National Service Framework for Mental Health*. London: Stationery Office.

Department of Health (2010). *A Vision for Adult Social Care: Capable Communities and Active Citizens*. London: Stationery office.

Dunn, M. (2011). "Discourses of Disability and Clinical Ethics Support," *Clinical Ethics*, 6(1): 32–8.

17.5

Response to Commentaries

Nancy Berlinger and Michael K. Gusmano

In our chapter, "Taking Seriously Ill People Seriously: Ethics and Policy Dimensions of the Chronic Disease/End-of-Life Care Continuum," we describe the various ways in which a person can be chronically ill, and argue that efforts to improve care for persons who are living with one or more chronic health conditions should start from a framework for thinking about ethical challenges arising in the chronic-care context. These challenges may overlap with "bedside" dilemmas involving patients near the end of life, and may also arise outside the acute-care setting and the end-of-life context. The scope of chronic illness, and of the chronic disease/end-of-life care continuum, is vast, and different health-care systems may reflect different values about how best to offer good care to persons who are living with (and often self-managing) different chronic illnesses. Chronic illness is about the experiences of the person living with chronic illness and about populations affected by different chronic conditions. It is also about how a society, through its health financing and other policies, expresses its support for these experiences—or else turns away from its chronically ill members. Our three commentators offered perspectives that included insights from South Korea, Japan, and the United Kingdom, and that focus on different aspects of our topic and arguments.

Dr. Ilhak Lee of the Bioethics Policy Research Center at Yonsei University in Seoul, South Korea, focuses on the "end-of-life" part of the continuum, and on the care of older patients with diseases that are both chronic and progressive, with a terminal prognosis. Dr. Lee describes the ethical uncertainty created when the cultural value often expressed in English as "filial piety" and characterized as a Confucian (or generically "Asian") virtue ethic expressed through the care of one's parents is interpreted in the context of progressive illness *as if* it meant: ICU care is the "best" care and is therefore consistent with the duty of filial piety owed to one's parents. As Dr. Lee points out, "ICU care cannot be the best type of care" when a patient's potential to benefit from intensive interventions is limited to narrow "biological" measures while the patient is "dying a miserable death on the ICU bed" (Lee in this chapter). The situation Dr. Lee describes does not comport with any ethically defensible notion of "the best" way to care for a person who is ill; in fact, this course of action could result in needless harm. And yet, this situation occurs frequently and is not limited to Asia or uniquely associated with the concept of filial piety. Clinicians in the United States also describe and write about families (and also, sometimes, patients) who want to start or continue intensive interventions that cannot change the patient's prognosis, have little or no potential for benefit, and are experienced by most patients as burdensome.

The ICU is a life-saving or life-sustaining setting for some patients. What is hazardous is making the ICU—or any treatment or technology in isolation—stand in for the good, and then using access to the ICU, or to ever more intensive interventions, to stand in for informed decision-making and family caregiving. And yet, as Dr. Lee makes clear, this can happen so easily, especially when no acceptable alternative presents itself through the health-care system. In Korea, for example, it is difficult for terminally ill patients to obtain hospice or palliative care services, while it is easy to arrange a funeral through a hospital. This structure supports a perception that the ICU is the proper place to die and makes it difficult to imagine, let alone try to arrange, another end-of-life setting for one's elders. It also, as Dr. Lee suggests, imposes terrible pressures on patients and their adult children:

Even [when] parents explicitly refuse aggressive medical care, children feel (or are expected to feel) guilty if they give up on providing every possible medical treatment. In modern Korea, offspring will sacrifice their jobs, houses, and savings to pay hospital expenses in order to allow their parents to remain in hospital longer...What becomes of these sacrifices? Many patients spend their last days in the ICU attached to ventilators...and children are forced to terminate treatments for which they are unable to pay. (Lee in this chapter)

Here is the basic problem again, in stark and startling detail. When the care of the sick or the dying is reduced to the consumption of treatment (without attention to what the patient wants, can benefit from, or be harmed by), devotion is reduced to payment for treatment, and money is the decision-maker. And yet, adult children either "feel" or "are expected to feel" as if they are doing wrong by their parents if they question this way of thinking and acting. Implicit in Dr. Lee's account is a question: What can bioethics do for the patient and family caught in this situation, experiencing these pressures? Because bioethics in the clinical setting addresses itself primarily to the clinician, it should aim to draw clinicians' attention to what Dr. Lee calls "the unexamined tradition" affecting patients and families every day, as well as offering clinicians new models for thinking about and organizing good care for dying people and their families.

Every culture has its "unexamined tradition." By describing how Korean families may interpret their tradition in the ICU setting and by encouraging health-care professionals to be prepared to challenge this tradition in the interests of their patients who may wish to spend their remaining days in a different way, Dr. Lee adds an additional cross-cultural dimension to our discussion.

Prof. Yukihiro Nobuhara of the University of Tokyo focuses on the psychological impact of living with chronic illness and on the need for physicians who care for chronically ill patients to be adequately prepared to recognize and support patients as they cope with the meaning of illness that is not curable and with the medical management of this illness. We may dispute Prof. Nobuhara's suggestion that a chronically ill person is "less likely" than a person with a sudden-onset disability or late-stage terminal diagnosis to lose a sense of life's meaning. These two contrasting examples are significantly different from each other, and the psychological impact of different chronic illnesses also differs, making generalizations difficult and perhaps unnecessary. We agree, however, with the conclusion, that physicians who care for patients who live with chronic illness should be attentive to patients' psychological needs, should know how to present treatment decisions, and should recognize cost as an ethical issue that requires physicians to have accurate knowledge of the costs of treatment options.

Dr. Michael Dunn of The Ethox Centre at the University of Oxford focuses on the values question implicit in the title of our chapter: what does it mean to take seriously ill people seriously? Dr. Dunn's proposal that one way to accomplish this would be "to understand chronicity as disability" is intriguing. We certainly agree with him that looking at chronicity from a perspective informed by the experiences of people living with chronic illness is essential. His suggestion that chronic illness is transformative of how a person functions, while acute illness (which may be part of chronic illness) is disruptive of how a person functions, seems a helpful way to capture how the accommodation of chronic illness shapes everyday life. However, we do not think his "chronicity as disability" proposal quite works. While it may be accurate to say that a chronic illness is a disability in some way, or becomes one at some point (for example, the point at which a chronically ill person reaches the threshold for a certain disability entitlement), the experience of chronicity may or may not be like the experience of disability. Some of this concerns how a person identifies himself or herself or is socialized by a diagnosis. A person with advanced breast cancer may, reasonably, identify more with this specific diagnosis—with how her life has been disrupted and is being transformed by this diagnosis—than with "cancer" in general, or with a still broader category such as "disability." "Disability" can carry specific connotations or even stigma in different societies, and this may make it difficult for persons with chronic illness to self-identify with "disability" as a social group to which they belong. Also, while some disabling conditions are not diseases, and some disabilities are caused by relatively stable or slowly progressing conditions that affect function gradually, chronic illness includes a range of conditions that, if not closely medically managed, will become life threatening or severely impairing. To point this out is not to draw a sharp distinction between "chronicity" and "disability"— we think that there is considerable overlap here—but is a reminder that some chronic diseases are diagnosed as life-threatening diseases (and may yet become life threatening if attempts at medical management fail). The person diagnosed with advanced breast cancer has immediate, ongoing, and specific medical needs that *must* be addressed if she is to have a chance to *live with* cancer as a chronic illness. To acknowledge that this is her reality does not reduce the lived experience of chronicity, including its psychological and social dimensions, to "medical need and symptom management." Another British sociologist, Dr. Tom Shakespeare, suggests a way to bridge the concepts of "chronicity" and "disability" that avoids the dichotomy (and polarizing politics) of a "medical" versus a "social" model (Shakespeare 2006: 62–5). Shakespeare argues that bodily impairment is more complex than the social model, which views impairment as problematic only insofar as a differently abled person experiences externally imposed barriers to full participation in society, suggests. He proposes thinking about impairment as a "predicament," explaining that "[t]o call something a predicament is to understand it as a difficulty, and as a challenge, and as something we might want to minimize but which we cannot ultimately avoid" (Shakespeare 2006: 63). Dr. Shakespeare's proposal seems to be a potentially productive way to think about the experience of living with some chronic illnesses, including the experience of relying on medical professionals and other professional caregivers to help one "self-manage" chronic illness. As Dr. Dunn recognizes, it is a lot of work to live with chronic illness, including those illnesses that are life threatening and those that are relatively stable, and we agree with his assertion that "the conception of the good in personal and social support [for chronically ill persons and their caregivers] remains, in contrast to medical care, under-theorized" in bioethics and related health policy (Dunn in this chapter).

References

Dunn, M. (2014). "Navigating the Twilight Zone," in A. Akabayashi (ed.), *The Future of Bioethics: International Dialogues*. Oxford: Oxford University Press, 618–23.

Lee, I. (2014). "End-of-Life Care in Korea: The Tradition of Filial Loyalty in the Area of High-Tech Medicine," in A. Akabayashi (ed.), *The Future of Bioethics: International Dialogues*. Oxford: Oxford University Press, 610–13.

Shakespeare, T. (2006). *Disability Rights and Wrongs*. Abingdon: Routledge.

18.1

Primary Topic Article
Ethics in Long-Term Care Practice: A Global Call to Arms

Tony Hope and Michael Dunn

Introduction

This chapter examines the practical ethical issues that arise in long-term care settings. Our attention focuses predominantly on the care provided to people with dementia, a condition which is expected to present a major challenge to countries around the world over the next few decades. By providing specific examples, we show how the bulk of problematic ethical issues arise in the context of day-to-day care practices, and consider how these issues become even more problematic when recent developments in transnational migration for the purposes of providing and receiving long-term care are taken into account. We argue, first, that that these ethical issues need to be addressed in ways that can command broad agreement across different cultures and, second, that whilst contemporary approaches to identify universal principles ought to be part of this process, these principles alone will be insufficient to foster ethical practice. Our claim is that there need to be processes at both the macro and micro levels that can facilitate discussion around, and enable the resolution of, context-specific ethical challenges. Such processes will require international collaboration between academics, policymakers and care providers, and will involve new interventions in practical settings.

1 Long-term care: a global challenge

An ageing population and improvements in the quality of health care are predicted to pose major demographic challenges to all parts of the world in the twenty-first century. One central component of this challenge is the almost certain increase in the number of people with dementia worldwide. Epidemiological studies have shown that, in developed countries, the prevalence of dementia will increase markedly in percentage terms (Groth, Klingholz, and Wehling 2011). In the US, the number of people with dementia is predicted to increase from 5 million in 2010 to 8.5 million in 2030; in Germany from 1.1 million in 2007 to 2.2 million in 2050; in Japan from 2 million to 4 million by 2040

(Ferri et al. 2006); and, in the UK, from 820,000 in 2010 (Luengo-Fernandez, Leal, and Grey 2010) to over 1.7 million by 2051 (Knapp and Prince 2007). The picture in developing countries is less clear, but, with increases in life expectancy growing rapidly in China, India, and Latin America, the most recent evidence from the 10/66 Dementia Research Group (Prince 2000) suggests an even greater increase in the number of people with dementia in these countries as the century progresses (Kalaria et al. 2008; Prince 2009). Another component is the less substantial—but still marked—increases that are predicted in the number of people with severe intellectual impairments (Emerson 2009).

Such developments will have marked effects. One effect will be the socio-economic difficulties that result from the need for a larger proportion of a country's population to devote their time to providing informal care to others. Another effect is the increased demand on public and private services designed to meet the varied health, social, and personal care needs of these individuals (Qiu, De Ronchi, and Fratiglioni 2007).

Whilst care services for people with dementia around the world remain underdeveloped (Prince et al. 2009), or are orientated towards acute hospital settings, it is recognized that the needs of people with dementia relate to their personal and social functioning as well as the need for health-care interventions. Accordingly, a significant proportion of the needs of these individuals is best met in supported residential or community-based settings, rather than in hospital environments, and there is a growing call for these services to become better established in all countries (Prince et al. 2009).

The solutions emerging to address the long-term care needs of an ageing population pose another kind of global challenge. There is evidence of a growing trend for people to migrate between countries to provide—and increasingly to receive—care. A significant number of the care workers employed in long-term care settings in the United Kingdom have moved from Eastern Europe, South East Asia, South Asia, and Africa in order to take such jobs (Cangiano et al. 2009; Hussein, Stevens, and Manthorpe 2010), and a similar pattern involving different migratory trends is documented in the US (Smith and Baughman 2007). Those requiring care may also move to another country. Older Japanese citizens, for example, move to Indonesia, Thailand, Malaysia, and the Philippines for the purpose of receiving care in elder-care communities (Toyota, Böcker, and Guild 2006; Ono 2008). Concern that such patterns of international migration are causing negative effects on the inter- and intra-national distribution of labour in health and long-term care services has been raised. This concern is partly captured by the fact that countries are increasingly opening up their borders to economic migrants specifically for the purpose of care provision, and partly because the countries from which these migrants are moving from are developing training that is specifically designed for international care markets, with knock-on effects on the ability of these countries to retain the labour needed to meet the care requirements of their own citizens.

2 Ethical issues in long-term care practice

Connected to these social and economic considerations are a number of ethical challenges associated with the increase in the global demand for long-term care. When people think about ethical issues in relation to long-term care it is often the 'big' issues that spring to mind. Medical ethicists, in particular, have analysed decisions about end-of-life care such as the withholding and withdrawal of life-sustaining treatment and the place, if any, for euthanasia. In light of the fact that (mainly female) care workers move from less economically developed countries to provide low-paid care for people in wealthier countries, bioethicists have also problematized these developments in light of arguments about social and transnational justice (Brown and Braun, 2008; Eckenwiler, 2009; Meghani and Eckenwiler 2009; Lee 2011). Questions of justice have also connected moral and political philosophical claims about the broader question of the obligations that societies have to their older and disabled members. These discussions have focused on questions of intergenerational justice, public strategies for enablement and empowerment, and the amount of resources that ought to be allocated to provide care for, and undertake research into, the needs of people with dementia and disabilities.

There is, however, another dimension to the ethics of long-term care that has received comparatively less attention: the ethical aspects of the practice of long-term care. Whilst there has been recent acknowledgement of the issues that arise in both family (Baldwin et al. 2005; Lindemann 2007; Baldwin 2008) and paid (Kane and Caplan, 1990; Hasselkus 1997; Powers 2001; Hughes and Baldwin 2006; Solum, Slettebø, and Hauge 2008; van der Dam et al., 2012) care settings, these studies have tended to be limited to the detailed analysis of issues in a small number of practical settings. There has been no attempt to situate these issues in the context of the wider social and demographic trends described above, nor has there been a move towards building international consensus on systematic ways for addressing such issues. This will be the aim of our chapter, and we begin by outlining the variety of issues that arise in the day-to-day provision of long-term care. This account will be illustrative rather than comprehensive, and our focus will predominantly be long-term care for people with dementia. It is important, however, to recognize that the issues we outline, and the proposals that we put forward, apply equally to other individuals who are in need of long-term personal and social support. Our central message is that the ethical issues in long-term care practice are many and varied, and that in order to address these, several complementary strategies must be pursued at local, national, and international levels. We wish to emphasize particularly that ordinary care, as practised throughout the world by relatives in their own homes, and by care workers working within community and residential care settings, involves making difficult ethical decisions on a daily basis.

2.1 Freedom of action versus risk to self

One set of ethical issues relates to person-orientated considerations. One respondent to the Nuffield Council on Bioethics consultation exercise concerning dementia wrote: 'For fear of risk, too many people with dementia have a poorer quality of life.' Another wrote: 'Anybody looking after someone with dementia would naturally make sure they are never put at risk' (Nuffield Council on Bioethics 2009: 100). Taken together, these quotations illustrate the dilemma facing carers.

Risk of harm comes in many forms: there are risks associated with wandering off and being vulnerable from road traffic or hypothermia; risks from misusing a cooker; or risks that arise from eating inappropriately stored food. To reduce risk, carers may judge it to be necessary to restrict the person's freedom.

How are the person's interests in remaining safe to be balanced against his desire for, and his enjoyment from, being free to go about, free from restraint?

2.2 New technologies: safety versus privacy

Assistive technologies have the potential to make substantial improvements to the lives of people with dementia and their carers, and it has been argued that such technologies are a way of avoiding the dilemma highlighted in the section above. Tracking devices can reduce the dangers from getting lost. Video surveillance methods (telecare) may enable carers to respond more quickly in case of need. But both these uses of technology raise questions of invasion of privacy and the availability of telecare also raises concerns that the possibility of such remote 'care' will lead to the acceptance of such care in place of personal visits (Hughes and Louw 2002; Pols, 2010; Ganyo, Dunn, and Hope 2011).

2.3 Balancing the person's previous wishes and values with their current interests

A different kind of issue arises in those conditions, such as dementia, in which the person may lose the capacity to make decisions. A dilemma can arise when a person had values, or made decisions, that seem at odds with what she currently enjoys and appears to value. This kind of situation, and the weight that should be given to 'advance decisions', has been much discussed in the setting of end-of-life decisions (Dworkin 1986; Dresser 1995; Treloar 1999; Berghmans 2000; Widdershoven and Berghmans 2001) but it is relevant to many other situations (Holm 2001; Hope, Slowther, and Eccles 2009). For example, what should care staff do if a person with dementia who was previously vegetarian is now in a care home and tries to take the meat off other residents' plates? Should care staff change the television channel if a person who identified himself as being an atheist prior to the onset of dementia is enjoying singing along to the hymns broadcast within a religious affairs programme, when doing so would cause him significant distress? In addition to the substantive dimensions of this issue, there are ethical questions relating to the process through which such decisions are made. Who ought to be involved, and why? How should disagreements between parties be resolved?

In care settings for people with lifelong impairments such as those with profound intellectual disabilities, the ethical issue will be a different one entirely: how should decisions be made for people who have never been able to develop values or express preferences? In medical ethics, this issue is often addressed through an objective account of the concept of 'best interests'. However, in long-term care settings, there is difficulty in substantiating this concept because, unlike health care, the purpose of providing long-term care is not to cure, treat, or manage disease. Instead, the focus is on enhancing a person's quality of life within a broad sphere of personal and social experiences. Should an objective account of this person's interests be endorsed (and what should an objective account consist of), or should decisions be made in line with the views, wishes, and values of a family member or those of the professional care workers with whom that person might have lived for many years?

2.4 Truth telling and deception

It is a widely held ethical principle that we should not tell lies and should generally tell the truth. Many long-term relationships are built on trust and truthfulness. What should carers do when, because of cognitive impairment, telling the truth causes distress to an individual? (Schermer 2007) For example, a person with dementia may keep forgetting that his wife has died. If every time he asks where she is he is told that she is dead he may mourn each time anew.

Three contrasting positions were given by different respondents to the Nuffield Council consultation.

1. 'I don't think it helps anyone to lie about anything.'
2. 'I felt fully justified in telling lies if it prevented my mother going through even more distress.'
3. A sensible balance of truth and 'white lies'. (Nuffield Council on Bioethics 2009: 104)

Even when relatives believe that it might be right to tell a 'white lie' to prevent distress, some find it very difficult to do so because it is at odds with the history of their relationship (Baldwin et al. 2005).

A similar problem arises when a person with cognitive impairment refuses to take medication important for health. When, if ever, is it right to secretly give the person the medication without their knowledge?

2.5 End-of-life issues

We have emphasized the point that there is a very wide range of ethical issues that arise in long-term care practice, in addition to end-of-life issues. This is not, of course, to diminish the significance of these issues. Family members and health professionals may be involved in difficult decisions about which, if any, life-extending treatments should be given.

2.6 Freedom of action versus the interests of others

A second set of ethical issues emerges out of the fact that, in long-term care, the person is often receiving support in a communal living environment, and, when this is not the case, the person's care will be situated within a community or neighbourhood setting. Dilemmas about acting in line with the interests of one person can become even more complex when other individuals might be at risk from the person's behaviour. This can occur, for example, when a next-door neighbour is at risk from a fire caused by misuse of a cooker or, more commonly, when the driving skills of a person with dementia deteriorate, potentially putting other road users at risk. For many, driving is not only a pleasure but a crucial source of the ability to go out and enjoy life. Until the later stages, people with dementia appear to be as safe drivers as many other groups who are allowed to drive (Dubinsky, Stein, and Lyons 2000). When should carers and professionals, such as the family doctor, alert relevant driving assessment authorities, and what criteria should those authorities use for preventing the person from driving?

It is not only physical risks but also the interests of others more broadly that are relevant. Within a nursing home, for example, one person's unfettered behaviour may interfere with the freedoms, or enjoyment, of other residents (Powers 2001). When should staff intervene to restrict the freedom of one resident for the sake of other residents?

2.7 Sexual relationships

Although younger people may prefer to think otherwise, intimate sexual feelings often continue into old age (Lindau et al. 2007). Care homes, and long-stay hospitals, do not in general cope well with sexual relationships partly because of the lack of facilities for the privacy needed. But, whatever the facilities available, situations will arise that pose complex ethical problems, some of which will be significantly affected by cultural expectations and religious values.

A problem that arises quite commonly in care homes that look after people with dementia is that two residents will form a close relationship with at least some physical intimacy (e.g. Parker and Dickenson 2001). Care-home staff may be asked by the spouse or other family to prevent such intimacy. This raises questions of the person's well-being, their likely previous wishes, the interests of the family, the role of the family in decision-making, and society's position on what sexual relationships citizens should be allowed to continue. Different cultures may take very different positions on these issues.

2.8 Balancing the interests of the person with the interests of the carer(s)

In non-institutional care settings, a third set of issues relates to the interests of the individual and the interests of those who have devoted time and effort to provide care to that individual. Friends or family carers continually face the problem of how to balance their interests, and those of others for whom they are responsible such as children, with the interests of the person for whom they are caring. Such carers often face enormous restrictions on what they can do and enjoy because of their caring responsibilities. Professionals involved in supporting such carers face issues of confidentiality—what information about the person's condition or about their care plan, for example, should be shared with the carer?

2.9 Impact of globalization on the ethical issues in long-term care practice

The ways in which the ethical issues that we have outlined are solved will, in practice, be influenced by the sociocultural expectations that undergird institutional routines, the actions that constitute caring activities, and context-specific accounts of the value base of such activities (e.g. Wu 2004). For example, attitudes to new sexual relationships being formed in the context where the person with dementia no longer recognizes his own spouse are likely to differ across cultures, and it is likely that care practices and decision-making processes will already reflect ways of managing this issue on the basis of such attitudes. The role of close family members in decision-making differs between cultures (e.g. Savishinsky 1991), and this will be highly significant in the setting of the care of people who are no longer able to exercise full capacity over their decisions.

End-of-life care decisions will be affected not only by differing attitudes but also by legal structures, and these differ between countries.

As care workers increasingly migrate to different countries in order to carry on their work, and as people are cared for in a country other than the one in which they have been acculturated, there are likely to be an increasing number of potential clashes between the sociocultural assumptions of the person and those providing care and support.

2.10 Conclusions

From these considerations of ethical issues in long-term care practice we come to two main conclusions. First, that in any long-term care setting there are many ethical issues, a large proportion of which arise in the ordinary aspects of day-to-day life, rather than the extraordinary situation in which a person is receiving health care. These issues are inevitably resolved in one way or another. The danger is that they are resolved without proper consideration of the ethical issues involved. Many carers will need support in tackling these issues. Second, as people move across national borders, both staff and residents, and as an increasing number of organizations providing care are international, these ethical issues will be affected in two main ways: the resolution will have to involve more consideration of cultural differences in how to balance the relevant ethical issues and come to a judgement, and there will be new ethical issues arising from the differences in culture.

Globalization will increase the number and complexity of the ethical issues that arise in long-term care practice. To tackle these issues effectively it will be necessary for the international community to work constructively towards the common goal of increasing the quality of care and of ethical decision-making in the practice of long-term care.

3 Fostering ethical practice in long-term care work

In order to improve the ethical standards of care there are three main issues to be addressed: the *prevention of abuse* and other practices in care that are clearly wrong; *establishing the appropriate standards of care* and addressing how these standards can be maintained and acted upon; and *enabling difficult ethical decisions to be made* through identifying and providing appropriate training and support to those involved in care work. We suggest that these three issues are best addressed by three processes, each of which roughly maps on to the respective issue. These three processes are: asserting human rights; agreeing principles; and applying principles to individual cases. We will consider in turn each of the stages required to set these processes in place.

3.1 Asserting human rights

Evidence of basic abuses taking place within long-term care settings is compelling, even in countries with well-established regulatory regimes. We believe that the most effective theoretical underpinning of all actions to prevent the abuse of people in long-term care, and to establish the basic minimum standards of such care, is through the notion of human rights. Human rights are the subject of several widely supported international declarations and agreements. These include the Universal Declaration of Human Rights and the Convention on the Rights of Persons with Disabilities by the United Nations, and the Convention for the Protection of Human Rights and Fundamental Freedoms (commonly known as the European Convention on Human Rights). These international agreements have not only attracted broad endorsement, but have affected the laws in many countries. They provide a basis on which nations and institutions can develop policy and guidelines, and they can set in place substantive resources to individuals in struggling against abuse and lack of support.

Article 2 of the Universal Declaration of Human Rights states that: 'Everyone is entitled to all rights and freedoms set forth in the Declaration, without distinction of any kind.' Article 7 states: 'All are entitled to equal protection against any discrimination in violation of this Declaration.' Article 22 states: 'Everyone ... has the right to social security and is entitled to realization ... of the economic, social and cultural rights indispensable for his dignity.' It is clear that these rights are not simply those negative rights to be free from problematic interference from others, including the state. They include also positive rights to be helped to enjoy the benefits of a free society.

The Cross-Party Group in the Scottish Parliament on Alzheimer's disease chose to strongly endorse a rights-based approach when working towards ensuring that high-quality services are available for those with dementia, and their carers. They have produced a Charter of Rights for People with Dementia and their Carers in Scotland (Cross-Party Group by Alzheimer Scotland 2009), and this charter is now a central part of the Scottish government's 2010 Dementia Strategy. In explaining why the Cross-Party Group thought that such a charter is necessary, they wrote: 'People with dementia have the same human rights as every other citizen. However, it is widely recognized that, in addition to the impact of the illness, they face cultural, social and economic barriers to fulfilling these' (Cross-Party Group by Alzheimer Scotland 2009). The same could be said of groups, other than those with dementia, who are receiving long-term care.

The Scottish Charter itself draws heavily on the United Nations Convention on the Rights of Persons with Disabilities. It is important to recognize that most of those in long-term care would fall within the definition of disability within this convention: 'Persons with disabilities include those who have long-term physical, mental, intellectual or sensory impairments which in interaction with various barriers may hinder their full and effective participation in society on an equal basis with others' (Article 1). This clearly includes people with dementia and, yet, in the Code of Practice to the 2010 Equality Act in England and Wales—the Act that effectively brings the United Nations Convention into English law—there is virtually no explicit mention of dementia.

In the preamble to the United Nations Convention on the Rights of Persons with Disabilities it is stated: 'Recognising the need to promote and protect the human rights of all persons with disabilities, including those who need more intensive support'. The preamble also emphasizes the 'importance of international cooperation for improving the living conditions of persons with disabilities in every country'. It also highlights 'the fact that the majority of persons with disabilities live in conditions of poverty, and in this regard recognizing the critical need to address the negative impact of poverty on persons with disabilities'.

The United Nations Convention places a general obligation on the state to undertake to ensure and promote the full realization of all human rights and fundamental freedoms for all persons with disabilities. The mechanisms for realizing such undertaking specifically mentioned in the convention include through appropriate legislation, promoting standards and guidelines, promoting research and development of assistive technologies, and providing accessible information, and to 'promote the training of professionals and staff working with disabilities in the rights recognized in the present convention so as to better provide the assistance and services guaranteed by those rights' (Article 4; 1i). The convention also places a responsibility on states to ensure that persons with disabilities have access on an equal basis with those without disabilities to the physical environment, transporting information and to 'other facilities and services open or provided to the public' (Article 9; 1).

In addressing these responsibilities, countries have focused on improving access for people disabled through physical impairments, for example in improving access by wheelchair users to transport, shops, and places of entertainment. Less recognition has been given to the ways in which mental impairment can reduce access, and how these barriers can be overcome. Article 30 specifically addresses enabling participation in cultural life, recreation, leisure, and sport, and again places on states responsibility, for example, to ensure that disabled people 'Enjoy access to places for cultural performances or services, such as theatres, museums, libraries and tourism services' (Article 30; 1c).

Whilst alternative approaches, such as the capabilities approach (Nussbaum 2006), have been developed recently to give shape to the processes that ought to be established in relation to providing real-world opportunities to people with disabilities, we think that human rights, rather than capabilities, are best placed to prevent abuses and to establish minimum standards in long-term care. Human rights are widely recognized as an ethical framework across the globe, and they enjoy high status in political circles that is not shared by the more narrowly academic-orientated discussions around capabilities. Whilst the capabilities approach might address some of the weaknesses that underpin the philosophical justification for rights-based claims in the context of long-term care for people with disabilities, the need for action to tackle abuses can, on pragmatic grounds, take instantaneous advantage of the pre-existing consensus on human rights.

3.2 Agreeing principles

Human rights can establish basic standards for how people should be treated and for the responsibilities of states in ensuring that their citizens are treated according to these standards. But once we go beyond these basic standards to think about the ethical duties owed to those in need of care, we can no longer rely on the concept of the universal rights possessed by all human beings. Various ethical principles may be relevant to a specific care situation, and different principles may pull in different directions. In deciding what is the right thing to do there may need to be some judgement as to how varying principles are relevant and how they are to be integrated, or balanced, in their application to a particular situation. This raises the question of what are the relevant principles and whether there can be international consensus on these principles.

In seeking to answer these questions, it is helpful to identify other areas that have sought to establish international agreement on ethical standards for particular kinds of activities. One area where there have been serious and sustained attempts to develop such consensus at the level of ethical principles is that of the regulation of medical research.

The Nazi abuses led to the Declaration of Helsinki by the World Medical Association, which remains an internationally agreed set of standards and principles for governing medical research relationships anywhere in the world. The need for international agreement is ever greater as more and more research is carried out across national borders; for example, research that is funded by one country or pharmaceutical company, might be carried out in other countries. The Declaration of Helsinki has had to be continually revisited and revised. In recent years, as the number of countries involved in international research has increased, there have been disagreements arising from differences in culture (e.g. Vastag 2000).

The experience of medical research shows that international agreement is not easy and may need continual discussion and revision. Nevertheless we believe that these attempts at such agreement, and the ensuing discussions, play an important role in promoting good ethical practice, and could be a model to apply in the context of long-term care.

In the context of long-term care, what might principles that can be internationally agreed look like? One strategy here is to ascertain whether well-established ethical principles in health care can be adopted within long-term care. Some commentators have argued that the ethical principles that ought to be applied in long-term care are different (Kuczewski 1999), whilst others have embraced philosophically nuanced readings of the principles that are drawn upon within medical ethics in ways that are carefully tailored to the realities of the long-term care environment (Agich 2003).

The Nuffield Council on Bioethics proposed an ethical framework for the care of people with dementia (Nuffield Council on Bioethics 2009). We believe that certain principles identified within this document could—when elucidated robustly—command broad agreement across cultures. At the individual level, the Nuffield Council Report advocates the promotion of both the autonomy and the well-being interests of the person needing care. These two principles have been very widely applied to issues in medical ethics (e.g. Beauchamp and Childress 2008), and autonomy is explicitly endorsed in the preamble to the UN Convention on the Rights of Persons with Disabilities (point n). Beyond the policy arena, a number of ethicists have advocated the principle of respect for human dignity as the foundational principle for guiding ethical practice in care work (Pullman 1999; McIntyre 2003; Gallagher 2004; Foster 2011). Whilst this principle has been drawn upon to shape, for example, UK policy in this context (Royal College of Nursing 2008; Social Care Institute for Excellence 2010), others have questioned whether such a principle can provide the kind of practical advice required to address the ethical issues outlined above (Agich 2007).

The Nuffield Report discusses the ways in which the principles of promoting autonomy and well-being might be understood within the setting of long-term care, and, importantly, endorses a reading of these principles that can respond to the critiques of the narrow and limited interpretations of such principles in the medical ethics literature. We agree with Agich (2003), for example, that elucidating the principle of respecting the autonomy of those in receipt of long-term care should be sensitive to a detailed understanding of the practical ways that people are able to live their everyday lives in such settings. No doubt a similar nuanced account of the principle of respect for human dignity would also need to be developed if it were to shape long-term care practice in the correct way. Such a project, we believe, might also show how the additional principles that have been put forward, such as respect for narrative integrity, could be subsumed within the principle of promoting autonomy or the principle of respecting human dignity.

At the international level, we call for extended discussion of the ethical principles that should underpin long-term care practice, and how these principles should be elucidated and defended in light of the different contexts in which long-term care is provided. This process should be separate from, but dovetail with, the process of fostering a rights-based approach to establishing minimum standards in long-term care settings.

3.3 Applying and interpreting principles to specific situations

Principles are not by themselves sufficient to determine what the ethically right thing to do is in any specific situation. Principles need to be interpreted, their application to the specific situation needs to be determined, and different principles may need to be integrated or balanced in order to make a decision. This is not an endorsement of ethical relativism as it is not about making moral judgements that are relative to values specific to particular care contexts. It is simply to acknowledge that, even with an internationally agreed set of principles, there will be further work that needs doing in order to foster ethical practice.

Principles will need to be *tailored* to context, and the ways in which this is done is also an international issue to some extent, if only because there may be people from different cultural backgrounds working together in the same care setting. Again this approach is not controversial; nor is it particularly novel. In research ethics regulations and governance, most of the current debate in policy and academic debates centres on how the principle of, for example, respect for research participants' autonomy ought to be implemented in different research activities across different local, national, and international research settings. The question then focuses on what is required of researchers in order to ensure that research practices are aligned with this principle. This might, for example, imply a duty to seek anticipatory individual written consent, or it might, alternatively, require community involvement in group decision-making about research participation. A similar approach is being advocated in the development of a global curriculum in education in bioethics that can be adopted within, and shaped to, the unique pedagogical settings in which the education materials will need to be adopted (UNESCO 2008).

This focus on tailoring, which again we think can be usefully translated from the research to long-term care context, raises the issue of what *processes* should be in place at the local level to enable this tailoring to take place such that the ethical issues discussed in the second section of the chapter can be addressed. In contrast with the research ethics model, we believe that the tailoring of ethical principles to the everyday decisions that arise in long-term care settings ought to be a bottom-up process, situated in the practical settings in which care is provided, led by those involved in care work, and facilitated by individuals with experience of undertaking ethical analysis in these settings.

In the context of professional care environments, we believe that the main process that ought to be put into place is a model of ethics support that can be implemented straightforwardly in the different settings in which care is provided, and that can incorporate skill development and training components within a self-reflective and formative approach to addressing ethical issues. Well established approaches to case consultation and clinical ethics support in health-care environments that are built upon a committee-based or consultant model are likely to be inadequate in long-term care, not least because these approaches enact solutions to ethical problems in health care that have been subject to extended and detailed analysis. In contrast, the development of networks of community practitioners in ethics (http://www.communityethicsnetwork. ca), deliberative meetings around ethical real cases (Abma, Molewijk, and Widdershoven 2009; van der Dam et al. 2012), and care forums for reflecting on difficult decisions (Dunn in progress) seem to be better placed to ensure that the tailoring of principles to practice is responsive to the issues raised by those working in these settings. In addition, such a bottom-up process can help to ensure that reasoning through ethical issues is sensitive to the governmental and institutional policies and procedures that must be adhered to in care settings, the requirements of local and national legal frameworks, and the perspectives and individual values of all those involved in the practice of care. Moreover, on a pragmatic point, such informal processes that can integrate seamlessly into the daily patterns of professional life in the care setting can help to ensure that ethics support of this form is welcomed as an adjunct to, rather than a distraction from, the working regimes of community- and residential-based care settings.

Within this process, the role of the facilitator of an ethics support meeting will be different from that of the clinical ethics committee member or the ethics consultant. His primary role will be to ensure that practical ethical issues experienced by those working in care are raised for discussion, that the relevant ethical principles are introduced in a suitable manner during discussions, and that all those participating are invited to contribute. As ethical issues are identified and discussed, this role will also involve adopting a set of ethical 'tools' that encourage care staff to reason carefully through practical problems. These tools might include the use of case comparisons and thought experiments, the ability to distinguish facts from values, and the balancing of principles and intuitions, and will equip the care staff with the skills to reason through ethical issues as they encounter them during their work. In the long term, such an approach is designed to help establish a culture of ethical awareness and inquiry in care settings (Bolmsjö, Sandman, and Andersson 2006), and the development of agreed ways to act when providing support to individuals in ways that are in alignment with the relevant ethical principles identified as the foundations for ethical practice in these settings.

The Nuffield Report also emphasizes the importance of providing support to family members who provide long-term care for people with dementia often without any professional input whatsoever. Given that the majority of the ethical issues documented above apply equally to family care settings, another process that we think is necessary to translate principles into good long-term care practice is the provision of training and support in ethics in family care settings. In those home environments where family carers receive input from social services or community care practitioners, ethics input should be an additional component of the support provided. When family carers do not receive such additional support, we advocate that information about ethical principles should form part of information made available within primary care, and that proactive efforts should be made by dementia charities and other non-governmental organizations to infuse an ethics component into the information that they provide about dementia.

4 Conclusions

The rapid growth in the number of people requiring long-term care poses a number of practical ethical challenges to societies around the world, and these challenges have a uniquely global character. One set of distinct but underexplored challenges relates to the everyday ethical issues that arise in the practice of long-term care and support within community and residential living environments. Addressing these issues and fostering good ethical practice within long-term care require, we have argued, three linked developments.

First, preventing significant abuses within long-term care settings (which continue to occur even in carefully regulated settings) and establishing a minimum baseline for the quality of care provided require the establishment and integration of human rights-based standards into care work. Second, fostering good practice requires the identification of a set of ethical principles that are appropriate for the aims of long-term care and are robust enough to gain universal acceptance across cultures. Finally, these principles need to be tailored to context using a model of ethics support that can support the resolution of practical ethical issues in ways that are sensitive to the relevant political, institutional, and legal aspects of practice in different settings. The first two of these three steps will largely take place at the international level, and require new collaborations and discussion between academics, policymakers, care providers, and governmental organizations. The final step will take place at the local level, and be driven by those working in long-term care supported by individuals with appropriate training in the relevant principles and procedures.

References

Abma, T. A., Molewijk, A. C. and Widdershoven, G. A. M. (2009). "Good Care in Ongoing Dialogue: Improving the Quality of Care through Moral Deliberation and Responsive Evaluation," *Health Care Analysis*, 17:217–35.

Agich, G. J. (2003). *Dependence and Autonomy in Old Age*. Cambridge: Cambridge University Press.

Agich, G. J. (2007). "Reflections on the Function of Dignity in the Context of Caring for Old People," *Journal of Medicine and Philosophy*, 32:483–94.

Baldwin, C. (2008). "Family Carers, Ethics, and Dementia," in G. Widdershoven et al. (eds), *Empirical Ethics in Psychiatry*. Oxford: Oxford University Press, 107–22.

Baldwin, C. et al. (2005). *Making Difficult Decisions: The experience of Caring for Someone with Dementia*. London: Alzheimer's Society.

Beauchamp, T. L. and Childress, J. F. (2008). *Principles of Biomedical Ethics*, 6th edition. New York: Oxford University Press.

Berghmans, R. (2000). "Advance Directives and Dementia," *Annals of the New York Academy of Sciences*, 913:105–10.

Bolmsjö, I.A., Sandman, L., and Andersson, E. (2006). "Everyday Ethics in the Care of Elderly People," *Nursing Ethics*, 13(3): 249–63.

Brown, C.V., and Braun, K. L. (2008). "Globalization, Women's Migration, and the Long-term Care Workforce," *Gerontologist*, 48(1): 16–24.

Cangiano, A. et al. (2009). *Migrant Care Workers in Ageing Societies: Research Findings in the United Kingdom*. Oxford: COMPAS.

Cross Party Group by Alzheimer Scotland. (2009). *Charter of Rights for People with Dementia and their Carers in Scotland*. http://www.dementiarights.org/ (accessed September 14, 2011).

Dresser, R. (1995). "Dworkin on Dementia: Elegant Theory, Questionable Policy," *Hastings Center Report*, 25:32–8.

Dubinsky, R. M., Stein, A. C. and Lyons, K. (2000). "Practice Parameter: Risk of Driving and Alzheimer's Disease," *Neurology*, 54:2205–11.

Dunn, M. (in progress). "Ethics Support Beyond the Clinic: Confessions of a Care Home Ethicist."

Dworkin, R. (1986). "Autonomy and the Demented Self," *Millbank Quarterly*, 64(Supplement 2): 4–16.

Eckenwiler, L. (2009). "Care Worker Migration and Transnational Justice," *Public Health Ethics*, 2(2): 171–83.

Emerson, E. (2009). "Estimating Future Numbers of Adults with Profound Multiple Learning Disabilities in England," *Tizard Learning Disability Review*, 14(4): 49–55.

Ferri, C. P. et al. (2006). "Global Prevalence of Dementia: A Delphi Consensus Study," *Lancet*, 366(9503): 2112–17.

Foster, C. (2011). *Human Dignity in Bioethics and Law*. Oxford: Hart.

Gallagher, A. (2004). "Dignity and Respect for Dignity: Two Key Health Professional Values: Implications for Nursing Practice," *Nursing Ethics*, 11(6): 587–99.

Ganyo, M., Dunn, M., and Hope, T. (2011). "Ethical Issues in the Use of Fall Detectors," *Ageing and Society*, 31(8): 1350–67.

Groth, H., Klingholz, R., and Wehling, M. (2011). *Future Demographic Challenges in Europe: The Urgency to Improve the Management of Dementia*. The WDA-HSG Discussion Paper Series on Demographic Issues.

Hasselkus, B. R. (1997). 'Everyday ethics in dementia care: Narratives of crossing the line', *The Gerontologist*, 37(5): 640–9.

Holm, S. (2001). "Autonomy, Authenticity, or Best Interests: Everyday Decision-Making and Persons with Dementia," *Medicine, Health Care, and Philosophy*, 4: 153–9.

Hope, T., Slowther, A., and Eccles, J. (2009). "Best Interests, Dementia, and the Mental Capacity Act (2005)," *Journal of Medical Ethics*, 35:733–8.

Hughes, J., and Baldwin, C. (2006). *Ethical Issues in Dementia Care: Making Difficult Decisions*. London: Jessica Kingsley.

Hughes, J., and Louw, S. (2002). "Electronic Tagging of People with Dementia Who Wander," *BMJ*, 325:847–8.

Hussein, S., Stevens, M., and Manthorpe, J. (2010). *International Social Care Workers in England: Profile, Motivations, Experiences, and Future Expectations*. London: Social Care Workforce Research Unit.

Kalaria, R. N. et al. (2008). "Alzheimer's Disease and Vascular Dementia in Developing Countries: Prevalence, Management and Risk Factors," *Lancet Neurology*, 7(9): 812–26.

Kane, R. A., and Caplan, A. L. (1990). *Everyday Ethics: Resolving Dilemmas in Nursing Home Llife*. New York: Springer.

Knapp, M., and Prince, M. (2007). *Dementia UK*. London: Alzheimer's Society.

Kuczewski, M. G. (1999). "Ethics in long-term care: Are the principles different?", *Theoretical Medicine and Bioethics*, 20(1): 15–29.

Lee, L. W. (2011). "International Justice in Elder Care: The Long Run," *Public Health Ethics*, 4(3): 292–6.

Lindau, S. T. et al. (2007). "A Study of Sexuality and Health in Older Adults in the United States," *New England Journal of Medicine*, 357:762–74.

Lindemann, H. (2007). "Care in Families," in R. E. Ascroft et al. (eds.) *Principles of Health Care Ethics*. 2nd ed. Chichester: John Wiley and Sons, 351–7.

Luengo-Fernandez, R., Leal, J. and Grey, A. (2010). *Dementia 2010: The Economic Burden and Associated Research Funding in the United Kingdom*. Cambridge: Alzheimer's Research Trust.

McIntyre, M. (2003). "Dignity in Dementia: Person-Centered Care in Community," *Journal of Aging Studies*, 17(4): 473–84.

Meghani, Z., and Eckenwiler, L. (2009). "Care for the Caregivers? Transnational Justice and Undocumented Non-citizen Care Workers," *International Journal of Feminist Approaches to Bioethics*, 2(1): 77–101.

Nuffield Council on Bioethics. (2009). *Dementia: Ethical Issues*. London: Nuffield Council on Bioethics.

Nussbaum, M. (2006). *Frontiers of Justice: Disability, Nationality, Species Membership*. Cambridge, MA: Harvard University Press.

Ono, M. (2008). "Long-stay Tourism and International Retirement Migration: Japanese Retirees in Malaysia," in S. Yamashita et al. (eds.) *Transnational Migration in East Asia: Japan in a Comparative Focus*. Osaka: National Museum of Ethnology, 3–13.

Parker, M. and Dickenson, D. (2001). *The Cambridge Medical Ethics Workbook: Case studies, commentaries and activities*. Cambridge: Cambridge University Press.

Pols, J. (2010). "The Heart of the Matter: About Good Nursing and Telecare," *Health Care Analysis*, 18(4): 374–88.

Powers, B. A. (2001). "Ethnographic analysis of everyday ethics in the care of nursing home residents with dementia: A taxonomy," *Nursing Research*, 50(6): 332–9.

Prince, M. (2000). "Dementia in Developing Countries: A Consensus Statement from the 10/66 Dementia Research Group," *International Journal of Geriatric Psychiatry*, 15(1): 14–20.

Prince, M. (2009). "The 10/66 Dementia Research Group: 10 Years on," *Indian Journal of Psychiatry*, 51: 8–15.

Prince, M. et al. (2009). "Packages of Care for Dementia in Low- and Middle-income Countries," *PLoS Medicine*, 6(11): e1000176.

Pullman, D. (1999). "The Ethics of Autonomy and Dignity in Long-term Care," *Canadian Journal of Aging*, 18(1): 26–46.

Qiu, C., De Ronchi, D., and Fratiglioni, L. (2007). "The Epidemiology of the Dementias: An Update," *Current Opinion in Psychiatry*, 20:380–5.

Royal College of Nursing. (2008). *Defending Dignity: Challenges and Opportunities for Nursing.* London: Royal College of Nursing.

Savishinsky, J. S. (1991). *The Ends of Time: Life and Work in a Nursing Home.* New York: Bergin and Garvey.

Schermer, M. (2007). "Nothing but the Truth? On Truth and Deception in Dementia Care," *Bioethics*, 21:13–22.

Smith, K., and Baughman, R. (2007). "Caring for America's Aging Population: A Profile of the Direct-care Workforce," *Monthly Labor Review*, 9:20–6.

Social Care Institute for Excellence. (2010). *Dignity in Care.* London: SCIE.

Solum, E. M., Slettebø, A., and Hauge, S. (2008). "Prevention of Unethical Actions in Nursing Homes," *Nursing Ethics*, 15: 536–48.

Toyota, M., Böcker, A., and Guild, E. (2006). "Pensioners on the Move: Social Security and Trans-border Retirement Migration in Asia and Europe," *Newsletter of the International Institute of Asian Studies*, No. 40: 30.

Treloar, A. (1999). "Advance Directives: Limitations upon Their Applicability in Elderly Care," *International Journal of Geriatric Psychiatry*, 14:1039–43.

UNESCO. (2008). *Bieothics Core Curriculum: Section 1—Ethics Education Programme.* Paris: UNESCO Division of Ethics of Science and Technology.

van der Dam, S. et al. (2012). "Here's my Dilemma: Moral Case Deliberation as a Platform for Discussing Everyday Ethics in Elderly Care," *Health Care Analysis*, 20(3): 250–67.

Vastag, B. (2000). "Helsinki Discord: A Controversial Declaration," *JAMA*, 284:2983–5.

Widdershoven, G., and Berghmans, R. (2001). "Advance Directives in Psychiatric Care: A Narrative Approach," *Journal of Medical Ethics*, 27:92–7.

Wu, Y. (2004). *The Care of the Elderly in Japan.* Abingdon: Routledge.

18.2

Commentary
Ethical and Policy Issues in Long-Term Care in China

Xiaomei Zhai

The aging of population in China

According to the 2011 national census, the number of Chinese elderly (60+ years old) was 0.178 billion, 13.26 percent of the total population. Of these, 19 percent are incapacitated or semi-incapacitated. China is the only country with more than 100 million elderly people (National Bureau for Statistics, PRC: 2011).

One of the characteristics of population aging in China is "aging before getting rich." The growth of the elderly population is five times more rapid than the growth of the general population.

In 2000, people aged 60+ and 65+ accounted for 10 percent and 7 percent of the population respectively, whilst GDP per capita was US$856. In 2010, this rose to US$4283 (ranked 95th in the world), and in 2011 to US$4382 (93rd). It is expected that in 2015 the number of people aged 60+ will be 0.221 billion, 16 percent of the total population; and in 2020, 0.243 billion, 18 percent of the total population (Zeng et al 2006).

Study of long-term care in Beijing

In 2005–6 our research team conducted a study in Beijing city and its suburbs. The study involved sampling, interview, recording interview, transcriptions, and analysis. Samples come from two basic types of long-term care (LTC) arrangements, home-based and institution-based LTC. We interviewed elderly persons, family members, assistant nurses, physicians working in different LTC settings, and administrators of LTC institutes. An analysis of the interview data gave us an overview of the following aspects: (1) quality and location of care; (2) decision-making; (3) financing of LTC; and (4) meaning of "dignity." "Quality and location of care" are defined as the location of care, the range of care, who is responsible for the care, family's responsibility, and government's responsibility. "Decision-making" refers to the people who make the key decisions concerning health and living arrangements. "Financing of LTC" refers to the division of responsibility for financing LTC among the elderly individual, family, and the government. Data on "meaning of 'dignity'" was generated by asking the respondents to describe, in their own words, what the word "dignity" means to them (Zhai 2005; Zhai and Qiu 2007).

Challenges to the model of family-based LTC

There are three models for LTC: family based, community based, and institution based. The traditional model of LTC in mainland China for thousands of years has been family based. The change in population structure and rapid aging raise serious challenges to the traditional, family-based LTC model, however. Let us review these challenges.

Challenge 1: increasing life expectancy. With improvements in public health and well-being, average life expectancy in China has been increasing. In 1960 life expectancy was about 40 years, rising to 75 years in 2011. This means that the lifespan of the elderly after retirement is much longer than before, which has several implications. One is that the burden of LTC for the elderly imposed on their children is heavier than before. Another is that the frequency of geriatric diseases such as Parkinsonism and Alzheimer's disease is higher in those aged between 70 and 80 than in the younger elderly. Such diseases require specialist care that cannot be provided by the family alone, and which may be difficult for the family to finance (Qiu 2002).

Challenge 2: the change of family structure. The most common type of family in China is the nuclear family. A nuclear family consists of a pair of adults and their children, and may be contrasted with the smaller single-parent family, and with the larger extended family. Indeed, the large family with three, four, or five generations living together (a Confucian ideal) is now a rare phenomenon. The number of single-parent families and childless families is also increasing, though still in a minority. The changing structure of the family has implications for LTC, since a nuclear family has fewer resources for such care than does an extended family.

Challenge 3: the result of restrictive population policy (in most cases, such as in areas populated by Han people, the policy permits couples to have only one child). The bitter fruit of this restrictive policy, coupled with the effects of aging, is that the superstructure of the family follows the pattern 4 + 2 + 1. As a result, each child has to support two parents and four grandparents, which is a burden too heavy for many families to afford.

These factors lead to serious problems for LTC. On the one hand, the size of the typical family has reduced, and along with it the resources for LTC; but LTC needs are growing. On the other hand, in a nuclear family, care for the elderly must compete for resources with care for the member of the third generation (the elderly's grandchild). Members of the second generation in a nuclear family must, then, not only support themselves, but also care for their child(ren) and their parents and grandparents. Whilst they may be keen to meet all of these needs, they may be unable to do so. Since economic and cultural development places the care of elders far beyond the resources of the typical Chinese family, the traditional model of family-based LTC is under threat.

As a result of all this, the function of the family in LTC has been diminishing. It is, therefore, imperative to develop socialized LTC, including community- and institution-based LTC (Wu 2006). Based on the findings of our study, we suggest that all models of LTC should be available to meet the different needs of different elders and their families, but it remains important to consider which model of LTC will best meet the needs of the majority of elders and their families. For example, everybody may agree that the model of institution-based LTC is unlikely to be dominant in the near future, but are we able keep family-based LTC dominant without making changes? Or must we turn to some kind of community-based LTC, or to a combination of family- and community-based care? We must now make efforts to increase the role of the community and government in LTC, and the traditional model of family-based LTC should be revised. The government's Long Term Care Programme (2011–15) plans to develop community- and institution-based LTC. In the case of institution-based LTC, up to the end of 2010, the number of beds in LTC institutes was 3.208 million, that is 18 beds per 1,000 elderly. (In contrast, there were 50–70 beds per 1,000 elderly in developed countries, and 20–30 beds per 1,000 elderly in some developing countries.) In 2015, beds per 1,000 elderly will rise to 30, making the total number of beds 6.63 million (The State Council, China: A Programme on System Building of Long Term Care Programme 2011).

This change will not be welcomed by proponents of familism. In research ethics, there is much debate about whether "family consent" should replace individual informed consent; and in the bioethics literature there is debate about whether the model of family-based LTC should still be seen as dominant (Fan 1997; Fan and Li 2004; Fan and Tao 2004; Fan 2007; Zhai and Qiu 2007; Zhai 2009; Cheng, Ming, and Lai 2012; Zhang 2012). The debate is not about the value of the family in research ethics or in LTC; but about whether familistic models, such as "family consent" in research ethics or family-based LTC, should always be dominant. The reality is that, within families, there are not only harmony and similarity, but also diverse interests and emotional conflicts between family members—especially in a Confucian family. Further, following the Confucian tradition gives rise to gender inequalities in society which should not be ignored. In all cases of family living organ transplantation, all donors are wives and all recipients are husbands. Family involvement in clinical decision-making or research projects is important in a culture with strong family ties, but the replacement of individual informed consent with "family consent" will violate the autonomy of, and may bring harms to, patients and research participants. In the case of LTC, familism would impose unaffordable burdens of care on nuclear families, which would harm the couple and their child(ren), as well as the elderly.

Who should provide long-term care?

A central tenet of contemporary Chinese family values is filial piety. So many Chinese people maintain that children have an obligation to care for their elderly parents, and the elderly can enjoy care at home that is even better than socialized LTC (Zhai and Qiu 2007). This view contrasts sharply with what has been argued by some US scholars (Hui 2004).

The US scholar Jane English (1991) argued that the obligation of children to their parents is something like an obligation to friends. This obligation comes from the love between them and their parents, but not from the recognition of the sacrifice their parents made to raise them. Meyers, Kipnis, and Murphy (1993) even rejected the claim that children have any special obligation towards their parents, whether based on friendship, filial piety, citizenship, etc. She and her co-authors argued that the idea of such a special obligation implies preferential treatment, which conflicts with the ethical requirements of impartiality and equal respect for people.

The crucial issue in China is that, owing to the challenges mentioned above, relying on children's obligations to provide their parents' LTC needs is unrealistic if those needs are to be met. The community and the state should assume the obligation for LTC. The Confucian ideal, "Let elderly be supported," is the goal of the Programme on Long Term Care. The Chinese support the idea that the government should take responsibility for LTC of the elderly.

This responsibility includes finding a way to finance LTC. At the end of 2010, US funds for LTC were about $19,000 billion; but China only has CNY 1,300 billion (2.3 percent of US funds) for LTC. The financing of LTC is a complicated issue, involving four categories of stakeholder: the government, employers, families, and elderly individuals. Although there is little disagreement among Chinese people that making it compulsory for individuals to save for LTC is a good idea, they disagree on how much it is appropriate to deduct from salaries for this purpose. It raises a question about which standards can be used to measure the appropriateness of compulsory individual savings for LTC, and how to justify this appropriateness (Zhai and Qiu 2007).

The same applies to the share of all four stakeholders in funding LTC. The Chinese agree that all four stakeholders should share the costs; but how can we best decide how much should be paid by each? Which standards can be used to measure, and to justify, the appropriateness of the share that each stakeholder must pay (Zhai and Qiu 2007)?

Intergenerational justice

Financing of LTC is an issue of intergenerational justice. In the US, the costs of medical care for those aged 65+ are much higher than for other age groups. Some US scholars (Preston 1984; Lamm 1987) pointed out that those aged 65+ amount to 12 percent of the overall US population, but to one-third of national individual medical costs; and that with a limited budget, aged persons are an easy target for reducing costs. For example, excluding those aged 55+ from renal diseases programs will save 45 percent of these programs' budgets. So they suggested that the proposed rationing system of medical care should be based on age, and resources should be shifted from the aged population to the younger population. They maintained that unless the costs of medical care are constricted in this way, the resources allocated to medical care for younger people and other social welfare will be exhausted. Their suggestion may work in the US, where the medical costs for elders may go far beyond what society can afford. In current mainland China, however, the problem is that much fewer resources are allocated to elders. The problem facing us is that more—not fewer—resources should be shifted to LTC. Many Chinese believe that the government should assume greater responsibility for LTC, including supporting family- and community-based LTC with wise policy and direct financing. To allay worries relating to intergenerational justice, we have to find a way to "three win"; that is, to benefit the elderly as well as younger people, and society at large.

LTC for billions of elderly people may be viewed as a great burden to society at large. However, it also provides a huge opportunity for the market and employment. It is estimated that in 2015 the size of the potential market for LTC of the elderly will reach CNY 450 billion, and will potentially require 500 million employees (The State Council, China: A Programme on System Building of Long Term Care Programme 2011). So what we need is a wise policy to ensure that we achieve the "three win."

References

Cheng, K.-Y., Ming, T., and Lai, A. (2012). "Can Familism be Justified?" *Bioethics*, 26(8): 431–9.

English, J. (1991). "What Do Grown Children Owe Their Parents?" in N. S. Jecker (ed.): *Aging and Ethics: Philosophical Problems in Gerontology*, Clifton, NJ: Humana, 147–54.

Fan, R. P. (1997). "Self-Determinations vs. Family-Determination: Two Incommensurable Principles of Autonomy," *Bioethics*, 11:309–22.

Fan, R. P. (2007). "Which Care, Whose Responsibility, and Why Family? A Confucian Account of Long Term Care for the Elderly," *Journal of Medicine and Philosophy*, 32(5): 495–517.

Fan, R. P., and Li, B. (2004). "Truth Telling in Medicine: The Confucian View," *Bioethics*, 29:179–93.

Fan, R. P., and Tao, J. (2004). "Consent to Medical Treatment: The Complex Interplay of Patients, Families, and Physicians," *Journal of Medicine and Philosophy*, 29:139–48.

Hui, E. (2004). "Personhood and Bioethics: A Chinese Perspective," in R. Z. Qiu (ed), *Bioethics: Asian Perspectives—A Quest for Moral Diversity*, Dordrecht: Kluwer, 29–44.

Lamm, R. D. (1987). "Ethical Care for the Elderly: Are We Cheating Our Children?" in M. Timothy et al. (eds), *Should Medical Care Be Rationed by Age?* Totowa, NJ: Rowman and Littlefield, xi–xv.

Meyers, D. T., Kipnis, K., and Murphy, C. F. (eds) (1993). *Kindred Matters: Rethinking the Philosophy of the Family*. Ithaca, NY: Cornell University Press.

National Bureau for Statistics, PRC: (2011). Bulletin of Major Data of the 6th National Census (1), April 28 http://www.ce.cn/macro/more/201104/28/t20110428_22390326.shtml (accessed January 18, 2013).

Preston, S. H. (1984). "Children and the Elderly in the U.S," *Scientific American*, 251(6): 44–57.

Qiu, R. Z. (2002). "Ethical Issues on Population Aging," in K. J. Chen (ed), *Aging China: Problems and Policies*. Beijing: PIMC Press, 65–89.

State Council, China (2011). A Programme on System Building of Long Term Care (2011–15). http://www.gov.cn/xxgk/pub/govpublic/mrlm/201112/t20111227_64699.html (accessed January 16, 2013).

Wu, J. (2006). "Socialized Long Term Care—How Can It Work?" *Beijing Daily*, November 2, p. 12.

Zeng Y. et al (2006). *21st Century Population and Economic Development in China*. Social Science Academic Press.

Zhai, X. M. (2005) "The *Status Quo* of Aging Population and Social Security System in Beijing, China," a background paper for the Long term care Project.

Zhai X. M. (2009). "Informed Consent in the Non-western Cultural Context and the Implementation of Universal Declaration of Bioethics and Human Rights," *Asian Bioethics Review*, 1(1): 5–16.

Zhai X. M., and Qiu, R. Z. (2007). "Perceptions of Long Term Care, Autonomy and Dignity, by Residents, Family and Care-givers: The Beijing experience," *Journal of Medicine and Philosophy*, 32(5): 425–45.

Zhang, X. Q. (2012). "Reflection on Family Consent Based on a Pregnant Woman Death in a Beijing Hospital," *Bioethics*, 12(3): 164–8.

18.3

Commentary
Whose Rights? Rights Protection in Long-Term Care

Shunzo Majima

Introduction

In their chapter, Tony Hope and Michael Dunn raise one of the most important ethical issues in the future of health care: the ethics of rights protection in long-term care practice for the elderly, especially those with dementia. As they point out, this issue has not been fully explored, despite the fact that the growing need for this type of care warrants an immediate and complete study. The increase in life expectancy, and accompanying rapidly aging population, will increase the percentage of elderly patients with dementia in the future. This is a parallel trend that many other countries will experience in the near future.[1]

After illustrating the global challenges facing long-term care, Hope and Dunn list a number of ethical issues surrounding the practice—including freedom of action versus risk to self, truth telling and deception, and sexual relationships—and suggest the need to foster ethical principles on the basis of fundamental human rights. They also suggest that these principles should be explored, agreed upon, and adjusted in order to be applicable to or interpretable for particular situations. Their chapter is informative and illuminating, and each of the ethical issues raised is worth detailed consideration.

Although Hope and Dunn raise several interesting points for further investigation, given limited space I will restrict my analysis to the topic of rights protection in long-term care settings, focusing on one particular aspect: the use of new technologies

---

[1] I am hesitant to call this a 'global trend' for fear of misleading readers with regard to our understanding of the current health situation in the world, because this health-care issue is certainly not universal. It is important to note that life expectancy in many parts of Africa is below 60, and even below 50 in some areas, according to the social indicator of life expectancy published by the United Nations Statistics Division (http://unstats.un.org/unsd/demographic/products/socind/health.htm, accessed February 3, 2012). Furthermore, many people worldwide are not in a position to receive long-term care despite their needs; however, this issue, although extremely important, is not part of the discussion in Hope and Dunn's chapter.

such as surveillance cameras. I will examine this aspect from the perspective of the rights of those who provide care (e.g. care workers) and those who receive care.

New technologies in rights protection: do they violate rights, or serve as double-edged swords or panaceas?

A key issue concerning the ethics of long-term care practice pertains to ethical tensions inherent in new technologies, or more precisely, in the *use* of such technologies. Any new technology has potential to bring about both positive and negative changes. Hope and Dunn point out that despite the possible benefits, implementation of tracking devices and video surveillance systems in the long-term/dementia care arena raises "questions of invasion of privacy." However, this type of problem is not new, as in the case of public safety and security, where issues regarding rights to privacy have been raised over surveillance cameras installed in public spaces for various purposes.

The fundamental issue is not new technologies per se, but the way they are used. In some cases, technological innovations such as surveillance cameras can be used to spy on innocent people, which can breach their right to privacy. Perhaps cameras in standard communal areas are a norm, but the idea of putting them into a bathroom cubicle is the issue which would cause fear or moral revulsion towards the constant monitoring of our behavior. This is an obvious scenario of an intrusion of privacy for two reasons: (1) we have, or believe that we have, little risk of harm in the bathroom, except for the extremely rare possibility of assault, stroke, heart failure, and so on; and (2) we can, or we believe we can, take care of our needs in the bathroom as rational, fully autonomous people.

Let us consider another case: the use of nanny cameras or nannycams, which are video-recording devices used to monitor babies or infants, as well as babysitters. One website posts a photo of a cute, purple stuffed toy called "stuffed animal puppy dog teddy bear with hidden camera," which is advertised for sale at the price of US$349. The description follows: "Whether you want to watch your child or even to make sure the babysitter stays out of trouble, no one will suspect that this harmless stuffed bear is watching them! If you have to be away all day yet you don't quite trust the new babysitter or want to keep an eye on your child (to ensure they're staying out of trouble or even to make sure they're sleeping throughout the night), then the popular talking stuffed animal puppy dog/teddy bear camera is the perfect device for you."[2] Compared to the imaginary scenario of cameras being installed in the bathroom, the moral revulsion many of us feel against nannycams might be substantially less (except for some people who might feel qualms or scruples about distrust toward babysitters). This is presumably based on our inclination to be concerned about the safety of babies/infants in our absence, and our belief that babies/infants are to be cared for.

---

[2] http://www.nannycam.com/Stuffed-Animal-Puppy-Dog-Teddy-Bear-with-Hidden-Camera-Purple-BB2BearGirl10.htm (accessed February 10, 2012).

Under certain circumstances, the use of surveillance cameras, such as nannycams for babies and monitoring devices for long-term care patients with severe dementia, can be considered beneficial, as such surveillance systems can provide protection for some of the fundamental human rights of vulnerable people. It is their right to be protected from cruel, inhumane, or degrading acts, or from the fear of being mistreated—physically, mentally, or both. Behind closed doors, the abuse of vulnerable people can easily be concealed, and in this sense, installation of surveillance cameras can virtually open up the space to enhance transparency in long-term care settings.

When considering surveillance systems in long-term health-care facilities, we are more likely to assume a situation where carers watch people under their care with cameras; however, there are also situations in which carers themselves are being monitored—by their colleagues, or by families or guardians of those receiving care. In these situations, it becomes important to consider and clarify who is monitoring the carers for quality assurance purposes. In other words, surveillance cameras could be used to monitor the carers in order to render care provision transparent. By monitoring care workers, better, more transparent long-term care can be practiced, at least to a certain degree. The degree and severity of dementia in patients, however, may affect the extent to which this scheme could function as a means of preventing, monitoring, and deterring the abuse of rights or malicious acts committed by problematic workers.

More importantly, surveillance cameras could bring another benefit to the effect that the rights of other vulnerable people are protected, namely, those who provide care. If cameras are installed in long-term care facilities to monitor and record the way care is being provided or received by care workers and residents, both the workers' colleagues and the residents' families can observe how care workers themselves are being treated. If care workers are abused or subjected to offence under video surveillance, their colleagues can intervene to prevent or stop further abuse or offence. If the case is serious, data recorded by surveillance cameras could be used as evidence in civil or criminal litigations, as well as to justify the proportionate measures taken against the perpetrators (for example, expulsion from the institution as the most severe measure). Furthermore, monitoring of care facilities could contribute to vindication of the rights of care workers, as recorded data can be used to defend them against false accusations of misconduct or rights abuses by residents. Indeed, since the manager of any care institution has an obligation to maintain a morally sound work environment without breaches of human rights, surveillance cameras could be used as leverage for management of facilities where the rights of employees as well as residents are protected.

Some might be concerned about the rights of carers who are under video surveillance. Indeed, the extent to which the rights of carers should be protected is still a matter of debate. I am not arguing that carers have no right to privacy in the workplace, or that cameras should be installed at every institution. Rather, my point is that at some institutions, such measures could be introduced that provide carers with an opportunity to decide whether to agree to the terms and conditions of video surveillance when they sign the employment contract. The rights of carers could then be secured, not by installing surveillance cameras in their workplace, but by allowing them to opt out by not signing the contract.

Conclusion

In this chapter, I briefly examined one of the ethical challenges facing long-term care practice from the perspective of rights protection for both care providers and receivers. I argued that one of the most urgent issues to be considered is the protection of vulnerable people in long-term care settings. In this brief discussion, I implied that the identity of the vulnerable parties—whose rights need to be protected—depends on the situation; in some cases, they represent people receiving care, and in others, people providing care. Under certain circumstances, care workers could potentially be put in a vulnerable position in relation to those who receive care. Under other circumstances, both parties are at risk of being forced into vulnerable positions. I argued that surveillance cameras could be used to protect the rights of both parties—in particular, the right to be protected from abuse and offense. Again, it is not to say that all surveillance systems are risk free; rather, despite the risks involved in implementing innovative tools, their merits could outweigh the risks in some cases. My argument is perhaps most convincing when considering the following point: surveillance cameras can contribute to the enhancement of safety and security of the vulnerable, whether those who provide or those who receive care.

18.4

Commentary
Listening to Voices that Are Difficult to Hear

Susumu Shimazono

This work highlights the ethical issues in health care related to the increasing population of older adults with dementia and the increase in migration of foreign health-care providers.

Prior work by Tony Hope and Michael Dunn offer detailed exploration of the gravity of ethical issues related to the increasing number of foreign health-care workers migrating to developed countries to address the nursing needs of a growing elderly population.

To date, most work in this field has focused on the major ethical issues surrounding suspension of end-of-life treatment and social justice for disadvantaged populations. However, there have been few studies examining the ethical issues faced daily by nursing staff in long-term care settings.

The nursing care of elderly populations in developed countries will likely become increasingly dependent on foreign labor, and it is necessary to consider ways to address the ethical issues faced in this setting, particularly those that result from cultural differences.

The following are ethical issues that will likely be of particular importance:

- Freedom of action versus safety and risk to self;
- New technologies: safety versus privacy;
- Balancing the person's previous wishes and values with their current interests;
- Truth telling versus deception;
- End-of-life issues;
- Freedom of action versus the interests of others;
- Sexual relationships;
- Balancing the interests of the patient with the interests of the carer.

While some of these issues relate specifically to elderly patients, and others apply more generally to a broader population of patients with disabilities, all involve ethical issues related to long-term nursing care. An evaluation of the ethical issues related to the care of older adults with dementia may prompt a re-evaluation of the ethical issues involved in nursing care in general. Such an ambitious aim may be concealed by the specific context of the discussion, but it is a topic of considerable significance. In Japan, awareness of these issues is growing, and studies that advance our understanding of the ethical challenges related to cultural differences in nursing are expected in the future.

Next, proposals to foster ethical practice in actual nursing care must be considered. To this end, a foundation of universal consensus is needed, and the authors of this paper propose the following three-step process: 1) affirmation of the importance of human rights, 2) attaining consensus on basic principles, and 3) applying principles to individual situations. Putting these processes into practice will be a future challenge.

A foundation of general ethical principles for nursing care may be attained by expanding on past consensus-building processes. Developing a consensus for a highly specific field such as the nursing care of elderly patients would be a significant achievement. Prior work to build international consensus regarding the ethics of cutting-edge medical research may serve as a model for this effort. While the example may be valid, its practical application will likely be difficult.

More than being a field of cutting-edge medical technology, the care of the elderly involves daily nursing tasks and confronting significant cultural issues. Attaining international agreement on ethical issues such as *in vitro* fertilization, surrogate pregnancy, abortion, and euthanasia has been difficult, and similar challenges can be expected in the field of nursing as well. Ethical considerations will likely first be considered at the level of individual countries and national coalitions. Consensus and discussion with countries providing large numbers of nurses will be especially important.

Of the consensus-building processes offered here, the third stage is perhaps the most consequential and significant. Real-world application of ethical principles with simultaneous feedback will be essential. Foreign nurses have a wealth of real-world experience confronting these issues, but they may have few opportunities to voice their knowledge and opinions. It is therefore essential that we emphasize the importance of their role and the value of their real-world experience as we work toward building ethical foundations in the nursing care of the elderly.

18.5

Commentary

On Universal and Particular: Guidance Seeking via Human Rights and Ethics Facilitating

Michael C. Brannigan

In their fine inquiry into establishing a moral basis for a global long-term ethic, particularly with respect to the substantively increasing rate of dementia among elderly, Professors Hope and Dunn nicely situate the conundrum of situational immanence and the possibility of principled transcendence. Their work deserves applause on various levels and constitutes a rich step forward in intercultural bioethical discourse. My own offering remains modest and will be in three parts. I will first acknowledge their account's more singular contributions; second, more closely examine the problematic regarding human rights as their proposed model of universal consensus; and third, further unpack questions surrounding the suggested role of ethics facilitating.

Of the many merits in their report, here are some of the more substantive. 1) In asserting the need for international discourse and dialogue while recognizing limits, they wisely broaden the matter of "health" beyond traditional biomedical models, underscoring the critical role of community support. At the same time, while we may often erroneously confuse "community" and "public," their insights prod us to explore more closely what may comprise elements of genuine community. 2) They sensibly steer our focus away from headline media topics, such as the penumbra of end-of-life questions, to the ordinary, day-to-day concerns that constitute the more prevailing and real matter of morality and ethics. Implicit in these day-to-day issues are those abidingly deep questions regarding, for instance, intergenerational justice and resource allocation on numerous micro levels. They do this while providing solid examples of conflicts regarding the scope of liberty rights, privacy, prior wishes, and truthful disclosure. 3) In view of the context of globalization, attendant with globalization's conceptual, pragmatic, and moral disquiet, their study provides further urgency to more critically inspect the prevailing though less examined rubric of "cultural competency."[3] 4) Professors Hope and Dunn prudently caution us against

---

[3] My most recent work addresses this more closely (Brannigan 2012a). Here, I argue that cultivating a "virtue of presence," presence in an embodied, interpersonal sense, is a necessary condition for genuine cultural competency.

reifying moral principles, instead urging us to consider them operative within specific cultural contexts. In doing so, they rightly ask whether such principles can be internationalized. 5) Finally, their "call to arms" entails sustained reasonable discourse, transparency, and sound, open debate.

The heart of my commentary will now more address two related issues, allied in that they share the generic theme of *guidance seeking*. On a universal level, this guidance seeking resorts to the notion of "human rights" as a likely ground for a global moral standard. On a particular level, guidance seeking utilizes a model of ethics facilitation as a more useful, unbiased approach toward consensus over moral conflicts.

In the matter of human rights

First, consider further what the authors refer to as a "pre-existing consensus on human rights." My principal question is: *Is there one?* If so, what is the nature of this consensus? To what degree does such consensus exist? How applicable is this consensus? More importantly, who reached this consensus, under what terms, and how? In highlighting human rights, Professors Hope and Dunn rightly call for international discussion and cooperation. However, does international cooperation necessarily presume international consensus? Two sub-issues unavoidably seep into the question: What do we mean by "consensus"? Tristram Engelhardt notes at least four types of consensus: as "authorizing," "hypothetical," "procedural," and "outcome" (Engelhardt 2006: 7). And when does "international" translate into "universal"?

In the authors' quoting Article 22 in the Universal Declaration of Human Rights, we read: "Everyone…has the right to social security and is entitled to realization…of the economic, social and cultural rights *indispensable for his dignity*" (italics added). While "human dignity" intuitively finds favor, appeals to human dignity open a wide door to discretionary interpretation. For example, are there limits to alleged medical enhancements, and, if so, where do we draw lines between medical and nonmedical? Does "human dignity" assume diverse meanings contingent upon contexts that tend to be, without overgeneralizing, more individualistic or more collective in disposition? That is, there inescapably appear to be fundamental ontological bearings regarding what we think of as constituting "human dignity." If so, then what relationship exists between matters of human dignity and nuanced versions of autonomy, self-determination resting on various notions of "self"?

Given the historical origins and unfolding of the Universal Declaration of Human Rights, how would the application of universal human rights as a basis for guidance seeking attend to the perennial friction between individual self-determination (personal autonomy) and state self-determination (state autonomy or sovereignty)? Again, on what grounds can we claim a "pre-existing consensus on human rights"?

Consider more closely this historical context (Ishay 2008: 211–43).[4] To begin with, recall the strident protest from less powerful countries in Latin America and elsewhere against the very idea of a "United Nations" and who felt that their sovereignty would be

---

[4] Micheline R. Ishay offers a thorough and insightful account in Ishay 2008.

threatened by the apparent hegemony and disproportionate reach of the more powerful states.[5] This protest in effect led to stronger emphasis upon human rights within the new international initiative. Nonetheless, underscoring universal human rights and dignity while at the same time prohibiting international intervention in member countries' domestic jurisdiction provided grounds for ongoing debate.

No doubt, the language of the Declaration appears universal, the consequence of various intellectual voices like Benedetto Croce, Mahatma Gandhi, Teilhard de Chardin, and Quincy Wright speaking on behalf of major philosophical and religious traditions. Nonetheless, friction as to whether human rights emphasize more individualistic or collective autonomy, and fears from nations like Poland, Czechoslovakia, South Africa, Saudi Arabia, and the former Soviet Union that individual self-determination rightly underscored considering the brutality of the Holocaust as the historical lynchpin for protection against further human rights abuses, may preempt national sovereignty eventually led to the two distinct human rights covenants in 1976: The International Covenant on Civil and Political Rights, and The International Covenant on Economic, Social and Cultural Rights (Ishay 2008: 223–4). Despite such effort to resolve this friction through forming these separate covenants, human rights scholar Micheline R. Ishay sharply describes this abiding tension:

While the architects of the United Nations certainly intended to create a venue that would peacefully resolve existing conflicts between nations and groups, its very structure, including its human rights mechanisms, excludes attention to the human rights violations of the major powers, which remain in critical instances protected by the veto privilege of the Security Council. The UN's guiding principle of national sovereignty would also limit its capacity to protect human rights. (Ishay 2008: 242–3)

In the matter of ethics facilitation

As for guidance seeking on more individual, micro levels, the authors suggest ethics facilitation as a more effective model to reach consensus regarding moral conflicts. As a start, in view of their fair-minded encouragement of a grassroots "bottom-up" process as a global ground to negotiate complex moral conflicts in long-term care settings, just how different is this approach, at least in principle, from the traditional model in hospital ethics committees and consultations? In my extensive experience working with and consulting hospital ethics committees, similar concerns also exist regarding institutional, civic, state, governmental, and legal parameters, part of which has brought about requirements to address issues in organizational ethics. As it now stands, ethics committees in the US face the daunting challenge of incorporating organizational ethics as well as cultural competency components to fulfill Joint Commission on Accreditation of Healthcare Organizations (JCAHO) standards. And though committee members either volunteer or are appointed, there continues to be an emphasis on both bottom-up and

---

[5] I more generically discuss this in my *Times Union* ethics column (Brannigan 2012b).

top-down direction with respect to ethics committees' three primary purviews: education, case review and consultation, and policy review.

The authors then go on to recommend that an ethics facilitator operate to facilitate discussion and resolution of moral conflict in the long-term care setting. At the same time, they stress that the facilitator's role is "different from that of the clinical ethics committee member or the ethics consultant." While agreeably distinct from an ethics committee member, particularly since members tend to represent assorted health-care sectors (medical, nursing, social work, psychiatry, clergy, lay representatives, etc.), it is less clear how the ethics facilitator is distinct from an ethics consultant, or even the committee "ethicist" (a term I continue to find problematic; Brannigan 1996: 206–18). It would help to more precisely delineate this distinction between ethics facilitating and ethics consulting. For instance, does this suggest that the ethics facilitator, given his or her background and training in ethics, its deliberative process, and its aim of seeking some degree of resolution, can, and more importantly *should,* maintain neutrality in the role of facilitator?

This somewhat resembles the ongoing dispute in the US as to whether there is, in substance, any clear difference between ethics consultation and ethics mediation. This concern is distinct from yet still related to questions establishing what constitutes sufficient skills in ethics. Though the American Society of Bioethics and Humanities (ASBH) has put forth a set of core competencies in ethics consultation, with increasing number of ethics programs awarding potentially premature certification in ethics training, the problem becomes rather intense. While this essay is not the appropriate forum to address this latter concern, the above analogy of bioethics mediation merits extended comment. Bear in mind, however, that one requirement for bioethics mediation not emphasized in ethics facilitation lies in familiarity with health-care law.

Bioethics mediation is not proposed in opposition to traditional bioethics consultation, but as complementary, contingent upon the issues that need to be addressed. There are, in other words, situations in which mediation is inappropriate and consultation necessary, particularly when no agreement can be reached or when clear legal rulings and/or ethical principles apply. Mediation seems more suitable over matters regarding, for instance, communication breakdown among health providers themselves, as well as between health providers, patients, and family members. In these sorts of cases, various options may not be clearly laid out for patients and family members, and there may appear to be some reluctance or inability to communicate more directly and openly with patients and family.

In similar fashion, ethics facilitation, as distinct from ethics consultation, may also make good sense if it is a matter of facilitating communication, communicative issues being the primary concern, rather than conflicting ethical principles and values. As we see in Hope and Dunn's disclosure example, among others, this case represents clear conflict among certain ethical principles as a sufficient ground for what ought to be done. Just as clear-cut ethical conflict is less appropriate for bioethics mediation, such conflict may not be fitting turf for ethics facilitation *if* facilitating, as distinct from consulting, requires neutrality.

Ardent proponents of bioethics mediation as an alternative to consultation, Nancy Dubler and Carol Liebman, nicely articulate its aims. Nonetheless, a vital feature is that whatever consensus is reached, it still must be grounded on a "principled resolution," which they describe as "compatible with the principles of bioethics and the legal rights of patients and families" (Dubler and Liebman 2004: 10). They explain further:

A principled resolution is a plan that falls within clearly accepted ethical principles, legal stipulations, and moral rules defined by ethical discourse, legislatures, and courts and that facilitates a clear plan for future intervention. (Dubler and Liebman 2004: 11)

Dubler and Liebman also acknowledge limitations to mediation and situations whereby mediation simply does not succeed. Along these lines, it would help in further clarifying the meaning and scope of ethics facilitation in asking the authors whether there may be situations in which proposed facilitation may also not succeed and why not.

While mediation aims at some measure of neutrality, the question remains whether this is intended to be the case for ethics facilitators. At the same time, the fact that mediators are often employed by their respective hospitals can easily contribute to marring patients and family members' perspectives regarding mediators' alleged neutrality. Thus, here is a further question to the authors: Along these lines, would ethics facilitators likewise be employed by the long-term care institutions in which they operate? If so, they may surely face the same challenges regarding perceptions of skewed institutional bias. There are, no doubt, benefits of ethics facilitators working as employees, such as their familiarity with the institution, its personnel, physicians, staff, residents, and patterns of practice. Questions will surface regarding a facilitator's impartiality, whether he or she will most likely side with institutional policy, practice, and professionals. If facilitators are to be employed by the institution, how can we address perceptions that the facilitator may be in effect acting as a rubber stamp?

In all this, it becomes more clear that complete neutrality is not possible. Even in the case of bioethics mediation, as Dubler and Liebman point out, the mediator also wears the hat of consultant should legal and/or ethical conflict come to the surface so that, while attempting to be "neutral" they are not, at the same time, "indifferent to the outcome" (Dubler and Liebman 2004: 77). As they put it, "They may and should, whenever appropriate, reformulate the options to satisfy the needs and the interests of the parties. They must be ever mindful, however, of the rights of the parties and be ready, when appropriate, *to act in support of the rights of patient and family*" (Dubler and Liebman 2004: 77; italics added). In the case of Hope and Dunn's disclosure to a demented, lone-surviving spouse, we still need to sort through these rights. When asked about the whereabouts of a deceased spouse, should the truth be given when conveying the truth brings about heavy anxiety and anguish, only to be forgotten later, so that the question will resurface? Here, there are clearly at least two moral principles at stake: telling the truth and minimizing harm. Herein lies the question regarding to what degree the ethics facilitator ought to be and/or can be neutral, if that is the facilitator's distinguishing quality. If the ethics facilitator aims at both enabling discussion and arriving at some resolution among parties through a set of ethics tools, there will eventually need to be some prioritization of these two principles. Depending upon the circumstance, one will trump the other, either truth telling or alleviating harm. The setting forth of the ethics tools, applying them, and facilitating the discussion in such a manner as to bring about prioritization in order to reach resolution requires more from the ethics facilitator than simply acting as facilitator. As the authors point out, the facilitator's role is to identify the moral issue(s), help sort out morally relevant facts, apply appropriate theory and principles, communicate all this to parties involved, and apply ethical tools of analysis. That is, the facilitator naturally also assumes the role of guide through this complex terrain. The guidance itself assumes the privileged position of going beyond a simple, neutral, and distanced role. Again, just what makes the facilitator's role distinct from the consultant's?

Here is one last related point, one which, though seemingly minor, carries ripple effects which merit extended research and analysis. Though there is little room for such in this essay, here is a starting point. Unpacking the role of ethics facilitator is all the more pressing in view of group dynamics that are naturally involved in group discussion and in the process of arriving at some recommendation or decision. From my experience in these group processes, there are often nuanced, subtle, and not-so-subtle power plays in process, a typical side effect of group dynamics in decision-making. Certain voices carry more authority than others. Yet the collateral damage can mar what may generally be considered fair process. Even in raising case comparisons, in view of the fact that no two cases are alike, a tyranny of precedence can bring about an *inherited* consensus, rather than a consensus arrived at through hard struggle, especially in the face of conflicting values and beliefs. In light of the ethics facilitator's role and reality along with this tensional subterfuge in group dynamics, reaching consensus as to resolution entails guidance from the trained, and this, in principle, continues to be the guidance sought from the consultant.

To close, I again applaud Professors Hope and Dunn's sterling work that encourages us to more closely examine grounds for the possibility of global discourse and dialogue regarding long-term care. So long as we continue to engage in open, honest, and sensitive dialogue with each other and with other cultures, there is always hope for growth in ways that will help to alleviate the suffering of so many elderly and their families.

References

Brannigan, M. C. (1996). "Designing Ethicists," *Health Care Analysis*, 4:216–18.

Brannigan, M. C. (2012a). *Cultural Fault Lines in Healthcare: Reflections on Cultural Competency*. Lanham, MD: Lexington Books.

Brannigan, M. C. (2012b). "Is There Consensus on Human Rights?" *Times Union*, March 12.

Dubler, N. N., and Liebman, C. B. (2004). *Bioethics Mediation: A Guide to Shaping Shared Solutions*. New York: United Hospital Fund of New York.

Engelhardt, T. H., Jr. (2006). "Global Bioethics: An Introduction to the Collapse of Consensus," in Tristram H. Engelhardt. Jr. (ed.). *Global Bioethics: The Collapse of Consensus*. Salem, MA: M and M Scrivener Press, 1–17.

Ishay, M. R. (2008). *The History of Human Rights: From Ancient Times to the Globalization Era*. Berkeley, CA: University of California Press.

18.6

Response to Commentaries

Michael Dunn and Tony Hope

We would like to thank all four commentators for their engaging perspectives on our chapter. Each of the commentaries connects with one or more of the key arguments that we put forward, and each offers novel insights in understanding the ethical dimensions of long-term care practice across national and transnational settings. There are two distinct themes that mark out the different contributions. The papers by Zhai and Majima develop and substantiate the context in which our arguments are designed to have effect. We begin by reflecting on the richness of the contributions that these two commentators offer for situating our arguments. The papers by Brannigan and Shimazono engage with, and offer a critical reading of, one or more of the three proposals we have put forward for fostering good ethical practice within long-term care settings. Our reflections on these two themes structure our response.

Clarifying the context

As Zhai observes, the ethical issues that arise in the day-to-day practice of long-term care must be situated within a clear understanding of the particular demographic trends and political make-up that give shape to the needs for, and realities of, long-term care in different countries. We could not agree more. Zhai gives a detailed account of the scope of the long-term care challenge in China, highlighting important aspects of the social, cultural, and political landscape in China relevant to the ethics of long-term care practice. In particular, Zhai draws our attention to the fact that Chinese society has endorsed a family-based model of long-term care, but that this model is being challenged by important changes within Chinese society. In particular, rapid increases in life expectancy, the gradual shift from an extended family to nuclear family structure that is accompanying rapid industrialization, and the additional pressures placed on young adults to provide care for parents and grandparents that have resulted from the imposition of the one-child policy in recent years.

For Zhai, these challenges give rise to a set of ethical questions about social justice and the distribution of obligation to provide care and support to an increasingly aged and disabled population. We agree that such questions ought to be exposed to ethical analysis, but they are a different set of questions from those upon which we have focused our attention in the chapter.

In light of our claim that the everyday practice of long-term care gives rise to a range of ethical issues that ought to be central to the ethical dialogue around this topic, we also believe that the insights provided by Zhai illustrate the context-specific difficulties in making sense of, and addressing, these ethical issues. For example, what kinds of processes need to be introduced at the local level in China to enable family members to receive appropriate support in addressing these ethical issues? There will also be clear tensions within a family-based model of long-term care about balancing interests of those family members who receive care against the interests of those family members who provide care. The interests of family carers will often have a place in ethical deliberations around particular kinds of issues in ways that the interests of professional carers will not. On the other hand, the emergence of community-based and institution-based long-term care services provides an excellent opportunity to facilitate discussions around the ethical principles that ought to be endorsed in such settings, and how these principles ought to be tailored to these new professional care contexts. In addition, the professional workforce that is now developing to meet the ever expanding long-term care needs in China should be situated at the very heart of how these ethical issues are tackled within the new spaces of care work.

Majima's contribution substantiates the context of our arguments in a different way. Rather than exposing the socio-demographic realities in which our 'global call to arms' is being made, Majima hones in on one specific ethical issue that we highlight in the everyday provision of long-term care work: the use of new video surveillance technologies. Majima's careful analysis of the use of such technologies draws attention to the fundamental tension that arises between the competing values of respect for privacy and the prevention of harm when these technologies are used either to monitor a person's actions in his or her home, or to monitor the quality of the care provided to that person.

In contrast to Majima, however, we believe that the resolution of the question of how video surveillance technologies ought to be used is a question that should be addressed within the practical settings of care work, rather than through an argument presented on the pages of a bioethics book. It is unclear to us whether such a decontextualized, philosophically orientated analysis can be tailored appropriately to the different contexts in which these technologies are being deployed such that a correct ethical judgement can be made. It is difficult to ascertain, for example, how the ethical importance of respecting the privacy of an ageing relative should be made sense of within a culture that, as Zhai observes, places a great emphasis on the interests of the family unit as a whole, rather than the interests of the individual. Whilst we commend Majima for putting forward the kind of analysis that ought to be facilitated far more frequently in long-term care settings, this analysis, we believe, cannot be distanced from the practice of care, and the practitioners of care, in such settings.

Transforming policy and practice in long-term care

The argument that ethical issues need to be resolved within practice in order to ensure that ethical principles and values are appropriately tailored to the specific contexts of care work is one that Shimazono strongly supports. He rightly points out that practitioners in long-term care—care assistants and nurses—are equipped with a broad range of real-world experiences that can be drawn upon to shape how ethical judgements in practice ought to be made. The cross-cultural and transnational nature of the long-term care workforce reinforces this claim; it is only likely to be in the specific spaces of particular care work settings that the unique interface between personal, social, cultural, and ethical values will be able to be clarified and negotiated.

For Brannigan, this process of tailoring and translating principles into long-term care practice through the development of novel ethics support mechanisms in situ needs to be given careful thought. We entirely agree with this point, and agree that the relationship between established framework for ethics support in clinical environments and the novel frameworks that we are calling for in the long-term care setting needs to be carefully worked through. The subtle but important distinctions between the role of ethics consultant, ethics facilitator, and ethics mediator to which Brannigan draws attention offer a good starting point for determining the structure and content of ethics support services in long-term care settings. We believe that determining how ethics support is provided in these settings depends fundamentally on clarifying the aims of such support, given the nature of the ethical issues and the unique social, cultural, and organizational tensions that are present in the care home, nursing home, and home-care environments.

We are quite clear that the role of the ethics facilitator—as we perhaps unhelpfully termed this individual—in the long-term care setting is not a neutral role. Thus, like the clinical ethics consultant or ethics committee member, this individual is tasked with supporting the process of making reasoned ethical judgements. The requirement to *support,* rather than *make,* judgements does, however, differentiate the task of the ethics facilitator from that of the consultant. It will be important that the facilitator is well versed in the foundations of ethical analysis and deliberation, but the role of this facilitator is to steer rather than determine the direction of ethical dialogue amongst staff members within the setting. As we emphasized in our chapter, this steering role into and through ethics in practice will have a major pedagogical component. This is because the evidence suggests that there are few long-term care settings in which formal ethics education or training programmes are well established, and a firm institutional footing for ethics in such settings is lacking.

We acknowledge that there will be an enduring tension between the practical goals of resolving the kind of ethical issues that we outlined in our chapter, and engaging staff members in the home in broader ethical and pedagogical goals. This is a tension that we believe ought to be addressed through a formative process of ethics education and support that will develop in situ, and take different forms within different long-term settings as it is tailored to the specific needs, and culture, of the workplace. The use of the word 'facilitator', then, aims to orientate the reader towards a focus on the facilitation of ethical understanding within the ethics support process, rather than as a term that defines the interactions between that individual and the staff within the long-term care environment. Such a role, if successful, will also, we believe, offset Brannigan's concerns about the power dynamics that will be at play in the ethics support process, and the risk that inherited consensus rather than careful reasoning will dictate how ethical issues are weighed up.

The manpower challenges associated with the development of such a process are, as Brannigan correctly observes, significant. We believe that the only feasible way in which such a model would be sustainable would be for the ethics facilitators to be individuals who were employed within the long-term care setting. This does, of course, raise concerns about institutional bias, and this would therefore need to be an issue that was addressed continually within the ethics support process. An additional question that would need to be addressed is how these 'in-house' ethics facilitators acquired the skills in ethics to be able to take on this role.

The model of ethics support we tentatively introduced in our essay does not place communicative issues at the centre of the process—as our use of the terem ethics facilitation would suggest it might—but this is not to deny that communication challenges will not be closely intertwined with the process of resolving the ethical issues that arise in the long-term care setting. Quite clearly, there will be challenges in communicating with residents and their family members about the difficult decisions that need to be made. These challenges may be exacerbated by the fact that the nature of the care provided relates closely to the provision of support within families, and therefore that family members may feel that their voice ought to be accorded extra weight. Our point here is that, whilst the ethics facilitation process might highlight such communicative issues in the decision-making process, the forum in which these issues are addressed ought to engage with communication challenges only in the sense that these challenges are judged to be relevant to determining the ethically right course of action, rather than because this forum has been established to do so.

We would also not support a shift from viewing this process as one of mediation. The clear-cut ethical conflict that defines much of the moral landscape of the long-term care setting, and the poor development of medical law outside the clinical setting, means that a definitive resolution of ethical issues will not be feasible. Again, this resists shifting the emphasis of the ethics support process from ethics to communication, and avoids moving to a neutral position with regards to the issues identified within the process.

Brannigan's second main concern focuses not on the practice of ethics support, but on the feasibility of drawing on human rights discourse to establish minimum standards in long-term care. Brannigan makes two separate points here that deserve a response. First, he observes that our claim about a pre-existing consensus on human rights is open to question, and argues that international cooperation does not presume consensus. Second, he interrogates the conceptual foundations upon which the relevant Articles of the Universal Declaration of Human Rights that we cite in out chapter are built, and links this point into his first by showing how competing interpretations of the conceptual basis of human rights are likely to divide people who hold different values.

We share Brannigan's concerns here, but must emphasize that we are endorsing only a limited role for human rights in international dialogue about the ethics of long-term care. We argue for a human rights-based approach to eradicating the most basic abuses of people receiving long-term care. Human rights, we believe, can provide the most effective theoretical underpinning of actions taken to prevent these abuses. A lack of universal consensus around the specific components of human rights laws or international declarations does not detract from the fact that human rights form a common language on the world stage, and are publicly endorsed by member countries of the United Nations.

Further, whilst there may be culturally determined disagreements about the values and concepts that make up human rights-based claims, we are confident that such disagreements do not extend to the issue that we are seeking to address here. No competing claims about human dignity as individualistic or collective, for example, will impact on an argument about the wrongness of the physical, sexual, psychological, and material abuse, or negligent care, provided to vulnerable adults receiving care in the long-term care setting. Such concerns will of course undermine attempts to adopt a human rights framework to address the ethical issues in long-term care that we have identified in our essay, and it is for this precise reason that we have limited our application of this framework to establishing the basic minimum standards of acceptable care. If Brannigan's concerns were such that human rights could not function to undergird action to prevent such abuses, then it is likely that transnational laws and policies relating to human rights would not have stood the test of time.

In conclusion, we wish to reinforce the point that our aim in the chapter was to set in motion a long-term process of developing a practical and theoretical framework within which the ethics of long-term care practice could flourish. We believe that the three-pronged structure of this framework: i) preventing abuse and other care practices that are wrong, ii) establishing the appropriate standards of care, and iii) enabling difficult decisions to be made, can substantiate a strategy for making progress at the local, national, and international scales. Clearly there is a great deal more theoretical and practical work to be undertaken for this framework to gain traction and to become established. We thank all of our commentators for continuing this work, and for signposting directions for future inquiry.

SECTION D

Rethinking Medical Professionalism

19.1

Primary Topic Article

A Virtue Ethics Analysis of Disclosure Requirements and Financial Incentives as Responses to Conflicts of Interest in Physician Prescribing

Justin Oakley

The pervasive and sometimes corrosive influence of the pharmaceutical industry on the prescribing behaviour of physicians raises significant ethical concerns about medical conflicts of interest. In response to these concerns, many bioethicists and policymakers have argued for greater disclosure requirements, such as public reporting of physician–industry relationships and industry-sponsored educational events. These sorts of transparency measures have now been implemented in a number of countries. These requirements offer a promising way to help curb certain professional vices, such as dishonesty and disrespect for patient autonomy, which can be exhibited by physicians in conflict of interest situations. However, a number of bioethicists have pointed to various shortcomings of increased disclosure requirements as an adequate solution to medical conflicts of interest, even where the information physicians are required to disclose about their industry relationships is very detailed and specific. In response to such deficiencies, some policymakers have proposed that physicians should be offered financial incentives to overcome industry bias in their prescribing decisions, but such proposals raise further ethical concerns about the impact of such incentives on doctor–patient relationships.

In this paper I argue that virtue ethics provides a deeper and more compelling analysis of the ethical problems raised by conflicts of interest in physician prescribing than do other ethical perspectives. I argue that disclosure requirements fail to address specifically medical vices, such as physician maleficence and betrayal, which are shown when physicians' industry ties lead them to engage in harmful prescribing behaviour, or to redefine their therapeutic relationships with patients as business relationships. I also evaluate proposals to use financial incentives for physicians to avoid biased prescribing, and I indicate how such an analysis can also help with the development of a virtue ethics model for regulatory interventions more generally. I do not here aim to provide a fully developed virtue ethics regulatory model, but rather to highlight a moral cost to the use of financial incentives here that, although justifiable in terms of utilitarian cost-effectiveness grounds, is a moral cost that on a virtue ethics approach to policy should not be paid in efforts to improve health outcomes.

1   Disclosure requirements as a response to conflicts of interest in physician prescribing

Physicians' interactions with the pharmaceutical industry range from receiving subsidized conference travel, entertainment, and other forms of hospitality, to being paid lucrative consulting fees, and owning shares in pharmaceutical companies. A comprehensive literature review concluded that many types of physician interactions with industry (including receipt of gifts, free meals, and honoraria) were associated with a greater likelihood of the clinician prescribing one of the company's products (Wazana 2000; see also Brennan et al. 2006: 431; Weber 2006, Devi 2011). Nearly one in five respondents to a survey of US obstetricians and gynecologists reported that they had a personal financial interest in a pharmaceutical or medical device company (Morgan et al. 2006: 561). And 'as many as 59% of the authors of clinical guidelines endorsed by many [US] professional associations have had financial relationships with companies whose drugs might be affected by those guidelines' (Blumenthal 2004: 1886). These problems can be magnified for clinicians working with the chronically ill, where there is likely to be an ongoing demand for the product, and the medical devices which are used extensively in this context tend to be less stringently regulated than are pharmaceuticals. And there is growing evidence that patients are becoming concerned about their doctors' relationships with industry (Edwards and Ballantyne 2009).

In response to these problems, many policymakers and bioethicists have argued for increasing physician disclosure requirements, such as public reporting of various physician–industry links (see e.g. Kassirer 2005). For example, the US Institute of Medicine's widely cited 2009 report *Conflicts of Interest in Medical Research Education, and Practice* recommended (3.4) that Congress require all payments to physicians and medical associations by pharmaceutical and medical device companies to be reported on a searchable public website (Lo and Field 2009: 94). These sorts of proposals are now being adopted. For example, the US Cleveland Clinic introduced a policy in December 2008 requiring their physicians to name on their websites any pharmaceutical companies from which they receive annual consulting fees of US$5,000 or more, and similar policies have subsequently been introduced by a number of other US clinics (Steinbrook 2009). The *Physician Payments Sunshine Act 2010,* enacted as part of President Obama's health reforms, requires details of all industry payments to US physicians to be collected and reported on a public website, scheduled to be launched in 2014. In Australia, the pharmaceutical industry body Medicines Australia introduced a Code of Conduct requiring companies to provide details of their sponsorship of medical events and associated hospitality, and these details are publicly available on Medicines Australia's website (http://medicinesaustralia.com.au/code-of-conduct/education-events-reports/member-company-reports/). These new industry–physician disclosure requirements reflect broader moves towards greater transparency and accountability in health care. For instance, mortality rates of individual cardiac surgeons have now been publicly available in the UK and some US states for a number of years (see Clarke and Oakley 2007).

These disclosure requirements can clearly be supported on grounds of informed consent and respect for patient autonomy, insofar as patients find their physicians' industry ties material to their decisions about taking prescribed medications. From a virtue ethics perspective, these sorts of disclosure requirements can also be seen as justified insofar as they help doctors to act in accordance with the virtue of honesty, which is important for respecting patient autonomy, and is a virtue for all professionals. These disclosure requirements therefore also offer some hope of curbing certain professional vices such as dishonesty, which can be exhibited by doctors in conflict of interest situations.

However, despite their merits, evidence is emerging that these sorts of disclosure requirements may not be very effective at curbing inappropriate prescribing due to industry influence (see Rodwin 2011: 215–19; Pham-Kanter, Alexander, and Nair 2012). For the effectiveness of such disclosure requirements is too reliant on patients reacting to such disclosures in certain ways, and such requirements in any case shift the burden of responsibility for overcoming such influences from physicians to patients. To begin with, it may be naïve for policymakers to assume that patients will check their physicians' websites. Further, patients who read their physicians' disclosures of industry relationships may not react to such disclosures in the ways that policymakers may expect them to. There are a range of factors that often make it difficult for receivers of such disclosed information to appropriately adjust their beliefs and actions in light of this information. One factor is the undue weight often given by people to decision-making 'anchors', such as a doctor's manner or other personal characteristics: 'Research on judgment suggests that the starting point in a judgmental process often holds undue sway over the eventual judgment, even when the anchors are known to be utterly irrelevant' (Cain, Loewenstein, and Moore 2005: 109). Thus, for instance, a Cleveland Clinic patient who learns through the clinic website about their physician's industry links may place more weight on their physician's appearance than they might on those links, in considering their physician's recommendations about what medication is appropriate for them. Furthermore, even when patients do have concerns about undue industry influence on their physician's prescribing, many patients are likely to be reluctant to query their physician about this. And in any case, patients are often ill equipped to judge for themselves which medication is best for them. Thus, more stringent disclosure requirements may not be very effective in achieving their aim of preventing biased prescribing decisions, given the reliance of such interventions on patients overcoming their likely reticence about such matters in the clinical setting. Indeed, Cain, Loewenstein, and Moore (2005) argue that greater disclosure requirements can sometimes be counterproductive, insofar as they can encourage a misplaced additional confidence in the trustworthiness of the person who is disclosing the information (see also Lowenstein, Sah, and Cain 2012). So these disclosure requirements may well fall short of fulfilling their intended goals.

But along with these practical problems, there are also theoretical concerns about the ethical adequacy of preventing biased physician prescribing by introducing greater disclosure requirements. Whatever effects more stringent disclosure requirements might be shown to have on physician prescribing behaviour, many commentators acknowledge that such requirements in any case fail to address the core ethical problem raised by medical conflicts of interest—that is, undue influence, rather than secrecy (Rodwin 1989, 1993, 2011; Elliott 2009; Lo and Field 2009). A conflict of interest is commonly defined as follows: P has a conflict of interest if and only if: (i) P is in a relationship with Q, requiring P to exercise judgement on Q's behalf; and (ii) P has an interest tending to interfere with the proper exercise of judgement in that relationship (Davis 1998). Thus, conflicts of interest lead to unethical behaviour when a physician is influenced unduly by an interest which undermines appropriate clinical decision-making in that context. And providing patients with more and more information in the hope of their making more informed decisions about their physician's prescribing behaviour is not an ethically adequate way of dealing with medical conflicts of interest, as such transparency measures fail to address the priorities that should be guiding physicians' prescribing decisions in the first place.

Virtue ethics evaluates decisions and actions according to the dispositions guiding the agents in question, and since the core ethical problem with conflicts of interest concerns the appropriateness of the interest *influencing* or *guiding* one's decisions and actions, virtue ethics seems to offer a particularly promising approach to analysing and addressing the problems here. That is, in judging someone's action as wrong in a conflict of interest situation, we are essentially concerned with what interest *guided* the person to perform this action, and the ethical acceptability or otherwise of this influence is determined by reference to what interest should, according to the proper goals of this person's role, be guiding them in this context (see Oakley and Cocking 2001). Thus, a central question here would be: What sort of person do doctors show themselves to be when they prescribe drugs on the basis of self-interest, rather than according to the best interests of patients? In allowing pharmaceutical gifts and shares to influence their prescribing in such ways, doctors seem to be redefining themselves and their roles. It is important to note that there is a difference between doctors exhibiting vices *qua professionals* and doctors exhibiting vices *qua doctors*. Certain virtues and vices in the professional lives of doctors have a special moral status, because these virtues and vices are directly connected with the proper goals of the medical profession (which the community has entrusted doctors to serve), and its distinctive brief, in the first place. While greater disclosure requirements may help doctors act in accordance with the virtues of honesty or truthfulness, these are *generic* professional virtues, rather than specifically *medical* virtues. We have seen that the vices of dishonesty and secrecy are not the core wrongs in conflicts of interest. Thus, disclosure requirements fail to *directly* address the causes of medical harm, medically corrupt relationships, and specifically medical vices.

Suppose a physician prescribes a drug because it is manufactured by a company in which they have shares. Where this drug does not result in foreseeable harm to patients, the physician is exhibiting the vice of *medical corruption,* because s/he is redefining a therapeutic relationship as a business relationship. But where this drug does result in foreseeable *harm* to patients, the doctor is exhibiting the vices of both *maleficence* and *medical corruption.* Unlike generic *professional* vices (such as dishonesty), maleficence and medical corruption are specifically *medical* vices, as they involve dispositions that run contrary to the distinctive ethical core of medicine. By contrast, a *virtuous* physician would be guided in their prescribing decisions by the virtue of medical *beneficence*, which involves a disposition to act in their patient's best interests. A virtuous physician would also have the virtue of trustworthiness, in that they are committed to having a therapeutic relationship with their patients. Unlike dishonesty and failures to respect patient or client autonomy, which violate generic ethical constraints applying to all professionals, maleficence and betrayal by physicians are deeper (and typically more serious) medical vices because they involve dispositions which run contrary to the proper goals of medicine.

Our evaluations of whether a professional has behaved in a morally acceptable way often depend not so much on whether welfare was maximized, or whether people's rights were upheld, but on an appeal (implicitly or explicitly) to some proper professional goal. For example, a doctor who takes 'personal wealth maximization' as their overarching governing condition in their relationships with patients has transformed the therapeutic nature of the doctor–patient relationship, and acts contrary to what professional integrity demands here. So, while greater disclosure requirements in medical conflicts of interest may help doctors to have a generic integrity in their professional role, which is to be expected of all professionals, these measures do not help doctors to act with professional integrity *qua doctors*. These vices are shown when physicians are influenced by their industry links to engage in harmful prescribing behaviour, or to *redefine* their therapeutic relationships with patients as business relationships.

2 The use of financial incentives to improve physician prescribing behaviour

Another approach which has been used to modify physicians' decision-making is the provision of various kinds of incentives. Financial incentives have been used by US government organizations, hospitals, and Health Maintenance Organizations (HMOs) to influence physician behaviour since the early 1980s. Initially such incentives were used to discourage over-servicing and to encourage frugality in physicians' clinical decision-making, in order to better utilize Medicare and Medicaid resources, or to increase the profitability of HMOs (Rodwin 1996). More recently, however, financial incentives have been offered to physicians to promote their patients' best interests by providing high-quality care—for example, in so-called 'pay-for-performance' schemes (see Rodwin 2011: 16–20), and in encouraging physicians to perform more regular preventative tests, such as pap smears. The apparent effectiveness of financial incentives in these contexts (see e.g. Campbell et al. 2007) could be seen by policymakers as a reason to provide physicians with such incentives to give greater priority to their patients' best interests in their prescribing decisions. Financial incentives could therefore appear to be a more promising way of countering pharmaceutical company influences on physician prescribing than are disclosure requirements, no matter how stringent such requirements are.

If financial incentives were found to be a cost-effective way of improving doctors' prescribing behaviour, then utilitarian approaches to regulation would presumably endorse such interventions here. However, Marc Rodwin (1996) and others have argued that using financial incentives to modify doctors' clinical decision-making can undermine professionalism and distort the overall orientation of doctor–patient relationships towards patients' best interests. Financial incentives also raise concerns about distorting doctors' values away from patient care and towards, in effect, doctors' own self-interest. These sorts of considerations are crucial for a virtue ethics analysis of such regulatory interventions in medical practice.

However, the development of virtue ethics approaches to evaluating regulatory interventions have faced obstacles which have often been thought insurmountable, because it has been assumed that such approaches rely on detecting the motives of the agents involved, yet those motives will not usually be apparent. For example, the 2009 US Institute of Medicine Report on medical conflicts of interests argues that policies in this area cannot investigate physicians' motives:

conflict of interest policies…do not focus on the motives in a particular case. First, reliably ascertaining or inferring motives in this context is usually impossible for those assessing whether a relationship constitutes a conflict of interest. Generally, medical research, patient care, and education involve multiple considerations and many small judgments and decisions that are impractical to review; and even if they were reviewed, they would likely not yield a clear picture of the underlying motivation…The motives behind institutional decisions are usually even more opaque. Second, any thorough effort to determine motivation in a particular case would be improperly intrusive and highly time-consuming. (Lo and Field 2009: 50–1)

This report then argues that regulatory interventions into conflicts of interest should instead focus on situational factors, such as removing circumstances where other interests might tempt doctors away from the primary interest they ought to have in serving their patients' health.

Some philosophers have suggested that a virtue ethics regulatory model is best developed by focusing on the motives and character traits exhibited by *regulators* or *legislators* themselves, when supporting a certain policy of legislative intervention, rather than the motives of individual agents (see Slote 2001: 100–3). Such an approach may lead to fruitful avenues for further research. However, the virtue ethics regulatory model I am proposing here considers what sort of person *those who are regulated* show themselves to be when they comply with or resist a particular regulatory intervention, such as attempts by policymakers to influence physicians' prescribing behaviour by providing them with financial or other incentives for prescribing in patients' best interests.

The above concerns about the inaccessibility of physicians' motives do not entail that regulators cannot realistically take into account any considerations regarding physicians' characters. A physician's character is shown not only by their *motives,* but also by what they are disposed to *prioritize* in their clinical decision-making, and the governing conditions that those priorities express. For instance, a doctor who regularly places their own financial interests ahead of their patients' best interests in their drug prescribing decisions clearly shows themselves to be more self-interested in such contexts than does a doctor whose priorities in such contexts are the reverse of this (even if the latter's underlying motivation in being a medical practitioner at all is largely because of its financial rewards). So another way of developing a virtue ethics model for regulation is to focus on the impact of a particular regulatory intervention on a practitioner's *priorities* and governing conditions, and on whether the intervention in question shifts those governing conditions away from what the practitioner has been entrusted by the community to take on. For in return for being granted a monopoly of expertise on the provision of key goods, doctors are expected not only to act in certain ways, but also to have certain professional character traits—to be guided by a disposition to serve their patients' best interests, and so to prioritize patient welfare in their decisions. Doctors made commitments when joining the profession to have a professional character of a certain sort, and to maintain therapeutic rather than commercial relationships with patients.

Thus, in evaluating certain regulatory interventions into physician prescribing behaviour, we can investigate the impact which those regulatory initiatives aimed at improving patient outcomes in conflict of interest (and other) situations have had on doctors' prioritizing of patients' best interests over other considerations in their prescribing decisions. Particular attention needs to be paid here to studies indicating changes in clinical practice due to such interventions, along with studies canvassing explanations of how such interventions seem to operate in altering doctors' decisions (see e.g. Lindenauer et al. 2007). If many doctors appear to place their industry ties second to patients' interests only when given financial incentives by government to do so, this raises questions about the compatibility of financial incentives and exemplifying professional virtue. What sort of character is demonstrated by a doctor who prioritizes their patients' best interests in prescribing decisions only when given a financial incentive to do so? How could such a disposition exemplify *professional* virtue? Behavioural change in doctors, and patients receiving better medication, should not be achieved at the cost of redefining the doctor–patient relationship from a therapeutic relationship into a commercial relationship. So, a virtue ethics regulatory model can focus on what the evidence suggests are doctors' reasons for altering their priorities in response to such interventions.

Utilitarians focus on whether a regulatory intervention improves outcomes, while Kantians focus on whether an intervention upholds patients' rights, e.g. to information about their doctors' industry ties. By contrast, the virtue ethics regulatory model proposed here examines the impact of a particular regulatory intervention on the conditions by which physicians govern their prescribing decisions, and whether those conditions would be consistent with the priorities that the community has entrusted medical professionals to have. Physicians betray the community not only when they harm patients or violate their rights, but also when they redefine their therapeutic relationships with patients as business relationships. A virtue ethics approach therefore highlights how certain regulatory responses, such as financial incentives, carry an ethical cost to which utilitarian and Kantian approaches to regulation are blind.

References

Blumenthal, D. (2004). 'Doctors and Drug Companies,' *New England Journal of Medicine*, 351:1885–90.

Brennan, T. A. et al. (2006). 'Health Industry Practices That Create Conflicts of Interest,' *JAMA*, 295:429–33.

Cain, D. M., Loewenstein, G., Moore, D. A. (2005). 'Coming Clean but Playing Dirtier: The Shortcomings of Disclosure as a Solution to Conflicts of Interest,' in Don A. Moore et al. (eds), *Conflicts of Interest: Challenges and Solutions in Business, Law, Medicine, and Public Policy*. Cambridge: Cambridge University Press, 104–25.

Campbell, S. et al. (2007). 'Quality of Primary Care in England with the Introduction of Pay for Performance,' *New England Journal of Medicine*, 357:181–90.

Clarke, S., and Oakley, J. (eds.) (2007). *Informed Consent and Clinician Accountability: The Ethics of Report Cards on Surgeon Performance*. Cambridge: Cambridge University Press.

Davis, M. (1998). 'Conflict of Interest,' *Encyclopedia of Applied Ethics*, Vol. 1, San Diego, CA: Academic Press, 589–95.

Devi, S. (2011). 'US Physicians Urge End to Unnecessary Stent Operations,' *Lancet*, 378:651–2.

Edwards, D., and Ballantyne, A. (2009). 'Patient Awareness and Concern Regarding Pharmaceutical Manufacturer Interaction with Doctors,' *Internal Medicine Journal*, 39:191–6.

Elliott, C. (2009). 'Industry-Funded Bioethics and the Limits of Disclosure,' in Denis G. Arnold (ed), *Ethics and the Business of Biomedicine*. Cambridge: Cambridge University Press, 150–68.

Kassirer, J. P. (2005). *On the Take: How America's Complicity with Big Business Can Endanger Your Health*. New York: Oxford University Press.

Lindenauer, P. K. et al. (2007). 'Public Reporting and Pay-for-Performance in Hospital Quality Improvement,' *New England Journal of Medicine*, 356:486–96.

Lo, B., and Field, M. J. (eds) (2009). *Conflicts of Interest in Medical Research, Education, and Practice*. Washington, DC: National Academies Press.

Lowenstein, G., Sah, S., and Cain, D. M. (2012). 'The Unintended Consequences of Conflicts of Interest Disclosure,' *JAMA*, 307:669–70.

Morgan, M. A. et al. (2006). 'Interactions of Doctors with the Pharmaceutical Industry,' *Journal of Medical Ethics*, 32:559–63.

Oakley, J., and Cocking, D. (2001). *Virtue Ethics and Professional Roles*. Cambridge: Cambridge University Press.

Pham-Kanter, G., Alexander, G. C., and Nair, K. (2012). 'Effect of Physician Payment Sunshine Laws on Prescribing,' *Archives of Internal Medicine*, 172:819–21.

Rodwin, M. A. (1989). 'Physicians' Conflicts of Interest: The Limitations of Disclosure,' *New England Journal of Medicine*, 321:1405–8.

Rodwin, M. A. (1993). *Medicine, Money, and Morals: Physicians' Conflicts of Interest*. New York: Oxford University Press.

Rodwin, M. A. (1996). 'Physicians' Conflicts of Interest in HMOs and Hospitals,' in R. G. Spece, D. S. Shimm, and A. E. Buchanan (eds), *Conflicts of Interest in Clinical Practice and Research*. New York: Oxford University Press, 197–227.

Rodwin, M. A. (2011). *Conflicts of Interest and the Future of Medicine: The United States, France, and Japan*. New York: Oxford University Press.

Slote, M. (2001). *Morals from Motives*. Oxford: Oxford University Press.

Steinbrook, R. (2009). 'Online Disclosure of Physician–industry Relationships,' *New England Journal of Medicine*, 360:325–7.

Wazana, A. (2000). 'Physicians and the Pharmaceutical Industry: Is a Gift Ever Just a Gift?' *JAMA*, 283:373–80.

Weber, L. J. (2006). *Profits before People? Ethical Standards and the Marketing of Prescription Drugs*. Bloomington, IN: Indiana University Press.

19.2

Commentary
Trust and Professionalism: A Perspective on Conflict of Interest Policy

Ilhak Lee

Introduction

Professor Justin Oakley tries to provide evidence for his virtue ethics approach to professional ethics, using the transparency clause to address conflict of interest issues. He argues that we are better in responding to many ethical issues we encounter during our lives. (Or, professionals taking a virtue ethics approach would be better prepared for the issues of professional life.) Professionals, with their professional ideals, are open to taking the professional ideal as their guidance for action ('regulatory ideals'). He also argues that voluntary discipline is preferable to legislative enforcement: he regards a justification in terms of virtue ethics as better than those in utilitarian or Kantian terms.

Regulative ideals and professional ethics

To evaluate Oakley's argument, it is necessary to reflect on his claim about the legitimacy of virtue ethics, especially the concept of 'regulatory ideals', and its relationship with the role of professionals and the aims of medicine (Oakley and Cocking 2004: 25–31). A regulative ideal is 'an internalised normative disposition to direct one's actions and alter one's motivation in certain ways' (Oakley and Cocking 2004: 25). For particular activities, this regulatory ideal guides the agent to perform specific actions. In medical practice this relationship is easily observed: 'it may be thought part of being a good medical practitioner that one has internalised a conception of what the appropriate ends of medicine are, and one is disposed to treat one's patients in ways which are consistent with those ends' (Oakley and Cocking 2004: 26).

Naturally one can ask how an ideal can bring about action, and here Professor Oakley answers:

having a particular virtuous disposition requires internalising a certain normative standard of excellence, in such a way that one is able to adjust one's motivation and conduct so that it conforms or at least does not conflict with that standard. (Oakley and Cocking 2004: 28)

For virtue ethicists, the aim of an institution is crucial to defining its standards of ethical analysis. Oakley presents the aim of medical professionals in the following way:

a good professional...is one which involves a commitment to a key human good, a good which plays a crucial role in enabling us to live a humanly flourishing life.

...health as the central goal of medicine...given a general practitioner's concern with the broad health needs of their patients/the GP's role within medicine would seem to count as a good professional role. (Oakley and Cocking 2004: 74)

Virtue ethics in conflict of interest policy

Professor Oakley's argument for conflict of interest (COI) management emphasizes professional self-regulation rather than enforcement of legal clauses, such as transparency clauses. His argument can be summarized as follows. In regulating COI, disclosure and transparency are required as measures to inform the patient, who can decide autonomously with sufficient information and freedom of choice (in terms of access to health care and lack of coercive influence). This method of managing COI is, however, based on the false belief that rational consumers of medicine will drive out improper health-care providers from the market. But since patients may fail for various reasons to use this information in their choice of physician, this requirement of disclosure seems to fail. Medical service is not based on a contract between rational and equal agents, but between people who are sick and people who can potentially cure them—between the needy and the needed—which means that the balance of power is tipped in favor of physicians, especially when they are hard to find. So, rethinking the concept of medical teleology may be an appropriate solution to COI. Medical professionals are highly independent, and their practices are highly personalized and contextual and cannot be standardized. From a policy perspective, physicians may be amenable to persuasion and inducement, but not to coercion. In short, to address this failure of transparency policy, we must develop a kind of policy that will preserve the goals of medicine and renewal of medical teleology. When physicians renew their understanding of their professional ideal, they will (try to) change their prescribing behaviour according to that renewed ideal.

Managing conflict of interest with legislation: the case of South Korea

COI management has become a headache for health-care administrators across the world. As the interdependence between the health-care industry (especially the pharmaceutical industry) and medical professionals becomes closer, concerns have grown about the potential for bias in physicians' clinical (and scientific) judgement. Traditionally, physicians have been seen as advocates for patients, which means their priority should be the welfare of their patients. But financial interests could prevent physicians from acting in this way.

The industry has long been responding to this concern: for example, the Pharmaceutical Manufacturer Association (PhRMA) developed their own code of ethics.[1] There has also been much legislation on this issue, including the US's Physician Payment Sunshine Act, and the UK's 'Blue Book' (UK). Some legal responses take a stricter form, such as Korea's so-called 'dual punishment', which was introduced in the Medical Practice Act of 2010. The newly introduced clause prohibits 'inappropriate financial interests' of medical professionals. It prohibits professionals—on pain of imprisonment[2]—from receiving any benefit (including financial benefits, goods, convenience, human labour, and entertainment) from industry.[3] Even though this clause leaves some exceptions, general application could be very broad. The legislation was regarded as humiliating by physicians, and opposed by medical professional bodies, ultimately without success. This opposition was related to the fact that it had long been customary for medical professionals to receive 'landing fees' or 'rebate (kickback)', which was accepted or at least overlooked. Further, even before this legislation, inappropriate relationships between professionals and industry were regulated by fair competition acts and could be punished as civil misbehaviour.

The humiliating 'dual punishment' legislation was introduced following the failure of earlier efforts to ensure that physicians did not develop inappropriate relationships with industry. Initially, there existed guidelines giving principles and particular action guidance. When this method failed to eradicate inappropriate relationships, legislation listing permissible financial support or sponsored research followed, with the aim of enforcing transparency from the parties involved. However, this was also ineffective.

It may be humiliating for physicians to have their every relationship placed under surveillance. But it is also worthwhile asking why physicians regard benefits from industry as their privilege, or as natural for medical professionals, especially in modern society where medicine is a social institution. This relationship between the pharmaceutical industry and physicians is deeply rooted in the very practice of medicine: it pervades institutional administration, education, self-development, scientific research, and even the dearly held idea of independent but beneficent physicians. Since the relationship is so inherent in medical practice, is it not natural that there should be a close relationship between providers and consumers?

The situation is more complicated than this, however. In addition to their relationship with the pharmaceutical industry, medical practice and institutions are funded by governments or other social finance run in large-scale organizations. As a result, medical practices and institutions are subject to a variety of influences, and the possibility that they may be impeded in performing their proper function as a result should be taken seriously.

Meanwhile, medical professionals are increasingly aware of the unfriendly atmosphere around them. Newcomers to their clinics and laboratories are suspicious of their relationship with old partners. Guidelines, regulations, and provisions have much to say on their, in some sense, very private and privileged relationships. Physicians have failed

---

[1] Code on Interactions With Healthcare Professionals. website: http://www.phrma.org/about/principles-guidelines/code-interactions-healthcare-professionals

[2] Medical Practice Act. 88-2.

[3] Medical Practice Act. 23-2.

to respond sensitively to these concerns, which has eroded society's trust in them, and along with it the funds of national health insurance.

In Korea, the issue of COI management policy has become more of a legal issue than an ethical one. Because physicians in general did not regard COI as a serious issue, the situation became difficult to control without strict enforcement. The concept of the virtuous physician could be useful here, by providing a standard by which to analyse professionally acceptable action. Rather than obsessing over the details of the differences between legally accepted and prohibited action, thinking about professional ideals could be more informative for physicians, and encourage them to consult ethical codes of relationships. In this respect, the following claim by Oakley is relevant:

for virtue ethicist…a doctor's doing X for a patient would be right because doing X is expressive of what the profession of doctoring actually is, considered as an activity which is committed to one important substantive human good (health). (Oakley and Cocking 2004: 114)

Trust rather than health

As we are trying to provide particular guidelines for 'lost' professionals, we should be more particular in our understanding of medicine. The important aspects of the relationship a physician bears to patients are taking responsibility and instilling trust. Professional physicians honour the trust of their patients. This trust is not a result of treatment, but of the 'decisional orientation' toward the well-being of patient that physicians show (Pellegrino and Thomasma 1981: 58–81).

There is a pitfall, however. As mentioned above, modern medicine involves stakeholders other than patients and physicians. Whilst patients and physicians are at the core, funding institutions such as health insurance play a role with reimbursement policies; and there are others to consider, such as the physician's future patients, who will also make demands on resources. Traditionally, it was considered sufficient for physicians to prioritize the best interest of their patients, but their health-care budgets may be unable to meet all the needs of all their patients, meaning that the best interests of each cannot all be prioritized. In such an environment, a call to return to the ideal does not solve the problem, and may add yet another ball to the juggling act that physicians must perform. This is partly because of the unclear, controversial definition of 'health' as ideal. Health seems too abstract for pragmatic analysis. We may need a more specific and particular standard.

If we schematize the medical relationship as responsibility and trust, conforming to the required standards relating to trust could be easier than conforming to an ideal of health. Gathering information about trust would be a more realistic objective than defining health in a manner that all relevant parties would accept, and could yield a more particular standard. It could be argued that the relevant concept of trust presupposes an ideal of health: that a patient's trust in his physician amounts to trust that she will try her best to promote the health of her patients. But the concept of trust has the advantage of figuring in sociological accounts of professionalism. Among the many theories of medical professionalism, social contract theory is persuasive ethically (Reid

2011). If the cornerstone of this contract is mutual trust, trust itself should be the very thing that defines our standards.

Conclusion

COI is a serious threat to medical professionalism. It undermines public trust in medical professionals, and its countermeasures are viewed as invasive and humiliating by those professionals. Effective COI management should work by encouraging professionalism of physicians, rather than by regulation or inducement. But this requires a clearer understanding of relevant medical relationships than has been reflected in attempts at regulating COI to date. We need more particular standards of action, and we could define these by focusing on trust rather than on the theoretical concept of health.

References

Oakley, J., and Cocking, D. (2004). *Virtue Ethics and Professional Roles*. Cambridge: Cambridge University Press.

Pellegrino, E. D., and Thomasma, D. C. (1981). *A Philosophical Basis of Medical Practice: Toward a Philosophy and Ethic of the Healing Professions*. Oxford University Press.

Reid, L. (2011). 'Medical Professionalism and the Social Contract', *Perspectives in Biology and Medicine*, 54(4): 455–69.

19.3

Commentary
Conflicts of Interest: Relationship between Japanese Physicians and the Pharmaceutical Industry

Masatoshi Nara

Conflict of interest is 'a set of conditions in which professional judgment concerning a primary interest (such as patient's welfare or validity of research) tends to be unduly influenced by a secondary interest (such as financial gain)' (Thompson 1993: 573). It often arises from undue relationships that exist between physicians and the pharmaceutical industry. Such relationships have recently received public attention in Japan. I present here an overview of the rules governing pharmaceutical industry–physician relationships in Japan, and argue for a virtue ethics approach to assess this relationship.

Promotional activities by pharmaceutical companies are now regulated by law and pharmaceutical industry practice codes. The Antimonopoly Act and Act Against Unjustifiable Premiums and Misleading Representations prohibit the use of expensive gifts and cash to induce an unfair trade practice.[4] Accordingly, the pharmaceutical industry has promulgated practice codes to limit transactions with health-care professionals. The Fair Competition Code prohibits pharmaceutical companies from offering premiums (i.e. gifts or monetary benefits) as a means to induce an unfair transaction.[5] Furthermore, the Japan Pharmaceutical Manufacturers Association (JPMA) Promotion Code prohibits offering any gift that affects the appropriate use of a drug.[6] Under the JPMA Promotion Code, 'promotion' involves the provision or dissemination by pharmaceutical companies of drug information to health-care professionals in an effort to promote proper drug use. Promotional activities are permitted, including providing drug samples and supporting seminars (i.e. meals and payments in cash for travel expenses).

---

[4] Act on Prohibition of Private Monopolization and Maintenance of Fair Trade (Act No. 54 of 14 April 1947). Act against Unjustifiable Premiums and Misleading Representations (15 May 1962).
[5] The Fair Trade Council of the Ethical Pharmaceutical Drugs Marketing Industry, *Fair Competition Code Concerning Restriction on Premium Offers in the Ethical Pharmaceutical Drugs Marketing Industry* (1 July 1984).
[6] The Japan Pharmaceutical Manufacturers Association, *JPMA Promotion Code for Prescription Drugs* (24 March 1993, revised, 23 May 2008). http://www.jpma.or.jp/english/isuues/practice.html

Pharmaceutical companies are also permitted to offer gifts with a minimal value of approximately 3,000 yen, medical utility items, and cultural courtesy gifts.

Professional medical associations have also expressed concerns over the relationship between physicians and pharmaceutical companies. The *Principles of Medical Ethics* of the Japan Medical Association (JMA) states that it is desirable for physicians to establish a good cooperative relationship with pharmaceutical representatives as this may lead to useful information about new medications. However, it prohibits physicians from giving priority to personal interest.[7] Policymakers have also expressed concern over conflicts of interest that exist in medical research. In 2003, the Ministry of Health, Labor, and Welfare (MHLW) published the *Ethical Guidelines for Clinical Studies,* which stated that research subjects should be informed of conflicts of interest that researchers may have with the pharmaceutical industry.[8] Furthermore, the Ministry of Education, Culture, Sports, Science, and Technology (MEXT) held a panel discussion, calling for the attention of universities, research institutes, hospitals, and academic societies. Such entities were urged to implement their own policies to manage conflicts of interest in medical research. In 2008, the MHLW published guidelines regarding the management of conflicts of interest for all research funded by them. Policymakers think that a fundamental problem resides in the proper management of conflicts of interest.

Medical societies and pharmaceutical companies introduced new guidelines in 2010 and 2011. For example, the Japanese Society of Internal Medicine (JSIM) developed the *Policy of Conflict of Interest in Clinical Research,*[9] which requires all authors of a manuscript to submit a form disclosing financial relationships with companies that have an interest in the research. If these financial relationships exceed a certain limit, authors are required to disclose detailed information,[10] and this information appears in the published article.

The JPMA also promulgated *Transparency Guideline for the Relation between Corporate Activities and Medical Institutions.*[11] This guideline required pharmaceutical companies to (1) develop their own policies to make their activities with medical institutions and health-care professionals transparent, (2) disclose information regarding the funding provided to such institutions and professionals, and (3) disclose this information on its corporate website.[12] The common feature between JSIM's policy and JPMA's guideline is that both require self-reporting to ensure transparency. The development of such policies and

[7] Japan Medical Association, *Principles of Medical Ethics* (2004, revised, 2008).

[8] The Ministry of Health, Labor, and Welfare, *Ethical Guidelines for Clinical Studies* (Public Notice of the Ministry of Health, Labor, and Welfare No. 255, amended in 2008).

[9] The Japanese Society of Internal Medicine, *Policy of Conflict of Interest in Clinical Research* (12 April 2010). http://www.naika.or.jp/coi/shishin_english.html

[10] Matters of 'interests' and 'limits' are specified below. (1) Employment, leadership position, or advisory roles (1,000,000 yen or more). (2) Stock ownership or options (profit of 1,000,000 yen or more, or ownership of 5 per cent or more of total shares). (3) Patent royalties or licensing fees (1,000,000 yen or more). (4) Honoraria (e.g. lecture fees) (500,000 yen or more). (5) Fees for promotional materials (e.g. manuscript fee) (500,000 yen or more). (6) Research funding (2,000,000 yen or more). (7) Others (e.g. trips, travel, or gifts, which are not related to research) (50,000 yen or more). http://www.naika.or.jp/coi/saisoku_english.html

[11] The Japan Pharmaceutical Manufacturers Association, *Transparency Guideline for the Relation between Corporate Activities and Medical Institutions* (19 January 2011).

[12] Disclosed matters are (1) research and development expenses, (2) academic research support grants, (3) manuscript authorship fees, (4) information provision-related expenses, etc.

guideline was prompted by the increase in industry–academic collaborative research, and the influence of the Physicians Payments Sunshine Act 2010 in the United States.

In Japan, conflicts of interest in clinical practice have attracted less attention compared to that in medical research. This issue has been extensively discussed among policymakers and academic institutions, and information disclosure was adopted as a mechanism to deal with conflicts of interest. While this disclosure mechanism will now be applied to clinical practice in Japan, a number of problems may arise. For example, the disclosure mechanism is grounded on informed consent and respect for autonomy, thereby giving those who are involved 'information they need to make their own decisions' (Thompson 1993: 575). However, many Japanese patients are still unwilling to make decisions by themselves. In general, clinical care rests on fiduciary relationships between health-care professionals and patients. Yet Japanese patients tend to place trust in physicians above their own autonomy. In such cases, the disclosure mechanism may not be effective. The mechanism is also based on the idea that 'when people divulge the interest they have, others can take this into consideration' while judging the validity of research (Lemmens 2008: 752). In the context of clinical practice, patients ultimately determine whether a physician's judgement is unduly influenced by financial gain. However, this can be difficult because patients often do not know how to assess the disclosed information. Indeed, disclosures may merely increase a patient's distrust towards health-care professionals.

Although gift giving and information provision-related payments (e.g. lecture fees and financial support for meetings) prevail in Japan, many physicians do not recognize the influence they have on their clinical judgement or prescribing behavior. A national survey conducted in Japan revealed that more than 60 per cent of practising physicians do not believe that gifts have an unfavourable impact on their prescribing behaviour (Saito, Mukohara, and Bito 2010: 5). This finding likely reflects a lack of education and awareness on this matter among Japanese physicians, residents, and medical students (Gohma 2011: 416). Although physicians should be more concerned with how patients feel about physician–pharmaceutical industry gift relationships, no studies exploring this relationship from the Japanese patient perspective have been published. In the United States, studies indicate that patients who perceive a physician–pharmaceutical industry gift relationship are likely to distrust the physician and/or health-care system (Grande et al. 2012: 278). Even if pharmaceutical companies disclose information about their financial relationship with physicians and/or hospitals, guidelines established to control such relationships will be ineffective without physician acknowledgement.

In the last decade, means to deal with conflicts of interest have developed from mere disclosure to 'more stringent as well as more structural approaches' (Lemmens 2008: 753). However, as discussed above, acknowledgement of conflicts of interest by Japanese physicians remains lacking. Physicians should increase their awareness about whether their clinical judgement and prescribing behaviour are influenced by gifts or financial gains provided by pharmaceutical companies.

A virtue ethics approach is a useful remedy for Japanese physicians and policymakers. This approach is effective for analysing and ameliorating conflicts of interest because 'the core ethical problem with conflicts of interest concerns the appropriateness of the interest *influencing* or *guiding* one's decisions and actions' (Oakley in this chapter). The virtue ethics approach does not focus on one's decisions and actions, but on the character of those who make such decisions and actions, and their underlying motivation. One advantage to this approach is that it helps physicians reflect on the sort of person they should be and what society entrusts them with. Regarding this issue, Oakley states that *virtuous* physicians are guided during clinical decision-making 'by the virtue of medical *beneficence,* which involves a disposition to act in their patient's best interests', and by 'the virtue of *trustworthiness,* in that they are committed to having a therapeutic relationship with their patients' (Oakley in this chapter). Some bioethicists may object and argue that regulation by law or other means (e.g. financial incentives) provides more assurance than the physician's good character. In my view, we need to focus on both, i.e. the physician's character and regulation by law. Many may question whether or not a virtuous physician would have financial ties to or accept gifts from a pharmaceutical company; yet, according to the Aristotelian definition of virtue, a virtuous physician has the practical wisdom to act appropriately in a given situation.[13]

Discussions concerning conflicts of interest and the prescribing behaviour of physicians have just started in Japan. Pharmaceutical companies have built a system to help deal with conflicts of interest in clinical practice and medical research. Physicians are now required to change their behaviour and implement self-regulation (Gohma 2011). While implementing guidelines and practice codes is important, the ethical problem raised by conflicts of interest must first be acknowledged by practising physicians. Should a physician receive gifts and/or financial gain from a pharmaceutical company? A virtue ethics approach provides a simple answer—a beneficent and trustworthy physician would not dare accept such gifts or financial gains.

References

Gohma, I. (2011). 'Medical Professionalism and Relationships among Pharmaceutical Industry and Physicians,' *Journal of Kyoto Prefectural University of Medicine,* 120(6): 411–18.

Grande, D., Shea, J. D., and Armstrong, K. (2012). 'Pharmaceutical Industry Gifts to Physicians: Patient Beliefs and Trust in Physicians and the Health Care System,' *Journal of General Internal Medicine,* 27(3): 274–9.

Lemmens, T. (2008). 'Conflict of Interests in Medical Research. Historical Development,' in E. J. Emmanuel et al. (eds), *The Oxford Textbook of Clinical Research Ethics.* Oxford University Press, 747–57.

---

[13] Virtue, then, is a state of character concerned with choice, lying in a mean, i.e., the mean relative to us, this being determined by a rational principle, and by that principle by which the man of practical wisdom would determine it. (Aristotle, *The Nicomachean Ethics:* 1107a. trans.)

Oakley, J. (2014). 'A Virtue Ethics Analysis of Disclosure Requirements and Financial Incentives as Response to Conflicts of Interest in Physician Prescribing,' in A. Akabayashi (ed.), *The Future of Bioethics: International Dialogues.* Oxford: Oxford University Press, 669–77.

Saito, S., Mukohara, K., and Bito, S. (2010). 'Japanese Practicing Physicians' Relationships with Pharmaceutical Representatives: A National Survey,' *PLoS ONE* (5)8; e12193.

Thompson, D. F. (1993). 'Understanding Financial Conflict of Interest,' *New England Journal of Medicine*, 329:573–6.

19.4

Commentary
Virtue Ethics and Conflict of Interest

Tom L. Beauchamp

For over 30 years I have defended the place of virtue theory in bioethics (starting with Beauchamp and Childress 1979: chap. 8), so it will come as no surprise that I welcome Justin Oakley's recent contributions to this area of bioethics (notably Oakley and Cocking 2001). My interest in the subject was originally stimulated by David Hume's celebrated virtue theory and by some writings on the virtues of physicians in the history of medical ethics (e.g. Percival 1803). Although Oakley and I do not come to the subject from an identical background, we agree that virtue theory deserves to be a leading area of investigation in bioethics.

Oakley says that he will 'argue that virtue ethics provides a deeper and more compelling analysis of the ethical problems raised by conflicts of interest in physician prescribing than do other ethical perspectives'. I will argue that he shows important virtues of virtue ethics, but that he has not shown that virtue ethics provides a deeper or more compelling analysis than do 'other ethical perspectives.' Oakley's analysis actually supplies us with good reasons to think that we need ethical perspectives that supplement and are not derivative from virtue theory. I will argue that we should be concerned about both the character and motives of persons and about conformity to rules in conflict of interest situations.

The language of virtue

The terms *virtue* and *vice* have been extensively used in the history of ethical theory— perhaps more than any other vocabulary, even if this language is today less common in our moral vocabulary than *obligations* and *human rights*. The idea behind virtue theory is intuitive and sensible: We commend and deeply respect persons who are honest, fair, respectful, just, or caring, or have various other admirable qualities. Likewise, we condemn and disrespect persons who are dishonest, malevolent, uncaring, unjust, or dishonourable, or have other vices.

Conceptually, a *moral virtue* is a morally good and commendable trait of character that makes persons morally reliable, whereas a vice is the converse. We do not always think of virtues in terms of character traits, because parts of our vocabulary include 'virtuous action' and 'virtuous person'. This terminology is perfectly acceptable, but a virtue itself is a character trait. Virtue theory proposes that we not start theorizing with right actions, as if the virtues were derivative from right actions. The idea is to construct a moral theory from character traits that enable and dispose a person to right actions (cf. Annas 2011). I accept this model, though not as having priority over a theory of principles of obligation.

Virtue theory and other types of moral theory

To what in moral theory is Oakley opposed, given his promotion of virtue theory? The answer is not clear. At the end of the article he separates his views from those of utilitarians and Kantians, but he offers no argument to show that virtue theory in general is superior to these moral theories. Few, if any, moral theories would deny the importance of the need for careful examination of the virtues, but few would grant this type of theory superiority or make it foundational for obligations and rights. Even if one thinks that a person disposed by character to have good motives and desires provides the model of the moral person and that this model determines our expectations of persons, it does not follow that rule-governed obligations of the persons are either derivative from virtues or less important in the moral life.

Moreover, the merit of actions often does not reside exclusively in motive or character. Actions must be gauged to bring about desired results and must conform to relevant principles and rules. For example, the physician or nurse who is virtuous in character and appropriately motivated to help a patient, but who violates moral rules or rights, does not act in a praiseworthy or acceptable manner.

Some virtue theorists maintain that virtues enable persons both to discern what they should do and be motivated to do it in particular circumstances without need for pre-existing rules. Oakley seems to fall into this class. According to an influential assessment by Rosalind Hursthouse:

Virtue ethics provides a specification of 'right actions'—as 'what a virtuous agent would, characteristically, do in the circumstances'—and such a specification can be regarded as generating a number of moral rules or principles (contrary to the usual claim that virtue ethics does not come up with rules or principles). Each virtue generates an instruction—'Do what is honest,' 'Do what is charitable,' and each vice a prohibition—'Do not…do what is dishonest, uncharitable.' (Hursthouse 2001: 170)

However, there is no reason to think that all specific rules will rely exclusively on underlying notions of virtue. For example, rules of informed consent may rely on values of autonomy beyond the virtue of respectfulness for autonomy. Virtue theory, from this perspective, does not prove that virtues have advantages over principles and rules of obligation as guides to action.

The limits of virtue theory

It is not easy to see how the notion of a morally worthy pursuit can be adequately built into a virtue theory without reliance on at least some non-virtue premises of what constitutes a morally good life and morally good conduct, which in turn may require reference to action guides and to the general objectives of morality. Many virtues are character traits that are compatible with the performance of morally wrong actions. Courage, wisdom, respectfulness, benevolence, and loyalty can lead to unethical actions if not checked by explicit moral rules of conduct. For example, the physician who acts kindly and loyally by not reporting the failure of a colleague to make proper disclosures to a patient acts unethically. Such a failure to report professional misconduct does not suggest that loyalty and kindness are not virtues, only that the virtues need to be accompanied by an understanding of what is right and good conduct, and of what deserves loyalty, kindness, generosity, and the like.

Virtue theory works less well for forms of moral encounter in which trust, intimacy, familiarity, and the like have not yet been established. When strangers meet, character may play a less significant role than principles, rules, and institutional policies. For example, when a patient first encounters a physician, the physician's conformity to moral rules may be essential in situations of obtaining consent and disclosing a conflict of interest. Likewise, physicians may welcome explicit and mutually agreed-upon rules of informed consent and conflict of interest, as well as codes of ethics.

Oakley notes that 'disclosure requirements can clearly be supported on grounds of informed consent and respect for patient autonomy'. He is correct, but this statement does not reflect a virtue-based analysis. He follows this claim by saying that 'From a virtue ethics perspective, these sorts of disclosure requirements can also be justified insofar as they help doctors to act in accordance with the virtue of honesty, which is important for respecting patient autonomy'. He is again right, but both virtues and specified principles are at work in this statement, and neither is 'deeper' or more foundational than the other.

Problems of conflict of interest and disclosure requirements

Much of Oakley's article is focused on the moral importance of virtues such as honesty and truthfulness and vices such as maleficence and corruption as a way of addressing situations of conflict of interest. He assesses conventional approaches that employ disclosure requirements as ineffective.

I will be using a definition of conflict of interest from a recent report of the Institute of Medicine that I think is slightly preferable to Oakley's formulation: A conflict of interest is 'a set of circumstances that create a risk that professional judgments or actions regarding a primary interest [such as patient welfare or objective research results] will be unduly influenced by a secondary interest [such as financial gain or a personal relationship]' (Lo and Field 2009: 45–6). The worry is that personal interests will create temptations, biases, and the like that will lead to a breach of role responsibilities through judgements, decisions, and actions other than those reasonably expected in the role.

Oakley's concern is that despite the apparent value of disclosure rules, their lack of effectiveness has to do largely with problems of information processing by patients, their reluctance to query physicians, and their misplaced confidence in the trustworthiness of physician disclosures. He acknowledges that 'greater disclosure requirements may help doctors act in accordance with the virtues of honesty and truthfulness', but he thinks that we still need to address, using virtue theory, 'the core ethical problem raised by medical conflicts of interest—that is, undue influence'.

I do not resist Oakley's important thesis about the virtue of honesty and the vice of medical corruption. However, his claim does not undermine the importance of tough-minded and carefully enforced rules of disclosure backed by penalties for non-conformity. I regard them as essential and as more likely to succeed than reliance on virtuous character. He says that the requirements laid down by rules 'fail to *directly* address the causes' of medically corrupt relationships. It is unclear what 'address the causes' means here, but rules do not do less to address the causes than do virtues and vices. Disclosure rules are only intended to address what should be done to prevent and remediate conflicts. To this end, disclosure rules have often been effective, and nothing in Oakley's article indicates otherwise.

However, I agree with him both that disclosure rules are often morally inadequate and that physician fidelity, beneficence, and honesty will be vital forces in preventing bias and temptation. I also agree that in many cases, disclosure is not the proper remedy. For example, one may need to recuse oneself from a decision, judgement, or recommendation because of a conflict of interest, but recusal is most likely to occur (and I think will only occur in many situations) if individuals are *required by rule to recuse* themselves for participation. In my experience, reliance on virtues is entirely ineffective for this purpose. Even virtuous people often lack the proper virtue of discernment when conflicts arise.

Different remedies are appropriate for the wide variety of problems of conflict of interest that occur in medicine, health care, biomedical research, and the review of grant proposals and articles submitted for publication. Rules for each have proved to be vital in some cases, while they work less well in others. Appeals to virtue have value, though often only limited value, in controlling situations of fee splitting, self-referring, accepting gifts, accepting fees for recruiting patients for a research protocol, appointing industry-based physicians to government regulatory agencies, and industry-paid lecturing on an industry product. At least as important are stringent regulations by institutions that govern gifting, the funding of programmes, grants and contracts, providing free samples, and the like. Deliberative assessments need to be made regarding ways to address such conflicts of interest. For example, we might eliminate them, manage or mitigate them, or require disclosure of conflicts directly to parties at risk. Each strategy is justifiable in some contexts, and each is preferable to the traditional convention of relying on professional or personal character to make the proper assessments.

Professionals sometimes view attempts to address conflicts of interest as negative judgements on their character and moral integrity, as if they might be corrupt and might act against the reasonable expectations of their professional roles. However, this assessment misses the point of conflict of interest rules. *Unconscious* and *unintentional* distortions of professional judgements, decisions, and actions are usually the chief concern. Accordingly, general rules and regulations can be essential normative structures in institutional contexts.

References

Annas, J. (2011). *Intelligent Virtue*. New York: Oxford University Press.

Beauchamp, T. L., and Childress, J. (1979). *Principles of Biomedical Ethics*. 1st ed. New York: Oxford University Press.

Hursthouse, R. (2001). *On Virtue Ethics*. Oxford: Oxford University Press.

Lo, B, and Field, M. J. (eds). (2009). *Conflict of Interest in Medical Research, Education, and Practice*. Washington DC: National Academies Press.

Oakley, J., and Cocking, D. (2001). *Virtue Ethics and Professional Roles*. Cambridge: Cambridge University Press.

Percival, T. (1803). *Medical Ethics: Or a Code of Institutes and Precepts, Adapted to the Professional Conduct of Physicians and Surgeons*. Manchester: S. Russell.

19.5

Commentary

Dealing with Conflicts of Interest: Is Virtue Ethics Tough Enough?

Alastair V. Campbell

Justin Oakley's paper raises a crucial ethical issue in current health care, one which grows in importance as pressures to apply market models to both health research and delivery of health care increase in virtually every country seeking to deliver a modern health service. The independence of the health-care professions and their ability to meet the basic ethical requirement to act solely in the best interests of the patient are clearly compromised by an all too cosy relationship with both the pharmaceutical industry and the medical technology and medical devices industries. Professional associations and medical licensing bodies have tried to grapple with this problem, with only limited success. A survey of all the various codes and practice guidelines internationally, including those drawn up by the industries themselves, reveal a certain amount of damage limitation, but hardly a tough and unambiguous stance against all forms of inducement to be influenced by advertising and advocacy rather than by an objective assessment of the patient's good.

In the midst of this ethical minefield Oakley offers a possible solution, based on the character of the individual practitioner, revealed, not in his or her motivations (since these can be opaque), but in the actual behaviour of physicians in prescribing and other uses of technology, revealing where their priorities lie. Using this virtue ethics (VE) approach, Oakley offers a critique of the moral adequacy of both disclosure requirements and attempts to alter physician behaviour through financial incentives. He concludes that, by exhibiting the medical professional vices of medical corruption and of risking potential harm to the patient (maleficence), physicians betray the trust which the community has placed in the profession. Disclosure of financial interests is not enough and accepting financial incentives to prescribe differently is a sell-out to the notion that medicine is no more than a business venture.

Since I have written quite extensively about VE in relation to health care (Campbell 1998; 2003; 2005), it will be obvious that I am supportive of Oakley's approach. In particular, I can see no merit in the idea that financial incentives will bring about better physician behaviour in this sphere, since this merely seems to accept and underscore the surrender of professional values to commercial ones. However, there are some problems inherent in VE itself that may undermine this attempt to make a significant change in physician behaviour. These are: idealism and elitism; cultural relativity; and a focus on the individual rather than on societal influences. I shall consider each in turn, whilst also suggesting a way forward.

Godlike doctors

VE can easily appear to be idealistic and elitist. With its emphasis on virtue, it can appear to single out some individuals as above the common herd, as exceptionally moral and well motivated, with a commitment greater than that of ordinary mortals. This kind of elevation of the medical profession has been subject to devastating critiques by some writers, notably Ivan Illich (1976) and Eliot Freidson (1975). They see such claims to superior moral commitment as merely a social device to gain power and prestige in society. So if this kind of supererogatory behaviour is what Oakley wants, then his project seems doomed to failure. Yet, in fact, VE seeks to portray not the exceptional human, but rather the human anyone can be if he or she fulfils the simple requirements of being human—and I shall return to this below. The virtuous doctor has to be seen as what any doctor can be, without superhuman effort or exceptional character.

Non-relative virtues?

A second problem in VE is its tendency to portray as universal what are merely esteemed social traits of a particular culture or era. Martha Nussbaum (1988) has a helpful discussion of this point. She suggests that, although there are 'thick' virtues, specific to each culture (an example would be cultural variation in the evaluation of suicide), there are also 'thin' virtues, which cross cultural divides in offering desirable traits in face of basic human challenges. Examples of such universal human challenges are our vulnerability, our desire to be creative or generative, and our awareness of our own mortality. While each culture may 'thicken' the traits needed to face these challenges in its own fashion, all humans need the characteristics that help them overcome them. An answer, then, to the relativity problem as it might affect medical virtues is that every culture needs practitioners who can be trusted to help us deal with these challenges. A businessman trying to market someone's products is simply not the person we need! That is why throughout the ages people of all cultures have sought out priests or healers (often both) to provide help at times of birth, illness, and death. It is not culturally relative to say that such helpers need to be genuine, not merely fakers of goodwill aiming for profit.

Cultural change

However, I would argue that the biggest challenge to the VE approach is that it seems to concentrate on the individual practitioner, rather than focusing on those social forces that induce individuals to act in certain (potentially vicious) ways. This is what I mean by the question in my title: 'Is Virtue Ethics Tough Enough?' From basic medical training (with its 'hidden curriculum') onwards we know that medical practitioners are influenced by peer pressure, and by the role models of good practice (and bad practice) found in their senior colleagues. Various factors influence medical choices towards an uncritical view of the profession's relationships with industry. The most obvious one is the way in which postgraduate medical education and much continuing professional education have been left to the industry to finance, rather than being seen as integral to the society's need to have competent and professionally motivated doctors. Moreover, an increasing emphasis on competition between health-care providers, in the name of efficiency, and the vast differences in status and financial reward between the different medical specialities also push recent graduates in the direction of the business model. Against these forces, the exhortation to be virtuous seems weak indeed!

Perhaps, however, some answers can be found in a return to the roots of VE in Aristotle's account. Rather than trying to make lists of medical virtues and vices, in the manner of later traditions in VE (such as the medieval Christian one), we can return to the core concepts of practical wisdom, the golden mean and human fulfilment (*eudaimonia*) found in Aristotle. To counter the forces of the marketization of medicine, we need to restore a balance between avarice and self-sacrifice in the golden mean of a just reward for the socially vital work of the profession. We need to fight the culture of greed with a return to those good role models of medical practice, instanced in the practical wisdom of practitioners who put the welfare of their patients above personal gain. But especially, if medicine is to survive as a genuine profession at all, we need young doctors to see where fulfilment lies, which is not in just making as much money as possible, but in finding that one's work, even in a small way, has helped the lives of others be fuller and richer, despite the major challenges of illness and imminent death. In summary, we need to rediscover the culture of medicine as, at its core, a moral enterprise, not a business one.

However, none of this can happen unless the professional and licensing bodies take a much tougher stance on the current major conflicts of interest between medicine and the health-care industries. The plea to be virtuous will never be enough to change the current trends. We know this already from the present worldwide financial crisis. Just as we have all seen how badly we need *real* controls on the banking industry, we require the same sense of urgency about safeguarding the future of medicine through stronger and clearer regulation. VE alone is simply not tough enough.

References

Campbell, A. V. (1998). 'The 'Ethics of Care' as Virtue Ethics,' in M. Evans (ed.), *Critical Reflection on Medical Ethics*. Vol. 4. Stamford, CT: Jai Press, 295–305.

Campbell, A. V. (2003). 'The Virtues (and Vices) of the Four Principles,' *Journal of Medical Ethics*, 29:292–6.

Campbell, A. V. (2005). 'A Virtue Ethics Approach,' in R. Ashcroft et al. (eds), *Case Analysis in Clinical Ethics*. Cambridge: Cambridge University Press, 45–56.

Freidson, E. (1975). *Profession of Medicine*. New York: Dodd Mead.

Illich, I. (1976). *Medical Nemesis*. New York: Pantheon.

Nussbaum, M. (1988). 'Non-relative Virtues: An Aristotelian Approach,' in P. A. French et al. (eds), *Ethical Theory: Character and Virtue*. Notre Dame, IN: University of Notre Dame Press, 32–53.

19.6

Response to Commentaries
Sketch of a Virtue Ethics Regulatory Model

Justin Oakley

In my primary topic article (Oakley in this chapter), I argued that virtue ethics' evaluation of actions in terms of the appropriateness of the dispositions *guiding* the agent provides a particularly compelling analysis, compared with other ethical perspectives, of what is recognized as the core ethical problem in conflicts of interest in medicine—namely, doctors being unduly *influenced* by interests other than those of their patients, such as doctors' own self-interest due to financial or other ties they may have with the pharmaceutical industry. I used the limitations of disclosure requirements in handling medical conflicts of interest as a way of making this point, by showing that such requirements are poorly targeted at peripheral aspects of what is ethically problematic about such conflicts. It should come as no surprise, therefore, that such disclosure requirements are turning out to be somewhat ineffective in curbing biased prescribing behaviour by doctors. I also outlined a virtue ethics analysis of the introduction of financial incentives as another way of combating biased prescribing. In doing so I highlighted some ethical concerns about financial incentives in this context, and I briefly sketched how a virtue ethics approach to regulation might be developed, taking such incentives in clinical practice as a case study. As the four commentaries on my article indicate, it is vital to devise appropriate regulatory responses to combat medical conflicts of interest, so I will here elaborate a little on how such an approach might work. The relative advantages of a virtue ethics analysis of what is most ethically problematic about such conflicts, compared with analyses from other ethical perspectives, needs to be explained in more detail, and that is something I aim to provide in subsequent work on this topic.

Tom Beauchamp, Alastair Campbell, Ilhak Lee, and Masatoshi Nara all acknowledge the relevance and usefulness of virtue ethics in addressing problems raised by medical conflicts of interest, and all four commentators mention the inadequacies of disclosure requirements as a solution to the problems created by such conflicts in clinical practice.[14]

[14] I wish to thank all four commentators for their reflections and insights on these issues. Thanks are also due to Norman Daniels, Mike Dunn, Tony Hope, Josh May, Tom Murray, and Rob Sparrow, for their very helpful comments on earlier versions of this paper. I also wish to thank Marco Antonio Azevedo, Chris Megone, and Katrien Devolder, for their useful feedback at the 2012 UK Society of Applied Philosophy annual conference, Oxford University, where I also presented a version of this paper.

Further, as several of the commentators point out, reliance on codes of ethics and exhortations to professional virtue are also insufficient remedies for these ethical problems. But while I believe ideals of medical virtue do help to illuminate where the most serious ethical problems in medical conflicts of interest lie, I do not regard virtue ethics as opposed to regulatory responses to such problems. Indeed, I believe that virtue ethics can play an important role in helping to devise effective and well targeted regulatory solutions to such problems. However, this is a question I took up only at the end of my paper, and I will say more about this issue shortly.

Masatoshi Nara and Ilhak Lee describe a series of recent regulatory initiatives in Japan and South Korea, respectively, which were introduced in response to problems that various physician–industry relationships have created with physician prescribing behaviour and other areas of clinical practice. I welcome such initiatives, including prohibitions of industry payments to physicians, as necessary steps in protecting patients in an era of increasing commercialization in medical practice. Lee comments that, while it is important to remind the medical profession that a virtuous physician serves patient health, he is concerned about the breadth and vagueness of such a goal. A more specific and perhaps achievable goal here, in Lee's view, is to remind physicians of the importance of the patient's and community's trust in them, and of the essential fiduciary nature of physician–patient relationships. Nara also emphasizes the significance of medical trust here, particularly given the inordinate level of trust he says patients in Japan often have in their physicians.

I agree that there is considerable merit in highlighting the value of trust in this context. Patients implicitly trust their doctors to make clinical decisions in the patients' own best interests, and the importance of this trust is often overlooked until it is breached. (And one only needs to think of the scandal in paediatric cardiac surgery at Bristol Royal Infirmary in the mid 1990s, and the 2001 Bristol Inquiry, to see how difficult it can be to restore public trust in the medical profession when this has been significantly breached.) However, I do not see this as at odds with a virtue ethics approach. Trustworthiness is another important medical virtue, along with beneficence and honesty, and it would be difficult to provide a satisfactory analysis of the nature and moral significance of medical betrayal without reference to the virtue of trustworthiness in this context. Nevertheless, one limitation I find with the trust-based approach Lee suggests to medical conflicts of interest is that it is not clear how such an approach could demonstrate the wrongness of a doctor acting from self-interest rather than medical beneficence, in cases where patients have no trust that doctors will act in their best interests in the first place (say, in a country where medical corruption is rife).

Masatoshi Nara is sympathetic to the virtue ethics approach to medical practice that Dean Cocking and I have developed (see Oakley and Cocking 2001). He shares my concerns about meeting conflict of interest problems with greater disclosure requirements, pointing out that 'many Japanese patients are still unwilling to make decisions by themselves' (Nara in this chapter), and that 'patients often do not know how to assess the disclosed information' (Nara in this chapter). Nara highlights how Japanese physicians are only now beginning to acknowledge the ethical problems that conflicts of interest can cause in doctors' prescribing behaviour, and he reminds us of the importance of raising doctors' awareness of how their industry ties can impact on their clinical decision-making in ways that are detrimental to patients. Nara argues that combating these problems through both regulation and the promotion of medical virtue are complementary strategies, which are both needed to assure patients that biases in their doctors' prescribing behaviour will be minimized.

Tom Beauchamp also regards such steps as complementary remedies to medical conflicts of interest. As a pioneer of applications of virtue theory in bioethics, Beauchamp recognizes the importance of medical virtues and vices for reaching a deeper understanding of the morality of medical conflicts of interest. Nevertheless, Beauchamp sees reliance solely on medical virtue as a 'traditional convention' that has been shown inadequate, and he therefore recommends the use of 'tough-minded and carefully enforced rules of disclosure backed by penalties for nonconformity…as more likely to succeed' (Beauchamp in this chapter). While Beauchamp agrees that disclosure rules are often 'morally inadequate', he argues that disclosure requirements have nevertheless been effective in preventing and remediating medical conflicts of interest. However, evidence is now emerging that the greater disclosure requirements recently implemented in response to conflicts of interest in physician–industry relationships have not been effective in improving physician prescribing behaviour (see Pham-Kanter, Alexander, and Nair 2012). Alastair Campbell is also concerned that issuing a plea to doctors to be more virtuous is a weak regulatory response to medical conflicts of interest, in the face of the various pressures on doctors to behave in a more commercial manner. Campbell argues that 'professional and licensing bodies [should] take a much tougher stance on the current major conflicts of interest between medicine and the health-care industries', and he suggests that 'stronger and clearer regulation' (Campbell in this chapter) is needed, as the recent failures in the banking industry illustrate.

I take this point made by Nara, Beauchamp, and Campbell about the importance of rules and well designed regulation in this context. However, I had not intended to suggest that reliance on professional virtue is a suitable professional or regulatory response to medical conflicts of interest. Rather, I was appealing to virtue considerations to help reveal the ethical problems lying at the heart of such conflicts, and my aim was to then draw on such considerations to indicate how a well targeted regulatory response might be devised. Let me therefore say a little more about how such an approach to regulation in this area could be developed.

I suggested that, in evaluating a certain regulatory intervention here, we could investigate the impact which such an initiative may have had on doctors' prioritizing of patients' best interests over other considerations in their prescribing decisions, in other, comparable sorts of cases. For example, consider a proposal which involves paying doctors a modest financial incentive to avoid being unduly influenced by their industry ties in their drug prescribing decisions. One way for regulators to evaluate such a proposal is by scrutinizing evidence showing that the introduction of financial incentives for doctors in *other* contexts has been a cost-effective way of improving health outcomes, as appears to be the case, for example, with certain pay-for-performance schemes. For instance, there is evidence that the introduction in 2004 of financial incentives for UK family practitioners to better manage patients with asthma and type-2 diabetes led to improvements in health outcomes for those practitioners' patients with those conditions (Campbell et al 2007). Where the evidence indicates such incentive schemes are a cost-effective way of improving health outcomes, regulators who adopt a straightforwardly utilitarian regulatory model would regard this evidence as providing decisive grounds in support of such initiatives (see e.g. Goodin 1995). By contrast, the crucial question here for the virtue ethics regulatory model would be: What impact does the evidence suggest such pay-for-performance schemes have on the conditions which the doctors involved might subsequently use to govern their relationships with patients? Where there is evidence that the doctors involved in such schemes are serving their patients' best interests only on condition of being paid additional financial incentives to do so, then those doctors have arguably redefined the therapeutic nature of their doctor–patient relationships as commercial relationships. This, according to a virtue ethics approach to policy, is too high a moral cost for us to pay, in improving health outcomes.

The distinctive contribution of a virtue ethics policy approach in this context can also be demonstrated by considering what policymakers can do to help professional associations in medicine meet their avowed goals of preserving the therapeutic orientation of doctor–patient relationships, at a time of increasing commercialization of medical practice, and in an environment where health researchers and policymakers are investigating how a variety of financial incentives might be used to bring about cost-effective improvements in health outcomes. Thus, for instance, the Australian Medical Association's (AMA) current *Code of Ethics* advises that doctors must 'Recognise that an established therapeutic relationship between doctor and patient must be respected' (1.1.14). It also advises doctors, 'If you work in a practice or institution, place your professional duties and responsibilities to your patients above the commercial interests of the owners or others who work within these practices'(1.1.23). And the 2010 AMA *Position Statement on Doctors' Relationships with Industry* states that 'The major principles guiding doctors' relationships with industry include the following: ...The doctor's primary obligation is to the patient. Considerations involving industry are appropriate only insofar as they do not intrude into or distort that primary obligation. The primary objective of relationships between doctors and industry should be the advancement of the health of patients. The patient's health needs should be the primary consideration when utilising products and services' (3.1). Suppose that regulators propose that doctors be given financial incentives encouraging them to prioritize their patients' best interests in drug prescribing decisions. Where regulators profess to share the AMA's commitment to preserving the therapeutic orientation of doctor–patient relationships, they have no choice but to consider what studies of doctors' responses to the introduction of previous financial incentive schemes—such as pay-for-performance schemes—might tell us about the conditions by which doctors govern their relationships with patients. For it is important to protect patient and community trust in the doctor–patient relationship as not only a transparent one, but also as beneficent and therapeutic in its guiding values and commitments.

The overarching focus of current research on various physician incentive policies is the question of how financial incentives to doctors to provide better patient care—or conversely, to limit their care in various ways—have impacted on doctors' clinical decision-making. This is a large and complex issue, as there is evidence that such incentive schemes have affected clinical decision-making in a variety of ways (on the clinical impact of pay-for-performance schemes, see Rodriguez et al. 2009; Doran et al. 2011; Kontopantelis et al. 2012). It is therefore important to focus more specifically on what such studies suggest about the effectiveness of proposals to use financial incentives to encourage doctors to prioritize their patients' best interests in their prescribing. (Studies of UK and Australian state-funded financial incentive schemes encouraging doctors to prescribe cheaper generic substitutes instead of brand-name pharmaceuticals will also be important sources here, particularly as such schemes may already be curbing the influence of doctors' industry ties on their prescribing, to some extent: see Löfgren 2009.) The following question would be crucial for the development of a virtue ethics regulatory model in this context: If there is good reason to believe that such financial incentives are likely to improve health outcomes for patients, how might such incentives impact on the nature of doctor–patient relationships? For example, the above-mentioned reactions of many UK family practitioners to the introduction of pay-for-performance incentives (Campbell et al. 2007) tell us something about the conditions under which those practitioners govern their relationships with patients, and so about the nature of those relationships. It is possible that those UK family practitioners who responded to such financial incentives by better managing their patients with asthma, heart disease, and diabetes have done so at the cost of transforming their relationships with the particular patients involved from therapeutic to commercial relationships. Thus, there needs to be an investigation into similar studies of the impact of financial incentives on medical professional behaviour, as an indication of the conditions such doctors apply to their relationships. Here it is important to consider evidence of the likely mechanisms by which certain pay-for-performance schemes have improved patient outcomes, and whether any such changes in clinical decision-making are compatible with maintaining the therapeutic orientation of doctor–patient relationships and professional virtue. This evidence will assist in the development of a central 'test question' which could be posed by a virtue ethics regulatory model. In this context, such a question might be put as follows: For any proposed policy aimed at improving patient outcomes, is this policy likely to transform doctors' relationships with patients from therapeutic relationships into a different sort of relationship, which has no inherent link with the proper goals of medicine?

An important underlying question here is whether *all* financial incentive policies in medicine are contrary to virtue, and so consideration also needs to be given to whether a virtue ethics regulatory model would be opposed to all financial incentives in medicine. For instance, paying doctors an incentive to work in rural areas might not conflict with professional virtue because such incentives arguably do not by themselves involve a corruption of the doctor–patient relationships that the rural doctor thereby takes on (and the individual prescribing decisions s/he thereby makes). After all, statements by professional associations (such as the AMA, above) exhorting doctors to always place their patients' interests above commercial interests clearly do not altogether preclude doctors making a profit from their activities, nor do they preclude doctors accepting incentives to work in rural areas. Also, doctors have not *already* committed themselves to filling gaps in rural medical services when they joined the profession. By contrast, doctors have already agreed, when joining the profession, to prescribe medication in their patients' best interests. Thus, a fully developed virtue ethics regulatory model would provide a plausible explication of the moral psychology of medical virtue, and of how any financial interests of doctors could consistently guide them within such a picture.

References

Beauchamp, T. L. (2014). 'Virtue Ethics and Conflict of Interest: A Comment on Oakley,' in A. Akabayashi (ed.), *The Future of Bioethics: International Dialogues*. Oxford: Oxford University Press, 688–92.

Campbell, A. V. (2014). 'Dealing with Conflicts of Interest: Is Virtue Ethics Tough Enough?' in A. Akabayashi (ed.), *The Future of Bioethics: International Dialogues*. Oxford: Oxford University Press, 693–6.

Campbell, S. et al. (2007). 'Quality of Primary Care in England with the Introduction of Pay for Performance,' *New England Journal of Medicine*, 357:181–90.

Doran, Tim et al. (2011). 'Effect of Financial Incentives on Incentivised and Non-incentivised Clinical Activities: Longitudinal Analysis of Data from the UK Quality and Outcomes Framework,' *BMJ*, 342:d3590.

Goodin, R. E. (1995). *Utilitarianism as a Public Philosophy*. Cambridge: Cambridge University Press.

Kontopantelis, E. et al. (2012). 'Family Doctor Responses to Changes in Incentives for Influenza Immunization under the UK Quality and Outcomes Framework Pay-for-performance Scheme,' *Health Services Research*, 47:1117–36.

Lee, I. (2014). 'Commentary on Justin Oakley's "A Virtue Ethics Analysis of Disclosure Requirements and Financial Incentives as Responses to Conflicts of Interest in Physician Prescribing"', in A. Akabayashi (ed.), *The Future of Bioethics: International Dialogues*. Oxford: Oxford University Press, 678–82.

Lindenauer, P. K. et al. (2007). 'Public Reporting and Pay-for-performance in Hospital Quality Improvement,' *New England Journal of Medicine*, 356:486–96.

Löfgren, H. (2009). 'Generic Medicines in Australia: Business Dynamics and Recent Policy Reform,' *Southern Med Review*, 2:24–8.

Nara, M. (2014). 'Conflicts of Interest: Relationship between Japanese Physicians and the Pharmaceutical Industry', in A. Akabayashi (ed.), *The Future of Bioethics: International Dialogues*. Oxford: Oxford University Press, 683–7.

Oakley, J. (2014). 'A Virtue Ethics Analysis of Disclosure Requirements and Financial Incentives as Responses to Conflicts of Interest in Physician Prescribing,' in A. Akabayashi (ed.), *The Future of Bioethics: International Dialogues*. Oxford: Oxford University Press, 669–77.

Oakley, J., and Cocking, D. (2001). *Virtue Ethics and Professional Roles*. Cambridge: Cambridge University Press.

Pham-Kanter, G., Alexander, G. C., and Nair, K. (2012). 'Effect of Physician Payment Sunshine Laws on Prescribing,' *Archives of Internal Medicine*, 172:819–21.

Rodriguez, H. P. et al. (2009). 'The Effect of Performance-based Financial Incentives on Improving Patient Care Experiences: A Statewide Evaluation,' *Journal of General Internal Medicine*, 24:1281–8.

20.1

Primary Topic Article

The Future of Clinical Ethics Education: Value Pluralism, Communication, and Mediation

Edward J. Bergman and Autumn Fiester

The traditional American approach to clinical ethics: consultation

In the United States, the traditional approach to resolving clinical ethics dilemmas in a hospital setting is the "clinical ethics consultation." The most common structure for this kind of work is the hospital ethics committee. Five years ago, 81 percent of American hospitals had ethics committees and another 14 percent were in the process of forming them (Fox et al. 2007). In fact, the national hospital accreditation board in the US, The Joint Commission, mandates that all hospitals provide some mechanism to resolve clinical ethics disputes (The Joint Commission 2011), and the ethics committee is typically the structure by which a hospital fulfills this mandate. The traditional process involves summoning the ethics committee, or a subset of it, to explore ethical issues, discuss the merits and drawbacks of the various positions being taken (or that might be taken), and, ultimately, offer recommendations to the clinical providers who requested the consult (Aulisio et al. 2000; Clinical Ethics Consultation Affairs Committee 2010).

We perceive many ethical problems with this approach to the resolution of a clinical ethics conflict (Caplan and Bergman 2007; Fiester 2007a; Fiester 2007b; Fiester 2011; Fiester 2012a; Fiester 212b; Bergman 2013). Here we seek to highlight only one—that clinical ethics consultation, in its traditional form, fails to recognize the value pluralism that exists in even the most homogeneous communities. To avoid engaging in a meta-ethical debate about the theoretical validity of value pluralism, we will simply define value pluralism in this context as the pedestrian claim that individuals engaged in a clinical ethics conflict bring their own values, moral commitments, and hierarchy of virtues to the conflict and that no third-party expertise exists which embodies the objective moral wisdom to adjudicate between them. When two parties hold incommensurate positions in an ethics dispute, there are deeply held values at the root of those positions. No ethicist possesses the moral wisdom to objectively rank the values at play in those conflicts. Thus, issuing recommendations, or offering verdicts, in such cases is tantamount to prioritizing some people's values over others, without the necessary moral authority or justification (Fiester 2011; Bergman 2013). Without social consensus on the community's hierarchy of values, and agreement on the moral authority of certain institutions to enforce them, no third party is justified in choosing some values over others when a pluralism of legitimate values is in play. Recommendations by ethics committees in traditional clinical ethics consults reflect the values of that committee rather than an objectively superior moral position.

A concrete case will illustrate the above point. One of the most prevalent types of clinical ethics conflict occurring in US hospitals involves withdrawal of life-sustaining therapies from a patient whose condition is deemed futile by the medical team. By "futile," clinicians mean that the patient has, in their view, no hope of significant improvement or of regaining substantial physical or cognitive function. Treatments offered will not be curative, though steady-state maintenance of current levels of function is certainly possible. In fact, that steady state could continue for a very long time. "Futile" does not mean that death is either imminent or predictable. The famous American end-of-life court and media battle involving a patient named Terri Schiavo is a prime example (The Terri Schiavo Case 2011). Not surprisingly, this paradigmatic kind of conflict—involving various permutations of physicians and family members in disagreement about whether life-sustaining therapy should be removed because it provides no therapeutic value (or that the associated quality of life is violative of the patient's dignity) and those who believe that all aggressive therapies should be implemented—is not uncommon. There may be multiple values at play for both parties, but let us imagine that, in this case, one family member believes that continuing care constitutes squandering the scarce resources of an intensive care unit (ICU) bed that could be used for a patient capable of deriving greater benefits, and that another believes the removal of life-sustaining therapies like breath, food, and water is the moral equivalent of murder. Clearly two legitimate moral values are at stake. If an ethics committee deliberates and decides in favor of one party, it has either prioritized the concern about scarce resources over the concern about murder or, alternatively, prioritized the concern about murder over the concern about scarce resources. But on what moral and objective grounds is that decision based? In a situation where more than one legitimate value is at stake—where there is "value pluralism" in our sense—the ethics committee has no legitimate moral standing to decide that one ethical stance trumps the other.

When clinical ethics consultation does not actually involve "*ethics*": the issue of communication

As outlined above, traditional clinical ethics consultations are inapposite when there really *is* a value-based disagreement. In many conflicts referred to an American ethics committee, there is no identifiable *ethics* conflict. At root, the stakeholders all agree on the ethical considerations relevant to the situation, and they agree on how to hierarchize them. Their disputes emanate, instead, from ineffective communication, partial or inaccurate information, personality clashes/relationship issues, psychological stress, and/or cultural differences.

The complex interactions, vulnerabilities, power differentials, and emotional stakes involved in health-care delivery inevitably lead to interpersonal conflict between, and among, providers, patients, surrogates, and family members. In American ethics consultations, it may well be the case that the majority of clinical disputes do not involve ethical conflict in the strict classical sense.

It is predictable that disputes of the aforementioned nature will occur regularly in an inpatient unit, given structural issues of health-care delivery in America. For example, inpatient units in American hospitals typically generate conflict in the context of fractured, inconsistent, and compartmentalized care. In the tertiary care center referred to as a "teaching hospital" in the US, there are caregivers at every level of training and credentialing in all aspects of health care. Patients and their families will encounter medical students, postgraduate physicians in training (called "residents"), and fully trained physicians (called "attendings"), in every specialty related to their care. In a typical stay in the ICU of a teaching hospital, in addition to members of the nursing staff responsible for much of the bedside care, a patient's primary attending physician will rotate off service every two–three weeks, when a new attending takes over. Many of the day-to-day communications with patients and their families won't even be with the attending physician, but with others in the above-described categories. Lack of continuity of care creates a situation ripe for communication breakdowns. When grueling work schedules—sometimes an 80-hour week for the most junior clinicians—are added to the stresses of high-pressure units like the ICU, interactions are bound to be less than ideal. On the patient and family side, fear, resentment, frustration, anxiety, distress, and emotional fragility are added to the mix. Interpersonal conflicts are inevitable.

Compounding these stressed interactions is a shift in the way contemporary American society views physicians and their expertise. The physician–patient relationship in the US has changed from the model of "physician-as-expert" to a model of shared responsibility, described variously as a "negotiated" relationship or one that embraces "shared decision making" (Green, Simms, and Blackall, 2009). Expectations on the part of patients and their families that they will be prime decision-makers for their own health care, or the care of their loved ones, magnifies problems in communication, given the vast disparity in clinical knowledge—patients and families have much of the control but not much of the medical expertise. A negotiated model of the physician–patient relationship requires very effective communication and the provision of complex information that is truly comprehensible, along with sensitivity to the particular values, priorities, and cultural concerns of patients and their families. That is a heavy burden to assume, and breakdowns in the physician–patient relationship are bound to occur. When they do, and the relationship ceases to function smoothly, the impasse generated often lands the parties before an ethics committee.

An innovative approach to clinical ethics: mediation

Given that standard American clinical ethics consultations are fraught with thorny issues such as the value pluralism previously described, coupled with the fact that many bedside disputes are not, strictly speaking, actual conflicts of values but are communication or relationship based, we advocate for an innovative approach to clinical ethics referred to as "clinical ethics mediation" or "bioethics mediation" (Bergman and Fiester 2009; Dubler and Liebman 2011; Bergman 2013).

Clinical ethics mediation is a descendent of the classical genre of mediation and negotiation used as a dispute resolution mechanism in the arenas of law, business, international relations, etc. It is a form of assisted negotiation needed when the stakeholders in a relationship find themselves in a dispute they cannot navigate without the aid of a third party. When a relationship is threatened by conflict, the assistance of a neutral third party—the mediator—may be sought to manage the conflict resolution process. Mediation has, indeed, been the fastest-growing dispute resolution mechanism in the United States for quite some time, and most state and federal courts have incorporated mediation programs as an alternative or complementary dispute resolution process.

Advocates of mediation have included both those who applaud its efficacy and those attracted to its humanistic approach (Casarett et al. 1998; Walker 1993). Not only does mediation work as a conflict resolution mechanism, but it works by being both non-adversarial and noncoercive. Classical mediation posits a neutral third party, unbiased both as to parties and outcomes. In other words, the mediator does not have a proverbial "dog in the fight." The mediator acts as a facilitator of dialogue, assisting parties to define the problem, determine their respective interests, and to identify, where possible, the compatibility of those interests. The mediator also serves as a translator of opaque information, a process manager, a catalyst for creativity, and a provider of information sources. Significantly, the mediator acknowledges and validates all parties through active listening, empathy, and non-judgmental responses, while providing a protected space for the candid exchange of thoughts, feelings, and ideas, in both global sessions and private caucuses. By encouraging the uninterrupted telling of each party's story, mediation promotes catharsis, which is often lacking in more formal, rule-driven processes, such as litigation or arbitration (Moore 2003). Due to its non-adversarial and noncoercive nature, mediation has also been viewed as the dispute resolution process most likely to preserve existing relationships (Stone, Patton, and Heen 1999). The inclusive, noncoercive and empowering aspects of a process in which all resolutions are consensual, rather than imposed by third parties, explains this signature characteristic.

All of these characteristics of classical mediation render it effective, not only for the management of communication- or relationship-based clinical conflicts, but for those that involve irreconcilable values or moral commitments. In all such cases, a facilitated dialogue can assist stakeholders in repairing a dysfunctional or broken relationship and forging a consensual solution that honors all parties' positions—the antithesis of an ethics committee taking a stand on what the resolution should be.

In the case of communication- or relationship-based conflicts, advocacy of mediation as a preferred process for clinical ethics consultation meets little resistance. However, the prospect of mediation for management of a true values dispute is often met with criticism. A principal argument offered is that "consultation" rather than "mediation" is required in values disputes to safeguard against the possibility that malevolently motivated stakeholders, under the supervision of a truly neutral mediator, might craft an ethically unsupportable solution (e.g. agreeing to withdraw care for a patient who is curable in order to reap some financial gain from the patient's early demise). But the mediation process is, by its inclusive nature, conducive to the ascertainment of self-interested motives which, once revealed, will extinguish any perception of good faith and fail to elicit consensus. That clinicians and family members so at loggerheads that they call for an ethics consult would engage in treacherous collusion to manipulate the mediation process strains plausibility. Nonetheless, the rebuttal to this objection is to identify the safeguards that inhere in classical mediation outside the clinic—mediators are constrained by laws or codes or policies applicable to the jurisdictions in which they function. In legal mediation, mediators are constrained by the law. In institutional settings, there are often regulations or policies that must be adhered to. Clinical ethics mediators are constrained in a parallel way. This is what advocates of clinical mediation refer to as "principled resolution" (Dubler and Liebman 2011). Clinical ethics mediators have the responsibility of understanding, in addition to knowing the techniques of conflict resolution, what constitutes a solution that runs afoul of the law, hospital policy, or the ethical scaffolding in the community that supports them. For example, in the United States, competent patients must give their informed consent to any invasive procedure, or they must waive their right to it. A mediator, consequently, cannot facilitate a solution that denies a competent patient access to this right or waiver. From our perspective, this objection is the proverbial "red herring." One is hard-pressed to find a real-world clinical ethics case that implicates such concerns. At best, this objection represents the kind of interesting conceptual conundrum philosophers are drawn to, rather than a real-world dilemma. At worst, the objection is motivated by a perceived threat to the authority of clinical ethics consultants, whose traditional role empowers them to exert significant control over the lives of parties with a personal stake in these conflicts.

We do not reject the utility of bioethics principles in the function, training, and skill set of prospective clinical ethics mediators. We suggest, however, that the relevance of that body of knowledge in the management of clinical conflict is, primarily, as a vehicle for the articulation and framing of competing values, each of which should be accorded legitimacy. This should not be surprising, as the principles at the core of American bioethics—patient autonomy, beneficence, non-maleficence, and justice (Beauchamp and Childress 2009)—do not direct outcomes in values disputes, but assist in framing the dilemma posed by legitimate, competing commitments and moral considerations. Said principles serve as a convenient springboard for a dialogue that elicits, and encourages respect for, value systems, each of which accord primacy to different, yet defensible, moral perspectives. Ultimately, it is the prospect of respect for value pluralism, rather than the prospect of moral conversion by force of will, or purported moral authority, that distinguishes a mediated approach to moral disagreement from the more authoritarian and adjudicatory models employed in conventional clinical ethics consultations.

Teaching mediation as clinical ethics consultation

Until now, distinctions have been drawn between clinical ethics consultation and clinical ethics mediation. The traditional consultation is viewed as authoritarian and hierarchical while the mediation approach is seen as inclusive and a product of self-determination. Various American working groups have recently been charged with the task of defining qualifications required of clinical ethics consultants that merge the skill sets applicable to traditional clinical ethics consultations with those of mediation (Dubler et al. 2009; ASBH 2011). We fear that these formulations may obfuscate, rather than clarify, the requisite skill set of a clinical ethics consultant by their continued focus on the paramount need for bioethical expertise, coupled with mere marginal support for process-oriented mediation skills (Dubler et al. 2009; ASBH 2011). No one denies that mediation skills are useful. The debate centers around how much prominence mediation skills should have, relative to other skills. This is not lost on the lead author of the prominent White Paper written by one such working group (Dubler et al. 2009). In the second edition of their book, *Bioethics Mediation,* Nancy Dubler and Carol Liebman write:

> The landscape has changed and mediation is an accepted part of Clinical Ethics Consultation. Our concern, however, is that this acceptance of dispute resolution and mediation has arrived without a robust and powerful commitment to the skills that the discipline demands. (Dubler and Liebman 2011, xiii)

To address that concern, we believe that clinical ethics mediation must become the explicit focus of clinical ethics education and clinical ethics consultation, not its handmaiden. In essence, we advocate a redefinition of clinical ethics consultation as delivered via a mediation model.

At the heart of clinical ethics mediation training is the use of role-plays based on clinical conflicts.[1] In simulated disputes, students assume the roles of disputants (including health-care professionals, patients, surrogates, and family members), as well as mediators. Enacting the disputant roles gives prospective mediators an understanding of what those positions, interests, values, and concerns might feel like. It helps create empathy through identification with those in provider, patient, and family roles. Those neither mediating nor enacting a disputant role observe the process unfold and, ultimately, participate in the debriefing process, bringing the perspective of individuals one step removed from the immediate pressures of performance. Both the observation and conduct of simulated mediations provide learning opportunities that cannot be replicated by more traditional teaching methods of lecture, discussion, and reading. Immersion in the mediation process is necessary to an appreciation of the dynamics of managing an interactive process, with its infinite number of variables, and to the self-discovery requisite to effective mediation skills.

While exposure to and participation in the clinical ethics mediation process are a critical aspect of training, repetition is insufficient without timely critical analysis of the experience. The role-plays, therefore, are followed by a debriefing dialogue between actors and observers, moderated by the instructor, which focuses on choices made by the mediator, alternative options that might have existed, communication issues that surfaced, interpersonal dynamics, emotions, relationships, cultural concerns, medical facts, legal issues, sources of disagreement, and competing value systems at play. The debriefing session provides a basis for self-examination, constructive feedback from all parties, and the internalization of mediation skills. We believe that repeated participation

[1] Two models of clinical ethics mediation training that exist in the United States are the Certificate in Clinical Ethics Mediation that we offer at the Perelman School of Medicine at the University of Pennsylvania (http://www.med.upenn.edu/mbe/students.shtml#Mediation), and the workshop offered by Nancy Dubler and Carol Liebman at Albert Einstein College of Medicine (http://www.einstein.yu.edu/masters-in-bioethics/page.aspx?id=30968&ekmensel=15074e5e_3686_4439_30968_1 - bioemediation).

in simulated mediation role-plays followed by debriefings constitutes the single most important aspect of training in clinical ethics mediation. As such, we have included a sample role play at the end of this essay.[2] We are, of course, mindful that role plays, however instructive, are pedagogical tools for use in a laboratory setting which we believe inherently lack verisimilitude. Nonetheless, we believe that their utilization provides optimal preparation for exposure to the open-ended complexity of real-world conflict.

Conclusion

Clinical ethics mediation borrows effective strategies of conflict resolution long employed by mediators of disputes in myriad contexts. These techniques have already been recognized as an important supplement to the training of individuals engaged in resolving clinical ethics disputes. We argue that mediation should replace consultation or become the model for its delivery and, as such, should constitute the focus of future clinical ethics training. Mediation is not only perfectly suited for the clinical ethics conflicts that are communication- or relationship-based, but it avoids ethically problematic aspects of traditional consultation that render judgments suspect in disputes emanating from a pluralism of legitimate values.

MIRACLES AND MEDICINE: A SAMPLE ROLE-PLAY

Four-person role play

Roles

Ann Fitzgerald, patient's daughter
Dr. Aaron Cook, patient's nephrologist
Olivia Fell, head nurse
Mediator

General instructions

An 80-year-old man named Bill Fitzgerald has been on hem dialysis for ESRD for the past five years and recently had a stroke. Bill has remained comatose for a week and the prognosis for neurological recovery is grim. He continues to receive dialysis three times per week and is physically stable. His physician, Dr. Cook, believes that further treatment is futile and that it is time to withdraw life support and dialysis. Nurse Fell, the head nurse on Bill's hospital floor, is in agreement with Dr. Cook that it is time to end treatment. On the other hand, Bill's very religious daughter Ann claims to believe that a miracle will occur to save her father. Consequently, Ann opposes withdrawal of life-support treatment.

Continued

---

[2] Other examples of published role plays can be found in the Dubler and Liebman book (2011).

Confidential information for Ann Fitzgerald, patient's daughter

(Do not share this information with others.)
You can't believe how pushy all of these doctors and nurses are being! They keep asking you if you want to consider withdrawing treatment from Dad, but they don't listen when you tell them that it clearly isn't his time yet. When God wants Dad's life to be over, He'll take control. You've been praying every morning and every night and you have faith that God will bring Dad back for at least a little bit of time so that you can talk to him one more time. Just this past Sunday at church, Kim Henderson was telling you about her mother's breast cancer that suddenly went into remission after she had begun praying four times each day. You prefer to let God control the fate of the world and not some know-it-all doctors and nurses. They appear not to have faith, but you do!

Confidential information for Dr. Aaron cook, patient's nephrologist

(Do not share this information with others.)
You have been Bill Fitzgerald's nephrologists for the past five years, ever since you diagnosed him with ESRD. Other than his kidney problems, Bill had been in good physical condition and was living a fairly happy life. His daughter, Ann, would visit him from time to time to keep him company during his dialysis and that always seemed to brighten his day. Unfortunately, the stroke he recently suffered put him into a coma. It doesn't look as if he'll be able to recover. It has been two weeks now and you think it's about time to stop dialysis. It is an expensive procedure and is always in high demand. You can understand if Ann wants to wait a little longer, though; they seem to have a great relationship and it must be hard for her to let go.

Confidential information for Olivia Fell, head nurse

(Do not share this information with others.)
This case has really gotten under your skin the past few days. It's always sad to see a happy man suddenly fall into a deep coma and watch his family struggle to accept the tragedy. But it's been two weeks now and most staff members think that it's time for the family to let go and withdraw all treatments. Bill's daughter, Ann, however, snaps at anyone who suggests this option. You are not trying to be disrespectful of her faith, but the reality is that her father is benefitting from valuable medical care that could help someone with a much more hopeful prognosis to survive.

Confidential information for Mediator

(Do not share this information with others.)
As a staff mediator you were referred this case by Dr. Cook. While Dr. Cook understands Ann's reluctance to withdraw care, he disagrees with her. Nurse Fell is adamant that care be withdrawn immediately but her basis for that position is unclear to you at this point. Facilitating effective communication among all three parties will be required in order to reach a consensual resolution.

References

American Society for Bioethics and Humanities. (2011). *Core Competencies for Healthcare Ethics Consultation*. 2nd ed. Glenview, IL: ASBH.

Aulisio, M. P., Arnold, R. M., and Youngner, S. J. (2000). "A Position Paper from the Society for Health and Human Values-Society for Bioethics Consultation Task Force on Standards for Bioethics Consultation. Health Care Ethics Consultation: Nature, Goals, and Competencies," *Annals of Internal Medicine*, 133(1): 59–69.

Beauchamp, T., and Childress, J. (2009). *Principles of Biomedical Ethics*. 6th ed. New York: Oxford University Press.

Bergman, E., and Fiester, A. (2009). "Bioethics Mediation," in V. Ravitsky, A. Fiester, and A. Caplan, (eds.), *The Penn Center Guide to Bioethics*. New York: Springer, 171–80.

Bergman, E. (2013). "Surmounting Elusive Barriers: The Case for Bioethics Mediation," *Journal of Clinical Ethics*, 24(1): 11–24.

Caplan, A., and Bergman, E. (2007). "Beyond Schiavo," *Journal of Clinical Ethics*, 18(4): 340–5.

Casarett, D. J., Daskal, F., and Lantos, J. (1998). "The Authority of the Clinical Ethicist," *Hastings Center Report*, 28(6): 6–11.

Clinical Ethics Consultation Affairs Committee. (2010). CECA Report to the Board of Directors, ASBH on Certification, Accreditation, and Credentializing of Clinical Ethics Consultants. http://www.asbh.org/uploads/files/ceca%20c-a%20report%20101210.pdf (accessed December 14, 2012)

Dubler, N., and Liebman, C. (2011). *Bioethics Mediation: A Guide to Shaping Shared Solutions*. Nashville, TN: Vanderbilt University Press.

Dubler, N. N. et al. (2009). "Charting the Future," *Hastings Center Report*, 39(6): 29–33.

Fiester, A. (2007a). "Mediation and *Aporia*," *Journal of Clinical Ethics*, 18(4): 355–6.

Fiester, A. (2007b). "The Failure of the Consult Model: Why 'Mediation' Should Replace 'Consultation,'" *American Journal of Bioethics*, 7(2): 31–2.

Fiester, A. (2011). "Ill-placed Democracy: Ethics Consultations and the Moral Status of Voting," *Journal of Clinical Ethics*, 22(4): 363–72.

Fiester, A. (2012a). "Mediation and Advocacy," *American Journal of Bioethics*, 12(8): 10–11.

Fiester, A. (2012b). "The 'Difficult' Patient Reconceived: An Expanded Moral Mandate for Clinical Ethics," *American Journal of Bioethics*, 12(5): 2–7.

Fox, E., Myers, S., and Pearlman, R. A. (2007). "Ethics Consultation in United States Hospitals: A National Survey," *American Journal of Bioethics*, 7(2): 13–25.

Green, M., Simms, S., and Blackall, G. (2009). *Breaking the Cycle*. Philadelphia, PA: American College of Physicians.

Joint Commission. (2011). Standards for acute care hospitals, revised December. 2010. http://www.cihq-hacp.org/images/pdf/2011_TJC_Acute_Care_Standards_-_Rev12.10.pdf.

Moore, C. W. (2003). *The Mediation Process: Practical Strategies for Resolving Conflict*. 3rd ed. San Francisco, CA: Jossey-Bass.

Stone, D., Patton, B., and Heen, S. (1999). *Difficult Conversations: How to Discuss What Matters Most*. New York: Penguin Books.

The Terri Schiavo Case. http://en.wikipedia.org/wiki/Terri_Schiavo_case (accessed December 14, 2012).

Walker, M. U. (1993). "Keeping Moral Space Open: New Images of Ethics Consulting," *Hastings Center Report*, 23(2): 33–40.

20.2

Commentary
Barriers to Clinical Ethics Mediation in Contemporary Japan

Atsushi Asai and Yasuhiro Kadooka

1 Importance of clinical ethics mediation

It goes without saying that mediation is important when dealing with clinical ethics problems. For those who need to cope with ethical difficulties or disagreements in the clinical setting, it is essential to understand the utility of mediation and learn effective communication skills. Antagonistic relations among all concerned and excessive self-assertion would only further complicate problematic situations. Negotiation (generating options for a solution and helping all parties understand their best alternative to a negotiated agreement), clarification (eliciting and clarifying the medical facts associated with patient care), neutralization (neutralizing the power imbalance among all concerned), and sympathy are all necessary elements (Watkins et al. 2007: 2328–41). Mediation would also contribute to the resolution of cognitive conflicts among those concerned (Wada and Nakanisi 2011: 2).

It is also essential that a person in charge of clinical ethics service or support maintains a neutral position. Craig (1996) reported that mediators are trained to be impartial and independent, and are equally concerned about the rights of all involved in the dispute; their concern is to have the views of all participants heard, discussed, and mutually reconciled, at least to the extent that participants reach an agreement on their own about resolving issues and determining outcomes. The author also argued that mediation is a noncoercive, gentle process that is well suited to patient decision-making, and that neutrality was considered more effective in achieving a balance in unequal and hierarchical power relations and promoting the primacy of patients (Craig 1996: 164–6).

We similarly claimed that in order to resolve clinical ethics dilemmas it is essential to clarify the problem at hand and rearrange medical facts and situations, to ensure communication, sharing, and understanding of relevant information and grasp the decision-making capacity of the patient, and to learn opinions and underlying reasons of the persons concerned. We further argued that those who need to cope with ethical difficulties in the clinical setting must discuss the problem at hand in a sympathetic manner, strive to understand different values or faiths, and make an effort to agree upon a course of action that is in the best interest of the patient (Clinical Ethics Support and Education Project 2009: 23–4).

Bergman and Fiester claim that traditional ethics consultation should be replaced with bioethics mediation, which will aid and support the legitimate decision makers in these cases, namely the patients and their families. Whether bioethics mediation should replace the conventional approach in the present American context or whether the former is better than the latter is difficult to determine given the limited knowledge on contemporary clinical settings and clinical ethics activities in America. Naturally, however, the legitimacy of ethical judgments presented by traditional clinical ethics consultation should be doubted if it imposes an alternative that fails to reflect the opinions of the persons concerned in an authoritarian manner.

Fiester also questioned whether the current ethics consultation service is qualified to mandate a course of action that will profoundly affect virtual strangers, whose values and priorities may be very different from those of the ethics consultation service members (Fiester 2007: 31–2). The answer to this important question would apparently be negative. Ethical uncertainty and deep value disagreements frequently exist in many hospital-based conflicts in most countries, and we agree that neither the ethical committee members nor an individual consultant has the dominative moral knowledge or ability for ethical judgments. Authoritarianism does not go hand in hand with being ethical.

2 Current situations in Japan

It is unclear as to what kind of impacts clinical ethics mediation, as proposed by Bergman and Fiester in their article, has on clinical ethics consultation and education in the Japanese context. This is because little is known about the present conditions of both ethics consultation and postgraduate clinical ethics education. However, to the best of our knowledge, there is only limited activity in this area, and paid employees who exclusively serve as ethics consultants do not exist in Japanese hospitals. The other problem, which may be contrary to the concern raised by Bergman and Fiester, relates to the authority of ethics committees. Here in Japan, we would claim that clinical ethics support activities do not have an authoritative power strong enough to affect the final decision-making in clinical cases. Indeed, there have been cases where the decisions of ethics committees permitting withdrawal of the respirator from dying patients in deference to the wishes of both the patient and the patient's family have been overturned by the hospital director. Given the aforementioned circumstances, we would like to examine several barriers that could prevent the effectiveness of clinical ethics mediation in current Japan.

3 Barriers to clinical ethics mediation in contemporary Japan: legal situations surrounding the clinical ethics approach in Japan

Bergman and Fiester argued that clinical ethics mediators have the responsibility of knowing not only the techniques of conflict resolution, but also what constitutes a solution that runs afoul of the law, hospital policy, or ethical scaffolding in the community that underpins them. According to their article, in the United States competent patients must give their informed consent for any procedure done to them, or they must waive their right to it; therefore, a mediator cannot craft a solution that denies a competent patient access to this right or waiver, no matter what level of agreement might be forged among others involved in the case.

According to Emanuel, for example, a patient has the legal right to refuse medical interventions; any and all interventions can be legally and ethically terminated; there is no difference between withholding life-sustaining interventions and withdrawing them; the views of a competent adult patient on terminating life-sustaining interventions prevail if there is a conflict between the patient and family; an appointed proxy or a legally designated hierarchy among relatives is in charge of the decisions regarding termination of life-sustaining interventions if the patient is incompetent; and advance care directives are legally enforceable (Emanuel 2012: 4–9). Such safeguards are essential for the clinical ethics mediation to be safe and effective.

In contrast, however, there are no ethical or legal safeguards surrounding decisions generated in the clinical ethics mediation process in Japan. In the Japanese context, for example, no written legal regulation concerning termination of medical intervention has existed to date, and health-care professionals, patients, and the patients' families are uncertain about which actions are forbidden (Asai et al. 2012). The Yokohama High Court declared in the Kawasaki Kyodo Hospital case that patient self-determination, family surrogate decision, or the limits of a physician's obligation to treat were not decisive grounds to support a legitimate termination of life support. They also claimed that withdrawal of life support would go against laws prohibiting murder at the victim's request and assisted suicide. In addition, no legally enforceable advance directives have existed in Japan. A relevant Bill was once presented to the Diet in 2007, but no further discussions have occurred. It can be argued that a patient's right to self-determination, particularly the right to refuse medical interventions, has not been established yet, except for the refusal of blood transfusion by an adult Jehovah's Witnesses believer.

4   Barriers to clinical ethics mediation in contemporary Japan: cultural factors

Confucianism has long had a strong impact on mentality, morality, conscience, and human relations of Japanese people, and its value systems place a lower significance on an individual's or patient's right to self-determination than collective decision-making. An Asian scholar also argued that the principle of patient autonomy may be of less significance in certain Asian cultures with ties to Confucian traditions, which place higher value on family cohesion, ancestor worship, and filial piety. Thus, the autonomy of an individual may not necessarily be the foremost consideration, particularly where the individual's choice may conflict with the family's wishes or pose a detriment to the family's greater welfare (Kim et al. 2010: 113–17). Together with the aforementioned lack of ethical, social, and legal safeguards, clinical ethics mediation could fail to respect and protect the best interest and dignity of the patient in a family-centered atmosphere.

Japanese culture also tends to consider conference and negotiation among all parties very important, often requiring unanimous decisions rather than individual self-determination or decisions under majority rule. Even today, "the principle of harmony (*Wa no Seishin*)" is stronger than respect for autonomy in human relationships, including the clinical setting (Izawa 2005: 404–37). However, respect for the principle of harmony through conference and negotiation in unequal human relationships could result in the imposition of collective decisions on unwilling individuals. At the end of life, those who are physically, mentally, or socially too weak to express and maintain their wishes are most damaged by the inappropriate medical intervention imposed by others (Tanida 2011: 55–75). In a number of cases, the family intervenes in the treatment plan against the patient's wishes (Imai 2011: 81–106). It is also claimed that because of the insistence on conference, negotiation, and unanimous conclusions, Japanese people often fail to make emergent decisions when necessary and tend to fail to reach any conclusions when faced with opponents (Izawa 2005: 404–37). Delayed decisions could cause physical and mental harm to the patient. In addition, when aiming toward unanimity, the patient as well as conference participants may be reluctant to express opinions that may differ from others' perspectives or can hardly be expected to gain social acceptance. Furthermore, the patient may not express his or her intention and may abide by the family's opinion even if he or she is not convinced.

Furthermore, Japanese culture traditionally permits a double standard in decision-making, which is often viewed as deep consideration or a caring attitude toward others. This difference in attitude has been recognized for a long time in the research and clinical experiences of doctors (Asai et al. 2012). A recent national survey conducted by the Ministry of Health, Labor, and Welfare revealed a consistent difference of about 20 percent between questions about life-sustaining preferences for oneself and preferences for others (Report of Committee Concerning End-of-Life, 2010). The extent to which clinical ethics mediation can satisfactorily work in Japanese culture is unclear. It would be extremely difficult to change long-established social and familial human relationships and individual mentalities.

5 Barriers to clinical ethics mediation in contemporary Japan: problems in clinical settings

In the Japanese context, although many other factors requiring critical consideration might exist, the closed and exclusive tendency of the health-care society, time constraint, and financial difficulty could become major barriers to the effective practical use of clinical ethics mediation. As for the exclusive attitudes of health-care professionals and institutions, thought processes (e.g. "There is no need to make a problem open and public," "It would be better to avoid a stranger and/or outsider, including a clinical ethics expert, and deal with problems only in the hospital"), psychology that attempts to avoid any conflict, and top-down workplace environments may block the resolution of ethical problems and introduction of mediation activities. We believe that the biggest obstacle among these is the self-respecting health profession that has little awareness of ethical problems (Asai 2010: 61–5).

In addition, in the current Japanese clinical setting, it is likely to be difficult to find enough time to spare for clinical ethics mediation where all the concerned parties participate. Furthermore, due to serious financial constraints, many medical institutions would not be able to employ a mediation specialist. As the next-best policy, they may educate existing health-care professionals as mediators. However, in this case it would be extremely difficult for the mediator, who is also a health-care professional employed by the hospital, to maintain a neutral outlook and position. Even if they can be truly neutral in their position, not many of those on the patient's side would be willing to trust their neutrality.

6 Some questions from the ethical standpoint

In the final section, we refer to and briefly consider a series of questions outside the realm of law, culture, and on-site problems, that is, what Bergman and Fiester described as classical bioethical disputes. This kind of dispute happens even when communication is exemplary, personality conflicts are not in evidence, and each party possesses all the relevant information (Bergman and Fiester 2009: 171–80). Furthermore, no emotional confrontation would exist in such cases. It can be argued that classical bioethical dispute is an authentic ethical dilemma.

The first of our concerns is a difficulty that one might experience in trying to remain truly ethically neutral. Can an individual in charge of clinical ethics mediation truly and forever maintain neutrality in the face of value-laden problems? We would argue that no one can completely escape the cultural or religious influences of the region where one has grown up. Everyone has his or her moral conscience. Mediators' behaviors and wordings could be affected by their cultural or personal values, and their ethical beliefs might surface even if their professional training, including role-playing, could largely prevent its occurrence.

Second, what should a mediator do when those concerned, such as patients, family members, or health-care professionals, ask for advice that includes substantial ethical dimensions? We assume that there are cases in which people are totally at a loss when confronting ethical dilemmas, but not in conflict against each other. Of course, one could respond by saying that offering practical or concrete ethical advice is not a part of their role. However, such a reply might fail to satisfy those who desperately want to know what others ethically think in a given case. Third, we would argue that non-coercive ethical opinion based on the third person's point of view is often useful for individuals mired in ethical dilemmas to arrive at well informed and well balanced conclusions on their own. In other words, it is an "ethical second opinion." Naturally, such an opinion should not be a mandate or a strong recommendation.

Finally, we wonder that, irrespective of the clinical ethics approach applied and regardless of traditional consultation or mediation, there are cases where all those concerned cannot agree on what should be done in order to achieve the best interest of the patient in a given case and no final agreement is reached. In such cases, no one might be satisfied or convinced. A commentator claims that it is often likely the case that the best course of action for the patient cannot be agreed upon because a single solution that would absolutely satisfy all parties' perceptions of what is best for the patient does not exist (DeAngelo 2000: 133–9). This situation is likely to occur particularly when the patient is incompetent or when he/she has not been informed of relevant medical information due to cultural reasons. Furthermore, in Japan where legally enforceable advance directives, appointed proxy, or a designated hierarchy among relatives has not existed to date, it could be sometimes difficult to protect the patient's wishes or interests even in an ideal process of clinical ethics mediation.

References

Asai, A. (2010). "Coauthor's Comment," *Kango kanri* 20:64.

Asai, A. et al. (2012). "Death with Dignity Is Impossible in Contemporary Japan," *Eubios Journal of Asian and International Bioethics*, 22:49–53.

Bergman, E. J., and Fiester, A. (2009). "Mediation and Health Care," in V. Ravitsky, A. Fiester, and A. L. Caplan (eds), *The Penn Center Guide to Bioethics*, New York: Springer, 171–80.

Clinical Ethics Support and Education Project. (2009). "Two-Step Clinical Ethics Approach," in A. Asai et al. (eds), *Tomoni Kangaerutameno Checklist*, Kumamoto, Japan: Department of Bioethics, Kumamoto University Graduate School of Medicine, 23–4.

Craig, Y. J. (1996). "Patient Decision-making: Medical Ethics and Mediation," *Journal of Medical Ethics*, 22:164–7.

DeAngelo, L. M. (2000). "Mediation in Health Care Settings: Some Theoretical and Practical Concepts," *Journal of Clinical Psychology in Medical Setting* 7: 133–9.

Emanuel, E. J. (2012). "Bioethics in the Practice of Medicine," in L. Goldman, and A. I. Schafer (eds), *Goldman's Cecil Medicine*. 24th ed. Philadelphia, PA: Elsevier, 4–9.

End-of-Life Committee. (2010). *Report of Committee concerning End-of-Life in Japan*, December, 2010. Tokyo: Ministry of Health, Welfare, and Labor.

Fiester, A. (2007). "The Failure of the Consult Model: Why 'Mediation' Should Replace 'Consultation,'" *American Journal of Bioethics*, 7:31–2.

Imai, S. (2011). "Kanja no Jikokettei to Support Taisei," in Keio University School of Medicine Medical Education Center (ed), Keio University School of Medicine Seimeirinri Seminar 2, Tokyo: Keio University Press, 81–106.

Izawa, M. (2005). *Gyakusetu no Nippon Rekisikan*. Tokyo: Shogakkan.

Judgment of the Yokohama High Court regarding Kawasaki Kyodo Hospital Euthanasia Case, February 2007.

Kim, S. et al. (2010). "A Korean Perspective on Developing a Global Policy for Advance Directives," *Bioethics*, 24:113–17.

Tanida, N. (2011). "Denial in Contemporary Japanese: From a Traditional View of Life and Death and Unrealistic Expectation of Modern Medicine," *Journal of Philosophy and Ethics in Health Care and Medicine*, 5:55–75.

Wada, Y., and Nakanisi, T. (2011). *Healthcare Mediation*. Tokyo: Shinyu.

Watkins, L. T., Sacajiu, G., and Karasz, A. (2007). "The Role of the Bioethicist in Family Meetings about End of Life Care," *Social Science and Medicine*, 65: 2328–41.

20.3

Commentary
Clinical Ethics After Morality: Mediation as Pure Procedure

H. Tristram Engelhardt, Jr.

The challenge is to provide a coherent account of education in clinical ethics against the background recognition that there is no common morality, no canonical morality, and therefore no canonical bioethics. Bergman and Fiester appear to recognize the disconnection of clinical ethics from morality as morality might have been understood in the dominant Western culture from the thirteenth century until the late twentieth century. Thirteenth-century western Europe sought to restore the centrality of the Greek vision of morality as a third thing supported by reason between God and man. Orthodox Jews and traditional Christians, including Orthodox Christians, recognized the God who commands and as a result had not seen a need for such a morality or a moral philosophy. However, the second-millennium West, especially after the translation of Aristotle into Latin in Paris in 1210, embraced the project of articulating a rationally grounded morality that continued into modernity. The presumption was that moral rationality was one, and that therefore one could provide univocal guidance in the face of a plurality of religious views.

Had such a project been possible, natural-law theorists would have been able to show how all humans should act, Kantians would have been able to establish right-making conditions morally constraining the actions of all persons, or consequentialists would have been able to compare various goods, pleasures, and satisfactions of preferences in order to establish a canonical account of how one should act in order to achieve the good. None of this has proven possible because there is no basis for an agreement regarding basic secular moral premises and rules of evidence. As Bergman and Fiester concede in their acknowledgements of moral pluralism, moral rationality is plural and cannot provide univocal moral guidance.

Against the background of the impending deflation of secular morality, and as a consequence of the increasing recognition of morality's foundationless character, Bergman and Fiester realize that the task of clinical ethics cannot be to ensure that one does the right, achieves the good, or acts virtuously because there is no agreement regarding the right, the good, or the virtuous. In the face of intractable moral pluralism and without canonical moral foundations to establish a canonical account of the good, the right, or the virtuous, one is left with the different freestanding clusters of moral intuitions sustained by diverse moral narratives, all of which are socio-historically conditioned. After God and after metaphysics, morality as well as the ethics of clinical ethics is intractably plural. There is no decisive, sound, rational argument to establish any one of the numerous moralities, bioethics, or practices of clinical ethics as normative (Engelhardt 1996). Against this background, there are at least three ways to understand clinical ethics as mediation:

1. Clinical ethics as a practice of mediation that focuses on bringing a patient and/or a patient's family, as well as health-care givers, to come into agreement regarding a therapy choice guided and/or constrained by a particular secular social-democratic vision of human rights, human equality, and human dignity.
2. Clinical ethics as a practice of mediation that focuses on bringing a patient and/or a patient/s family, as well as health-care givers, into agreement regarding a therapy choice guided and/or constrained by the dictates of a particular religious moral vision, such as Roman Catholic bioethics as this bears on the provision of health care in a Roman Catholic hospital.
3. Clinical ethics as a practice of mediation that focuses on helping a patient and/or a patient's family, as well as health-care givers, to come to agreement regarding a therapy choice guided and constrained by what happens to constitute the "law, hospital policy, or the ethical scaffolding [of a particular] community" (Bergman and Fiester in this chapter).

Bergman and Fiester appear to embrace clinical ethics as mediation in the third sense. However, insofar as secular social-democratic moral commitments or the constraints of the Roman Catholic church define hospital policy or the ethical scaffolding of a particular community and its hospital, they should be at peace with these understandings of mediation as well. Bergman and Fiester appear to understand that there is no canonical secular morality that *sub specie aeternitatis* can guide clinical ethics in the engagement of mediation. Of course, those who ideologically embrace ethics consultation as mediation in the first sense or who out of religious conviction embrace mediation in the second sense will find the other approaches wrongheaded.

Bergman and Fiester's account of ethics consultation appears fully at peace not only with the secular moral deflation of the traditional Western morality of sexual, reproductive, and end-of-life choices into matters of lifestyle and death-style preferences, but also by implication with the deflation as well of social-democratic moral commitments concerning human rights, human equality, and human dignity into macro lifestyle choices. Prescinding from any ultimate points of moral orientation or from any deontological constraints, mediation becomes the equivalent to a process of bargaining placed within limits set by law and public policy. Bergman and Fiester correctly realize that they can therefore best present only a procedural account of clinical ethics. Mediation values and catalyzes the effective communication of individual concerns, values, perspectives and feelings—all of which are essential to the clinical ethics consultation process (Bergman and Fiester in this chapter). In this circumstance, the concrete meaning of "effectiveness" will be determined by social-historical considerations, which as Bergman and Fiester concede are simply "the law, hospital policy, or the ethical scaffolding in the community" (Bergman and Fiester in this chapter). Ethics consultation as mediation is thus purely a "skill set" that can facilitate difficult conversations, including decisions in emotionally (but not necessarily morally controverted) laden situations. Clinical ethics, in a culture without God and without metaphysics, that is, in a secular culture without ultimate moral norms, becomes a clinical ethics evacuated of strong moral significance (i.e. asserting norms that rational persons as such must follow). For the now-dominant, secular culture, Bergman and Fiester implicitly recognize that there is no canonical secular moral narrative or ethics to guide.

In this context, clinical ethics education is not education in normative ethics. Clinical ethics is not a form of normative instruction or counseling. Instead, as Bergman and Fiester recognize, clinical ethics functions as a skill set for mediators who within certain constraints facilitate health-care decisions. In this context, education in traditional normative ethics will likely remain for clinical ethics education, something like a course in old-time osteopathy within schools of osteopathic medicine, which schools have become materially equivalent to what are now generally accepted as medical schools. Given the centrality of the constraints imposed by law and public policy on all clinical decision-making, clinical ethics education will need as a central element education in law and public policy as this applies to clinical decision-making. This is the case because clinical ethicists usually act as quasi-lawyers. They mediate on analogy with lawyers. They inform patients, families of patients, and health-care professionals of the legal and public policy constraints on clinical decisions, thus often helping to resolve the controversies that elicit health-care ethics consultations (Engelhardt 2009; 2011).

References

Bergman, E., and Fiester, A. (2013). "The Future of Clinical Ethics Education: Value Pluralism, Communication, and Mediation," in A. Akabayashi (ed), The Future of Bioethics: International Dialogues. Oxford: Oxford University Press, XXX–XXX.

Engelhardt, H. T. Jr. (1996). The Foundations of Bioethics. 2nd ed. New York: Oxford University Press.

Engelhardt, H. T. Jr. (2009). "Credentialing Strategically Ambiguous and Heterogeneous Social Skills: The Emperor without Clothes," HEC Forum, 21(3): 293–306.

Engelhardt, H. T. Jr. (2011). "Core Competencies for Health Care Ethics Consultants: In Search of Professional Status in a Post-modern World," HEC Forum, 23(3): 129–45.

20.4

Commentary
Bioethics Mediation and Narrative Consultation

Takanobu Kinjo

Introduction

I was hired by the University of the Ryukyus Hospital as an ethicist. I was said to be the first full-time ethicist to be employed at a Japanese health-care institution, and as a result, beginning work was not easy. Nobody really seemed to know what an ethicist even was, and I had a difficult time explaining my role in a university teaching hospital. After a while, I started to plan an ethics consultation service aimed exclusively at health-care workers. I made flyers, posted contact information, and so forth. Finally, I submitted the proposal at the department council meeting. Several clinical professors, however, strenuously objected to the establishment of individual-based ethics consultation. They recommended instead a more systematic, committee-based ethics consultation service. The reasons behind their objection were, in my view, quite legitimate. During the meeting, one professor asked me a critical question: "Dr. Kinjo, forgive me for asking you this question, but are you licensed to work in clinical settings?" I answered: "Well, I earned a PhD, but no, I don't have a license …" It was obvious that the legitimacy of my professional expertise as an ethics consultant was in question. Again and again, the same recurring question was raised: Who is qualified to be an ethics consultant?

Medical mediation in Japan

Verdict- and majority decision-based ethics consultation have come under considerable criticism in recent years, most notably by Autumn Fiester. Fiester points out that the ethics consultation system in the United States does not work, and vigorously proposes that it must be replaced with what she calls "bioethics mediation" (Fiester 2007: 31–2).

In fact, it seems like a good idea to adopt the model of "mediation" into clinical ethics in Japan, because medical mediation is becoming much more pervasive and popular than ethics consultation in Japanese clinical settings. The year 2005 saw the launch of the first medical mediator training program as an official course of the "Japan Council for Quality Health Care." In 2008, the Japan Association of Healthcare Mediators was founded, followed by the establishment of two other mediation organizations. Currently, these three organizations offer either direct or supervised medical mediator training programs in Japan, educating over 2,000 people every year (Wada and Nakanishi 2011: iv–vii). Since 2007, the total number of accredited medical mediators in Japan has reached 1,788, reflecting the spread of medical mediation in Japanese clinical settings (Japan Association of Healthcare Mediators). It is clear that accredited medical mediators far outnumber ethics consultants in Japan.

In light of this situation, it may indeed be wise to abandon ethics consultation and instead promote ethics mediation in Japan. Indeed, given the prevalence of medical mediation in Japan, ethics mediation might be expected to take root much more rapidly than ethics consultation.

Concerns about incorporating "mediation" into ethics

Above all, Fiester is absolutely right to criticize ethics consultation that is verdict based and seems to "take sides," as unethical. This makes her proposal to replace ethics consultation with bioethics mediation very convincing (Fiester 2011). However, I contend that we should be very careful when replacing ethics consultation with bioethics mediation for the following reasons.

My major concerns stem from the term "mediation." Although mediation has long been recognized as an important role of ethics consultants in the context of clinical ethics settings (Orr and deLeon 2000), the term "mediation" has its own history, purposes, and practices. Therefore, we must consider very carefully the implications of introducing "mediation" into clinical ethics.

First of all, because medical mediation is heavily influenced by the legal science tradition, I am anxious about the possibility that bioethics mediation may be viewed as simply an alternative method of legal dispute resolution.

Second, I suspect that medical mediation, consciously or unconsciously, presupposes that our differences in values, beliefs, and perception are in conflict. In order for a conflict to be mediated, at least two parties must be involved. Now, when integrating medical mediation into clinical ethics, there is the concern that health-care workers will have the mistaken impression that ethical dilemmas must always occur between two (or more) parties. The result is that they unconsciously look for two or more conflicting parties as a sign that intervention is needed, while easily overlooking an ethical dilemma quietly and secretly occurring inside a patient, family member, or health-care worker.

My last concern is related to mediation skills. Because medical mediation comes with a well established and defined set of skills and knowledge that can be measured during the accreditation process, I am concerned that bioethics mediation may also be subject to accreditation in the near future. It is not my intention, of course, to suggest that accreditation itself is problematic. But we should carefully examine why medical mediation in Japan has three professional organizations along with a well established accreditation system, while ethics consultation in Japan has no official organization or accreditation system.

The reason that ethics consultation should not, in my opinion, have an accreditation system is that it is a service intended to meet the needs of people facing a genuine ethical dilemma that cannot essentially be resolved or mediated by the mere application of a certain set of skills. I shall call such non-accreditable ethics consultation "narrative-based ethics consultation," the consultation most distinctively practiced, I think, by Richard Zaner.

What is narrative-based ethics consultation?

Given that the fundamental premise of the narrative approach is that we are all gifted storytelling animals (MacIntyre 1984), narrative-based ethics consultation is well summarized in the following statement by Zaner:

> The individuals whose situation is at issue have their own stories that need telling. Clinical ethics is in this sense a way of helping patients, families, and, yes, health providers to discover and give voice to those stories. In this way, clinical ethics is an evoking of meaning. (Zaner 2006: 655)

Narrative consultation can be defined as a service that provides patients, family members, and health-care professionals with opportunities to tell their own stories in a way that gives them the power to get through, cope with, and persist in the morally difficult times that they face in clinical settings. Borrowing Zaner's words, narrative consultation aims at "helping each other get through bad times and good" (Zaner 2006: 658) by telling, listening to, and sharing personal stories with one another.

The basic premise of narrative consultation is that morality is expressed in accepting responsibility toward one's own narratives and those of others (Walker 2007). In clinical settings, Zaner emphasizes that the ethicist is and ought to be "invited into the situation and conversation" (Zaner 1996: 272). The result of such an invitation is "responsive and responsible ethics." A responsive and responsible ethics consultant does not necessarily need to provide an ethical recommendation or an ethically ideal, "ought to be" narrative, but according to Zaner, "being present as an ethicist is itself a trigger for very crucial conversations" (Zaner 1993: 46). The role of the responsive/responsible narrative consultant is to "listen, question, listen, encourage further details, and listen still again" (Zaner 1996: 272) and to spontaneously respond to patients' and family members' stories. The objectives are to: 1) understand what matters most to them, 2) help them think carefully about their situation in light of their own beliefs, 3) help them restore and reconstruct their fractured illness narratives, and 4) help them make their illness experiences meaningful.

There are three distinctive features of narrative consultation: 1) helping prepare to tell a narrative in future, 2) narrative as an end in itself, and 3) genuinely listening to narratives with an attitude of "not knowing."

The first distinctive feature of narrative consultation is that it does not aim to provide verdict-based ethical recommendations, but instead helps patients, family members, and health-care professionals prepare to tell their own narratives in the future. When facing an authentic and unresolvable ethical dilemma (or aporia), we cannot know with certainty in advance which choice is right and which is wrong. Consequently, the least we can do is strive to think through the problem seriously and sincerely, so that in the future we can be satisfied that, in fact, the choice we made was the best possible one under the difficult conditions faced, regardless of whether the end result was what we intended. What an ethics consultant can do, then, is to help ensure that the decision-making process will be worthy of retelling as a narrative in the future. This is made possible by engaging in attentive, genuine, and sincere listening, ongoing dialogue, questioning, and giving thorough consideration to the issues raised by patients and family members.

The second distinctive feature of narrative consultation is the importance of regarding narratives as ends (gifts) in themselves. In clinical settings, narratives are typically viewed as a means to other ultimate ends. Generally speaking, the more the degree of your expertise increases, the more you are likely to listen to someone's story as a means to some other ends, ends that are defined and pursued by your area of specialization. For example, a physician listens to a patient's narrative, using it as grounds on which to base a diagnosis. In contrast, a narrative consultant listens to each patient's narrative as an end in itself. That is, a narrative consultant listens to their narrative not because s/he must make an ethical recommendation, but rather because he or she simply sees and responds to the intrinsic value and goals within the patient's narrative. In other words, for a narrative consultant, patient/family narratives are indeed a valuable gift. As Zaner points out below, the duty of narrative consultants is to respond to the gift in a responsible way. This means "genuine narrative listening," which is the third feature of narrative consultation:

My gift to Jim and Sue was listening; their gift to me was their story, the one they slowly understood took care of them when they desperately needed to be cared for. (Zaner 2004: 9)

Genuine narrative listening differs from attentive listening in two respects. In order to engage in such narrative listening, Zaner points out that a consultant is required to have "disciplined self-knowledge …followed by a rigorously disciplined suspension of it—a kind of practical distantiation that undergirds the act of compassion or affiliative feeling" (Zaner 1994: 220). In the narrative approach, "practical distantiation" could be characterized as an attitude of "not knowing" (Anderson and Goolishian 1992). Because the narrative consultant consciously tries to maintain an attitude of "not knowing" about the world that patients live in, s/he is no longer a privileged expert in possession of an esoteric truth, but instead simply feels privileged to bear witness to their lives (Charon 2006: 177–86). As Zaner explains below, a narrative consultant bears witness to the patient's struggle to search for an end, the end that gives a meaning to their illness experience, thus making their narratives worthy of telling and retelling in the future:

I honestly believe that I've been a privileged witness, time and again, to astonishing insights into what the moral order is all about by those who've allowed me into their lives to listen and question, perhaps at times even to talk, as they struggle to make sense of their lives. (Zaner 1996: 263)

Conclusion

Given the current controversy over whether ethics consultation should be replaced with bioethics mediation, my concern is that the controversy utterly misses a crucial point, as it seems to be limited to the debate over whether the ideal role of ethicists in clinical settings should primarily involve consultation or mediation. I was stunned to find that ethics consultation in the United States may not be functioning. It is furthermore outrageous to consider that verdict-based and/or majority decision-based ethics consultation may become dominant, as Fiester points out (Fiester 2007). The proper action, then, is not to rush into a decision of what ought to replace ethics consultation, but rather first try to correct misconceived notions about ethics consultation; for example, we should tell people that the authority of ethics consultants is never a function of their status as an expert on ethics, but instead is based on trusting relationships with patients and family members through ongoing dialogue with them (Agich 2000). It should be made known that the role of an ethics consultant is to help patients and family members clarify things and understand their situation, not to be the decision maker.

I think that the true reason the ethics consultation service may not be working in the United States or Japan is not because ethics consultation itself is a defective service, but because educating highly competent ethics consultants is simply very difficult. After all, I have come to believe that the future of clinical ethics depends upon establishing excellent programs to educate responsive and responsible genuine listeners who are determined to tread the path alongside patients/family members through morally aporetic situations. This indeed represents a very difficult but very worthy challenge that the future of clinical ethics education must face.

References

Agich, G. J. (2000). "Why Should Anyone Listen to an Ethics Consultant?" in H. T. Engelhardt, Jr. (ed), *The Philosophy of Medicine: Framing the Field*. Dordrecht: Kluwer, 117–37.

Anderson, H., and Goolishian, H. (1992). "The Client is the Expert: A Not-Knowing Approach to Therapy," in S. McNamee, and K. J. Gergen (eds), *Therapy as Social Construction*. Newbury Park, CA: Sage, 25–39.

Charon, R. (2006). *Narrative Medicine: Honoring the Stories of Illness*. New York: Oxford University Press.

Fiester, A. (2007). "The Failure of the Consultant Model: Why 'Mediation' Should Replace 'Consultation,'" *American Journal of Bioethics*, 7(2): 31–2.

Fiester, A. (2011). "Ill-placed Democracy: Ethics Consultations and the Moral Status of Voting," *Journal of Clinical Ethics*, 22(4): 363–72.

Japan Association of Healthcare Mediators. Website. http://jahm.org/ (accessed March 1, 2012).

MacIntyre, A. (1984). *After Virtue: A Study in Moral Theory*. 2nd ed. Notre Dame, IN: University of Notre Dame Press.

Orr, R. D., and deLeon, D. M. (2000). "The Role of the Clinical Ethicist in Conflict Resolution," *Journal of Clinical Ethics* 11(1): 21–30.

Wada, Y., and Nakanishi, T. (2011). *Iryo Mediation: Conflict Management he no Narrative Approach [Medical Mediation: Narrative Approach to Conflict Management]*. Tokyo: Signe.

Walker, M. U. (2007). *Moral Understandings: A Feminist Study in Ethics*. 2nd ed. Oxford: Oxford University Press.

Zaner, R. M. (1993). *Troubled Voices: Stories of Ethics and Illness*. Cleveland, OH: Pilgrim Press.

Zaner, R. M. (1994). "Experience and Moral Life," in E. R. DuBose, R. Hamel, and L. J. O'Connell (eds), *A Matter of Principle? Ferment in U.S. Bioethics*. Valley Forge, PA: Trinity Press International, 211–39.

Zaner, R. M. (1996). "Listening or Telling? Thoughts on Responsibility in Clinical Ethics Consultation," *Theoretical Medicine*. 17:255–77.

Zaner, R. M. (2004). *Conversations on the Edge: Narratives of Ethics and Illness*. Washington, DC: Georgetown University Press.

Zaner, R. M. (2006). "On Evoking Clinical Meaning," *Journal of Medicine and Philosophy*, 31(6): 655–66.

20.5

Commentary
The Functions and Limitations of Clinical Ethics Mediation

Ji-Yong Park

1 Introduction

The clinical ethics consultation, especially the hospital ethics committee, is the traditional approach to resolve medical ethics problem in a hospital. Bergman and Fiester address the question about availability of the traditional model on clinical ethics dilemmas. Central to Bergman and Fiester's article are two ideas: the clinical ethics consultation in traditional form fails to recognize value pluralism, and clinical ethics mediation is an effective alternative that could reflect value pluralism.

I basically agree with Bergman and Fiester's point of view about the usefulness and accessibility of the clinical ethics mediation. However, I also have questions about the possibility of the practical implementation of mediation model. This is because the hospital ethics committee has various roles that the mediation model does not have, and the clinical ethics mediation has limitations due to the characteristics of the mediation system itself.

2 Definition of ethics consultation

To begin with, it is imperative to clarify what the clinical ethics consultation is. In fact, because of the ambiguity of "consultation," clinical ethics consultation is a difficult concept to figure out in the context of various situations. However, according to the ASBH report, clinical ethics consultation is a service provided by an individual or group to help patients, families, surrogates, health-care providers, or the other involved parties address uncertainty or conflict regarding value-laden issues that emerge in clinical cases.

In defining the clinical ethics consultation, it may be useful to start out by examining the main issues of the clinical ethics consultation case, the nature of the dispute, and the subject of resolution. I would like to approach problems of the mediation model from these conceptual analysis frameworks.

3 Main issues of the clinical ethics consultation case

Clinical ethics consultation deals with a variety of ethical issues. It may involve such topics as: beginning-of-life decisions (e.g. abortion, the use of reproductive technologies), end-of-life decisions (e.g. withholding or withdrawing treatment, assisted suicide), organ donation and transplantation, genetic testing. These issues have moral and legal dimensions that may involve patient autonomy, informed consent, health-care provider rights of conscience, medical futility, resource allocation, confidentiality, or surrogate decision making.

It means that we should consider not only ethical issues but also legal issues in clinical ethics consultation. In particular, many cases are concerned with the relationship between ethics and law. For example, in Korea, abortion is prohibited in principle by a criminal Act. There are very narrow exceptional provisions to this rule in the Mother and Child Protection Act (e.g. biological problem, rape). It is doubtful whether ethics mediation is possible in this legal system. I think that biomedical mediation has a limit of application in many real cases due to the positive law or judicial precedent. In other words, if there are strong legal restrictions, the range of mediation will be reduced. In cases of this type, an authoritarian model (e.g. hospital ethics committee) could be advantageous rather than the mediation model.

4 Distinction between communication issue and pure ethical issue

The real cases that give rise to clinical ethical issues frequently also have complex interpersonal and affective features, such as guilt over a loved one's sickness or impending death, disagreement among health-care providers, conflicts of interest, or distrust of the medical system.

Strictly speaking, many of these cases are not conflicts of ethical value, but are communication issues or interpersonal conflicts. Theoretically, it could be distinguished between ethical grounds and others.

I entirely agree that mediation is an effective form for the management of communication issues, because it provides the opportunity to communicate for each party. However, in the case of pure ethical issues, it requires further examination whether it is applicable, although mediation has theoretical justification—value pluralism.

Mediation, a kind of negotiation, is originally a traditional form of dispute resolution in the area of law, Alternative Dispute Resolution (ADR). Mediation in legal proceedings has its roots in the game theory of economics. I think that it is essentially the exchange of interest. At this point I wonder if it serves as an available means in ethical issues of actual cases. Because there is only narrow room for compromise in these issues.

5 The subject of ethics consultation

In the United States, the ethics committee is the most typical way to resolve clinical ethics disputes. Bergman and Fiester (this chapter) say that "clinical ethics consultation, in its traditional form, fails to recognize ...value pluralism ...[C]linical ethics mediation is an effective alternative that could reflect value pluralism ...Mediation should replace consultation."

In general, there are three basic models of clinical ethics consultation: individual consultant, small-group consultation team, and ethics committee. Especially, the individual consultant model is linked to the mediation program in its form and functions. However, I suggest that the ethics committee should have important roles in the individual model. For instance, there is the obligation to report cases and activities from individual consultants or mediators.

Due to the complexity of clinical ethics issues, we could consider a variety of ethics consultation approaches and forms. I think that it is important to find an appropriate approach and form to ethics consultation by cases in cultural context. Although mediation would be a very useful way to resolve clinical ethics issues, the ethics committee has still unique functions. In conclusion, we should consider various forms of dispute resolution about clinical ethics cases.

In this regard, the ethics committee also is not the only way to resolve clinical ethics cases. For example, in Korea, like the United States, most hospitals have an ethics committee. However, it does not work well. This is because it was not to meet substantial needs but to meet a hospital evaluation standard. To my regret, people are not familiar with ethical discussions. They prefer to raise a lawsuit than to resolve conflict through compromise. It is a structural problem that there is only one approach; that is a full ethics committee.

6 Conclusion

Mediation is a very useful, effective way to communicate with stakeholders in clinical conflict, especially in Korea. However, no one model of ethics consultation serves every case optimally. In this regard, it might be more useful that mediation is not a replacement but a complementary measure for traditional ways of working, especially hospital ethics committees.

20.6

Response to Commentaries

Edward J. Bergman and Autumn Fiester

The commentary by Atsushi Asai and Yasuhiro Kadooka raises important issues emanating from comparative differences between United States and Japanese legal doctrines, cultural values, and clinical practices. In the legal sphere, we are told that the concept of self-determination, or patient autonomy, so central to American health-care decision-making, has not been embraced in Japan. In consequence, end-of-life disputes of the kind we address are largely non-existent because withdrawal of life support violates laws against self-elected euthanasia and assisted suicide. While this distinction would impact clinical ethics mediation in the sense that it removes an important class of cases from reference to mediation, our proposed model is applicable to the entire universe of clinical disputes, many of which do not concern withdrawal of life support, and the majority of which do not necessarily involve disputes classified as ethical in the traditional sense. For example, while one may reasonably argue that a physician is ethically bound to communicate medical facts, diagnoses, prognoses, and treatment options clearly and comprehensively, disputes over communication or interpersonal issues are not traditionally characterized as ethical in nature.

We are sensitive to the reality and magnitude of cultural factors on decision-making in clinical medicine, as noted by Asai and Kadooka. Confucian traditions and the principle of harmony will certainly impact the entire decision-making process and may present the problem, noted in this commentary, that weaker participants in the process may be disenfranchised by more powerful ones. Though the mediation process is imperfect, in our view it presents the best opportunity to mitigate such power imbalances by its inclusiveness and advocacy for mutual respect. The holders of power, especially in a society that embraces a harmony model, may well be drawn to a universally acceptable resolution in preference to a determination based on the exercise of power. Mediation, in the United States and elsewhere, always occurs in a context where, in the absence of consensual agreement, exercise of power by the party possessing it represents the alternative to consensus. We agree that how this particular cultural factor plays out in the Japanese experience can only be appreciated and addressed over time.

The practical concerns articulated by Asai and Kadooka regarding resistance from health-care professionals, and the impact of time and financial constraints, are not dissimilar to issues confronting implementation of clinical mediation in the United States. We view these as problems to be solved rather than intractable obstacles. For example, two decades ago, mediation in the context of legal disputes in the United States was largely opposed by legal practitioners who mistakenly, out of perceived threat to their role as litigators, were dismissive of its value. In the ensuing years, the legal culture has dramatically changed with regard to its acceptance of mediation, as exposure to the process has revealed benefits from the standpoints of client satisfaction, efficiency, and humanism. We believe that, over time, health-care professionals and institutions will similarly reconsider, leading to a more balanced view of the benefits and problems associated with widespread acceptance of clinical ethics mediation.

Finally, we address Asai and Kadooka's concerns, first with regard to neutrality and second, for situations in which concerned parties explicitly seek substantive advice on ethical issues.

First, neutrality is always a concern, especially when the mediator is likely to be compensated by the hospital and where, inevitably, the mediator will be charged with ensuring that any consensual resolution is within permissible legal requirements. There are two dimensions to this problem. Mediators must first overcome the subjective perception of bias. Anecdotally, experienced and effective mediators appear capable of surmounting this obstacle by earning the parties' trust through their demeanor, statements, and actions. As to *de facto* lack of neutrality, or prejudice, our answer comes in the form of a question. How does a judge, who is also an individual with values and a personal point of view, achieve neutrality? Through commitment to the legal process, judges, at their best, strive to apply the law, as they understand it, to the facts as they perceive them. Neutrality is an aspiration, not a guarantee. Mediators must also be committed to the virtues of a process, albeit a different one. The mediator's role is not to prescribe and evaluate, but to facilitate communication; to assist parties in understanding their respective interests and the extent to which those interests may be compatible; to promote mutual respect for persons and for the legitimacy of opposing perspectives; and, to serve as a catalyst for creative options which the parties may find preferable to the alternatives. Again, these are aspirational criteria. The better trained and more experienced mediators are, and the better the quality control measures adopted for oversight, the more likely it is we can approach these aspirations. Mediation, as a process, and mediators, as its practitioners, are subject to the frailties of all systems created and implemented by humans. Potential pitfalls do not invalidate the process but implore its practitioners to improve and evolve so as to approximate its ideals. Parenthetically, ethical decision-making by consultants functioning on a juridical model is at least, if not more, likely to run afoul of neutrality concerns. Individuals trained as neutrals may be less likely to substitute their own value systems for those of another than individuals empowered to make value-laden determinations on others' behalf.

Individuals who seek the substantive advice of an ethicist are free to elicit such advice. One hopes that the chosen consultant is inclined to present alternative ways of thinking about a problem, rather than one who deals in definitive answers. Indeed, one might imagine a case in which a participant in mediation sought to clarify her own views by seeking such a consultation. But that same individual may find it equally helpful, within or outside the mediation, to consult her priest, rabbi, psychotherapist, or uncle.

We read with great interest H. Tristram Engelhardt, Jr.'s commentary, which focuses on the concept of "mediation as pure procedure."

In many respects, we embrace Engelhardt's notion that "moral rationality is plural and cannot provide univocal moral guidance." We similarly agree that "the task of clinical ethics cannot be to ensure that one does the right, achieves the good, or acts virtuously because there is no agreement regarding the right, the good, or the virtuous" and that "[t]here is no decisive, sound, rational argument to establish any one of the numerous moralities, bioethics, or practices of clinical ethics as normative."

We are uncertain, however, that we subscribe to Engelhardt's conclusion that clinical ethics becomes..."purely a 'skill set' that can facilitate difficult conversations, including decisions" and that "Clinical ethics...in a secular culture without ultimate moral norms, becomes a clinical ethics evacuated of strong moral significance."

Our differences with Engelhardt may be purely semantic but can also be interpreted more broadly. While we agree that clinical ethics mediation embodies a primary commitment to process, we understand the process we advocate to be more than a "skill set." A "skill set" is certainly a precondition for effective implementation of the mediation process, but its ethical component resides in the moral dialogue that ensues between and among its participants. While the analogy is imperfect, the Platonic notion of moral dialogue—in which the dialogue itself, rather than the ethicist, is the teacher—is helpful. Like mediation, the positions articulated in the Socratic dialogues are subject to in-depth cross-examination (the "*elenchus*"), leading to catharsis and the prospect of reciprocal respect for opposing, yet legitimate, moral concerns. The process holds out the hope of a moral consensus, possibly having altered each other's moral perspective through the mechanism of dialogue and argument. Given this parallel, we believe that the process itself, and any ensuing moral consensus, possesses strong moral significance, in contrast to Engelhardt's view. Again, we understand that the differences may be semantic if, indeed, Engelhardt simply means that mediation does not purport to achieve norm-prescriptive outcomes through application of precedent.

Kinjo's commentary presents a problem for us because, ironically, we have little disagreement with the core of his perspectives. Nonetheless, we draw different conclusions from those perspectives, in large part, because of the cultural and socio-historical differences between the United States and Japan also posited by Asai and Kadooka.

Kinjo begins with a summary of the evolution and current status of "medical mediation" and "ethics consultation" in Japan. If Kinjo is accurate, and we have no reason to assume otherwise, the two countries are polar opposites as to the respective dominance of mediation and consultation in a clinical health-care context. While Kinjo cites the establishment of various curricula and health-care mediation organizations in Japan and advises that organizations educate in excess of 2,000 people annually as medical mediators, clinical ethics mediation training in the United States is extremely rare and no national organizations exist for health-care mediators. Indeed, Kinjo concludes that "accredited medical mediators far outnumber ethics consultants in Japan."

In light of those facts, we are not surprised that Kinjo is highly sensitive to issues raised by the introduction of mediation into Japanese clinical ethics. This is not to suggest that Kinjo's theoretical concerns regarding the widespread adoption of medical mediation in Japan are misguided. Nonetheless, we perceive that the comparative national contexts are so different that the very elements championed by Kinjo are more likely to develop within the nascent field of clinical ethics mediation in the United States than in conjunction with our long-standing, hierarchical system of bioethics consultation which, in direct opposition to Kinjo's criteria, demonstrates that the authority of an ethics consultant is primarily "a function of their status as an expert on ethics."

In the United States, obstacles to the adoption of narrative-based approaches to ethics are presented by the documented dysfunction, practice traditions, and turf protection associated with our widely employed system of bioethics consultation. While, in some instances, contemporary focus on patient autonomy, information technology, patient's rights, and consumer protection, along with the literature on clinical ethics mediation, have resulted in greater incorporation of patients and their families into the process, and some mitigation of the juridical, verdict-based approach associated with clinical ethics consultation, changes of the sort envisioned by Kinjo are unlikely to occur in the United States.

Alternatively, the narrative processes favored by Kinjo are fundamentally consistent with the clinical mediation process despite the reality that, as of today, neither the literature on narrative medical ethics nor clinical ethics mediation has indicated a recognition of their significant conceptual convergence.

In sum, we believe that more extended dialogue with Kinjo would reveal a surprising level of agreement once the two nations' respective obstacles to change in the practice of clinical ethics were more fully analyzed.

Finally, we respond to the interesting comments from Ji-Yong Park, who writes about the Korean context. One of Park's central concerns is the way in which mediation must function as a process inside the strictures of the legal system of the jurisdiction in which clinical ethics consultation takes place. We completely agree with Park that clinical ethics mediation operates within the boundaries of the law, and also within the confines of the policies of the particular hospital in which the consultation takes place. For example, in the United States, parents may not refuse lifesaving medical care for their children based on religious views, even if the minor child shares in that religious practice. A mediation between the parents and the clinical staff could not result in the withholding of lifesaving medical care, regardless of whether the parties would all agree to that outcome. Similarly, if a Catholic hospital has a policy that no abortions may be permitted in their institution, a mediation cannot result in a woman receiving an abortion, even if she and the provider agree that this is the best course of medical care for her. But we do not view these restrictions as an indictment of mediation as a process. We accept them as the rules that inherently govern any type of dispute resolution. Park is absolutely correct that the legal system will create the range of outcomes that are possible in any area in which the law speaks.

On Park's final point—that mediation cannot assist with conflicts that are truly values based—we do find ourselves in disagreement. Park's rationale for his claim is that each party in a true values-based conflict is so wedded to the value commitments that generate the conflict in the first place that there is no room for compromise. First, we do not take this claim as a truism. Parties can disagree on particular values claims and yet find overlap and consensus on other principles or values that can create common ground. Additionally, shifts in perspective can take place inside a mediation that could not be predicted or foreseen prior to the facilitated conversation, so the outcome is never pre-determined, and despair that a resolution cannot be found is unwarranted. Dialogue and conversation can overcome many seemingly insurmountable obstacles and barriers, which is why we are such passionate advocates of mediation.

21.1

Primary Topic Article
Informed Consent Revisited: A Global Perspective

Akira Akabayashi and Yoshinori Hayashi

1 Introduction

Informed consent is fundamentally grounded in the idea of respect for individual autonomy. However, health-care workers, patients, and their families sometimes encounter complicated situations regarding the interpretation and practice of informed consent. This is particularly true in cases of poor prognosis and the subsequent decisions regarding care. To illustrate the difficulty implementing informed consent as it has been traditionally interpreted, two cases, one from Japan and one from the US, were presented by one of the authors in previous publications (Akabayashi, Fetters, and Elwyn 1999; Akabayashi and Slingsby 2006). We proposed that a family-facilitated approach to informed consent could be equally appropriate to the first-person approach that has been commonly regarded as the standard method of ensuring patient autonomy.

The family-facilitated model of informed consent was discussed earlier as an alternative to the first-person approach rather than as a replacement for it. This reconceptualization of informed consent, while adding some complexity, takes into account cultural norms and different ways of thinking about the self. Specifically, a patient with an independent self-construction is one who identifies her/himself as an autonomous individual with an independent set of values, and is thus highly consistent with the conventional paradigm of autonomy and the standard approach to informed consent. In contrast, we suggest that many patients have an interdependent view of themselves, thus perceiving themselves as more connected and responsive to others. Thus, the patient with an interdependent self-construal is likely to identify her/himself first as a component of the family unit, in which case the family-facilitated approach may be more appropriate.

An article published in the 2006 *American Journal of Bioethics* (AJOB) by one of the authors (in collaboration with others) addressing this issue provoked a variety of reactions. Many of the responses shared some common misinterpretations of our position. We believe there were two reasons for these misunderstandings. Firstly, the premises for the argument promoting the use of the family-facilitated approach were not adequately communicated. Secondly, we asserted that the family-facilitated approach is compatible with respect for autonomy but did not adequately explain the reasoning behind the assertion. In this paper, we provide a more detailed description of the proposed family-facilitated approach to informed consent and present arguments establishing that this approach is not inconsistent with patient autonomy.

In the following two sections, we will review the previously published cases and clarify the characteristics of a family-facilitated approach. To further explain the family's role in proxy decision-making and differentiate the family-facilitated approach from other models of informed consent, we present an additional case that took place in Japan in 2010. We then go on to develop new models of informed consent. We call these the "soft proxy" approach and the "hard proxy" approach. We argue that the family-facilitated approach is supported by *a form of autonomy* that differs from some conventional views. This argument invokes the idea of *tacit consent* by a patient, as the family-facilitated approach does not require explicitly expressed consent. We defend the family-facilitated approach by describing a form of autonomy that is consistent with the original intent as governance of the self. We argue that the family-facilitated approach excludes the possibility of paternalism by the physician and undue influence by the family. We reassess the relationship between the family-facilitated approach and these new models in light of *relational autonomy*. Finally, we review the philosophical basis of the family-facilitated approach, and suggest that it is applicable to other topics. We assert that the first-person approach and family-facilitated approach to informed consent can be useful in many cultural settings beyond the borders of Japan and the US.

2 Case 1: a Japanese patient in the late 1980s

Case 1 was previously published in the *Journal of Medical Ethics* (JME).[1] The patient, while still healthy, had indicated to her family that she did not want to know the diagnosis if she ever developed cancer. At the time of her diagnosis the family requested that the physician not disclose the news to the patient.

---

[1] The full description of Case 1 is as follows (Akabayashi, Fetters, and Elwyn 1999: 296).
A 62-year-old Japanese woman presented to a Tokyo hospital with a fever and severe back pain. Diagnostic work-up included serological tumor marker testing and abdominal computed tomography. This revealed advanced gall bladder cancer metastatic to the liver and back. Since her expected survival was less than three months and she was not a candidate for surgery or chemotherapy, a regimen of comfort measures and pain control was needed. The diagnosis was first revealed to her family members, namely her husband and her son, separately from the patient. The husband and son discussed it with the daughter, and together the family requested that the patient not be told. The family explained that while still healthy the patient had mentioned to them her wish not to be told if she developed cancer. This mention of her preference may have been stimulated by intermittent media coverage of the issue in Japan and seemed plausible. After initial treatment for pain and fever, the patient stabilized and was competent to participate in decision-making, though she was a little withdrawn and dependent. The treating physician and family met with the patient and in the family's presence, the treating physician told her: 'You don't have any cancer yet, but if we don't treat you, it will progress to a cancer.' In response, the patient asked for no further details. An aggressive pain-control regimen was continued and though she was intermittently drowsy, she died four months later without apparent suffering from physical pain. The physician never explicitly discussed the diagnosis with her.

2.1 The custom of first notifying the patient's family of a diagnosis with poor prognosis

In Japan, until the 1980s, bad news such as a diagnosis of advanced-stage cancer was delivered first to the family rather than to the patient, because the family was thought to be in the best position to understand the patient's ability to comprehend the diagnosis and make the best decisions to promote his or her welfare. Physicians and family members were also often concerned that the patient would be traumatized by the diagnosis. Acknowledging the importance of family support, physicians often sought the family's consent before disclosing a cancer diagnosis to patients, even when the patient was clearly competent (Akabayashi, Fetters, and Elwyn 1999). This approach is not exclusive to Japan. In Italy, for example, bad news was also disclosed to the family, not to the patient (Surbone 1992).

2.2 "Something close to autonomy" and its implications

"Family consent, communication, and advance directives for cancer disclosure: a Japanese case and discussion," discusses the idea of "something close to autonomy," as described by the North American medical ethicist Edmund Pellegrino. Pellegrino argues that autonomy, or something close to autonomy, is a universal principle, not just a cultural artifact. However, he challenges the commonly held view of first-person consent as essential through his description of cases in which a patient is not apprised of his/her actual diagnosis, and shows how this nonetheless might be consistent with a form of autonomy.

In many cultures clinicians encounter patients who are fully aware of the gravity of their condition but choose to play out the drama in their own way. This may include not discussing the full or obvious truth. This is *a form of autonomy,* if it is *implicitly and mutually* agreed on, between physician and patient. (Pellegrino 1992a: 1735; italics added)

He continued thus:

Autonomy is still a valid and universal principle because it is based on what it is to be human. The patient must decide how much autonomy he or she wishes to exercise, and this amount can vary from culture and culture. It seems probable that the democratic ideals that lie behind the contemporary North American concept of autonomy will spread and that *something close to it* will be the choice of many individuals in other countries as well. (Pellegrino 1992a: 1735; italics added)

What Pellegrino is suggesting is that patient autonomy or something close to it is applicable across cultures, and moreover that this particular notion of autonomy should be respected because it is based on patient preference. However, he rejects the strict interpretation of autonomy used in North America as universal, instead recognizing diverse beliefs about the interpretation and implementation of autonomy in different cultures.[2]

---

[2] Further arguments discussed in the JME article are as follows: Yet when considering this issue in the international context, the term 'autonomy' should be used carefully since it is not a concept with only one meaning. Pelligrino does not specify whether his notion of a North American concept of autonomy refers to the definition of autonomy or the degree of exercise of autonomy, or both. Surbone's remark that autonomy is often synonymous with isolation in Italy illustrates that the exercise of autonomy differs in Italy and North America, even though the definition may be very similar (Akabayashi, Fetters, and Elwyn 1999: 299).

In this context, the fundamental question becomes: How is autonomy understood in other countries?

Our analysis of Case 1, described above, concludes that the patient's autonomy was respected based on the following criteria: 1) the patient's prior declaration of her wishes; 2) the physician's vague explanation, which did not reveal the cancer diagnosis to the patient, respected the patient's wishes; and 3) the patient, who was competent and had the opportunity to question the physician but chose not to do so. However, when discussing the case in question we did not discuss specifically what form of autonomy was being respected and in what way.

3   Case 2: an American patient in the 1990s

Case 2, previously presented in AJOB, involved a patient in the US.[3] This is a case in which, at the time of the onset of cancer, the patient's family asked the physician not to disclose the diagnosis to the patient. The patient was alert, oriented, and competent; therefore, it is not clear why the family received information before the patient herself. Because the practice of informing the family first is not typical in the US, we assume this is a case involving an ethnic minority.

3.1   Defining the family-facilitated approach and its premises

In the paper referred to above the family-facilitated approach was proposed as an alternative to the traditional first-person approach to informed consent.

A family-facilitated approach to informed consent where family and patient function as a single unit differs from the more popular first-person approach. In this paper, we define a family-facilitated approach as a process of informed consent in which a patient's family communicates with the attending physician and medical staff and often makes treatment-related decisions. This differs from acting as a proxy in that the patient does not officially appoint his or her family. (Akabayashi and Slingsby 2006: 11)

The validity of a family-facilitated approach is based on two premises: 1) a patient–family fiduciary relationship, and 2) a patient who identifies her/himself more as a component of the family unit than as an independent individual. This kind of fiduciary

---

[3] The full description of Case 2 is as follows (Akabayashi and Slingsby 2006: 9).
A 74-year-old woman was admitted for increased blood sugar and fever. A CT scan revealed multiple liver masses. A biopsy revealed a squamous cell carcinoma. The patient's family (a daughter and two sons) was told the diagnosis and insisted that the patient not be told. They were afraid that the knowledge would decrease her will to live and thus shorten her life. The patient was very close to her family as she spent most weekdays with her daughter and the weekends at home with her unmarried son. By all accounts, the patient was alert and oriented.

The nursing staff were not willing to tell the patient her diagnosis without the attending physician's permission (and the patient had never asked, though she was upset about being in the hospital). The attending said that he had seen patients for over 30 years and that if the patient did not ask what was wrong, he would not tell them. He thought that patients "usually figure out what is wrong anyway and adjust quite well." The attending said that he understood that it was "in fashion" to tell patients what is wrong with them, but that he disagreed with this silly trend.

The family became extremely upset when again approached about informing the patient and questioned the justification for the 'hospital policy' that patients should be told their diagnosis.

relationship is one in which decisions regarding the patient as made by the family are assumed to be in their own best interests.

3.2 Self-construction and the binary approach

The binary model, in which both the first-person approach and family-facilitated approach can be used, takes into account divergent concepts of self-construction—independent and interdependent. A person with an independent view identifies her/himself as an autonomous individual with an individual set of values and a unique perspective.[4] In the health-care setting, a patient with an independent view would naturally prefer a first-person approach to informed consent—free to make his or her own decisions based on careful consideration of the fully disclosed risks and benefits of each treatment option. In contrast, an individual with an interdependent self-construction will tend to identify her/himself as part of a larger unit consisting of family, friends, and others.[5] Accordingly, such patients may be more comfortable with a collaborative process in which disclosure of risks and decision-making regarding treatments involve important members of that unit. In Case 2, it is apparent that the patient had a more interdependent view of self and therefore she would have preferred a family-facilitated approach.[6]

3.3 The relationship to autonomy in Case 2

Our discussion of Case 2 in our previous paper concluded that the family-facilitated approach was not inconsistent with respect for patient autonomy.[7] However, as with Case 1, we did not describe the philosophical basis for this conclusion. Both cases show situations in which the family plays an important role in decision-making, even though the patient did not explicitly designate any particular family member as his or her legal representative. However, in our earlier work we did not explain why the family is

---

[4] The independent view was originally described as follows: This view of the self derives from a belief in the wholeness and uniqueness of each person's configuration of internal attributes...The essential aspect of this view involves a conception of the self as an autonomous, independent person (Markus and Kitayama 1991: 226).

[5] The interdependent view was originally described as follows: This view of the self and the relationship between the self and others features the person not as separate from the social context but as more connected and less differentiated from others (Markus and Kitayama, 1991: 226).

[6] Explanation in the article was as follows: In this case, we need to ask whether or not the patient was willing to entrust her decision-making to her family. This depends largely, however, on her relationship with her family and her self-construal. The patient was "alert and oriented" (competent), "very close with her family," and she never asked her attending physician about her diagnosis. Judging by these facts, if she had not been willing to entrust her decisions to her family, she more than likely would have asked her family or attending physician directly about her disease. Deducing from the fact of her competence combined with her silence on the matter intimates that she indeed held an interdependent view (Akabayashi and Slingsby 2006: 12).

[7] The analysis in the article was as follows: Moreover, a family-facilitated approach does not necessarily contradict with the general ethical principle of respect for autonomy in the United States. In fact, a family-facilitated approach to informed consent may be respecting a patient's individual choice. That is, if a patient who holds an interdependent view has a propensity to prefer a family-facilitated approach, providing this approach to informed consent may indeed be respecting patient autonomy (Akabayashi and Slingsby 2006: 13).

entitled to perform such a role in such situations, or how the family-facilitated approach differs from use of a legal proxy. We will clarify these points below.

4 Case 3: Mr. K, a Japanese patient in 2010

Thus far, we have summarized some arguments for recognizing the validity of the family-facilitated approach in two previously published case studies. In this section, we present a third case to further elucidate the characteristics of the family-facilitated approach. Although fictitious, this example is based on an actual case from 2010.

4.1 Case presentation: Mr. K

Mr. K was a 61-year-old corporate executive who presented with cervical adenopathy in 2010. Stage 4 metastatic squamous cell cancer was diagnosed by biopsy. The prognosis was unclear, but assumed to be very poor because the cancer was of unknown primary origin. Mr. K was informed of the diagnosis by the physician and presented with a choice of chemotherapy, radiation therapy, or surgery. His wife was present during the consultation. Mr. K had been married for more than 30 years and had an excellent relationship with his wife. They had no children. Mr. K's siblings included an older sister and younger brother; however, both were married and he was not close to either of them.

Mr. K told his physician and wife, "I am shocked. I cannot make this decision by myself." This reaction and apparent loss of decision-making capacity made his wife uneasy, and she turned to the physician for advice. However, the physician would not recommend a specific treatment, replying that the patient and family must make the decision. The wife consulted with a family member who was a medical practitioner, and gathered information from the Internet. After careful consideration, she arrived at the following conclusion: Begin treatment with chemotherapy and then, if necessary, pursue radiation therapy or surgery. After consulting with the physician to confirm the appropriateness of her decision, Mrs. K told her husband in the presence of the physician, "I spoke with the doctor and decided to start with chemotherapy. I hope that's OK," to which Mr. K nodded, and, without inquiring about the details of the chemotherapy or the pros and cons of the treatment alternatives, he was subsequently admitted to the hospital for treatment.

4.2 A new type of informed consent in contemporary Japan

Mr. K's case illustrates a new way of thinking about informed decision-making in contemporary Japan. Our analysis is based upon three central points. Firstly, Mr. K says that he is shocked by the diagnosis. Nonetheless, he exhibits no sign of difficulty making other types of decisions such as giving work-related instructions to those at his company. In that sense, he is competent enough to participate in the decision-making regarding his treatment. However, he explains that he regresses when emotionally taxed, and therefore cannot make these difficult medical decisions on his own.[8] Secondly, Mr. K and his wife have a long-standing relationship and get along well. Thus, we may assume that a fiduciary relationship exists between him and his wife as a family unit. Because he explains that he is unable to make the decision alone and wants to rely on others, it

---

[8] The human tendency to withdraw in difficult situations or weakened conditions is an important psychological defense mechanism necessary for survival.

is reasonable to assume that he holds an interdependent view of himself. Finally, Mr. K nods in agreement with his wife's explanation of her decision regarding his treatment. Mr. K was given the opportunity to disagree with his wife's decision and refuse hospitalization or treatment.[9]

Cases like the one described above whereby a family member takes leadership in the decision-making on behalf of a competent patient still occur. The question remains: What type of approach is appropriate for a patient who is emotionally withdrawn? Mr. K has shown that he has an interdependent view of himself. The two conditions described above required for a family-facilitated approach are in place. Therefore, we consider it appropriate that his wife, in consultation with the physician, makes the therapeutic decisions on his behalf.

The interdependent view does not compel strict self-determination for a patient who is emotionally withdrawn. In contrast, a strictly first-person approach requires that, unless the patient is clearly incompetent and requires legal representation, the patient must take responsibility for decision-making based on comprehension and consideration of fully disclosed information.

4.3 The use of proxy decision-making in Case 3

Mr. K did not officially appoint his wife as a proxy. His wife saw that her withdrawn husband was not able to make important decisions about his own treatment. She therefore used her own judgment based on her understanding of her husband's best interests to choose a treatment strategy after consultation with his physician and finding additional information on her own. She informed her husband by telling him, "I talked with the doctor and decided to start with chemotherapy. I hope that's OK." The husband just nodded without apparent interest in the process by which his wife reached the decision and without requesting any details about the treatment options.

Although Mr. K approved his wife's decision, he did not officially appoint her as a proxy. We wish to use the term "soft proxy" approach for the way in which Mr. K's wife is entitled to make decisions in such a case. The soft proxy approach can be defined in the following way: despite no official request by the patient, the family and physician decide on a treatment strategy independently of the patient, and this decision is ultimately confirmed by the patient. The soft proxy approach is congruent with the Japanese idea of *omakase* (patient leaving the decision to others, especially family members or physicians). In contrast, a conventional autonomous proxy is a third party, such as a lawyer, who is explicitly and officially appointed by the patient. This "hard proxy" approach is based on the assumption of an independent perception of the self. The process of integral family involvement in informed consent and decision-making may be easier to understand through these concepts of soft proxy approach and hard proxy approach.

[9] In Japan, enforcement of a new Personal Information Protection Act in 2003 enabled patients to obtain information from their medical records. It is reasonable to assume that Japanese physicians have directly informed patients of their diagnoses in almost all cases since that time. However, results of surveys have revealed that the decision to fully disclose the actual *prognosis* to a patient is still left to the best judgment of the health-care worker. According to the survey, physicians tended to disclose the patient's prognosis to his/her family pessimistically, but reveal the same prognosis to the patient rather optimistically. See Akabayashi et al. (1999).

5   In what sense is the family-facilitated approach consistent or inconsistent with patient autonomy?

So far we have described what we call the family-facilitated approach in the context of Cases 1 and 2. We believe that a family-facilitated approach is appropriate in cases such as these where patients have an interdependent self-construal and the two above-mentioned requirements are met. We have also suggested that taking a family-facilitated approach in such cases is not inconsistent with patient autonomy. However, some might believe that the approach is in conflict with a strict interpretation of patient autonomy, which would require direct discussion with patients, an assessment of their competence, full disclosure of information, and respect for patient self-determination based on adequate comprehension of the benefits, burdens, and risks of all reasonable alternatives. Some may argue that patient autonomy in this strict sense was not adequately respected in the two cases described above. In this section we defend the family-facilitated approach by considering arguments asserting that a family-facilitated approach is consistent with respect for patient autonomy.

5.1   Is the family-facilitated approach compatible with the conventional view of autonomy?

To see why we believe a family-facilitated approach is compatible with patient autonomy, let us revisit our conclusions from our analysis of Case 2. In Case 2, the argument was: if a patient who holds an interdependent view has a propensity to prefer a family-facilitated approach, providing this approach to informed consent may indeed be respecting patient autonomy (Akabayashi and Slingsby 2006: 13). The line of reasoning behind this argument begins with our assumption that patient autonomy is being respected when a patient's preferences are fulfilled. We then argue that a patient with an interdependent view of himself is highly likely to be more comfortable with a family-facilitated approach, thus taking a family-facilitated approach is consistent with the patient's preference. Therefore, we conclude, a family-facilitated approach is consistent with the patient's autonomy in that it is in accord with the patient's preferences.

We believe that it is safe to assume that patients in cases such as these two examples can be assumed to have interdependent view of themselves and prefer that the family make the decisions. The patient in Case 2 did not consult the physician despite the opportunity to do so, nor did she oppose her exclusion from the decision-making process. The patient in Case 1 was also given the opportunity to consult the physician and did not refuse the involvement of the family in the decision-making process. Thus, in both cases, the patient *tacitly* consented to the family making the medical decisions. In effect the patient ultimately authorized this process. Thus, the family-facilitated approach is consistent with the preference of patients who have an interdependent view of themselves.[10]

When consent is tacit, some doubt may remain as to whether patient autonomy can be said to be truly respected. Autonomy as conventionally interpreted requires explicit, rather than tacit, consent. We shall return to this question below.

---

[10] By comparison, in Case 3 it may seem that the wife consulted with the physician and made the medical decision without Mr. K's permission. However, despite being able to confer with his wife or the physician, he

	Self-construal	Premise 1 fiduciary relationship	Premise 2 Identification as part of a unit	Conception of autonomy	Degree of ideal vs. local practice respected
First-person approach	Independent	Not necessary	Not necessary	Completely conventional	Ideal practice (respect for conventional autonomy)
Hard proxy approach	Independent	Required	Not necessary	Completely conventional	
Soft proxy approach	Interdependent	Strongly required	Required	Somewhat conventional (omakase)	
Family-facilitated approach	Interdependent	Strongly required	Strongly required	"Something close to autonomy"	Local cultural practice (respect for family-oriented decisions)

Figure 21.1   Four models for informed consent

5.2 A comparison of four models for informed consent with regard to patient autonomy

To address the potential concerns stated in the previous paragraph, as well as to see how our conclusions could be applied in broader contexts, it will prove helpful to make a brief summary of the landscape as described thus far. Let us now review the four models that have been presented (Figure 21.1).

The first-person approach is a decision-making process with expressed consent and is in accordance with the conventional view of patient autonomy. It is consistent with an independent self-construal. When applying the hard proxy approach, the patient does not actively make the medical decisions, but officially and explicitly appoints a legal representative of his/her own choosing. The legal proxy may be a third party outside the family, such as an attorney. In this case, the patient is also likely to have an independent construction of him/herself. His/her relationship to the legal representative is a fiduciary one.

By contrast, the soft proxy approach used in Case 3 is consistent with an interdependent construal of the self and satisfies the two premises needed for a family-facilitated approach. In addition, a close relative can act as the representative without being explicitly designated as such by the patient. Here, decisions made by the family are ultimately

did not do so. In effect, he did not use his veto power. Moreover, he provided explicit rather than tacit authorization by nodding. In Case 3, the conventional view of autonomy supports either (1) that the patient should make decisions himself or (2) that the legal representative has to be designated by the patient with explicit authorization (in which case the scenario would fit with the hard proxy approach model).

confirmed by the patient. There is some expression of consent by the patient. In the family-facilitated approach, the decisions are made by the family without explicit designation of proxy by the patient, and the patient undergoes the chosen treatment, giving only tacit consent. The family-facilitated approach is consistent with the notion of an interdependent construal of self and requires the two premises of patient–family fiduciary relationship and patient primary identification as part of a family unit to be satisfied.

The differences among the four models can be summarized as follows: 1) whether the patient or another party makes decisions with regard to specific treatments (first-person approach vs. all others), 2) whether the patient provides tacit or expressed consent (family-facilitated approach vs. all others), and 3) the degree of voluntariness when deciding the level of proxy (soft proxy approach vs. hard proxy approach).

When we consider the issue of autonomy within these four approaches, the first-person approach and hard proxy approach are consistent with the idea of respecting patient autonomy as traditionally understood. The same cannot be said for the soft proxy approach and family-facilitated approach. However, because the patient expresses their consent in the soft proxy approach, it does not lack due respect for patient autonomy as understood traditionally. The family-facilitated approach requires only tacit consent, and therefore may appear not to respect the patient's autonomy. Thus, the family-facilitated approach is not acceptable within the scope of this conventional view of autonomy.

This analysis might strengthen questions about whether or not patient autonomy is respected in the family-facilitated approach. Our aim in the following section will be to address the way in which the family-facilitated approach can be compatible with patient autonomy.

5.3 What sort of autonomy is compatible with the family-facilitated approach?

In what sense can we claim that the family-facilitated approach is still compatible with patient autonomy? In answering this question, we wish to emphasize that in the family-facilitated approach, physician paternalism and any undue influence from the family are excluded as points of contention. In the family-facilitated approach, the patient's desire for family decision-making, authorized by tacit consent, is respected, and the possibility that the physician will make decisions against the will of the patient is removed. It is important to remember that the rejection of physician paternalism is the original issue in contemporary bioethics regarding respect for patient autonomy. Thus, the family-facilitated approach addresses arguments criticizing potential paternalism.

It is true that strong family involvement in medical decision-making may appear oppressive and in conflict with patient autonomy. However, in the family-facilitated approach, it is the patients who *want* their family to make the medical decisions, as they see themselves first as part of a family unit, and family decision-making is preferred by the patients themselves. Therefore, family involvement is not an undue restriction to patient autonomy.

Based on these considerations we conclude that the family-facilitated approach is compatible with the motive behind the conventional view of autonomy, although the family-facilitated approach is not compatible with autonomy in the strictest conventional sense of the word. However, we maintain that it is consistent with some particular sort of autonomy, which fits well with the Japanese clinical settings and any other settings where the family's role in treatment choice is considered more significant, including certain Italian, Chinese, and some American subcultures. This is congruent with Pellegrino's expression "something close to autonomy," "a form of autonomy." Pellegrino, who first stated that a form of autonomy was used in the case of a patient in Italy, did not offer a clear definition (Pellegrino 1992a: 1735). We claim that the crux of what Pellegrino calls "something close to autonomy," "a form of autonomy" might best be understood as the minimization of physician paternalism and respect for patient preference.

6 Relational autonomy and the family–facilitated approach

To further clarify the concept of autonomy in the family-facilitated approach, it is useful to compare it to the concept of relational autonomy. According to Catriona Mackenzie and Natalie Stoljar, "[t]he term 'relational autonomy'…does not refer to a single unified conception of autonomy but is rather an umbrella term, designating a range of related perspectives" (Mackenzie and Stoljar 2000: 4). However, these perspectives share "the conviction that persons are socially embedded and that agents' identities are formed within the context of social relationships and shaped by a complex of intersecting social determinants, such as race, class, gender and ethnicity" (ibid).

Stated simply, the exploration of relational autonomy is characterized as an attempt to facilitate the reconsideration of contemporary philosophical accounts of autonomy based on this view of identity formation. As Susan Sherwin stated: "Under a relational view, autonomy is best understood to be a capacity or skill that is developed (and constrained) by social circumstances. It is exercised within relationships and social structures that jointly help to shape the individual while also affecting others' responses to her efforts at autonomy (Sherwin 1998: 36)."

Reexamination of the concept of autonomy from a relational perspective has a range of implications for bioethical problems. We will focus on the arguments of Anita Ho, which address the connection between respect for patient autonomy and family influence from a relational standpoint. By focusing attention on the patient's vulnerability and relational identity, she suggests that we need to reevaluate the role of family and respect for patient autonomy in situations of medical decision-making.[11]

6.1 Patient's consent, family's role, and relational autonomy

According to Ho (2008), when a patient's relational identity is understood, family involvement is not necessarily in conflict with respect for patient autonomy. In fact, in certain cases it may actually enhance it. In the health-care setting, patients can feel isolated and in such circumstances they may (1) prefer preservation of identity through family connections to self-determination, and (2) prioritize intimate relationships and the welfare of loved ones over their individual interests. Respecting the autonomy of

---

[11] For other attempts to discuss the role of family in decision-making in connection with the idea of relational autonomy, see Lee (2007) and Turoldo (2010).

the patient may be considered equivalent to respecting the patient's needs and wishes, which are influenced by the family.[12]

The fundamental issues explored in the study of relational autonomy by feminist bioethicists correspond with the core philosophical issues upon which the family-facilitated approach is based. First, the family-facilitated approach is founded on a construction of self similar to that found in writings about relational autonomy. Both consider carefully the importance of human relationships. In addition, the goal of the family-facilitated approach to reevaluate the conventional definition of autonomy and pursue alternatives shares a great deal with the feminist analysis of relational autonomy. Finally, Ho acknowledges that the family has an important role in medical decision-making, and asserts that family intervention does not necessarily infringe respect for patient autonomy. The family-facilitated approach also recognizes this assertion.

6.2 Oppression and the feminist interpretation of autonomy

Nonetheless, we disagree with Ho's interpretation of respect for patient autonomy when she describes what *kind* of patient consent is needed. We have argued that within the family-facilitated approach tacit consent is the minimum requirement of respect for patient autonomy. Ho, on the other hand, still considers the patient's explicit expression of wishes a strict condition of respect for autonomy. In her commentary on the AJOB article in which the Case 2 was originally published, she states:

I argue that, in cases where patients defer decision-making to family members, unless there is clear evidence of neglect or abuse, caregivers should follow the patients' *expressed* wishes. (Ho 2006: 26; italics in the original)

Additionally, in another paper, Ho further contends that "professionals' default position should be to trust the patient's own final expressed wishes" (Ho 2008: 133). While Ho believes it is important that some patients prefer preservation of identity through family connections to self-determination, she nonetheless insists upon expressed consent.

What underlies Ho's insistence on the expressed intent of the patient, we believe, is concern about the potential for oppression that is shared by other feminist writers. Indeed, Ho states that "One concern that may arise here is that patriarchal and other oppressive relationships often disguise manipulation, exploitation, control and abuse as love and familial bond" (Ho 2008: 133). Requiring the patient's expressed consent may therefore be the last safeguard against manipulation and exploitation.

6.3 Expressed consent or tacit consent: do they truly differ?

The concern that oppression gives rise to manipulation and exploitation is well founded. We suspect, however, that expressed consent may not be sufficient in itself for removing

---

[12] Ho argues as follows. "In this context of parenthood, dependency or family involvement may preserve rather than violate autonomous agency—it can help to maintain a range of identifications that can promote patients' own sense of integrity and worth. Because it is reasonable to assume that intimates generally care deeply about the patient's interest and well-being, such that their choices would probably match the patient's overall goals, family involvement can be compatible with or even enhance the patient's autonomy" (Ho 2008: 131). Further, she argues: "For those whose family is at the centre of their existence, consideration of their advice, needs and mutual interests is part of their autonomous agency" (Ho 2008: 132).

the potential risk of manipulation and exploitation of a patient with a relational identity. If in fact it is impossible to save the patient from exploitation and undue influence of the family based on their tacit consent to medical procedures, then it should prove to be impossible to do so with the patient's expressed consent as well.

To understand this point, let us compare Case 3 (the soft proxy approach), in which the patient expresses his consent, with Case 2 (the family-facilitated approach), in which there is only tacit consent. Although the patient in Case 3 expressed his consent to treatment by nodding, this alone does not ensure that there is less risk of exploitation or undue pressure from the family than in Case 2. For this to occur, more is needed such as the empowerment of the individual exposed to oppression, as suggested by Susan Sherwin (Sherwin 1998: 34–9). However, in situations requiring medical decisions, such decisions cannot wait for the patient's empowerment. While there are complicated social and institutional issues that make it very difficult to realize the empowerment of individuals in need, medical problems need concrete solutions appropriate to the circumstances and are subject to time and resource constraints.

Hence, if we take seriously the reality of such severe clinical situations like those presented in the cases under discussion, we conclude that there is no substantial difference between obtaining the patient's expressed consent and acknowledging the patient's tacit consent when considering the patient's vulnerability to exploitation or undue pressure from the family.

7 Informed consent: a global perspective

The arguments above suggest that the unique conditions of a clinical setting as well as the relationships of a patient placed therein have to be taken into consideration in establishing what we call "a form of autonomy" (i.e. a concept of autonomy for which obtaining the patient's expressed consent is not an essential criterion). Of course, even in this instance, the patient's wishes are made known by his tacit consent. It is for this reason that we consider the family-facilitated approach as "a form of autonomy."

In developing this family-facilitated approach model, we sought to balance respect for patient autonomy and the cultural importance of the family in decision-making. Restrictions of time and resources often influence the process of medical decision-making, and there are situations in which the ideal practice of informed consent is not possible or may be inappropriate. In addition, problems directly related to life and death demand immediate solutions. Thus, we acknowledge the importance of taking this reality into account in order to arrive at practical and ethical solutions.

Using the example of informed consent, we acknowledge the significance of the family's role in decision-making in local cultures. On the one hand, we attempt to pay due respect to local cultural values to the extent that they are compatible with the concept of autonomy that underlies the ideal practice of informed consent. On the other hand, we expand the interpretation of autonomy while shedding light on the interdependent construal of self that underlies the value of family decision-making in local cultural practices. Through attempting to reconcile apparently conflicting abstract ideals and local realities without giving either of them absolute status, we have developed the family-facilitated approach as a solution.

Such complexity cannot be reduced to a simple algorithm. Nonetheless, this method can provide a starting place for practical solutions that avoid the pitfalls of parochial ethnocentrism and arrogant universalism. This may provide a methodology for developing better solutions in a progressively globalized world.

The methodology and philosophy described here may also be applicable to other problems in clinical/medical ethics, given that hard questions in medical ethics often involve conflicts among universal and local values. For example, the process can be used to examine how to deal with different definitions and criteria of death or to reveal the merits and problems of living donor organ transplantation.

Using informed consent as an example, we developed four models of informed consent, which have here been discussed in the context of Japan and the US. We have argued that the family-facilitated approach is not a replacement for the first-person approach. Patients should be able to choose the approach best suited to them, and this may change for the same individual over time.

It is possible that these models could become choices for patients outside Japan and the US. Further, we hope our flexible methodology will be applied in different regions and cultures. This in turn may engender other informed consent models that are sensitive to the diversities of clinical realities[13]. As Pellegrino says, "this question of balancing autonomy is today a necessary part of any transcultural dialogue in medical ethics. The ethics of medicine offers a fruitful point for beginning a larger cultural dialogue

---

[13] For example, in a series of papers, Ruiping Fan and his colleagues employ the Confucian perspective to defend a family-determination model of informed consent that is familiar within a Chinese clinical context (Fan 2000; Fan and Li 2004; Fan and Tao 2004; Wang, Lo, and Fan 2010). This family-determination model is similar to the family-facilitated approach in that it recognizes situations in which it is more appropriate for the family, rather than the patient, to make decisions, regardless of the patient's decision-making capacities.

Fan and Tao (2004) also suggest that theoretical explanations for the family-determination model of informed consent may be provided by appealing to the concept of tacit consent.

The difficulty is to provide an adequate moral-theoretical account of the role of families and physicians in decision-making [in China and Hong Kong]....For contemporary bioethics, the theoretically least challenging approach is to account for the role of the physician and the family *by appealing to a background authorizing tacit consent.* (Fan and Tao 2004: 141–2; italics added)

Nevertheless, rather than choosing to provide explanations that appeal to tacit consent, Fan and Tao defend the family-determination model by highlighting the importance of the family's role in decision-making within the cultural context of Confucianism. Their unique views of the concept of autonomy may underlie this approach. According to Fan (1997), the Western conception of autonomy as a 'self-determination-oriented principle' and East Asian conception of autonomy as a 'family-determination-oriented principle' are disparate concepts; 'there is a different principle of autonomy implicit in the cultural and ethical traditions of East Asian countries which is incommensurable with Western principle of autonomy' (Fan 1997: 313). Rather than expanding the concept of autonomy as we do, Fan attempts to explain the propriety of family decision-making through the importance of the family's role from a Confucian perspective.

Thus, the conclusions of Fan et al. are similar to our conclusions, but the approaches taken to arrive at these conclusions differ. Whereas Fan et al. enthusiastically argue the importance of the family's role in decision-making based on Confucian concepts, we argue that decision-making by the family can be interpreted as respect for patient's autonomy using the interdependent construal of self. Notably, the concept of autonomy in this case refers to 'a form of autonomy,' an alternative concept of autonomy that stands alongside the conventional construction of autonomy that underlies first-person approach.

We have not aggressively demonstrated or defended the importance of the family's role, but this should not be interpreted as a denial of the family's importance. Rather, we choose to refrain from making direct moral judgments regarding the importance of the family's role, and argue that the family-facilitated approach gains support from the principle of autonomy as long as the concept of autonomy can be understood in the way explained in this paper.

between and among the world's major cultures" (Pellegrino 1992b: 18). We believe that our models and our way of thinking described here mark an important milestone in the reassessment of informed consent on a global scale.

References

Akabayashi, A. et al. (1999). "Truth Telling in the Case of a Pessimistic Diagnosis in Japan," *Lancet*, 354(9186): 1263.

Akabayashi, A., and Slingsby, B. T. (2006). "Informed Consent Revisited: Japan and the U.S.," *American Journal of Bioethics*, 6(1): 9–14.

Akabayashi, A., Fetters, M. D., and Elwyn, T. S. (1999). "Family Consent, Communication, and Advance Directives for Cancer Disclosure: a Japanese Case and Discussion," *Journal of Medical Ethics*, 25: 296–301.

Fan, R. (1997). "Self-Determination vs. Family-Determination: Two Incommensurable Principles of Autonomy," *Bioethics*, 11(3–4): 319–22.

Fan, R. (2000). "Informed Consent and Truth Telling: The Chinese Confucian Moral Perspective," *HEC Forum*, 12(1): 87–95.

Fan, R., and Li, B. (2004). "Truth Telling in Medicine: The Confucian View," *Journal of Medicine and Philosophy*, 29(2): 179–93.

Fan, R., and Tao, J. (2004). "Consent to Medical Treatment: The Complex Interplay of Patients, Families, and Physicians," *Journal of Medicine and Philosophy*, 29(2): 139–48.

Ho, A. (2006). "Family and Informed Consent in Multicultural Setting," *American Journal of Bioethics*, 6(1): 26–8.

Ho, A. (2008). "Relational Autonomy or Undue Pressure? Family's Role in Medical Decision-Making," *Scandinavian Journal of Caring Sciences*, 22:128–35.

Lee, S. C. (2007). "On Relational Autonomy: From Feminist Critique to Confucian Model for Clinical Practice," in S. C. Lee (ed), *The Family, Medical Decision-Making, and Biotechnology: Critical Reflections on Asian Moral Perspectives*. Dordrecht: Springer, 83–93.

Mackenzie, C., and Stoljar, N. (2000). "Introduction: Autonomy Refigured," in C. Mackenzie, and N. Stoljar (eds), *Relational Autonomy: Feminists Perspectives on Autonomy, Agency, and the Social Self*. New York: Oxford University Press, 3–31.

Markus, H. R., and Kitayama, S. (1991). "Culture and the Self: Implications for Cognition, Emotion, and Motivation," *Psychological Review*, 98:224–53.

Pellegrino, E. D. (1992a). "Is Truth Telling to the Patient a Cultural Artifact?" *JAMA*, 268(13): 1734–5.

Pellegrino, E. D. (1992b). "Prologue: Intersections of Western Biomedical Ethics and World Culture: Problematic and Possibility," in E. D. Pellegrino, P. Mazzarella, and P. Corsi (eds), *Transcultural Dimensions in Medical Ethics*. Frederick, MD: University Publishing Group, 13–19.

Sherwin, S. (1998) "A Relational Approach to Autonomy in Health Care," in S. Sherwin (ed), *The Politics of Women's Health: Exploring Agency and Autonomy*. Philadelphia, PA: Temple University Press, 19–47.

Surbone, A. (1992). "Truth Telling to the Patient: Letter from Italy," *JAMA*, 268(13): 1661–2.

Turoldo, F. (2010). "Relational Autonomy and Multiculturalism," *Cambridge Quarterly of Healthcare Ethics*, 19:542–9.

Wang, M., Lo, P.-C., and Fan, R. (2010). "Medical Decision and the Family: An Examination of Controversies," *Journal of Medicine and Philosophy*, 35(2): 493–8.

21.2

Commentary
Medical Practice and Cultural Myth

Carl Becker

An appreciative overview

Over the past two decades, Dr. Akira Akabayashi has established himself as a leading expositor of medical ethics in Japan. I am honored to have been a colleague of his at Kyoto University, and am deeply thankful to be invited to continue our dialogue through this series of conferences and articles. His latest article is one in a series which explains the Japanese position on informed consent and autonomy. I admire and agree with his description of the Japanese situation, and I should like to further develop some of the issues.

Dr. Akabayashi's first article depicted a cancer patient who did not want to be informed of her cancer; her doctor's mere oblique allusion to the word "cancer" allowed her to choose her own interpretation of whether she had it or not. His second article illustrated a cancer patient whose family and doctor collaborated not to tell the patient her fatal diagnosis, arguing that the family's decision-making could be considered a form of autonomy in place of the legal proxy expected in many Western medical settings.

His third and latest presentation depicts a "soft proxy," in which the terminal patient himself abjures responsibility for decision-making, but nods in apparent assent to his wife's decision that is based on her Internet research and conversations with relatives working in medicine.

His cases suggest that (1) when patients ask not to be told their diagnoses, (2) when families ask doctors not to tell patients their diagnoses, or (3) when patients refuse to deal with their own diagnoses—then decision-making by doctors and/or relatives is within the scope of "something like patient autonomy," because it respects the wishes of the patients. Through this series of case studies, Dr. Akabayashi's greatest contribution is his Figure 21.1, clearly comparing four models of informed consent.

I tend to agree with these Japanese ways of uninformed consent, or consent to others' decision-making, but I question whether they are indeed "something like patient autonomy." Particularly Case 2, where the family insists that their mother not be informed, and the physician readily sidesteps what he calls the "silly trend" of informed consent, is more a case of familial if not medical paternalism, than "something like patient autonomy."

Dr. Akabayashi's cases are ethically as well as culturally acceptable, *not* because they somehow approximate "patient autonomy," but *because they have apparently unobjectionable outcomes.* If the same patients had died screaming in agony; if their doctors' collusion with families had changed their treatments for the sake of inheritance or organ transplant without the patient's approval; if their nod of apparent assent were found to be actually suppressed disagreement or rage, then the same procedures would seem less ethically acceptable. Nothing innate to soft proxy or family-facilitated decision-making inherently minimizes these dangers to the patient.

Western myths of informed consent and autonomy

We should respect each culture's way of decision-making, even if autonomy is not central to its worldview. At the same time, we should seek ways to avoid immoral abuses which a cultural system might permit. When a cultural system, confronting new medical alternatives, risks significant increases of mental pain or physical abuse, then it needs to contemplate ethically as well as culturally acceptable ways of reducing that pain or abuse (Kitayama et al. 2010).

Informed consent has become an international topic, *not* because the whole world supports patient autonomy but because the mushrooming range of medical decisions leaves doctors legally and ethically liable to justify their choices.

There is substantial evidence that informed consent is an artificial substitute for trust, designed to reduce lawsuits (Hoshino 1995; Becker 1999); that autonomy is a misguided fiction (Fox and Swazey 2008; Wolff et al. 2009); that doctors remain paternalistic even in countries which chant the mantra of autonomy (Boisaubin 2004; Sypher, Hall, and Rosencrance 2005; Chew-Graham et al. 2006; Veerapen 2007); and that patients readily abjure responsibility, signing forms they do not understand in order to get medical treatment (Mueller, Reid, and Mueller 2010).

The notion of an autonomous decision maker is not only a legal fiction—even if it *were* possible, it would be unacceptably myopic and puerile. From the viewpoint of many traditional societies, the more adult and aware one becomes, the wiser and more compassionate one becomes. For a considerate adult, the ultimate grounds for decisions are *not* self-preference, but rather a consideration of the good for all people conceivably affected. Beauchamp and Childress's sole focus on the value of the life of the patient, for the patient, and by the patient, effectively ignores the value of the lives of those who must care for her and live on after her departure. For adults *not* thinking of all people affected, Wolff and others (2009) have concluded that the Western focus on "patient-centered" autonomy is inappropriate to long-term geriatric care, for example, where involvement of the family and community may be more important than the sporadic or specious preferences of a semi-senile patient. This does not mean that everyone should reject the ideal of patient autonomy, but rather that "something like patient autonomy" is not a necessary precondition for ethical medical practice.

Dr. Akabayashi's cases provide Western readers a valuable explanation of Japanese decision-making. However, his defense of their similarity to "autonomy" is questionable. *If* Japanese-style decision-making is unproblematic, then whether it chants the mantra of autonomy is secondary. However, *if* Japanese-style decision-making leads to danger or damage, then it should be reexamined, not because it is weak on autonomy (as are so many Western doctors and patients), but rather because of the other harms it may cause. Readers may respect the decision-making in Dr. Akabayashi's paradigm cases not so much because they are autonomous as because they produced apparently acceptable outcomes.

Dangers of defending practices without procedures

However, in discussing ethical acceptability, we need to look less at typically easy cases and more at troubling borderline cases. The interesting question for bioethics is less whether Japanese cases show "something like patient autonomy" than whether they pose moral hazards. Here we need to consider the potential dangers of uninformed tacit consent, and of "soft proxy" third-party decision-making.

The danger of ambiguity in uninformed tacit consent

Dr. Akabayashi is clearly correct that *trust* is central to this decision-making. Yet how can we distinguish a patient's nod of trusting agreement from a nod of resignation or abnegation? Dr. Akabayashi tells us there is no big difference between tacit and expressed consent, as in Case 3. But does the nod of an uninformed elderly Japanese patient unmistakably signify consent? Would the tacit consent of an elderly nod extend also to allowing her tissues and organs to be used later for scientific research? For medical procedures, would it not be more desirable to have at least a written expression of trust?

Determination of adequate trust and the danger of disputes

"Soft proxy" (family) decision-making is certainly an acceptable norm in a wide range of cultures (Blackhall et al. 1995), and Dr. Akabayashi is again correct that it presupposes a *very strong* level of trust. The next problem becomes: How can the physician *know* that such trust indeed exists between the patients and the family members who purport to represent them? When the family disagrees with their doctors, disputes between family and hospital often arise; conversely, when the family follows the doctors' advice, but are later unwilling to accept the outcome, the dangers of future lawsuits and bad publicity increase. This is precisely the reason that informed consent became standard practice in the West: not because Westerners all worship at the shrine of autonomy, but because legal liability to families and patients is too costly.

The danger of family feuds in the absence of legal proxy

A far more troubling issue arises when decision-making divides the family itself. I have personally witnessed all too many cases where half of the family favors extensive invasive treatment to prolong the patient's biological functions, while the other half of the family prefers a less disfiguring approach, such as palliation or "death with dignity" even if biological life were shortened. No matter which course is taken, such families often remain bitterly divided for many years after the patient dies: "It's all your fault because you chose such and such." If the medical profession does *not* know the patient's real wishes— *neither* about treatment, *nor* about whom the patient really trusts to make those decisions in her place—then there is no end to the potential for conflict *among* the so-called "soft proxy" family decision-makers. This violates most patients' real intentions; for most patients who refuse to decide their own medical treatments do not intend to cause family feuds lasting generations after their death.

In other words, allowing soft proxy appears unproblematic when the family decision makers and medical staff agree upon what course to take. However, when the decision makers disagree with the medical staff, or the decision makers themselves are divided, there arise strong reasons to ask patients themselves to document what they would like—or at least document *whom* they trust to represent them—by more than a nod of the head.

In sum, we should try to maintain and support traditional Japanese (and other non-Western) decision-making procedures that involve families and are sensitive to cultural values (Blackhall et al. 1995). At the same time, the increasing range of complicated decisions in medical care requires *some* kind of procedures—not to guarantee atomistic patient autonomy, but to provide the care that patients and families (as well as medical staff) can accept, both during and long after its provision. While I doubt whether universal principles are necessary or even possible, I am concerned that practical procedures be implemented to confirm whether patients really want to remain uninformed, and to whom they would prefer to designate decision-making authority (Asai 1995; Becker 2003).

Similarities and differences

Dr. Akabayashi and I agree on many fundamental issues, including that medical ethics and procedures need to allow room for variation in decision-making, since not all people share identical values. We agree implicitly on the need for consistency, on the rule of law, and on the need to make each nation's grounds for judgment understandable to other nations. Dr. Akabayashi's many years of clinical practice in Japan—and the case studies that he valuably introduces to his readers—demonstrate that Japanese decision-making rather differs from Western textbook cases of the "rational independent individual" decision-making.

Both Dr. Akabayashi and I recognize that Japanese practices of medical decision-making differ from Americans'. Both of us understandably want to avoid ethnocentric Americans' condescension towards other cultures that do not yet share their enlightenment values. Dr. Akabayashi's rightful concern to defend Japanese practices in terms that Western bioethicists can understand drives him to use principlist language, as if that principlist mantra had not been relativized nor deconstructed in the 40 years since its instantiation. Rather than proposing that Japan might have different but equally valid values, Dr. Akabayashi reinterprets Japanese procedures so that they seem compatible with Western enlightenment mantras, as if "something like autonomy" were a value that spans all cultures. I fear that the search for so-called "universal" values may force non-Western cultures into the Procrustean bed of trying to justify themselves on the basis of myopic monocultural "universals." Indeed, the fact that many languages traditionally cannot even translate the term "individual autonomy" demonstrates how ethnocentric and non-intuitive this "principle" is (Kitayama et al. 2010).

Indeed, it was Kant who advanced the notion of autonomy in order to reinforce social ethical responsibility, but Kant's focus on social responsibility was subsequently confused with or transformed into existential self-determination. The prioritization of "individual" ethical autonomy over social ethical autonomy is reminiscent of Spencer's misinterpretation of Darwin; as if survival of individuals were prior to survival of the species.

Dr. Akabayashi defends Japanese decision-making within the overarching framework of *individual* autonomy, whereas I would defend Japanese decision-making within a framework of *cultural* autonomy, which may or may not require individual autonomy. Dr. Akabayashi believes that latitude for decision-making should be maintained on a personal-individual level, something close to modern American autonomy. I believe that this latitude in decision-making can be left on a personal level in cultures which subscribe to the doctrine of personal autonomy, but that this same latitude in decision-making should allow other cultures to place decision-making in the hands of families or other culturally recognized agencies, rather than forcing all cultures to subscribe to the same theory of individualist autonomy.

Both Dr. Akabayashi and I want Japanese practices of medical decision-making to be transparent as well as philosophically acceptable. Dr. Akabayashi's concern seems to be to fit Japanese practices into a Western language frame (previously non-existent in East Asia); I seek other language to describe legitimate decision-making processes occurring in non-Western cultures, as well as *procedures* to guarantee that patients' wishes will be respected—even if those wishes were to ask someone else to decide on their behalf (Asai 1995).

Appendix

An English translation of Becker, "The Dilemma of Informed Consent" © 1999: The Underlying Problem: Trust vs. Adversarialism.

The ultimate scandal of informed consent is that it often pretends to tell the patient what she needs to know, but in fact conceals precisely that information. To wit, the patient is told the "success rate" of a given operation. But that is the rate reported for the nation, or the world, over the last decade or two. This information is completely irrelevant to any sane patient. The patient does not care about national averages. She does not care about local hospital averages. The only thing she really cares about is the success or failure rate of her own surgeon. This is precisely the information she is least likely to receive.

Every doctor learns on a curve. Fresh out of medical school, many surgeon-interns harm a quarter of their patients. By their second ten operations, they only mistake

20 percent, and by their third ten operations, they only mistake one, or 10 percent. No doctor wants to admit the number of patients he has lost in difficult operations. If patients knew the inexperience of young doctors, they would never go to those doctors, creating a vicious circle in which those doctors would never increase their experience. Bluntly speaking, if doctors publicize their failures, they will rarely be trusted. People will flock to the experienced doctors, and new doctors will only be able to practice on the poorest and those who can least afford to protest. However, doctors' failures constitute the information most critically relevant to the patients' informed consent. The irony of informed consent is that what the patient really needs to know is what she is least likely to be told: just how good her doctor is at curing her kind of case.

All in all, this is hardly surprising, because from the very outset informed consent is an attempt to legislate trust within an adversarial system. If there were genuine trust between doctor and patient to begin with, there would be no lawsuits, no fear of reprisals, and no need for standardized procedures of informed consent. Since the patient fears the doctor may weaken or injure her, and the doctor fears the patient may sue him, the informed consent contract sets up a businesslike relationship. The doctor gives the patient information and choice; the patient pays her money and makes her choice, and neither sues the other thereafter. This informed consent procedure strengthens the very adversarial relationship between doctors and patients that it was designed to ameliorate.

Conversely, in hospitals where patients already trust their doctors implicitly, or cultures where lawsuits are unheard of, informed consent is a fish out of water, a disingenuous uncalled-for attempt at an artificial trust. Many Western patients would like to spend more time with their physicians, to know more about their conditions. If informed consent moves them in that direction, it may be a good policy. But the additional costs, in time, in money, in patients' health and privacy, and in doctors' and pharmacists' income and respect, indicate that it is far from a panacea.

In fact, studies demonstrate that few patients understand their consent forms to begin with, and most follow what they think their doctors want to do anyway. In short, the whole procedure is a facade. The real reason many Western patients like informed consent is not because they make more autonomous or intelligent decisions; it is rather because they feel more respected than without the procedure. Informed consent is really all about making patients feel respected and cared for. In some cultures, information and legal forms to sign give the patient a feeling of being respected. In others, they may not. Surely there may be other even more effective ways of satisfying patients.

As it stands, informed consent succeeds in rendering doctors safe from lawsuits and in making patients feel more respected. It allows doctors to remain relatively empowered and immune, and gives patients an impression of being cared about, even within modern mass-produced health-maintenance organizations. Thus informed consent elevates medical paternalism to a higher level of abstraction, while often hiding the information which the patient most needs to know. Ideally, doctors should study interpersonal communication techniques and should devote substantially more time to each patient to gain their patients' trust and confidence. Conversely, if this level of education and communication were achieved, formal consent procedures would become superfluous, at least in non-litigious societies.

References

Akabayashi, A., and Slingsby, B. T. (2006). "Informed Consent Revisited: Japan and the U.S.," *American Journal of Bioethics*, 6(1): 9–14.

Asai, A. (1995). "Should Physicians Tell Patients the Truth?" *Western Journal of Medicine*, 163(1): 36–9.

Becker, C. (1999). "The Dilemma of Informed Consent," (in Japanese) in K. Takeyasu (ed), *Living Logic, Living Ethics*. Kyoto: Kyoto University Press, 111–25.

Becker, C. (2003). "Good Clinical Practice? Can East Asia Accommodate Western Standards?" in M. Barnhart (ed), *Varieties of Ethical Reflection*. Lanham, MD: Lexington Books, 317–27.

Blackhall, L. J. et al. (1995). "Ethnicity and Attitudes toward Patient Autonomy," *JAMA*, 274(10): 820–5.

Boisaubin, E. V. (2004). "Observations of Physician, Patient and Family Perceptions of Informed Consent in Houston, Texas," *Journal of Medicine and Philosophy*, 29(2): 225–36.

Chew-Graham, C. et al. (2006). "Informed Consent? How Do Primary Care Professionals Prepare Women for Cervical Smears: A Qualitative Study," *Patient Education and Counseling*, 61(3): 381–8.

Fox, R. C., and Swazey, J. P. (2008). *Observing Bioethics*. New York: Oxford University Press.

Hoshino, K. (1995). "Autonomous Decision-making and Japanese Tradition," *Cambridge Quarterly of Healthcare Ethics*, 4(1): 71–4.

Kitayama, S. et al. (2010). "Independence and Interdependence Predict Health and Wellbeing: Divergent Patterns in the United States and Japan," *Frontiers in Cultural Psychology*, 1:163.

Mueller, L., Reid, K. I., and Mueller, P. S. (2010). "Readability of State-sponsored Advance Directive Forms in the United States: A Cross Sectional Study," *BMC Medical Ethics*, 11:6.

Sypher, B., Hall, R. T., and Rosencrance, G. (2005). "Autonomy, Informed Consent, and Advance Directives: A Study of Physician Attitudes," *West Virginia Medical Journal*, 101(3): 131–3.

Veerapen, R. J. (2007). "Informed Consent: Physician Inexperience Is a Material Risk for Patients," *Journal of Law and Medical Ethics*, 35(3): 478–85.

Wolff, J. L. et al. (2009). "Optimizing Patient and Family Involvement in Geriatric Home Care," *Journal for Healthcare Quality*, 31(2): 24–33.

21.3

Commentary

Whose Interest Is It Anyway? Autonomy and Family-Facilitated Approach to Decision-Making

Anita Ho

This insightful paper by Akabayashi and Hayashi builds on a 2006 article by Akabayashi and colleagues that discussed how the first-person approach of informed consent is suitable for patients with an "independent construction of the self" but not for those with "a more interdependent view of personhood." For the latter group of patients who perceive themselves "as more connected and responsive to others" (Akabayashi and Hayashi in this chapter), Akabayashi and Hayashi argue that the family-facilitated approach is an alternative model as valid as the first-person approach.

I agree with the authors that this reconceptualization of informed consent is an attractive alternative to the first-person approach when we work with patients who consider themselves an integral component of the family unit. Akabayashi and Hayashi suggest that sometimes a "soft proxy" approach, which invokes the idea of tacit consent by a patient, is supported by "a form of autonomy" or "something close to autonomy" (Akabayashi and Hayashi in this chapter). As they explain, the conventional first-person approach fails to consider situations where patients hold a patient–family fiduciary relationship, "in which decisions regarding the patient as made by the family are assumed to be in their own best interests" (Akabayashi and Hayashi in this chapter).

So how may families make decisions in the patient's best interests? It is interesting to note that Akabayashi and Hayashi's family-facilitated approach bypasses the substituted judgment standard. In the North American bioethics literature, substitute decision makers (SDMs) are generally expected to make the health-care decision the competent patient would have made if capable (Beauchamp and Childress 2009). Under this approach, it is only when the incompetent person's specific health-care preferences are unknown that the SDM would appeal to the best-interests standard. It is also noteworthy that the cases considered by Akabayashi and Hayashi involve patients who are *capable* of making decisions and making their wishes known, marking an important distinction between their view of substitute decision-making and that of the conventional North American model, which generally only supports proxy decision-making when the patient is incapable of deciding.

I will return to the question of whether competent patients ought to be directly consulted regarding deferral of decision-making. At hand is the issue of how we can determine the patient's best interests. Beauchamp and Childress (2009) argue that best-interests judgments are meant to focus attention *entirely* on the value of the life for the patient who must live it, not on the value the patient's life has for others. In other words, SDMs follow what Akabayashi and Hayashi call the first-person approach. This approach focuses on the autonomy of the patient almost to the exclusion of the interests of anyone else (Sherwin 1998). It appears to apply to those who hold an independent view of the self, and imposes constraints on how the family may decide on behalf of the patient. Under the conventional model of substitute decision-making, family SDMs are seen mostly as a means to the patient's clinical ends (Nelson 1992). This model asks SDMs to be objective bystanders and interpret how the patient would view the value of their life, and how various health-care decisions may facilitate such a view. It appears to make no difference if the patient had no family members, or that the decision is made by others who have no relationship to the patient, such as public guardians or the legal equivalents. Family relationships under the first-person approach of substitute decision-making serve little or no inherent value or symbolic meaning. In fact, in some situations, families are seen as potential barriers to promoting the patient's interests. In warning against families from making decisions based on how the patient's life can serve the family's interests, the conventional approach to substitute decision-making suggests that the patient's interests and those of the family are distinct and potentially incompatible.

Given Akabayashi and Hayashi's (in this chapter) focus on patients who identify themselves as "part of a larger unit consisting of family, friends and others," the prominent North American model of distinguishing patients' interests from those of the family may not work well in situations "where family and patient function as a single unit" (Akabayashi and Hayashi in this chapter). The authors do not see the family's and patient's interests as pitting against each other. They point out that some patients prefer "a collaborative process in which disclosure of risks and decision-making regarding treatments involves important members of that unit" (Akabayashi and Hayashi in this chapter), suggesting that they are focusing on harmonious families that are not looking to override the patient's best interests.

While I agree that we need to take families' role and inherent value seriously, involving family members in the decision-making process does not by itself suggest that a patient holds an interdependent view of the self or relational identity. After all, even the conventional first-person approach of autonomy and the "hard proxy" approach allow the patient to officially appoint a family representative in times of stress. None of the cases put forth by Akabayashi and Hayashi explicitly proposes that the family's interests are *equivalent to* or at least *part of* their interests. In Case 1, for example, the family asked the physician not to disclose the cancer diagnosis to the patient because the latter had indicated to the family that she did not want to know the diagnosis. The patient opted for nondisclosure for her own self-regarding interests, not due to any particular concerns for the family. The family, while undoubtedly loving, acted as the surrogate and used the substituted judgment standard in abiding by the patient's desires. And in the case of Mr. K, the patient deferred decision-making because he was in shock and did not think that he could make the decision on his own without the help of others. While he reportedly had a good relationship with his wife, Mr. K's reaction to the treatment situation does not challenge, nor does it support, the assumption that he holds an interdependent view of the self, or that he saw his interests as intertwined with those of his wife. It would seem that even if Mr. K had an independent view of the self, he could still have requested help to make the difficult decision. After all, the conventional first-person approach to autonomy does not require patients to make their decisions on their own— the right to decide implies the right to solicit assistance or even defer to others if one wishes to do so, particularly when one determines that another may be more equipped in making the judgment at hand.

As I have argued elsewhere (Ho 2008), patients who hold a relational identity and see their lives as intertwined with those of their loved ones often do not separate their significant interests from those of their family's, such that a decision based on the family's best interests can also be in the patient's overall best interests. Contrary to the first-person approach, some patients prefer to not only defer decision-making to their family members, but also consider their interests extensively in the planning process. Their interests involve a dynamic balance among interdependent people who have overlapping concerns. These others-regarding interests are often part of the patient's consideration. The communal decision-making under this notion of relational identity may thus be a group effort to consider and nurture the patient's and family's *mutual* interests. In situations where reciprocal concern and sympathy underlie the familial relationship, our understanding of the patient's relational identity can help to determine how family involvement can respect, support, or even enhance the patient's autonomy.

This last point brings up my uneasiness with the soft proxy approach in *some* cases where we do not have the patient's explicit consent for proxy decision-making. Akabayashi and Hayashi (in this chapter) argue that the "soft proxy" approach, where "the family and physician decide on a treatment strategy independently of the patient," can allow the family to make decisions on behalf of the patient despite "no official request by the patient." In response to my argument elsewhere (Ho 2008) regarding the importance of seeking patients' expressed consent to proxy decision-making in situations that involve complex family dynamics, Akabayashi and Hayashi (in this chapter) argue that "within the family-facilitated approach tacit consent is the minimum requirement of respect for patient autonomy." When the patient holds an interdependent view of the self, the soft proxy approach is allegedly congruent with requirements of autonomy because it allows the decision to be "ultimately confirmed by the patient" (Akabayashi and Hayashi in this chapter).

However, some practical questions remain. For example, how do we verify or know if a patient adopts an independent or interdependent view of the self, particularly given that independence and interdependence come in degrees? It seems that even someone who adopts one or the other view may still be fluid in their decision-making depending on the context. For example, a person who holds an independent view of the self may still want to involve loved ones or consider their interests in certain important matters. Even those who want to decide on their own where to invest their money or consider it their right to make final determinations about various matters may nonetheless incorporate the interests and preferences of others in their choices and actions. This is, for example, often the case when people make decisions regarding where to live, where to spend important holidays, how to support family members' financial needs, how to distribute one's wealth after death, etc.

Given that the soft proxy approach does not seek explicit consent, it may not be easy to determine which notion of the self a patient holds and how that particular view of the self applies to health-care decisions. Certainly, in cases where the family appears to be harmonious and the family members appear to be on equal grounds and strive for mutual support, we may not need to actively seek the patient's explicit approval. However, in situations where the patient sees himself/herself as part of a larger unit, but potential conflicts and manipulation are involved, we may have a situation of co-dependency rather than interdependency, characterized by imbalances of power and expectations. In these cases, we may need further exploration of whether the soft proxy approach is appropriate. Without asking various questions or knowing a lot more about the patient's background, how he/she makes other important decisions, etc., it may also be difficult to affirm the patient's ultimate confirmation of consent.

Perhaps Akabayashi and Hayashi believe that given the clinical realities (e.g. patient vulnerability) and family histories, reliance on family decision-making is still most appropriate regardless of explicit patient consent. While I agree with them that it may not be possible "to save the patient from exploitation and undue influence" even with expressed consent (Akabayashi and Hayashi in this chapter), such dialogues can at least give health-care providers a better understanding of the patient's decision-making framework, family dynamics, etc. It may also help clinicians to find ways to best support the patient in cases of suspected manipulation or exploitation.

In closing, what makes Akabayashi and Hayashi's family-facilitated approach particularly convincing and insightful is that it recognizes the clinical realities and relational complexities that patients face in grim health-care situations. The conventional first-person approach, which is often considered the ideal approach to respect patients, seems to presume that patients hold perfect information and are not affected by emotional stress or influences by others. It is perhaps against this approach that Akabayashi and Hayashi consider the soft proxy and/or family-facilitated approach as "something close to autonomy" or "a form of autonomy." However, such language implies that the family-facilitated approach is short of being ideal, or that the first-person approach is the appropriate yardstick. But given the clinical reality and patient distress, it seems that the family-facilitated approach is not short of being ideal. It is not even simply as valid as the first-person approach. In fact, in many situations, particularly where patients hold an interdependent view of the self that emphasizes mutual or reciprocal support, it is perhaps *the* better way of respecting the person. The conventional approach may, in fact, be short of ideal or less valid, since it does not consider the complexities.

References

Akabayashi, A., and Hayashi, Y. (2014). "Informed Consent Revisited: A Global Perspective," in A. Akabayashi (ed.), *The Future of Bioethics: International Dialogues*. Oxford: Oxford University Press, 735–49.

Beauchamp, T., and Childress, J. (2009). *Principles of Biomedical Ethics*. 6th ed. New York: Oxford University Press.

Ho, A. (2008). "Relational Autonomy or Undue Pressure? Family's Role in Medical Decision-making," *Scandinavian Journal of Caring Science*, 22: 128–35.

Nelson, J. L. (1992). "Taking Families Seriously," *Hastings Center Report*, 22: 6–12.

Sherwin, S. (1998). "A Relational Approach to Autonomy in Health Care," in S. Sherwin (ed.), *The Politics of Women's Health: Exploring Agency and Autonomy*. Philadelphia, PA: Temple University Press, 19–47.

21.4

Commentary
How Should We Defend a Family-Based Approach to Informed Consent?

Ruiping Fan

Informed consent has become a universal norm in contemporary medical practice over the world. However, there are two different approaches to informed consent: while the individual-based, first-person approach has been promoted by Western bioethicists, a family-based approach is upheld by Asian bioethicists and is still practiced in Eastern societies. For example, the chapter developed by Professors Akira Akabayashi and Yoshinori Hayashi in this volume lays out what they call "a family-facilitated approach," attempting to provide an alternative to the Western first-person approach. They contend that their approach is appropriate to the kind of patients who hold an interdependent view of personhood, identifying themselves as persons inseparable from their families ("interdependent self-construction"). In this approach, "a patient's family communicates with the attending physician and medical staff and often makes treatment-related decisions" (Akabayashi and Slingsby 2006: 11). Such decisions made by the family on behalf of the patient are generally taken to be in the best interests of the patient (Akabayashi and Hayashi in this collection). Moreover, Akabayashi and Hayashi reject the idea that medical practices under this approach would support physician paternalism; rather, "the possibility that the physician will make decisions against the will of the patient is removed" (Akabayashi and Hayashi in this collection). Importantly, in terms of their argument, this approach "does not lack due respect for patient autonomy" because the patient has given tacit consent to family decision-making (Akabayashi and Hayashi in this collection). They conclude that this approach, as well as its underlying notion of autonomy, "fits well with the Japanese clinical settings and any other settings where the family's role in treatment choice is considered more significant, including certain Italian, Chinese, and some American subcultures" (Akabayashi and Hayashi in this chapter).

I think this approach is valuable, their view clearly made, and their argument insightful. I agree that their approach is eventually similar to the family-based approach for which I have argued in recent years. As they point out,

The conclusions of Fan et al. are similar to our conclusions, but the approaches taken to arrive at these conclusions differ. Whereas Fan et al. enthusiastically argue [for] the importance of the family's role in decision-making based on Confucian concepts, we argue that decision-making by the family can be interpreted as respect for patient's autonomy using the interdependent construal of self. (Akabayashi and Hayashi in this collection)

However, if it is true that their approach and my family-based approach have reached similar conclusions regarding informed consent, I am afraid that the argument they have offered in terms of patient autonomy cannot work to support their conclusion. In particular, I think they will have to make a distinction between two types of patient autonomy, personal autonomy and moral autonomy, in order to fulfill their goal. Eventually, I would argue, their approach (as well as my approach) can only be supported by a concept of moral autonomy, not personal autonomy. The reason is as follows.

Contemporary societies, including China and Japan, have witnessed fewer and fewer cases in which the patient does not want to know anything about his/her medical condition but leaves everything to his/her family to decide. Such cases have become unusual or special in today's medical practices. A useful approach to informed consent should not only take account of such unusual or special cases. Instead, it must take account of typical cases. At least in contemporary Hong Kong and mainland China, typical cases are those in which patients and their close family members make shared medical decisions. What usually takes place is that when a severe diagnosis or prognosis is involved, the patient's close family member who companies the patient to the hospital will be informed of it in the first place by the physician, and then the physician will talk to the patient together with the family member. Authoritative medical decisions will be made by both the patient and the family—because the family member will consult other family members and achieve a consensus. What is crucial in such cases is that if the patient and the family disagree about what treatment should be conducted, neither the patient nor the family is solely in authority to make a final decision. Rather, they must reach agreement before physicians can carry out therapeutic interventions, except in emergent or otherwise special situations in which physicians have therapeutic privileges. If Akabayashi and Hayashi's approach does cover such typical cases and support the ethical rationale embodied in them, then their approach cannot be supported by respect for personal autonomy. It cannot even be compatible with respect for personal autonomy, because personal autonomy is a robust liberal individualist concept, under which autonomous individuals (including competent adult patients) have a robust sense of self-sovereignty and a right to self-determination, including medical determination. For many liberal individualists, personal autonomy is an intrinsically valuable ideal on its own. Although relevant others (including physicians and family members) are welcome to offer medical advice or suggestions, it is patients themselves, as long as they are competent, who are solely in authority to make final decisions regarding their own lives or health. This, however, is not true in the typical cases we face in East Asian and relevant other cultures, in which patients and their families make shared medical decisions. Accordingly, I do not think the approach proposed by Akabayashi and Hayashi can be supported by any account of "respect for personal autonomy."

However, their approach can be supported by a concept of moral autonomy, such as a Confucian concept of moral autonomy. The Confucian concept of moral autonomy can be understood as including four elements as Joseph Chan lays out: voluntary endorsement, reflective engagement, importance of the will, and willing, not free choosing (Chan 2002). Importantly, the moral will recognized by Confucianism is not the free expression of an individual's arbitrary will. It is rather the expression of a determination to will what is grounded in the way of Heaven (天道 *tien dao*), such as the virtues of benevolence (仁 *ren*) and righteousness (義 *yi*). Accordingly, Confucian moral autonomy is not reducible to what individuals would choose given their desires and preferences. It is rather focused on an intention to make one's decisions consistent with the way of Heaven as appreciated in terms of the virtues. Based on this understanding, Confucian tradition does not grant the individual sole authority about certain important decisions regarding individual life or health, such as medical decisions. Instead, the family is granted authority to make such decisions. In clinical contexts, individual patients are never left alone to possess an exclusive decision power. It is both patients and their close family members who make shared decisions, with each side carrying a veto power in the normal situation. This family-based approach to medical decision-making can be supported by at least two reasons. First, the family stands crucially important in medical decision-making in that, as Akabayashi and Hayashi have indicated, individual patients identify themselves interdependently with their family members in relevant cultures. Since one is understood to be ontologically and ethically inseparable from one's family members, family members naturally possess a right to join one's medical decision-making. Second, if one is seriously ill, one can easily be overridden by one's passions. In making medical decisions, one may tend to require too much, too little, or too radical medical treatment than should be done properly. As a result, one's decisions will not be in one's best or long-term medical interests. Accordingly, if decisional authority is granted solely to the patient, it would easily lead to a deviation from the manifestation of what is grounded in the normal way of Heaven, namely the proper, virtuous mutual care and interdependence of family members. Family members joining in medical decision-making can help patients prevent or correct such deviations, accomplishing appropriate determinations in conformity with the way of Heaven. That is why I think Akabayashi and Hayashi's approach can be supported by the Confucian concept of moral autonomy.

What role should the physician play in the family-based or family-facilitated approach, especially when the patient and the family disagree about treatment choices? Indeed, such an approach rejects physician paternalism, as Akabayashi and Hayashi have correctly pointed out. However, this does not mean that the physician should not play a crucial role in medical decision-making. At least in the following contexts, the physician should actively participate in decision processes. First, when the physician finds that a decision held by a patient is evidently against his/her medical best interest, the physician should not willingly accept the decision. Rather, the physician should stand with the patient's family to persuade the patient to change the decision in order to meet his/her medical best interest (Chen and Fan 2010). For example, currently foot amputation is still medically better than limb-sparing procedures for patients with late-stage diabetic foot complications. The physician should join those patients' family members to talk to the patients and acquire their consent to amputation, although these patients may—perhaps due to emotional reactions—initially ask for limb-sparing procedures.[14] Moreover, in a special case in which a patient's family requests the physician to hide the medical truth from the patient, the physician cannot reasonably follow the family's request unless both of the two following conditions are satisfied: (1) the physician finds evidence of manifest mutual concern of the family members for the patient; and (2) the family's wishes are not egregiously in discord with the physician's professional judgment regarding the medical best interests of the patient. In other words, if either of these two conditions are unmet, the physician should directly talk to the patient (Fan and Li 2004: 189). Again, the role of the physician in such cases can be supported by the Confucian concept of moral autonomy, but is incompatible with a liberal individualist concept of personal autonomy.

In short, I think Akabayashi and Hayashi should have appealed to moral autonomy (such as Confucian moral autonomy) rather than patient autonomy to defend their approach. This does not mean that people in East Asian societies should be required to follow a concept of moral autonomy, not personal autonomy. Rather, the fact is that people in such societies still share what is essentially like the Confucian concept of moral autonomy, not personal autonomy, even when they hold otherwise different religious and non-religious beliefs. Accordingly, the family-facilitated approach presented by Akabayashi and Hayashi or the family-based approach presented by myself is defensible for these societies. There is no need to change relevant health-care policy. If some patients in these societies do not accept such a concept of moral autonomy as well as the related family-based approach to informed consent, the burden is on them to announce it clearly at the very beginning of their clinical settings, so that they can be treated according to the concept of personal autonomy as well as the related first-person approach to informed consent.

References

Akabayashi, A., and Hayashi, Y. (2014). "Informed Consent Revisited: A Global Perspective," in A. Akabayashi (ed.), *The Future of Bioethics: International Dialogues*. Oxford: Oxford University Press, 735–49.

Akabayashi, A., and Slingsby, B. (2006). "Informed Consent Revisited: Japan and the U.S.," *The American Journal of Bioethics*, 6(1): 9–14.

Chan, J. (2002). "Moral Autonomy, Civil Liberties, and Confucianism," *Philosophy East and West*, 52: 281–310.

Chen, X., and Fan, R. (2010). "The Family and Harmonious Medical Decision Making: Cherishing an Appropriate Confucian Moral Balance," *Journal of Medicine and Philosophy*, 35: 573–86.

Fan, R., and Li, B. (2004). "Truth Telling in Medicine: The Confucian View," *Journal of Medicine and Philosophy*, 29: 179–93.

---

[14] I thank Professor Alastair Campbell for offering me this example based on his clinical ethical experience in Singapore.

21.5

Response to Commentaries
Informed Consent, Family, and Autonomy

Akira Akabayashi and Yoshinori Hayashi

When we submitted a paper to AJOB in 2006, we received comments from a number of researchers. One particularly remarkable trend stood out among the comments. Namely, those who are sympathetic to the family-facilitated approach emphasized that it was culturally appropriate. Conversely the opponents of the family-facilitated approach tended to focus on cultural oppression of the patient and respect for the patient's will. These entrenched positions lead to the tired old schema of universalism versus ethnocentrism. A discussion that gets mired in this pattern of conflict reaches an impasse and cannot advance the debate in a constructive or subtle way.

Too obsessed with autonomy?

Upon reviewing Carl Becker's comments on our Primary Topic Article, we felt the need to break the impasse. Becker commented that "Dr. Akabayashi's cases are ethically as well as culturally acceptable, *not* because they somehow approximate 'patient autonomy,' but *because they have apparently unobjectionable outcomes*" (Becker in this chapter; italics in the original), and further stated that, "[w]e should respect each culture's way of decision-making, even if autonomy is not central to its worldview. At the same time, we should seek ways to avoid *immoral abuses* which a cultural system might permit" (Becker in this chapter; italics added).

However, Becker offers no explanation at all as to the kind of reasoning that lay behind his judgment of our work as "unobjectionable" or "immoral." Certainly to Becker, or to those who have sympathy for Japanese culture, the family-facilitated approach presented in Case 2 may seem intuitively unobjectionable. To a Westerner, however, it is unclear just how self-evident it is that the family-facilitated approach is indeed unobjectionable.

The claim that there exist culture-specific values, that is, values that are only accepted within the culture that produces them, is frequently used in arguments to defend cultural practices (which is evident in Ruiping Fan's comments). However, this argument is problematic as it simply insists on one's own viewpoint: it is closed off to criticisms from other points of view.

Our purpose in writing our article was to advance debate. Rather than basing our arguments on incommensurable values, we sought to explain and critically scrutinize these practices by introducing concepts and terminology for those unfamiliar with Japanese culture and practice. Without finding such common ground, it is doubtful that further dialogue can be sparked between people from different cultural backgrounds.

Accordingly, we used the concept of "a form of autonomy" to explain a mode of Japanese decision-making, as this model is also commensurable with values in the West. We believe that this approach enabled us to present a practice specific to Japan in a manner that is easily comprehensible to Westerners, while preserving openness to criticism. The argument that the family-facilitated approach is compatible with autonomy was aimed at providing a foundation for the family-facilitated approach. However, it was also our intention to reopen the discussion on truth telling and informed consent in order to find a way out of the dead-end debate over universalism versus ethnocentrism.

We might be missing the point of Becker's objection to our argument. Becker, who states that it is *unnecessary* to evoke the conception of autonomy in order to defend the family-facilitated approach, may go as far as to claim, as Fan did, that it is *impossible* to support the family-facilitated approach based on the conception of autonomy.

In fact, Becker comments that "Dr. Akabayashi's cases provide Western readers a valuable explanation of Japanese decision-making. However, his defense of their similarity to 'autonomy' is questionable" (Becker in this chapter). We contend, however, that our attempt to defend the similarity to autonomy is by no means questionable. We clearly articulated the substance of a form of autonomy, such as 1) rejecting paternalism, and 2) complying with patient preferences. We then addressed how, in the context of contemporary biomedical ethics, these two points had the potential to be applied broadly beyond the bounds of the Japan–US binary opposition within the discipline.

With respect to autonomy, Anita Ho commented that the notion of "something close to autonomy" or "a form of autonomy" "implies that the family-facilitated approach is short of being ideal" (Ho in this chapter). We do not, however, concur. We would like to remind Ho that the phrases "something close to autonomy" and "a form of autonomy" were quoted from the writing of Pellegrino, an American medical ethicist. From the perspective of an ethicist who has adopted the conventional autonomy-centered bioethics approach, the family-facilitated approach may appear non-ideal. Yet we are not attempting to debate the relative merits of the family-facilitated approach over the first-person approach, or to state that the conventional conception of autonomy is superior, or inferior, to "something close to autonomy." Rather, we are satisfied if we succeed in presenting our culturally specific practice as one of those decision-making models that can be adopted in different cultural settings.

Implications for clinical practice

Besides the discussion on the relationship between conceptions of autonomy and the family-facilitated approach—the original purpose of our paper—all three commentators shed light on the clinical implication of the family-facilitated approach. Here we provide some insights.

Becker states that "we need to look less at typically easy cases and more at troubling borderline cases" (Becker in this chapter). Contrary to this statement, we believe that each of our three cases represents a complex and difficult story. Perhaps Becker and Ho share a concern over the issues that might arise in applying the idea of tacit consent and the soft proxy approach to actual cases. These concerns are understandable.

However, our goal in this discussion was to show that, in some cases, the family-facilitated approach is more appropriate than the first-person approach. We must reaffirm the fact that this argument is constructed based on an ideal situation where two premises have been presumably met: 1) a patient–family fiduciary relationship exists, and 2) a patient identifies her/himself more as a component of the family unit than as an independent individual.

Therefore, the question of what the best response might be in a non-ideal situation, where these conditions have not been met, or where it is difficult to know whether these conditions have been met, falls outside our framework. Notwithstanding, we would like to address these concerns.

First, in contrast to Becker's understanding, we regard the "nod" in Case 3 as an expression of active and expressed consent rather than tacit consent. To begin with, our assertion that there is no difference between tacit consent and expressed consent is directed at Ho, who in our view thought that there was a danger of exploitation in tacit consent cases. If the two premises do not hold true, that is, in cases where there is no trust, the hard proxy approach and first-person approach should be adopted.

The first concern about the soft proxy approach, as Becker and Ho point out, relates to the problems that the physicians face in determining the best course of action when they do not know if there is trust between the patient and his/her family. In other words, how do we know, or verify, that a patient holds an independent or interdependent view of her/himself?

We are very positive about the significance of this concept, and hope that in the future, tests will be developed through advances in psychological analysis methods to ascertain a person's beliefs. Physicians could then use these psychological tests to judge whether there is trust, or whether a patient holds an independent or interdependent view.

Without these tests, however, it is somewhat difficult to make such judgments with any degree of certainty. There are, in reality, patients who have an interdependent view of themselves, but the only option is to make inductive inferences, as Ho suggests, by asking questions or learning more about the patient's background to identify these patients.

The second concern, which Becker and Fan raise, is how to handle situations in which the opinions of family members are divided.

We did not anticipate the possibility that disagreements may arise within the family, and there is a potential problem if there is a wide divergence of viewpoints. In such cases, the family would lack capacity to make decisions on behalf of the patient. The point raised by Becker and Fan is extremely astute, in that the family-facilitated approach would not be valid or effective. Therefore, it may be necessary to add a third premise: namely, that the family should possess decision-making capacity. Under this premise, if the patient still desired to have someone else make decisions in his/her stead, then the physician might be permitted to decide. This issue, however, requires further study.

Finally there is an unscrutinized clinical issue that should be mentioned before closing this section. We arrived at an important realization while reading Ho's comment. When we constructed the informed consent model, we only focused on the question of "who decides," i.e. the individual making the decisions. As a result, we did not clarify our position on problems that arise after the "who decides" issue has been resolved. In other words, problems regarding the standards for surrogate decision-making, of how the patient or proxies, such as family members, specifically decide. We did not comment at all, for instance, on the debate over substituted judgment standard/best-interests standard (Beauchamp and Childress 2009: 135–40) that arises in surrogate decision-making and is occasionally discussed in the bioethics literature.

There are reasons why we did not discuss this issue in depth. First, in the cases we have focused on thus far, that is, in cases where the family makes decisions for the patient even though he/she possesses decision-making capacity, the question of why it is appropriate for the family rather than the patient to make decisions is a serious dilemma. Once this problem is resolved and the decision-making authority is delegated to family members, it can be safely expected that the family's decision regarding the patient's treatment strategy will not cause any particularly negative results for the patient. At the very least, if the patient–family fiduciary relationship and patient–family interdependent identity, which formed the premise of our discussion, are taken as givens, it would be inconceivable that the family would make decisions that prioritize their own interests over those of the patient. Nor would they make decisions that unjustly oppress the patient. Therefore, our position is that the family's decision-making regarding the patient's treatment, irrespective of how those decisions were reached, would be for the patient's good.

Based on such considerations, we defined the family-facilitated approach as follows:

The validity of a family-facilitated approach is based on two premises: 1) a patient–family fiduciary relationship, and 2) a patient who identifies her/himself more as a component of the family unit than as an independent individual. This kind of fiduciary relationship is one in which decisions regarding the patient as made by the family are assumed to be in *their own best interests*. (Akabayashi and Hayashi in this chapter; italics added)

Yet the expression "their own best interests" is misleading. Ho interpreted the above definition of family-facilitated approach to mean "bypass the substituted judgement standard" (Ho in this chapter). However, the above definition makes no mention of the standards for surrogate decision-making. Because family decisions are assumed to be in the patient's own best interests, one must not make the mistake of thinking that the family-facilitated approach adopts the best-interests standard over the substituted judgment standard. Nonetheless the phrase "in their own best interests" might be revised to read "for the patient's good" or "for the patient's benefit."

A closer look at convergence and divergence for opening international dialogue

We shall end with a few remarks on the significance of international dialogue and its implications for our paper. To this end, we introduce the English philosopher Onora

O'Neill's argument about the conception of autonomy and its application to informed consent. She criticizes contemporary conceptions of autonomy in bioethics, and proposes an alternative interpretation that is derived from Immanuel Kant.

The concept of autonomy or (the principle of) "respecting autonomy" occupies a vital place in contemporary bioethics. It is remarkable that the conceptions of autonomy that appear in bioethics discussions share certain common features: commitment to individualism and independence. In the field of bioethics, autonomy "is generally seen as a matter of independence or at least as a *capacity for independent decisions and action*" (O'Neill 2002: 23; italics in the original). However, according to O'Neill, as long as autonomy is understood as a matter of individual independence, these conceptions of "individual autonomy" cannot serve as a convincing basis for the ethical framework of bioethics, because "they may encourage ethically questionable forms of individualism and self-expression, and may heighten rather than reduce public mistrust in medicine, science and biotechnology" (O'Neill 2002: 73). Thus, O'Neill tries to revitalize an older Kantian view of autonomy, which she calls "principled autonomy."

Kant is mostly regarded as the source of the concept "individual autonomy." However, O'Neill denies that this view is correct. For Kant, autonomy was not a matter of individual independence: "it is a matter of acting on certain sorts of principles, and specifically on principles of obligation" (O'Neill 2002: 84). Following this, we may wonder about the sorts of principles we should act on. The answer is summarized in the following remarks: "[P]rincipled autonomy is expressed in action whose principle could be adopted by all others. Any conception of autonomy that sees it as expressing individuality—let alone eccentricity—or as carving out some particularly independent or distinctive trajectory in this world is a form of individual rather than of principled autonomy" (O'Neill 2002: 85).

The conception of principled autonomy may seem highly abstract and far removed from contemporary styles of thinking. It might, therefore, seem unhelpful in deriving solutions to complex, modern bioethical issues. However, principled autonomy is not a useless, abstract relic. Indeed, O'Neill tries to argue that some substantially basic ethical principles or requirements can be identified using this conception of autonomy. She states: "Committing to principled autonomy—that is, commitment to principles that can be adopted by all—entails [the rejection of] setting aside, destroying, injuring, coercing or deceiving others, and rejecting influence to others' capacities to survive and to act" (O'Neill 2002: 149).

However, she also suggests that we cannot "expect to find any *timeless* account of the more narrowly specified human rights and human obligations that would express and implement these principles" (O'Neill 2002: 95; italics in the original). To paraphrase: we cannot think of the conception of principled autonomy, or the basic principles derived from it, as a simple algorithm for finding definite answers to bioethical issues. Rather, we are assigned the strenuous task of "identify[ing] ways of living up to these principles in actual circumstances, with their historically contingent but determinate configuration of medical, scientific and biotechnological resources and environmental constraints" (O'Neill 2002: 95). Our concern here is, specifically, what can we learn about informed consent from principled autonomy?

O'Neill begins by identifying the ethical importance of the informed consent procedure. According to O'Neill, informed consent is ethically important not "because it secures some form of individual autonomy," but because "[i]t provides reasonable assurance that a patient...has not been deceived or coerced" (O'Neill 2003: 5). It is worth noting that the refusal to deceive or coerce others is one of the basic ethical requirements that follow from the Kantian conception of principled autonomy. Consequently, when it comes to informed consent, the commitment to principled autonomy leads to the following proposition: "Patients...give genuine consent only if they are neither coerced nor deceived, and can judge that they are not coerced or deceived" (O'Neill 2003: 6).

How then can it be ascertained that patients provide *genuine* consent, or that there is no deception or coercion? O'Neill suggests that "[g]enuine consent is apparent where patients can *control* the amount of information they receive, and what they allow to be done" (O'Neill 2003: 6; italics in the original). It is worthwhile to highlight the two important points included in the short statement above. First, patients are not deceived if they are permitted easy access to additional accurate information: "even a patient who decides on the basis of limited information has judged that the information was enough to reach a decision, and is not deceived" (O'Neill 2003: 6). Second, as long as patients are aware of the right to rescind their consent at any time, they are not coerced. In effect, according to O'Neill, "Patients who know they have access to *extendable information* and that they have given *rescindable consent* have in effect *a veto* over what is done...Where these standards are met, there are reasonable assurances that nobody is coerced or deceived" (O'Neill 2003: 6; italics in the original).

Based on this idea, as long as it is ensured that the patient has reasonable opportunities to request explanations, and has opportunities to rescind consent at any time—to borrow O'Neill's words, the patient possesses a veto—it is possible to obtain genuine consent, even if the physician does not provide the patient with a point-by-point explanation of all information. In considering the cases presented in our article, in which the main topics were the family-facilitated approach and the soft proxy approach, it is apparent that these patients were by no means given all available information. Yet, at the same time, the patient's right of access to all information was guaranteed, and the patients knew they could rescind their families' consent at any point. In other words, as O'Neill puts it, the patients had a veto. We argued that the family-facilitated approach and soft proxy approach are compatible with autonomy. Furthermore, we can also say that our conception of "something close to autonomy" compatible with the family-facilitated approach and soft proxy approach is not necessarily heresy when viewed against the diverse historical interpretations of autonomy in the Western philosophical tradition.

We have realized through the commentaries on this article that we do not share the same conception of autonomy as Fan and Ho, and there are slight differences in both semantic meanings and points of emphasis.

Fan holds that shared decision-making between the patient and his/her close family members cannot be explained within the Western style of autonomy, for in the West only the patient him/herself possesses decision-making authority. Yet if, as O'Neill argues, the crucial point for commitment to autonomy is the absence of coercion, then, how can it be concluded that the Asian style of family-shared decision-making is incompatible with autonomy?

Furthermore, Ho states that the conventional first-person approach to autonomy does not require patients to make decisions on their own—the right to decide implies the right to solicit assistance or even defer to others if one wishes to do so. According to our definition, however, the right to defer to others is congruent with the hard proxy approach.

Ho also writes that Mr. K can be said to be independent. However if Mr. K were indeed independent, he might have delegated the decision-making authority to his physician, family, or someone else. Yet Mr. K said, "I cannot decide" and withdrew. This is one form of proof that Mr. K was actually interdependent.

In conclusion we will elucidate why we adhered to our concept of autonomy.

Using the concept of autonomy to explain the family-facilitated approach is significant in two ways. First, it opens up new possibilities, not just for the family-facilitated approach and the soft proxy approach, but for a new informed consent model that can be meaningful even for those who do not necessarily share the Japanese cultural approach. Second, it suggests a potential alternative to the conception of autonomy as commonly expressed in the Western tradition.

It is true that the family-facilitated approach and the soft proxy approach discussed here may seem somewhat strange to those sympathetic to the idea of individual autonomy, and perhaps to the three commentators. As Becker suggests, there is no reason to cling to the concept of autonomy. Or, as Fan noted, the family-facilitated approach and the soft proxy approach may seem incompatible with Western autonomy. Yet the family-facilitated approach and the soft proxy approach do have an affinity for the Western conception of *principled autonomy* that O'Neill employs. In fact, if one keeps in mind O'Neill's conception of principled autonomy and understanding of informed consent, rather than "individual autonomy," then it is clear that the family-facilitated approach and the soft proxy approach are not necessarily at odds with the concept of autonomy.

Initially, the family-facilitated approach may appear distinct and limited to Japan. With respect to the two points discussed above, however, this topic has universal application. Although the need for international dialogue and cooperation in bioethics is frequently emphasized, there have been few attempts to truly address this need and set agendas in such a way that people from diverse cultural backgrounds can participate. The intention of this article was to spark further dialogue and participation. That is why the title of our article advocated a global perspective. By broadening the scope of the concept of autonomy, we hope that it will be possible to open up new global developments in bioethics.

References

Akabayashi, A., and Hayashi, Y. (2014). "Informed Consent Revisited: A Global Perspective," in A. Akabayashi (ed.), *The Future of Bioethics: International Dialogues*. Oxford: Oxford University Press, 735–49.

Beauchamp, T. L., and Childress, J. F. (2009). *Principles of Biomedical Ethics*. 6th ed. New York: Oxford University Press

Becker, C. (2014). "Medical Practice and Cultural Myth," in A. Akabayashi (ed.), *The Future of Bioethics: International Dialogues*. Oxford: Oxford University Press, 750–6.

Ho, A. (2014). "Whose Interest Is It Anyway? Autonomy and Family-Facilitated Approach of Decision Making," in A. Akabayashi (ed.), *The Future of Bioethics: International Dialogues*. Oxford: Oxford University Press, 757–61.

O'Neill, O, (2002). *Autonomy and Trust in Bioethics*. Cambridge: Cambridge University Press.

O'Neill, O. (2003). "Some Limits of Informed Consent," *Journal of Medical Ethics* 29(1): 4–7.

Index